SUMMARY MEASURES
OF POPULATION HEALTH

Description of the cover artwork: The cover illustration is based on a simple graphical heuristic illustrating the key elements of summary measures of population health (see p. 16). From left to right, the segments of the graph represent time lived in full health, time lived in less than full health and time lost due to premature mortality.

SUMMARY MEASURES
OF POPULATION HEALTH

CONCEPTS, ETHICS, MEASUREMENT
AND APPLICATIONS

EDITED BY

CHRISTOPHER J.L. MURRAY, JOSHUA A. SALOMON,
COLIN D. MATHERS AND ALAN D. LOPEZ

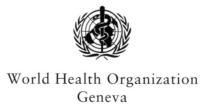

World Health Organization
Geneva

WHO Library Cataloguing-in-Publication Data

Summary measures of population health : concepts, ethics, measurement
and applications/ edited by Christopher J.L. Murray ... [et al.].

  1. Health status indicators 2. Population surveillance
  3. Life expectancy 4. Disability evaluation 5. Cost of illness
  6. Quality of life 7. Ethics 8. Social justice
  9. Data interpretation, Statistical 10. Analysis of variance
  I. Murray, Christopher J.L.

  ISBN 92 4 154551 8   (NLM classification: WA 950)

Design and production: Digital Design Group, Newton, MA USA
Typeset and printed in Canada
Cover: Upper right-hand picture credit: JHU/CCP; lower left-hand picture credit:
Patrick Coleman JHU/CCP. Pictures are courtesy of M/MC Photoshare at
www.jhuccp.org/mmc.

CONTENTS

ACKNOWLEDGMENTS

A key goal for this book was to solicit contributions from numerous authors to ensure that a wide diversity of views about summary measures of population health were reflected. We are extremely grateful to the many experts who contributed chapters to this book for their discipline in meeting production deadlines and their patience with the editorial process. In addition, we thank all of the other participants at the Marrakech conference that gave rise to this book. The debate and discussions at that conference have without doubt enriched and informed the final contributions that appear in this volume. We give special acknowledgment to the various peer reviewers of the chapters in this book, whose valuable comments have helped ensure the scientific integrity of the volume.

We are indebted to Nankhonde Kasonde for managing the production process and keeping the publication on schedule. Her contribution to the style and presentation of the book are also gratefully acknowledged. We wish to thank Marc Kaufman for his efficient and professional management of a challenging publication process. We would also like to thank Gabriella Covino for organizing the Marrakech conference and Sue Piccolo for administrative assistance.

We gratefully acknowledge financial support for this project from the National Institute on Aging (Research Grant No. P01 AG17625-01).

PREFACE

The epidemiological transition, characterized by a progressive rise in the average age of death in virtually all populations across the globe, has necessitated a serious reconsideration of how the health of populations is measured. Average life expectancy at birth is becoming increasingly un-informative in many populations where, because of the non-linear relationship between age-specific mortality and the life expectancy index, significant declines in death rates at older ages have produced only relatively modest increases in life expectancy at birth. At the same time there is considerable uncertainty in many populations as to whether—and to what extent—gains in life expectancy have been accompanied by improvements in health status. Such considerations are critical for the planning and provision of health and social services. Separate measures of survival and of health status among survivors, while useful inputs into the health policy debate, need to be combined in some fashion if the goal is to provide a single, holistic measure of overall population health.

Summary measures of population health (SMPH) are measures that combine information on mortality and non-fatal health outcomes. Interest in summary measures has been rising in recent years, and the calculation and reporting of various measures have become routine in a number of settings. With the proliferation of work on summary measures, there has been increasing debate about their application in public health, ranging from the ethical implications of the social values incorporated in these measures, to technical and methodological issues regarding the formulation of different measures, to concerns about distributive justice and the use of summary measures as an input to resource allocation decisions. Given these developments, and the diverse opinions about the construction and uses of summary measures, the World Health Organization's Global Programme on Evidence for Health Policy convened a conference in Marrakech, Morocco, in December 1999, to provide a forum for discussion and debate over the scientific, ethical and policy issues around summary measures of population health.

One key objective for WHO, in addition to advancing the technical work on summary measures, has been to promote greater transparency and understanding of the inputs to calculate summary measures and their appropriate application. The Marrakech Conference provided a unique opportunity to challenge existing notions and advance the conceptual and methodological research agenda on summary measures. Leading experts from a range of disciplines addressed the current state of the art, from basic concepts and uses, to detailed considerations on conceptual frameworks for measurement of population health, description and valuation of health states, as well as social values and key ethical arguments. The meeting engendered a rich debate about conceptual, technical and measurement issues and addressed a number of implications for the uses of summary measures.

The various papers presented at the Marrakech meeting form the basis of this volume, supplemented by additional chapters that arose from the discussion or were commissioned to fill important gaps in the debate. All chapters have been peer-reviewed to ensure their suitability for publication in this volume.

ORGANIZATION OF CONTENTS

The chapters in this book provide elaborations of these various themes, issues and concerns. Part 1 of the book begins by describing the framework adopted by WHO for the assessment of health system performance in countries and the specific role of SMPH within this framework. Some of the key issues in the development and critical appraisal of summary measures, and their foundations in the measurement of individual health, are then introduced. Part 2 presents a series of viewpoints on the uses of summary measures, from the perspectives of both researchers and policymakers. These uses range from comparisons of the health of populations (or of the same population over time), quantification of health inequalities and priority-setting for health services delivery and planning, to guiding research and development in the health sector, improving professional training, and analyzing the benefits of health interventions in cost-effectiveness studies.

BASIC CONCEPTS

Given the array of potential uses of summary measures, the chapters in part 3 address many of the fundamental concepts underlying their definition and construction. How broadly, for example, should the concept of "health" be defined? Is health separable from other components of well-being? Quite apart from such philosophical considerations, how should health be measured and aggregated across individuals in order to construct population indices? Other chapters in part 3 consider issues arising from the need to quantify both levels and distributions of health in populations. Several contributions in this section consider the question of whether summary measures should assess simultaneously both the average level of health, and health inequalities, or whether separate measures are required.

HEALTH EXPECTANCIES, HEALTH GAPS AND CAUSAL ATTRIBUTION

Summary measures of population health fall into two broad categories: health expectancies and health gaps. A wide range of health expectancies has been proposed since the original notion was developed. The chapters in part 4 review the basic components of health expectancy measures, including the methods used to calculate life expectancy (period or cohort) and the methods used to incorporate non-fatal health experience in health expectancies (for example, prevalence-rate life tables and multi-state life tables). Of key concern are the consequences of using different definitions and measurements of health status in the calculation of health expectancies, and, perhaps most importantly, the implications of basing health expectancy measures on dichotomous versus multi-state valuations of health states.

Of the different summary measures that have been widely used, none simultaneously includes information on both incidence and prevalence. There are long-standing arguments in health statistics about the relative merits of incidence-based and prevalence-based measures, but simple evaluative criteria suggest that summary measures should include information on both for the purpose of comparing the health of different populations. The final chapter in this section addresses the need for, and construction of, summary measures that include both incidence and prevalence information.

As a complement to health expectancies, health gap measures are critical to understanding the comparative importance of diseases, injuries and risk factors for population health levels. A variety of health gap measures have been proposed and calculated, following the tradition of mortality gap measures developed over the last half-century. Health gaps extend the notion of mortality gaps to include time lived in health states worse than ideal health. Part 5 of the book develops this notion further, with chapters addressing questions such as the choice of implicit or explicit population targets and other issues around the specification of normative goals for health gaps, and providing examples of different alternative health gap measures. The implications of the age-dependent formulation of typical gap measures, which is not an issue for health expectancies, are also discussed, and criteria are advanced and debated for desirable properties of health gap measures.

Given that one of the fundamental goals in constructing summary measures is to identify the relative magnitude of different health problems, including diseases, injuries and risk factors, an appropriate framework is required which will be both coherent and readily interpretable. There are two dominant traditions in widespread use for causal attribution: categorical attribution and counterfactual analysis. In categorical attribution, an event such as a death is attributed to a single cause according to a defined set of rules (in the case of mortality, the International Classification of Diseases). In counterfactual analyses, the contribution of a disease, injury or risk factor to overall disease burden is estimated by comparing the current levels of a summary measure with the levels that would be expected under some alternative hypothetical scenario. Chapters in part 6 discuss the relative advantages and disadvantages of these two approaches and the implications for comparability, of using the two approaches in the same analysis.

HEALTH STATUS DESCRIPTION AND CLASSIFICATION

Standardized assessments of multiple health domains are increasingly being used to describe the health states of individuals, both as quantities of interest in their own right, as well as critical inputs in the construction of summary measures. All efforts at measuring health state valuations and the subsequent calculation of severity weights incorporated within summary measures of population health depend on using meaningful, complete and comprehensible health state descriptions. Two key issues in describing health states are: (i) what constitutes a complete description of a health state, and (ii) how to convey this information effectively to an individual undertaking valuations. For the purposes of developing a valid and reliable approach to eliciting health state valuations, descriptions of health states must be standardized to provide information on the major domains considered important for individual valuation, and they must be comprehensible by individuals with widely varying levels of educational attainment and from different socio-economic, professional and cultural backgrounds. In addition to traditional psychometric criteria such as reliability and validity, it is also critical to ensure that measures of health levels are comparable across different populations. Chapters in parts 7 and 8 address these and other theoretical and empirical issues in the measurement of health states. Part 7 addresses various questions relating to the choice of domains in different health state classification systems and the presentation of health states to survey respondents, and part 8 describes different strategies for improving the cross-population comparability of survey results on health domain levels.

HEALTH STATE VALUATION

Any summary measure of population health, by definition, requires the quantification or explicit valuation of states of health worse than perfect health, given that, at any one time, a large number of individuals are likely to be in sub-optimal health. There has been extensive debate in the health economics literature on a number of fundamental issues relating to health state valuations, including: (i) whose values should be used; (ii) the advantages and disadvantages of various value elicitation techniques; (iii) the mode of presentation of health states as stimuli for valuations; and (iv) the combination of multiple methods, multiple states and deliberative processes in the development of standard data collection instruments and protocols. The empirical basis for the calculation of summary measures would be improved considerably through the collection of population-based data on individual valuations of a wide range of health states. The chapters in part 9 address many of the important conceptual and methodological issues that form the foundation for these data collection efforts.

Regardless of the resources available, it is clearly not feasible to measure health state valuations in a population for every possible health state. For the calculation of summary measures of population health, a predictive model that allows indirect estimation of health state valuations from information on domain levels would be invaluable. Several major efforts to develop such mapping functions have been undertaken, and the chapters in part 10 present the most prominent examples to date, describing the major characteristics of different approaches and outlining a broad research agenda for further work in this area.

One of the major empirical questions relating to health state valuation concerns the extent to which values may vary within and across populations. There are a number of arguments as to why health state valuations might be expected to vary between populations that have different cultural beliefs on disease causation, individual responsibility, fatalism, social roles and functioning or expectations for well-being, etc. Further, individual variation in valuations according to age, sex, education, income and other socio-demographic variables might also be expected. To date, however, there has been little empirical evidence that health state values vary markedly within and across populations. Part 11 examines concepts and methods for modelling the determinants of variation in health state valuations within and between populations, and includes examples of empirical studies relating to this question.

GOODNESS, FAIRNESS AND SOCIAL VALUE CHOICES

A key concern in the use of summary measures for resource allocation is that policies and programmes are chosen based on several considerations, and not only on the concern to maximize health outcomes. Level of health, in other words, constitutes one component in the overall goals for social policy, but there are compelling moral arguments that support additional desiderata for health policy. Should we give moral priority to the worst-off? Or should we attach greater significance to large benefits than to the sum of many small benefits, with life-saving interventions counting the most of all? Might we attach lower importance to life extension beyond a normal lifespan, thus attaching greater moral weight to achieving what has been described as a "fair innings"? Cutting across these moral choices are two methodological issues which have broad implications for measurement. One is whether our judgments on these moral trade-offs should be explicitly incorporated into the summary measures themselves, via weighting, or rather should be regarded as an altogether separate set of considerations in the allocation debate. The other issue is whether these questions of resource allocation should ideally be settled by processes of democratic deliberation and the elicitation of the public's values, or by the best of moral argumentation and theory. Chapters in parts 12 and 14 lay out some of the key debates regarding this moral arithmetic in detail, including tradeoffs between goodness and fairness and the role for empirical ethics.

The calculation and specification of summary measures of population health also involves several explicit social value choices. One key issue is whether or not to differentially weight healthy years of life lost at different ages, and if so, on what basis. Even if most people consider the period of young adulthood (e.g. the early childbearing years) as more valuable than years lived at the beginning or end of life, this view may be objectionable if the basis is the societal value of young adults compared to other people. Secondly, the choice of a discount rate for health benefits, even if technically desirable, may entail morally unacceptable allocations between generations. Are there other widely held values, and on what basis should we decide to incorporate social values into the summary measure, if at all? If they are to be incorporated, should these values be determined at the local or national level for country analyses and/or at the international level for cross-national comparisons? The debate on social value choices, as well as their application in summary measures, is the focus of part 13 of the book.

In the final section of the book, a series of conclusions and recommendations relating to the application of summary measures of population health are presented as a guide for the construction and use of these measures in practice. These conclusions represent the consolidated opinions of the editors, based on careful consideration of the issues and viewpoints raised in the preceding chapters, about the specific formulation of summary measures for various uses. Recommendations are provided not only on measurement issues and methodological choices in the construction of the measures, but more broadly on the types of information that need to be developed in order to calculate these measures reliably.

* * *

The chapters which follow will, we hope, provide a comprehensive and coherent treatise on the many complex but critical considerations which underly the construction and use of summary measures of population health. It is hoped that this volume—in drawing on the contributions of leading scientists in the area—will bolster the scientific and ethical foundations for the widespread promotion and use of summary measures. We believe that the publication represents an important contribution to the continuing evolution of health metrics, and hope that it will serve as a useful resource in guiding national and international applications in the coming decades.

Christopher J.L. Murray

Joshua A. Salomon

Colin D. Mathers

Alan D. Lopez

List of authors

Arnab Acharya
The Institute of Development Studies
University of Sussex
Brighton, BN1 9RE, UK
Tel: +44 1273 877 261
Email: a.acharya@ids.ac.uk

Rob M.P.M. Baltussen
Global Programme on Evidence for Health Policy
World Health Organization
20, Avenue Appia
1211 Geneva 27, Switzerland
Email: baltussenr@who.int

Jan J. Barendregt
Department of Public Health
Faculty of Medicine
Erasmus University of Rotterdam
PO Box 1738
3000 DR Rotterdam, The Netherlands
Tel: +31 10 408 7714 Fax: +31 10 408 9449/9455
Email: barendregt@mgz.fgg.eur.nl

Gouke J. Bonsel
Institute of Social Medicine/Public Health
Academisch Medisch Centrum
Meibergdreef 9
Postbus 22660
1100 DD Amsterdam, The Netherlands
Tel: +31 20 566 9111
Email: g.j.bonsel@amc.uva.nl

John Brazier
Sheffield Health Economics Group
University of Sheffield
Regent Court, 30 Regent Street
Sheffield S1 4DA, UK
Tel: +44 114 222 0715
Email: j.e.brazier@sheffield.ac.uk

Dan W. Brock
Department of Clinical Bioethics
Warren G. Magnuson Clinical Center
Building 10, Room 1C118
National Institutes of Health
Bethesda, MD 20892-1156, USA
Tel: +1 301 435 8717
Fax: +1 301 496 0760
Email: dbrock@mail.cc.nih.gov

John Broome
Department of Philosophy
Oxford University
10 Merton Street
Oxford OX1 4JJ, UK
Tel: +44 1865 276926 Fax: +44 1865 276932
Email: john.broome@philosophy.oxford.ac.uk

Somnath Chatterji
Health Financing and Stewardship
World Health Organization
20, Avenue Appia
1211 Geneva 27, Switzerland
Email: chatterjis@who.int

Eileen M. Crimmins
Andrus Gerontology Center
University of Southern California
3715 McClintock Avenue
Los Angeles, CA 90089-0191, USA
Tel: +1 213 740 1707
Email: crimmin@usc.edu

Norberto Dachs
Pan American Health Organization
Pan American Sanitary Bureau
Regional Office of the World Health Organization
525 Twenty-third Street, N.W.
Washington, DC 20037, USA
Tel: +1 202 974 3228 Fax: +1 202 974 3675
Email: dachsnor@paho.org

Paul Dolan
Sheffield Health Economics Group
Department of Economics University of Sheffield
Regent Court, 30 Regent Street
Sheffield S1 4DA, UK
Tel: +44 114 222 0670 Fax: +44 114 272 4095
Email: P.Dolan@shef.ac.uk

Marie-Louise Essink-Bot
Department of Public Health
Erasmus University
PO Box 1738
3000 DR Rotterdam, The Netherlands
Tel: +31 10 408 7714 Fax: +31 10 408 9455
Email: essink@mgz.fgg.eur.nl

Majid Ezzati
Center For Risk Management
Resources For the Future
1616 P. Street, N.W.
Washington, DC 20036, USA
Tel: +1 202 328 5004 Fax: +1 202 939 3460
Email: ezzati@rff.org or ezzatim@who.int

David Feeny
Institute of Health Economics
#1200, 10405 Jasper Avenue
Edmonton, AB T5J 3N4 Canada
Tel: +1 780 448 4881 Fax: +1 780 448 0018
Email: dfeeny@pharmacy.ualberta.ca
Web: http://www.ihe.ab.ca

Elizabeth Frankenberg
264 Haines Hall
Department of Sociology
University of California at Los Angeles
375 Portola Plaza
Los Angeles, CA 90095-1551, USA
Tel: +1 310 825 1313 Fax: +1 310 206 9838
Email: efranken@ucla.edu

Julio Frenk
Minister of Health, Mexico
Secretaría de Salud de México
Lieja 7, Col. Juárez, 06696 Mexico, D.F.
Email: Jfrenk@mail.ssa.gob.mx

Sander Greenland
University of California at Los Angeles School of Public Health
Department of Epidemiology
16-035 Center for Health Sciences
PO Box 951772
Los Angeles, CA 90095-1772, USA
Tel: +1 310 825 5140 Fax: +1 310 825 8440
Email: lesdomes@ucla.edu

James Griffin
Department of Philosophy
Oxford University
10 Merton Street
Oxford OX1 4JJ, UK
Tel: +44 1865 276926 Fax: +44 1865 276932

Daniel M. Hausman
Department of Philosophy
University of Wisconsin-Madison
600 N. Park Street
Madison, WI 53706-1474, USA
Tel: +1 608 263 5178 Fax: +1 608 265 3701
Email: dhausman@facstaff.wisc.edu
Web: http://philosophy.wisc.edu/hausman

Adnan A. Hyder
Department of International Health
Johns Hopkins University School of Public Health
615 North Wolfe Street, Suite E-8132
Baltimore, MD 21205, USA
Tel: +1 410 955 3928 Fax: +1 410 614 1419
Email: ahyder@jhsph.edu

Frances P. Kamm
Department of Philosophy
New York University
100 Washington Square East, 503K
New York, NY 10012, USA
Tel: +1 212 998 8331 Fax: +1 212 995 4179
Email: fmk1@is4.nyu.edu

Alan D. Lopez
Global Programme on Evidence for Health Policy
World Health Organization
20, Avenue Appia
1211 Geneva 27, Switzerland
Email: lopeza@who.int

Mathew McKenna
National Center For Chronic Diseases, Prevention and Health
Promotion
Centers for Disease Control and Prevention
4770 Burford Highway, N.E.
Mailstop K40, Atlanta, GA 30341, USA
Tel: +1 770 488 4227
Email: mtm1@cdc.gov

Prasanta Mahapatra
Institute of Health Systems
HACA Bhavan
Hyderabad-500004, AP, India
Tel: +91 40 321 0136
Email: pmahapat@ihsnet.org.in

James Marks
National Center for Chronic Diseases, Prevention and Health
Promotion
Centers for Disease Control and Prevention
4770 Burford Highway, N.E.
Mailstop K 40, Atlanta, GA 30341, USA
Tel: +1 770 488 5403 Fax: +1 770 488 5971
Email: jms1@cdc.gov

Colin D. Mathers
Global Programme on Evidence for Health Policy
World Health Organization
20, Avenue Appia
1211 Geneva 27, Switzerland
Email: mathersc@who.int

Laurien Metz
The Netherlands Red Cross
PO Box 28120
2502 KC The Hague, The Netherlands
Email: lmetz@redcross.nl

Gavin Mooney
Social and Public Health Economics Research Group
Department of Public Health and Community Medicine
University of Sydney
Sydney, New South Wales 2006, Australia
Tel: +61 2 9351 5997 Fax: +61 2 9351 7420
Email: g.mooney@curtin.eedu.au

Kim Moesgaard Iburg
Department of International Health
University of Copenhagen
Blegdamsvej 3
DK-2100 Copenhagen, Denmark
Tel: +45 35 32 7472 Fax: +45 35 32 7736
Email: k.m.iburg@pubhealth.ku.dk

Richard Morrow
Department of International Health
Johns Hopkins University School of Public Health
615 North Wolfe Street, Room E-8148
Baltimore, MD 21205, USA
Tel: +1 410 955 3928 Fax: +1 410 614 1419
Email: rmorrow@jhsph.edu

Christopher J.L. Murray
Evidence and Information for Policy
World Health Organization
20, Avenue Appia
1211 Geneva 27, Switzerland
Email: murrayc@who.int

Lipika Nanda
Institute of Health Systems
HACA Bhavan
Hyderabad-500004, AP, India
Tel: +91 40 321 0136 Fax: +91 40 324 1567
Email: lipika@ihsnet.org.in

Erik Nord
National Institute of Public Health
PO Box 4404
Torshov, 0403 Oslo, Norway
Tel: +47 22 04 2342 Fax: 47 22 04 2595
Email: erik.nord@folkehelsa.no

K.T. Rajshree
Institute of Health Systems
HACA Bhavan
Hyderabad-500004, AP, India
Tel: +91 40 321 0136 Fax: +91 40 324 1567

Juergen Rehm
Addiction Research Institute
University of Zürich
Rämistrasse 71
8006 Zürich, Switzerland
Tel: +41 01 634 1111 Fax: +41 01 634 2304
Email: jtrehm@isf.unizh.ch

Jeffrey Richardson
Health Economics Unit
Centre for Health Program Evaluation
PO Box 477
West Heidelberg, Victoria 3081, Australia
Tel: +61 3 9496 4441 Fax: +61 3 9496 4424
Email: jeff.richardson@buseco.monash.edu.au

Nigel Rice
Centre for Health Economics
University of York, Heslington
York, YO10 5DD, UK
Tel: +44 1904 433718 Fax: +44 1904 433644
Email: nr5@york.ac.uk

Jennifer Roberts
Sheffield Health Economics Group
University of Sheffield
Regent Court, 30 Regent Street
Sheffield S1 4DA, UK
Email: J.R.Roberts@sheffield.ac.uk
Web: http://www.shef.ac.uk

Jean-Marie Robine
INSERM Démographie et Santé
Centre Val d'Aurelle Parc
Euromédecine 34298 Montpellier Cedex 5, France
Tel: +33 467 61 30 43 Fax: +33 467 61 30 47
Email: Robine@valdorel.fnclcc.fr

Anthony Rodgers
Clinical Trials Research Unit
The University of Auckland
Private Bag 92019
Auckland, New Zealand
Tel: +64 9 373 7599 Fax: +64 9 373 1710
Email: a.rodgers@ctru.aukland.ac.nz

Ritu Sadana
Research Policy and Cooperation
World Health Organization
20, Avenue Appia
1211 Geneva 27, Switzerland
Email: sadanar@who.int

Joshua A. Salomon
Global Programme on Evidence for Health Policy
World Health Organization
20, Avenue Appia
1211 Geneva 27, Switzerland
Email: salomonj@who.int

Mamadou Sanon
Centre de Recherche en Santé de Nouna
BP 02
Nouna, Burkina Faso
Email: sanon@pra.bf

Rainer Sauerborn
Department of Tropical Hygiene and Public Health
Ruprecht-Karls-Universität Heidelberg
Im Neuenheimer Feld 324
D-69120 Heidelberg, Germany
Tel: +49 6221 565038 Fax: +49 6221 565948
Email: rainer.sauerborn@urz.uni-heidelberg.de

Kiyotaka Segami
Department of Public Health Policy
National Institute of Public Health, 2-3-6 Minami
Wako-city, Saitama Prefecture, 351-0197, Japan
Email: segami@iph.go.jp

Johannes Sommerfeld
Special Programme For Research and Training in Tropical Diseases
World Health Organization
20, Avenue Appia
1211 Geneva 27, Switzerland
Email: sommerfeldj@who.int

Edward Sondik
National Center for Health Statistics
Centers for Disease Control and Prevention
6525 Belcrest Road
Hyattsville, MD 20782, USA
Tel: +1 303 458 4636 Fax: +1 301 436 8459
Email: ESondik@cdc.gov

Ajay Tandon
Global Programme on Evidence for Health Policy
World Health Organization
20, Avenue Appia
1211 Geneva 27, Switzerland
Email: tandona@who.int

Duncan Thomas
Bunche Hall 9365
Department of Economics
University of California at Los Angeles
PO Box 951477
Los Angeles, CA 90095-1477, USA
Tel: +1 310 825 5304 Fax: +1 310 825 9528
Email: dt@ucla.edu

Aki Tsuchiya
Centre for Health Economics
University of York, Heslington
York, YO10 5DD, UK
Tel: +44 1904 433651 Fax: +44 1904 433644
Email: a.tsuchiya@sheffield.ac.uk

Bedirhan T. Üstün
Health Financing and Stewardship
World Health Organization
20, Avenue Appia
1211 Geneva 27, Switzerland
Email: ustunb@who.int

Paul J. van der Maas
Department of Public Health
Erasmus University Rotterdam
P.O. Box 1738
3000 DR Rotterdam, The Netherlands
Tel: +31 10 408 7714 Fax: +31 10 408 9482
Email: vandermaas@facb.fgg.eur.nl

Theo Vos
Health Outcomes Section
Public Health Division
Department of Human Services
18-120 Spencer Street
Melbourne, Victoria 3000, Australia
Tel: +61 3 9637 4236 Fax: +61 3 9637 4763
Email: Theo.Vos@dhs.vic.gov.au

Michael C. Wolfson
Analysis and Development
Statistics Canada
RH Coats Building 24A
Ottawa, Ontario, Canada K1A 0T6
Tel: +1 613 951 8216 Fax: +1 613 951 5643
Email: wolfson@statcan.ca

Chapter 1.1

SUMMARY MEASURES OF POPULATION
HEALTH IN THE CONTEXT OF THE WHO
FRAMEWORK FOR HEALTH SYSTEM
PERFORMANCE ASSESSMENT

CHRISTOPHER J.L. MURRAY AND JULIO FRENK

INTRODUCTION

This volume addresses the conceptual, ethical, empirical and technical challenges in summarizing the health of populations. This is critical for monitoring whether levels of population health are improving over time and for understanding why health differs across settings. At the same time, it is also important to recognize that improving population health is not the only goal of health policy and to understand the way health improvements interact with these other goals. For that reason, we briefly review the World Health Organization (WHO) framework for assessing the performance of health systems and the role of summary measures of population health (SMPH) in this framework. Following the recent peer review of the methodology used for health system performance by WHO (Anand et al. 2002), this framework will continue to evolve in response to the detailed recommendations of the scientific peer review group and to ongoing scientific debates and research.

Health systems vary widely in performance, and countries with similar levels of income, education and health expenditure differ in their ability to attain key health goals. The performance of health systems has been a major concern of policy-makers for many years. Many countries have recently introduced reforms in the health sector with the explicit aim of improving performance (Collins et al. 1999; Maynard and Bloor 1995). There exists an extensive literature on health sector reform, and recently there have been debates on how best to measure performance so that the impact of reforms can be assessed (Smith 1990). Measurement of performance requires an explicit framework defining the goals to which a health system contributes, against which the outcomes can be judged and the performance quantified (Goldstein and Spiegelhalter 1996).

In a recent paper (Murray and Frenk 2000), we defined health system performance in a way that enables the performance in different countries to be compared and the performance within a country to be monitored over a period of time. This WHO framework for assessment of health system performance was used in the *World Health Report 2000* (WHO 2000) to assess the levels of goal attainment and health system performance of 191 WHO Member States. In Figure 1, which illustrates the concept, the goals of the health system are measured on the vertical axis while the inputs to producing the goal are on the horizontal axis. The upper curve represents the maximum possible level of health goals that could be obtained for a given level of inputs.

A farm's output, for example, would be zero in the absence of any inputs, but in the field of health the output levels would not be zero (i.e. the entire population would not be dead) even in the absence of health expenditures and a functioning health system. The lower curve in Figure 1 presents the output level that would occur in the absence of the system. Assume that a country is observed to have achieved (a+b) units of health (see Figure 1). Murray and Frenk have defined the health system's performance as b/(b+ c). This indicates what the system is achieving compared to its potential. The challenge for health system reform is to find a way of measuring health system performance in a systematic way, which allows comparison between countries and within countries over time (Tandon et al. 2000; Evans et al. 2001).

This concept is very similar to the concept of efficiency in economics— the output per unit of input. For that reason, in the rest of this paper we use the term efficiency to describe the ratio b/(b+c), and health system performance assessment is defined as all the activities involved in measuring inputs, goal attainment and efficiency, and linking variations in outcomes to variations in the ways the critical functions of the system are undertaken.

Figure I   Health system inputs and achievement

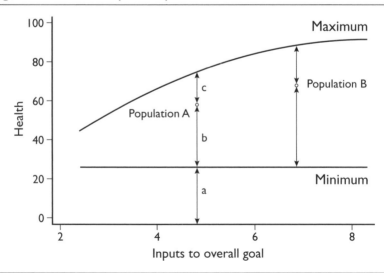

The analytical framework used for characterizing the social goals to which a health system contributes is derived from Murray and Frenk (2000). We differentiate intrinsic goals from instrumental goals. In this framework, an intrinsic goal is one: (a) whose attainment can be raised while holding other intrinsic goals constant (i.e. there is at least partial independence among the different intrinsic goals), and (b) the attainment of which is in itself desirable, irrespective of any other considerations. Instrumental goals, on the other hand, are goals that are pursued to attain the intrinsic goals. We may identify three intrinsic goals to which the system should contribute—health of the population, responsiveness of the system, and fairness in financial contribution (Figure 2).

These three intrinsic goals should be routinely monitored by all countries and form the main basis for the assessment of health system performance facilitated by WHO. Therefore, the work of operationalizing the measurement of goal attainment is focused on measuring attainment on these three goals as well as relating goal attainment to resource use in order to evaluate efficiency. The first goal is improvement in the health of the population (in terms of the levels attained and distribution). The second is enhanced responsiveness of the health system to the legitimate expectations of the population. Responsiveness in this context explicitly refers to the non-health-improving dimensions of the interactions of the population with the health system, and reflects respect of persons and client orientation in the delivery of health services, among other factors. As with health outcomes, both the level of responsiveness and its distribution are important. The third intrinsic goal is fairness in financial contribution which is significantly related to financial risk protection. The aim is to ensure that poor households should not pay a higher share of their non-subsistence expenditure for health than richer households, and all households should be protected against catastrophic financial losses related to ill health.

The measurement of efficiency relates goal attainment to the resources available. Variation in goal attainment and efficiency is a function of the way in which the health system organizes four key functions: stewardship (a broader concept than regulation); financing (including revenue collection, fund pooling and purchasing); service provision (for personal and non-personal health services); and resource generation (including personnel,

Figure 2   Health system goals

	Level	Distribution	
Health	✓	✓	
Responsiveness	✓	✓	Efficiency
Fairness in financial contribution		✓	
	Quality	Equity	

facilities and knowledge). By providing empirical evidence of the relationship between health system outcomes, efficiency and these four functions, WHO will begin to build an evidence base for not only understanding the proximate determinants of health system performance, but also for responding to major policy challenges.

INTRINSIC GOALS

This section discusses more precisely the content of each of the three intrinsic goals.

A. HEALTH

The first goal, health, is the defining goal for the health system—to improve the health of the population. Health of the population should reflect the health of individuals throughout the life course and take into account both premature mortality and non-fatal health outcomes as key components. In other words, WHO believes that the measurement of average levels of health and the distribution of health across individuals should use summary measures that reflect the full range of an individual's health experience. It is important to note that in the framework, we have proposed separate measures of the average level of population health and the distribution of health across individuals within a population. This distinction between measures of average population health and inequalities in health is central to the development of SMPH. It is consistent with the practice in other arenas such as national income accounting. GDP per capita is a measure of average income in the population, and the Gini coefficient is a measure of the distribution of income across households or individuals.

B. RESPONSIVENESS

The second intrinsic goal is to enhance the responsiveness of the health system to the legitimate expectations of the population for the non-health-improving dimensions of their interaction with the health system. Responsiveness expressly excludes the expectations of the public for the health-improving dimensions of their interaction, as this is fully reflected in the first goal of population health. The term "legitimate" is used because we recognize that some individuals may have frivolous expectations for the health system, which should not be a part of the articulation of this goal.

Responsiveness has two key components—respect of persons and client orientation. *Respect of persons* includes such elements as dignity, autonomy, confidentiality and communication, those aspects of the interaction between individuals and the health system which often have an important ethical dimension. *Client orientation* includes four elements: prompt attention, access to social support networks when receiving care, quality of basic amenities, and choice of provider.

As with the health goal, we are here concerned not only with the average level of responsiveness but also with inequalities in its distribution. A concern for the distribution of responsiveness across individuals means that we are implicitly interested in differences related to social, economic, demographic and other factors.

C. Fairness of household financial contributions

The third goal is also one of the common goals for all systems, namely, fairness in regard to households having to bear the burden of payments to the health system. We argue that fairness has at least three aspects. First, households should not have to pay a catastrophic proportion or share of their effective income after paying for their subsistence needs (capacity to pay) in order to obtain needed health interventions. Second, households in similar circumstances should pay a similar share of their capacity to pay. Third, poor households should pay less towards the health system than rich households. These three aspects can be captured by examining the health financing contribution of each household. This contribution should include contributions through all mechanisms: taxes, social security payments, private insurance, and out-of-pocket payments. Contributions of the household should be assessed in terms of their capacity to pay.

Figure 2 shows that we are interested in the level and distribution of both the health and responsiveness goals, but only in the distribution of the financing burden. The average level of financing is not an intrinsic goal for the health system. Rather, the level of health financing is one of the key policy choices for society. The level of resources invested in the health system is the variable against which goal attainment is compared in order to measure performance.

Composite goal attainment

Efficiency describes how well we achieve the socially desired mix of the five components of the three goals in relation to the available resources (see Murray and Frenk 2000).

Societies may differ on the weights that they attach to the five components shown in Figure 2. Nevertheless, we believe that for the purposes of global comparison, it is useful to develop a consensus weighting function so that a composite measure of health system goal attainment can be calculated, as well as a composite measure of efficiency. The consensus weighting function for global comparisons used in the World Health Report 2000 was based on a WHO survey measuring individual preferences for the different goals in a large convenience sample of people from over 120 countries (Gakidou et al. 2000). More recently variations in weights were explored in a representative random sample of respondents in over 60 countries (Üstün et al. 2001). Ultimately, the use of such a composite measure of goal attainment will be limited but, as with the

Human Development Index, it may spark increased attention to the performance of health systems and the factors explaining this performance.

INSTRUMENTAL GOALS

Absent from the parsimonious list of three main goals for health systems are many that have been prominently featured in discussions of health system performance, such as access to care, community involvement, innovation or sustainability. While we do not doubt their importance, these are instrumental goals whose attainment will raise the level of attainment of health, responsiveness and fairness in financing. For example, consider the goal of access to care. If we fix the level and distribution of health, responsiveness, and fairness in financing and change the level of access, we argue that this would not be intrinsically valued. Improved access to care is desirable insofar as it improves health, reduces health inequalities and enhances responsiveness. Access to care is an important instrumental, but not intrinsic, goal for health systems. If measurement of the attainment of the three intrinsic goals is carried out adequately, we will fully reflect the impact of access to care and other instrumental goals on the outcomes that are valued by society. Likewise, coverage of many effective public health programmes, such as DOTS for tuberculosis, immunization or use of impregnated bed-nets for malaria, are instrumental goals whose impacts would be captured in the measurement of health and responsiveness.

The scientific peer review group (Anand et al. 2002) has recommended that WHO collect information on the instrumental goals of coverage, access and participation in addition to monitoring the three intrinsic goals of health, responsiveness and fairness of financing. Measurement of instrumental goals will provide explanatory variables in the analysis of the determinants of health system performance, and such analyses will inform policy-makers on the role of factors such as access and coverage in achieving intrinsic goals.

EFFICIENCY OF HEALTH SYSTEMS

With a clearly defined set of goals and their measures, we can compare the level of goal attainment for different health systems. There is a long history of comparing measures of health across countries. The concept of efficiency, however, is more complex than simply recording the level of goal attainment. It involves relating goal attainment to what could be achieved. In other words, efficiency is a relative concept. A rich country has a higher level of health than a poor one, but which country has a higher level of efficiency relative to the health system's resources? We argue that efficiency should be assessed relative to the worst and best that can be achieved for a given set of circumstances. Figure 1 illustrated the concept of efficiency with respect to the goal of improving population health. The *y*-axis shows overall goal attainment, and the *x*-axis shows the resources spent on the health system. The top curve shows, for populations A and B, the maximum attainable level of health for each level of health expenditure, given the non-health system determinants such as the level of education or environmental pollution. It is clear from the Figure that efficiency is related to the level of health expenditure; for example, population A has a lower level of goal attainment than population B, but the two have approximately the same level of efficiency.

Measuring health system performance is intricately related to the question: Should one consider the health system to be accountable for the level of key determinants of health that are not entirely the responsibility of the health system, but can be influenced by it? We argue that the answer must be yes. The health system should be held accountable for these broader determinants of health to the extent that the best health system can influence them as compared to the worst health system. Some might argue that we should not judge the performance of a health system to be poor simply because the population level of tobacco consumption is high and leads to low levels of health. The implication of this argument is that health systems should not be held accountable for the levels of such determinants as tobacco consumption, diet or physical activity. Yet the counter-argument is strong: a good health system should pay attention to the level of tobacco consumption or the composition of the population's diet. In operationalizing the concept of performance, careful attention should be paid to the determinants (or the fraction of determinants) for which the health system should be routinely held to be accountable and those for which it should not. For example, health systems should be held to be substantially accountable for the levels of tobacco consumption; the health system should probably be held much less accountable for levels of educational attainment.

The criterion that should be used to determine the extent to which the health system should be held accountable for a determinant of health is the degree to which the best health system can change the level of that determinant. This degree is related to the time frame of the analysis. What the health system can achieve in one year to reduce tobacco consumption is different from what the health system can do in five or ten years. Should assessments of efficiency be made compared to what the best health system could do in one year relative to the starting point at the beginning of the year? We argue that efficiency assessment should be undertaken with a longer time horizon. The maximum level of goal attainment achievable at a given level of health expenditure should include what can be achieved over many years. Otherwise, health systems are never held accountable for past mistakes, nor rewarded for past successes. As one of the purposes of performance assessment is to provide a firmer empirical basis for the analysis of key organizational factors influencing attainment and efficiency, the measurement should not be overly sensitive to the starting point for a given year. Many health sector reforms and institutional changes may take several years to have their full effect, requiring a longer term perspective for assessment.

Attainment and efficiency can be assessed for each of the five components of the three goals. In the face of scarce resources, societies will choose explicitly, or more often implicitly, the relative importance of these goals. In other words, by choice, a society may perform poorly on responsiveness but well on health inequality because more resources from the total budget are assigned to addressing health inequalities than to enhancing responsiveness. Ultimately, a single budget for the health system is used to achieve all the goals. Because there will be implicitly or explicitly tradeoffs between some of the goals, performance in achieving the composite of the three goals is also a useful construct. In economics, the concept of efficiency means producing a desired output at least cost or producing the maximum quantity for a fixed budget. In this sense, composite goal performance—i.e. how well a health system achieves the desired outcomes, given the available resources—also indicates the efficiency of the health system.

As noted in the section on health system goals, societies may value the five components of the three goals differently. The function relating attainment on each goal to overall goal attainment represents an important policy choice which each society must make for itself. Nevertheless, the empirical evidence to date does not show any great variance in the importance attached to different goals by people according to age, sex, socioeconomic status, or region (developed versus developing countries).

DISCUSSION AND CONCLUSIONS

By clearly distinguishing the intrinsic goals of health systems from the organization of different functions of the health system and the technical content of the provision of health services, WHO hopes to facilitate a more constructive dialogue on health policy. There has long been a debate over whether health system architecture matters more or less than the intervention mix delivered by the systems. Interventions must be delivered by health systems, and a health system without effective interventions is useless. These two worldviews should not be seen as competitive but rather as complementary. By introducing clear measurements of (i) health system goal attainment and efficiency, (ii) key aspects of the organization of health system functions, and (iii) the technical content of health service provision, WHO hopes to facilitate a more reasoned and informed debate on the interaction of system architecture and intervention mix.

Much of the debate on health system design is couched in claims and counterclaims about what works and what does not work. Few decision-makers or health system experts have access to information on many different systems and their levels of attainment. The implementation of this WHO framework for health system performance assessment, we hope, will lay the basis for a shift from ideological discourse on health policy to a more empirical one. Over time, we should be able to provide empirical answers to such questions as the relationship between the organization of health financing and the level and distribution of health and responsiveness. This line of work should make it possible to ascertain the extent to which, for example, competition among purchasers or providers enhances responsiveness. If the framework encompasses the main intrinsic goals for health systems and the key candidate factors for explaining the variations in performance, it will lay the basis for a more scientific discourse on health policy.

Regular assessments of health system performance will focus attention on the policy options available to governments for improvement. Global institutionalization of performance assessment may contribute to the ongoing reflections on the role of the state in health systems. What are the policies that can enhance performance? What evidence is there that the state can enhance performance through the adoption of these policies? An enlightened role for the state would then be to enhance performance where the evidence supports its potential to do so.

In addition, by describing the levels of health system goal attainment, regardless of the reasons that explain them, national and world attention will be brought to bear on which countries have done well in improving health, reducing health inequalities, enhancing the level and distribution of responsiveness, and developing a fair means of financing.

The release of the World Health Report 2000 engendered considerable interest and debate, from governments, policy-makers and the academic community. This debate resulted in considerable refinement and revision of the health system performance assessment framework (WHO 2001) even prior to the detailed recommendations of the scientific peer review of health systems performance methodology carried out during 2001 and 2002 by a group chaired by Professor Sudhir Anand (Anand et al. 2002). The scientific peer review group endorsed the framework for health system performance assessment and made many detailed comments and recommendations on how it could be further developed (Anand et al. 2002). In particular, they endorsed the importance of using SMPH in the measurement of average levels of population health. In addition, they welcomed the development of the World Health Survey together with new methods to ensure cross-population comparability of self-reported health status used in the construction of SMPH. They also highlighted the importance of developing methods to measure health service provision and coverage to better understand the determinants of health system performance.

In conclusion, SMPH are important in their own right in monitoring levels of population health over time, and identifying reasons why health might vary across settings. However it is important to recognize, and this is shown clearly in the WHO health system performance framework, that improving the level and distribution of population health is not the only consideration for resource allocation. There has been some confusion in the past about the purpose of summary measures of population health and it is worth clarifying this. To say that population A is healthier than population B is not the same as saying we should allocate resources so as to maximize whatever we are measuring. We would argue that there are many other considerations that may go into the resource allocation maximand which are very appropriate and reflect other health system goals, such as responsiveness and fairness of financial contributions, or other concerns like fair chances, but they may not be relevant to the question of whether population A is healthier than population B.

The health system performance assessment framework separates the measurement of average level and inequality in population health, and separates them from the measurement of other intrinsic goals that are included in the resource allocation maximand. So in examining the various issues relating to the conceptual bases, ethical issues, and the development and assessment of SMPH, we suggest that it is important to keep in mind the dominant objective in the use of summary measures: Is population A healthier than population B?

REFERENCES

Anand S, Ammar W, Evans T et al. (2002). Report of the scientific peer review group on health systems performance assessment. World Health Organization, Geneva. Available on the world wide web at http://www.who.int/health-systems-performance/

Collins C, Green A, Hunter D (1999) Health sector reform and the interpretation of policy context. *Health Policy*, **47**(1):69–83.

Evans DB, Tandon A, Murray CJL, Lauer A (2001) Comparative efficiency of national health systems: cross national econometric analysis. *British Medical Journal*, **323**(7308):307–310.

Gakidou EE, Frenk J, Murray CJL (2000) *Measuring preferences on health system performance assessment*. (GPE discussion paper no 20.) World Health Organization/Global Programme on Evidence for Health Policy, Geneva.

Goldstein H, Spiegelhalter DJ (1996) League tables and their limitations: statistical issues in comparisons of institutional performance. *Journal of the Royal Statistical Society, Series A, Statistics in Society*, **59**(3):385–409.

Maynard A, Bloor K (1995) Health care reform: informing difficult choices. *International Journal of Health Planning and Management*, **10**(4):247–264.

Murray CJL, Frenk JA (2000) A framework for assessing the performance of health systems. *Bulletin of the World Health Organization*, **78**(6):717–731.

Smith P (1990) The use of performance indicators in the public sector. *Journal of the Royal Statistical Society, Series A, Statistics in Society*, **153**(1):53–72.

Tandon A, Murray CJL, Lauer J, Evans D (2000) *Measuring overall health system performance for 191 countries*. (GPE discussion paper no 30.) World Health Organization/Global Programme on Evidence for Health Policy, Geneva.

Üstün TB, Chatterji S, Villaneuva M, et al. (2001) *WHO multi-country household survey study on health and responsiveness, 2000–2001.* (GPE discussion paper no 37.) World Health Organization/Global Programme on Evidence for Health Policy, Geneva.

World Health Organization (2001). Proposed strategies of health systems performance assessment: Summary document. Global Programme on Evidence for Health Policy, World Health Organization, Geneva. Available on the world wide web at http://www.who.int/health-systems-performance/consultation.htm

WHO (2000) *The World Health Report 2000. Health systems: improving performance.* World Health Organization, Geneva.

Chapter 1.2

A CRITICAL EXAMINATION OF SUMMARY
MEASURES OF POPULATION HEALTH[1]

CHRISTOPHER J.L. MURRAY, JOSHUA A. SALOMON
AND COLIN D. MATHERS

INTRODUCTION

Summary measures of population health (SMPH) combine information on
mortality and non-fatal health outcomes to represent the health of a par-
ticular population as a single numerical index (Field and Gold 1998).
Efforts to develop such measures have a long history (Chiang 1965;
Fanshel and Bush 1970; Ghana Health Assessment Project Team 1981;
Katz et al. 1973; Piot and Sundaresan 1967; Preston 1993; Sanders 1964;
Sullivan 1966; 1971). In the past decade there has been a marked increase
in interest in the development, calculation and use of summary measures.
The volume of work from members of the *Réseau de l'Espérance de Vie
en Santé* (REVES) offers one indication of the activity in this field (Robine
et al. 1993; Mathers et al. 1994). Applications of measures such as active
life expectancy (ALE) (Katz et al. 1983) have been numerous, especially
in the USA. Calculations of related summary measures such as disability-
free life expectancy (DFLE) have also appeared frequently in recent years
(Bone 1992; Bronnum-Hansen 1998; Crimmins et al. 1997; Mutafova and
et al. 1997; Sihvonen and et al. 1998; Valkonen et al. 1997). Another type
of summary measure, disability-adjusted life years (DALYs), has been used
in the Global Burden of Disease Study (Murray and Lopez 1996a; 1996b;
1996c; 1997a; 1997b; 1997c; 1997d) and in a number of national burden of disease studies (Ministry of Health, Colombia 1994; Fundacion
Mexicana para la Salud 1995; Bobadilla 1998; Bowie et al. 1997; Concha 1996; Lozano et al. 1994; Lozano et al. 1995; Murray et al. 1998;
Murray and Acharya 1997; Ruwaard and Kramers 1998). The World
Health Organization (WHO) is committed to routine measurement and
reporting of the global and national burdens of disease (Brundtland 1998;
WHO 1999). The United States Institute of Medicine (IOM) convened a
panel on summary measures and published a report that included recommendations for enhancing public discussion of the associated ethical as-

sumptions and value judgements, establishing standards, and investing in education and training to promote the use of such measures (Field and Gold 1998).

We review below the range of options for summary measures of population health, and the main challenges and debates underlying them. Because there are many options, we propose criteria that can be used to evaluate different SMPH. The intended use of a measure may have important implications for its design, and we therefore outline the major uses of summary measures. A brief discussion of the information requirements for all summary measures is followed by a typology of summary measures in terms of health expectancies and health gaps. We outline key issues of importance for all summary measures. A number of criteria and other properties are proposed which can be used to evaluate different summary measures. We discuss some of the broad implications of this framework for choosing summary measures and consider the prospects for future progress.

This paper should be understood in the context of work under way in WHO on the development of an analytical framework for measuring health system performance (Murray and Frenk 2000). We consider one critical element of this framework, namely the need for measures of population health that capture the average levels of fatal and non-fatal health outcomes in a population. WHO is also developing measures that summarize health inequalities in populations (Gakidou et al. 2000; Murray et al. 1999). Assessments of health systems thus depend on both summary measures of the average level of population health and measures of the distribution of health among individuals.

Uses of summary measures

The design of a summary measure may depend on its intended use. Some potential applications are indicated below.

1. *Comparing the health of one population with that of another.* Such comparisons are an essential input into evaluations of the performance of different health systems, along with information on health inequalities, responsiveness, and fairness in financing (Murray and Frenk 2000). Comparisons may allow decision-makers to focus their attention on health systems with the worst achievement for a given level of resources. Comparative judgements also provide the dependent variable in analyses of the independent variables that contribute to health differences between populations.

2. *Monitoring changes in the health of a given population.* Monitoring changes in health status over time is essential in the evaluation of health system performance and progress towards stated goals for a given society.

3. *Identifying and quantifying overall health inequalities within populations.*

4. *Providing appropriate and balanced attention to the effects of non-fatal health outcomes on overall population health.* In the absence of summary measures, conditions that cause decrements in health state levels but not mortality tend to be neglected in favour of conditions that primarily cause mortality.

5. *Informing debates on priorities for health service delivery and planning.* A summary measure can be combined with information on the contributions of different causes of disease and injury or risk factors to the total. Such information should be a critical input to debates on the identification of a short list of national health priorities that will receive the attention of senior managers in public health agencies and of government leaders.

6. *Informing debates on priorities for research and development.* The relative contributions of different diseases, injuries and risk factors to the total summary measure also represent a major input to the debate on priorities for investment in research and development (WHO 1996).

7. *Improving curricula for professional training in public health.*

8. *Analysing the benefits of health interventions for use in cost-effectiveness analyses.* The change in some summary measures of population health offers a natural unit for quantifying intervention benefits in these analyses.

Consideration of the intended use of summary measures of population health, whether for simple comparative purposes or more tailored policy debates, can be expected to Figure centrally in the development of criteria for evaluating alternative summary measures. Nevertheless, in examining the properties of various summary measures it is important to recognize that all applications, even simple comparative ones, can influence the policy process (Field and Gold 1998). Because of their potential influence on international and national decisions relating to the allocation of resources, summary measures should be considered to be normative. As stated by the IOM panel, all measures of population health involve choices and value judgements in both their construction and their application. Great care must be taken in the construction of summary measures precisely because they may have far-reaching effects. Normative aspects of the design of summary measures continue to be the subject of extensive debate (Anand and Hanson 1998; Brock 1998; Daniels 1998; Murray 1996; Williams 1997; 1999).

INFORMATION REQUIREMENTS FOR SUMMARY MEASURES

It is important to distinguish clearly between the nature and quality of various inputs to summary measures and the properties of the measures themselves. Information on age-specific mortality and the epidemiology of non-fatal health outcomes provides a basic input to any type of summary measure. Another critical input is information on the values attached to various health states relative to ideal health or death. Instruments for the measurement of health states, such as SF-36 (Ware and Sherbourne 1992), can be used to describe health states in terms of performance in various domains of health. This information could be combined with valuations of health states in order to calculate the non-fatal health component of many different summary measures, but SF-36 and other instruments for the measurement of health states are not in themselves summary measures of population health. The occasional confusion surrounding the distinction between data inputs to summary measures and the summary measures themselves may be exacerbated when summary measures are linked by definition to particular health status instruments, as in years of healthy life (YHL) (Erickson et al. 1995).

A TYPOLOGY OF SUMMARY MEASURES

A wide array of summary measures has been proposed. On the basis of a simple survivorship curve they can be divided broadly into two families: health expectancies and health gaps. The bold curve in Figure 1 is an ex-

Figure 1   The survivorship curve

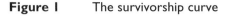

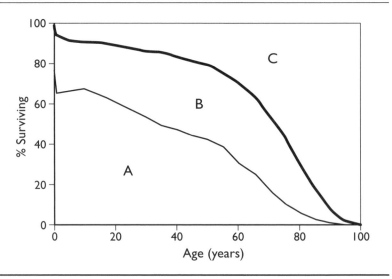

ample of a survivorship curve for a hypothetical population. This curve indicates, for each age along the x-axis, the proportion of an initial birth cohort that will remain alive at that age.

Area A + B under the bold survivorship curve represents life expectancy at birth. Health expectancies are measures of this area which take into account some lower weights for years lived in health states worse than full health, represented as area B in the diagram. More formally:

$$\text{Health expectancy} = A + f(B),$$

where $f(\bullet)$ is a function assigning weights to health states less than ideal health, using a scale on which full health has a weight of one.

A wide range of health expectancies has been proposed since the original notion was developed (Sanders 1964), including ALE (Katz et al. 1983), DFLE (Robine et al. 1993; Mathers et al. 1994), disability-adjusted life expectancy (DALE) (Murray and Acharya 1997), YHL (Erickson et al. 1995), quality-adjusted life expectancy (QALE) (Fanshel and Bush 1970; Wilkins and Adams 1992), dementia-free life expectancy (Ritchie et al. 1993), and health capital (Cutler and Richardson 1997; 1998).

In contrast to a health expectancy, a health gap quantifies the difference between the actual health of a population and some stated norm or goal for population health. The health goal implied in Figure 1 is for everyone in the population to live in ideal health until the age indicated by the vertical line enclosing area C at the right. The health gap shown in Figure 1 can be interpreted either as the life table health gap, i.e. the health gap of a hypothetical birth cohort exposed to a set of currently measured mortality and non-fatal health outcome transition rates, or as the absolute health gap of a stable population with zero growth.

Since the work of Dempsey (1947), there has been extensive development of various measures of the years of life lost attributable to premature mortality (e.g. Murray 1996; Romeder and McWhinnie 1977). Measures of years of life lost are all measures of a mortality gap, i.e. the area between the survivorship function and an implied population norm for survivorship, represented as area C in Figure 1. Health gaps extend the notion of mortality gaps to account for the time lived in health states worse than ideal health. The health gap, therefore, is a function of areas C and B, or, more formally:

$$\text{Health gap} = C + g(B),$$

where $g(\bullet)$ is a function assigning weights to health states less than full health, using a scale on which a weight of one implies that the time lived in a particular health state is equivalent to the time lost because of premature mortality. Various health gaps have been proposed and measured (Ghana Health Assessment Project Team 1981; Hyder et al. 1998; Murray 1996; WHO 1999), and many others could be derived.

Key issues in the design of summary measures

There are at least four sets of issues that cut across all summary measures of population health: technical issues of calculation, the definition and measurement of health states, the valuation of health states, and the inclusion of other social values.

Calculation methods

Absolute and covariate-independent forms of summary measure

While the survivorship function in Figure 1 provides a convenient heuristic illustration of the difference between health expectancies and health gaps, it is important to recognize that summary measures may take either an absolute or an age-independent form. For example, the number of deaths in a population is an absolute measure, while a period life table does not depend on the age distribution in a population. By their construction, all health expectancies are measures that do not depend on the particular age structure of a population. Health gaps, on the other hand, are usually expressed in absolute terms and as such are dependent on age structure. For example, a health gap may be expressed as the total number of healthy years of life that have been lost in a population; this varies with the age distribution of the population. A life table health gap, as illustrated in Figure 1, can be calculated easily and is independent of the age structure of the population. It is also possible to conceive of health expectancies that depend on age structure, e.g. total healthy years lived in a population, but these measures have not been developed thus far.

Most discussions of health statistics have focused on the development of measures that are independent of age structure. Clearly, age is only one of innumerable covariates of health outcomes, and we might therefore imagine developing sex-independent, race-independent or income-independent forms of summary measure, just as we have forms that are independent of age structure. There are, however, arguments for paying special attention to the latter:

- Age is one of the most powerful determinants of health outcomes, so that comparisons based on measures that are not independent of age structure may be dominated, in some cases, by variation in this variable.

- Age cannot be changed by an intervention.

- Age is unique in that all individuals belong successively to every age until they die.

Although it is possible to imagine applying at least some of these arguments to other factors, such as sex and race, there will probably always be a particular interest in summary measures that are independent of age structure. The design of a summary measure and the range of covariate-independent forms of the measure that might be developed depend ultimately on its intended use.

Calculation of health expectancies

As with standard life tables (Shryock and Siegel 1971), health expectancies can be calculated for a period or for a cohort. The first method, which is more common, calculates the health expectancy for a hypothetical birth cohort exposed to currently observed event rates (e.g. rates of mortality, incidence and remission) over the course of its lifetime. We are not aware of any calculations of cohort health expectancies for real populations, although longitudinal studies may provide such opportunities (Longnecker 1999). Deeg et al. (1994) projected disability transition rates based on longitudinal data for the Netherlands but did not convert them into cohort health expectancies. Barendregt and Bonneux (1994) calculated changes in cohort disease-free life expectancy attributable to hypothetical interventions in a simulation model.

Health expectancies may also be distinguished by the use of incidence or prevalence information on non-fatal health outcomes. The pioneering efforts of Sullivan (1971) and others to estimate health expectancies involved applications of the prevalence rate life table borrowed from working life, marriage and education life tables (e.g. Wolfbein 1949). Katz et al. (1983) proposed that calculations of active life expectancy should be based on double-decrement life tables, in which individuals can move into two absorbing states: limited function and death. More recently, multistate life tables have been estimated for health expectancies (Branch et al. 1991; Mathers and Robine 1997a; Rogers et al. 1989). Robine et al. (1992) and Barendregt et al. (1994) argued that the multistate method was required logically so that health expectancy would be based only on currently measured mortality, incidence and remission, and not on prevalence. Robine et al. (1992) argued that prevalence was not a period measure; it was a stock variable rather than a flow. In real populations there may not be much difference between health expectancies calculated using the prevalence, double-decrement or multistate approaches (Mathers and Robine 1997b).

Calculation of health gaps

The most fundamental consideration in the calculation of health gaps is the choice of a target or norm for population health. Health gaps measure the difference between current conditions and a selected target. The explicit or implicit target is a critical characteristic of any health gap. Despite the obvious importance of choosing the health target, in some cases the population target is neither stated nor easily calculated. This was true of one of the first health gaps proposed by the Ghana Health Assessment Project Team (1981). The original formulation of many mortality gaps was constructed in terms of the loss to each individual. The aggregate population implications of the loss due to premature mortality for each individual have been poorly appreciated. For example, Murray (1996) has shown that for many mortality gap measures and health gaps the implied target may change as the mortality level changes, making direct comparisons between communities impossible.

As with health expectancies, health gaps may be calculated in various ways that reflect differences between the period and cohort perspectives and the incidence or prevalence perspectives. For example, DALYs in the Global Burden of Disease 1990 Study (Murray and Lopez 1996a) have been calculated in two ways: using the incidences of mortality and non-fatal health outcomes, and using the incidence of mortality and the prevalence of non-fatal health outcomes. Still other combinations are possible. Healthy life years (HeaLYs) for a given time period are calculated on the basis of the incidence of pathological processes and the future non-fatal health outcomes and mortality from those processes (Hyder et al. 1998). A pure prevalence health gap could be constructed based on the prevalences of non-fatal health outcomes and of individuals who have died in the past and would have lost years of life in the present time period.

DEFINITION AND MEASUREMENT OF HEALTH STATES

There is an important source of variation across summary measures in the definition and measurement of health states worse than perfect health. How should the different health states comprising area B in Figure 1 be described? Critical issues have to be considered even before the psychometric properties of different measurement instruments for health are analysed. Among them are the domains of health which are measured, the difference between performance and capacity in a domain, and the determinants of discrepancies between self-reported and observed performance or capacity in a domain.

Many domains of health have been proposed, ranging from each of the senses, to pain, mobility and cognition, and finally to complex functions related to health, such as social interaction or usual activities (McDowell and Newell 1996). The International Classification of Impairments, Disabilities and Handicaps (Bickenbach et al. 1999) attempts to classify this broad range of health domains into body functions, activities and participation. Measurement instruments also vary as to whether they focus on the capacity of individuals to perform in a domain, as with the Health Utilities Index (see chapter 7.2), or their actual performance. As many commonly used instruments depend largely on self-reporting, the individual social, economic and cultural factors that influence expectations for performance or capacity on each domain can lead to substantial deviations between self-reported values and observed values (Murray and Chen 1993).

Many health expectancies are linked to a particular instrument for the measurement of health status. ALE is linked to variants of the activities of daily living. The YHL measure is linked to two questions collected in the United States National Health Interview Survey, concerning activity limitations and perceived general health (Erickson et al. 1995; Erickson 1998). QALE (Wilkins and Adams 1992) is linked to a question on activity restriction in the Canada Health Survey. In other cases, such as dementia-free life expectancy, health expectancy is linked to a particular diagnosis or a single domain of health. DFLE is often calculated from data on long-term disability and includes the duration of a condition in its definition of disability. Data on self-assessed general health have been used in the calculation of health capital (Cutler and Richardson 1997), although the measure is not, by definition, linked strictly to this instrument. Clearly, wherever a health expectancy is defined with reference to a particular instrument, the summary measure depends critically on the reliability and validity of the instrument. All of the particular instruments mentioned here represent very limited conceptions of health, emphasizing a restricted set of physical domains. This contrasts with other health status instruments more widely applied in current practice, such as EuroQol (EuroQol Group 1990) or SF-36 (Ware and Sherbourne 1992), which capture multiple dimensions of health. Direct linkages are not required in the construction of summary measures, so they may complicate evaluation of the properties of summary measures unnecessarily.

VALUATION OF HEALTH STATES

Once the health states represented in area B of Figure 1 have been described in various domains the next step in calculating either health expectancies or health gaps is to determine the value of time spent in each state relative to full health and death. This allows these non-fatal health outcomes to be combined with information on mortality.

Many health expectancies, such as ALE and DFLE, apply dichotomous valuations (Figure 2). Up to an arbitrary threshold the valuation is zero (i.e. equivalent to the valuation of death); beyond this threshold the valuation is one (i.e. equivalent to full health). Dichotomous valuations make the measure extremely sensitive to variation in the arbitrary threshold definition, which creates significant obstacles to cross-national comparisons and assessments of changes over time. Other health expectancies and health gaps such as YHL, DALE, health capital, and DALYs use polytomous or, in principle, continuous valuations (Figure 2).

For those summary measures that do not use arbitrary dichotomous schemes the valuation approach can be distinguished further on the basis of:

- The persons whose values are used, e.g. individuals in health states, relatives of these individuals, the general public, or health care providers.

- The type of valuation question that is used, e.g. the standard gamble, time trade-off, person trade-off, or visual analogue.

Figure 2   Valuations of time spent in health states worse than perfect
                 health

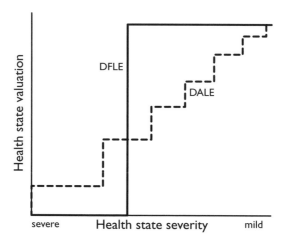

The solid line indicates dichotomous valuations, as in disability-free life expectancy (DFLE), while the dashed
line indicates categorical valuations, as in disability-adjusted life expectancy (DALE).

- The manner of presenting health states for the elicitation of valuations, i.e. with what type of description and what level of detail, including some selection of domains.

- The range of health states, from mild to severe, valued at the same time.

- The combination of valuation questions, and, more generally, the type of deliberative process undertaken, if any.

The relative merits of each of these choices continue to be debated extensively in the health economics literature.

OTHER VALUES

Values other than health state valuations also may be incorporated explicitly into summary measures. For example, health capital (Cutler and Richardson 1997; 1998) includes individuals' discount rates for future health. In addition to discounting, some variants of DALYs (Murray and Lopez 1996a; Murray and Acharya 1997) have included age weights, which allow the years lived at different ages to take on different values. Equity weights have also been proposed (Williams 1997) in order to allow the years lived by one group or another to take on different values. Incorporating other values into the design of a summary measure usually requires strong assumptions about the separability of health across both persons and time. Such separability has been challenged in the literature on quantifying the benefits of health interventions, as in the debate on healthy year equivalents and quality-adjusted life years (Culyer and Wagstaff 1993; Johannesson et al. 1993; Mehrez and Gafni 1989).

CRITERIA FOR EVALUATING SUMMARY MEASURES

Given the extensive interest in summary measures and the range of health expectancies and health gaps, one way to proceed is to propose a minimal set of desirable properties that summary measures should have and to evaluate the available summary measures against these criteria. The minimalist set of desirable properties for summary measures is likely to vary with the intended use. Thus a summary measure most appropriate for comparisons of population health over time may not be the most appropriate, or even acceptable, for reporting on the contribution of diseases, injuries and risk factors to ill health in a population. We consider the choice of an appropriate summary measure for comparative purposes, and then take up the question of choosing a summary measure that can be decomposed into the contributions of different diseases, injuries and risk factors. The objective is to begin to define an explicit framework for making these choices.

There is a common-sense notion of population health according to which, for some examples, everybody could agree that one population is healthier than another, or that the health of a particular population is becoming worse or better. For instance, if two populations are identical in every way except that infant mortality is higher in one, it is to be expected that everybody would agree that the population with the lower infant mortality is healthier. On the basis of this type of common-sense notion we can develop some very simple criteria for evaluating summary measures of health. However, even simple criteria lead to some rather thought-provoking conclusions.

Much of the discussion on the design of summary measures has been linked closely to the goal of maximizing gain in a summary measure in the face of a budget constraint. Inevitably, this has led to methods for constructing summary measures that emphasize the myriad value choices involved in the allocation of scarce resources, for example the use of the person trade-off technique for measuring health state valuations (Murray 1996; Nord 1995). Many authors have rightly focused on a range of values relevant to the allocation of scarce resources that may enhance the health of individuals (Nord et al. 1999). However, many of these considerations bring us far from the common-sense statement that one population is healthier than another. At least for the purposes of comparative statements on health it may be necessary to distance the development of summary measures from the complex values that have to be considered in the allocation of scarce resources. In other words, we can quite reasonably choose to measure population health in one way and conclude that scarce resources should not be allocated strictly to maximize population health as so measured. Indeed, implicit in the WHO framework for measuring health system performance (Murray and Frenk 2000) is the notion that resources should at least be allocated to maximize some socially desired mix of:

- average levels of population health;
- reductions in health inequalities;
- responsiveness of the health system to the legitimate expectations of the public—regarding the non-health dimensions of its interaction with the system; and
- fairness of health system financing.

Tentatively, we believe that we can construct summary measures for comparative purposes based on an application of Harsanyi's principle of choice from behind a veil of ignorance (Harsanyi 1953). In this construct, an individual behind a veil of ignorance does not know who he or she is in a population.[2] We propose that the relation "is healthier than" can be defined in such a way that population A is healthier than population B if, and only if, an individual behind a veil of ignorance would prefer to be one of the existing individuals in population A rather than an existing individual in population B, holding all non-health characteristics of the two populations to be the same.[3] We emphasize that the principle of choice behind the veil of ignorance does not mean choosing to join one of the populations as an additional member. A person must choose between two populations knowing that he or she would be one of the current members of either population, but not knowing at the moment of choice which particular member he or she would be in either population. Implementing the veil of ignorance approach to selecting the criteria for a summary measure of population health would have many far-reaching implications. On the basis of the veil of ignorance argument and consonant with common-sense notions of population health we argue that there are, minimally, five criteria that a summary measure should fulfil. These criteria are presented below with examples of comparisons between two populations at an instant in time.

- *Criterion 1.* If age-specific mortality is lower at any age, everything else being equal, then a summary measure should be better (i.e. the health gap should be lower and the health expectancy should be higher). Strictly speaking, this criterion refers to mortality rates among individuals in health states that are preferred to death. This criterion could be weakened to say that if age-specific mortality is lower at any age, everything else being equal, then a summary measure should be the same or better. The weaker version would allow for deaths beyond some critical age to leave a summary measure unchanged. Measures such as potential years of life lost would then fulfil the weak form of the criterion.

By inspection, all health expectancies fulfil the strong form of this criterion, but some health gaps do not. For health gaps, satisfaction of this criterion depends critically on the selection of the normative goal for population survivorship. For example, it can be demonstrated that the use of local life expectancy at each age to define the gap associated with a death at that age, as proposed by several authors (Ghana Health Assessment Project Team 1981; Williams 1999), leads to a violation of this criterion. For the purposes of illustration, let us imagine two hypothetical populations with linear survivorship functions, as represented by the bold diagonals in Figure 3. For the population represented in the first diagram, life expectancy at birth (the area under the survivorship function) is 25 years, while the second population has a life expectancy at birth of 37.5 years. Based on the survivorship function, $s(x)$, we can compute, for each population, the life expectancy at each age, $e(x)$, namely the area under the survivorship function to the right of age x divided by $s(x)$. The implied population norm, $G(\bullet)$, is defined so that $G(x + e(x)) = s(x)$. In Figure 3, $G(\bullet)$ is the diagonal boundary of the shaded area in each diagram. In the population with a life expectancy of 37.5, which has a lower mortality rate at every age than the population with a life expectancy of 25, the health gap shown as the shaded area has actually increased.

- *Criterion 2.* If age-specific prevalence is higher for some health state worse than ideal health, everything else being equal, a summary measure should be worse. Let us imagine two populations, A and B, with identical mortality, incidence and remission for all non-fatal health states but with a higher prevalence of paraplegia in population A. Be-

Figure 3   Health gaps based on local life expectancy

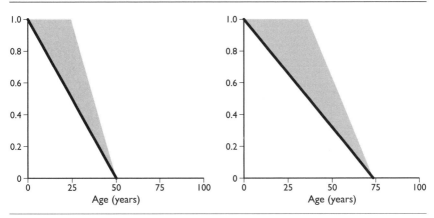

The first graph indicates a population with life expectancy at birth of 25 years, while the second graph indicates a population with life expectancy of 37.5 years. In each graph, the bold diagonal represents a survivorship curve. The shaded areas reflect survivorship norms in each population which are based on actual life expectancy at each age.

hind a veil of ignorance an individual would be expected to prefer to be a member of population B. Likewise, the common-sense notion of population health leads us to conclude that B is healthier than A. Health expectancies and health gaps calculated only on the basis of incidence and remission rates for non-fatal health states do not fulfil this criterion, whereas prevalence-based health expectancies and health gaps do fulfil it.

- *Criterion 3.* If age-specific incidence of some health state worse than ideal health is higher, everything else being equal, a summary measure should be worse. Let us imagine two populations, A and B, with identical mortality, prevalence and remission, but with a higher incidence of blindness in A than in B. We must conclude that B is healthier than A. Incidence-based health expectancies and health gaps would fulfil this criterion.

Taking criteria 2 and 3 together, we are led to the conclusion that no existing summary measure fulfils both of them. According to conventional wisdom in health statistics, incidence-based measures are better for monitoring current trends and are more logically consistent for summary measures because mortality rates describe incident events. Prevalence measures are widely recognized as important for planning current curative and rehabilitative services, while incidence-based measures are more relevant to the planning of prevention activities. These long-standing arguments have their merits but do not answer the question as to what it means for one population to be healthier than another at a given point in time. It seems undeniable that the common dichotomy between incidence-based and prevalence-based measures does not reflect the composite judgement that an individual behind a veil of ignorance would make on which population is healthier.

As one possible solution to this dilemma we could estimate cohort health expectancy at each age x, which would reflect both incidence and prevalence.[4] Thus the health expectancy of 50-year-olds depends on the current prevalence of conditions among individuals in this age cohort as well as on the current and future incidence, remission and mortality rates facing the cohort. A period health expectancy at each age x which reflects incidence and prevalence could also be constructed to provide a measure based only on currently measurable aspects of health. A summary measure for the population could then be based on some aggregation of the cohort or period health expectancies at each age, such as a simple average across all individuals in the population. This aggregate measure would reflect both incidence and prevalence and would be dependent on age structure. Although the mechanics of constructing this measure require further development, we believe that it offers a potential solution to the problem posed jointly by criteria 2 and 3.

- *Criterion 4.* If age-specific remission for some health state worse than ideal health is higher, everything else being equal, a summary measure should be better. The argument for this criterion is essentially identical to the argument for criterion 3.

- *Criterion 5.* If two populations, A and B, include individuals in identically matched health states except for one individual who is in a worse health state in population B, everything else being equal, then a summary measure should be worse in B. Here we refer to health states that are described completely in all domains. Any reduction or improvement in any domain would define a new health state. In practice, measurement instruments assign individuals into a finite number of discrete health states in which there is still heterogeneity of levels in each domain of health. At the extreme, measures that categorize the population into only two states, e.g. disabled and not disabled, are insensitive to substantial changes in the true health state of individuals. This criterion is particularly important for assessing the performance of health systems where much of the health expenditure in high-income countries may be directed to interventions that improve the health states of individuals without changing mortality. DFLE, impairment-free life expectancy and dementia-free life expectancy, which all use arbitrary dichotomous weights, do not fulfil criterion 5.

OTHER DESIRABLE PROPERTIES OF SUMMARY MEASURES

Summary measures for comparative purposes are meant to inform many policy discussions and debates. The intended widespread use of summary measures leads to several desirable properties in addition to the basic criteria described above. The appeal of these properties is not based on formal or informal arguments about whether one population is healthier than another, but rather on practical considerations.

- Summary measures should be comprehensible and their calculation should be feasible for many populations. It is of little value to develop summary measures that will not be used to inform the health policy process. The nearly universal use of a very complex abstract measure, namely period life expectancy at birth, demonstrates that comprehensibility and complexity are different. The interest of the popular press in DALE (Brown 2000; Crossette 2000), probably because health expectancies build on life expectancy, is one indication of the comprehensibility of health expectancies. Health gaps are perhaps less familiar to many but the concept is reasonably simple and communicable.

- It would be convenient if summary measures were linear aggregates of the summary measures calculated for any arbitrary partitioning of subgroups. Many decision-makers, and very often the public, desire information characterized by this type of additive decomposition across subpopulations. They would like to know what fraction of the summary measure is related to health events in the poor, the uninsured, the elderly, children and so on. Additive decomposition, which also often has appeal for cause attribution, can be achieved for health gaps but not for health expectancies. For example, we can report the number of DALYs in a population for ages 0 to 4 years and for ages 5 years and above, and the sum of these two numbers equals the total health gap in the population. On the other hand, it is not clear how to combine the DALE for everybody aged 0 to 4 years with that for everybody aged 5 years and older to obtain a meaningful number. Techniques for estimating the contribution of changes in age-specific mortality rates to a change in life expectancy have been developed (e.g. Arriaga 1984), but they do not have the property of additive decomposition.

CALCULATING THE CONTRIBUTION OF DISEASES, INJURIES AND RISK FACTORS TO SUMMARY MEASURES

Another fundamental goal in constructing summary measures, which may explain the increasing attention being given to them, is to identify the relative magnitude of different health problems, including diseases, injuries and risk factors, corresponding to uses 5, 6 and 7 above. There are two dominant traditions in widespread use for causal attribution: categorical attribution and counterfactual analysis. There has been little discussion of their advantages and disadvantages or of the inconsistency of using both approaches in the same analysis. An example of the latter is provided by the Global Burden of Disease 1990 Study (Murray and Lopez 1996a). Burden attributable to diseases and injuries has been estimated using categorical attribution whereas burden attributable to risk factors or diseases such as diabetes, which act as risk factors, has been estimated using counterfactual analysis.

CATEGORICAL ATTRIBUTION

An event such as death or the onset of a particular health state can be attributed categorically to one single cause according to a defined set of rules. In cause-of-death tabulations, for example, each death is assigned to a unique cause according to the rules of the International Classification of Diseases (ICD), even in cases of multicausal events. For example, in ICD-10, deaths from tuberculosis in HIV-positive individuals are assigned to HIV. This categorical approach to representing causes is the standard method used in published studies of health gaps such as the Global Burden of Disease 1990 (Murray and Lopez 1997c).

A classification system is required in order that categorical attribution may work. Such a system has two key components: a set of mutually exclusive and collectively exhaustive categories and a set of rules for assigning events to them. The ICD relating to diseases and injuries has been developed and refined over nearly 100 years. No classification system has been developed for other types of causes such as physiological, proximal or distal risk factors.

COUNTERFACTUAL ANALYSIS

The contribution of a disease, injury or risk factor can be estimated by comparing the current level and future levels of a summary measure of population health with the levels that would be expected under some alternative hypothetical scenario, for instance a counterfactual distribution of risk or the extent of a disease or injury. The models used in counterfactual analysis may be extremely simple or, in the case of some risk factors with complex time and distributional characteristics, quite complex. The validity of the estimate depends on that of the model used to predict the counterfactual scenarios. Various types of counterfactuals may be used for this type of assessment.

- The effect of small changes in the disease, injury or risk factor can be assessed and the results expressed as the elasticity of the summary measure with respect to changes in the disease, injury or risk factor, or as a numerical approximation of the partial derivative of the summary measure (Hill et al. 1996; Mathers 1999).

- Another form of counterfactual analysis assesses the change in a summary measure expected with complete elimination of a disease or injury. A number of studies have presented results on cause-deleted health expectancies (Colvez and Blanchet 1983; Mathers 1992; 1997; Nusselder et al. 1996; Nusselder 1998). Wolfson (1996) calculated attribute-deleted health expectancies (i.e. deleting types of disabilities rather than causes).

- More generally, Murray and Lopez (1999) have developed a classification of various counterfactual risk distributions that can be used for these purposes, including the theoretical minimum risk, the plausible minimum risk, the feasible minimum risk and the cost-effective minimum risk. The examples of tobacco and alcohol have been used to explore the implications of using these different types of counterfactual distribution to define attributable burden and avoidable burden.

- In intervention analysis the change in a summary measure from the application of a specific intervention is estimated.

Counterfactual analysis of summary measures has a wide spectrum of uses—from the assessment of specific policies or actions to more general assessments of the contribution of diseases, injuries or risk factors. Two important factors are independent of the type of counterfactual used: the duration of the counterfactual and the time during which changes in population health under the counterfactual are evaluated. The complexity of defining the duration of the counterfactual and the time during which change is evaluated can be illustrated with tobacco. A counterfactual for tobacco consumption in which the population does not smoke for one year, followed by a return to the status quo at the end of this year, could be traced out in terms of changes in future health expectancies or future health gaps. Because of time lags and threshold effects, removing a hazard for such a short duration may lead to little or no change in a summary measure of population health over time. Alternatively, the counterfactual change in tobacco could be longer, such as a permanent change to a state of no tobacco consumption.

Models have been developed (Gunning-Schepers 1989; Gunning-Schepers et al. 1989; Gunning-Schepers and Barendregt 1992) that facilitate counterfactual analyses with varying durations. Changes in the counterfactual distribution of exposure in a population may have an impact on summary measures of population health over many years in the future. Logically, all changes in future population health should be included. For reasons that are debated elsewhere one could argue that changes in the distant future should be weighted as less important than more proximal changes, i.e. future changes should be discounted. One method that has been used is to apply a dichotomous discount rate, such that changes up to time t are counted equally and changes after time t are given zero weight. Although discounting is controversial (Cropper et al. 1994; Redelmeier and Heller 1993; Sen 1967; Viscusi and Moore 1989), choices on the duration of a counterfactual are linked intimately to whether future changes in population health are discounted. For example, a permanent shift in exposure could lead to an infinite stream of future changes in health expectancies or health gaps in the absence of discounting.

As part of its work on comparative risk assessment, WHO is trying to facilitate a debate on the standardized definition of counterfactuals and the duration of evaluation for a counterfactual change in exposure.

ADVANTAGES AND DISADVANTAGES

There are three possible ways of analysing the contribution of diseases, injuries or risk factors (see Table 1). Population health can be summarized using health expectancies and health gaps, and cause attribution for diseases and injuries can be assessed using categorical attribution or counterfactuals. Because there is no classification system for risk factors they can only be assessed using the counterfactual approach. Even for diseases and injuries it is not possible to use categorical attribution with a health expectancy, as positive health cannot be assigned to specific diseases or injuries. What are the advantages and disadvantages of the three options in Table 1?

The advantage of categorical attribution is that it is simple, widely understood and appealing to many users of this information because the total level of the summary measure equals the sum of the contributions of a set of mutually exclusive causes (i.e. categorical attribution produces additive decomposition across causes). The disadvantage is well illustrated by multicausal events such as a myocardial infarction in a diabetic, or liver cancer resulting from chronic hepatitis B. If additive decomposition is a critical property, the contribution of diseases and injuries can only be assessed using health gaps.

The counterfactual method for calculating the contribution of diseases, injuries and risk factors has different advantages. It is conceptually clearer, solves problems of multicausality and is consistent with the approach for evaluating the benefits of health interventions (Wolfson 1996).

How can causal attribution be used to inform debates on research and development priorities, the selection of national health priorities for action, and health curriculum development? It can be argued that a method of causal attribution should give an ordinal ranking of causes which is identical to that of the absolute number of years of healthy life gained by a population through cause elimination (or appropriate counterfactual change for a risk factor). This means that the absolute numbers attributable to a cause are important where cause decomposition is intended to inform public health prioritization.

DISCUSSION

In this paper we have put forward a basic framework for characterizing and evaluating different types of summary measures. In choosing summary measures for a range of different uses it is critical not only to understand the important differences between the various types of available summary measures, but also to distinguish clearly between the range of measures and the different types of instruments and data that may be used as inputs for estimating them. We have defined five basic criteria that may be used as a starting point in evaluating summary measures. We hope that they will provoke further debate on other possible criteria that may be useful

Table I   Approaches to analysing the contributions of diseases, injuries or risk factors to summary measures of population health

	Categorical attribution	Counterfactual analysis
Health expectancies	—	Diseases Injuries Risk factors
Health gaps	Diseases Injuries	Diseases Injuries Risk factors

to analysts and policy-makers in choosing summary measures for policy applications.

It is worth noting a few examples where even our basic criteria lead to the rejection of certain methodological approaches. For example, the calculation of health gaps using local life expectancy (Ghana Health Assessment Project Team 1981; Williams 1999) violates criterion 1, which requires that as mortality declines, a summary measure should improve. According to criterion 5, we should also reject measures that are based on categorizing individuals into two health states, e.g. disabled and not disabled, with arbitrary zero and one weights as in DFLE, ALE and dementia-free life expectancy. A number of remaining health expectancies and health gaps fulfil four of the five criteria, but no measure fulfils the prevalence and incidence criteria at the same time. For comparative uses it may be necessary to develop a new class of measure that reflects both prevalence and incidence, as with the average age-specific health expectancy described above. It is very important to recognize that, for other uses of summary measures, different criteria may be formulated with different implications for the design of such measures.

Causal attribution is a key aspect of summary measures for several important uses outlined above. For diseases and injuries, ICD allows a choice between categorical attribution and counterfactual analysis. The desirability of additive decomposition strongly favours the use of categorical attribution. However, the magnitudes from counterfactual analysis have a more direct and theoretically cogent interpretation. We suggest that in practice the only solution to this tension is routine reporting of both categorical attribution and counterfactual analysis for diseases and injuries. All issues of multicausal death, as with diabetes mellitus, would be well captured in counterfactual analysis even if categorical attribution tends to underestimate the problem. There is no classification system for risk factors, whether physiological, proximal or distal, and consequently the only option is counterfactual analysis. There are many options for defining counterfactuals, and substantial work is needed to understand more fully the implications of adopting different approaches.

Improving the estimation of summary measures of population health depends on designing the most appropriate measures for particular purposes. It also requires improvement of the empirical basis for the epidemiology of fatal and non-fatal health outcomes, including attribution by cause, and for health state valuations. One critical requirement is an improved understanding of the determinants of differences between self-reported and observed measures of performance or capacity in selected domains of health.

In proposing this framework for choosing summary measures we have invoked both a common-sense notion whereby, in some cases, everybody could agree that one population was healthier than another, as well as a more formal mechanism for defining this choice, using Harsanyi's notion of choice behind a veil of ignorance. There are some potentially important implications of the veil of ignorance framework for choosing a summary measure of population health for comparative purposes. For example, the current methods used to measure preferences for time spent in health states may not be entirely consistent with this framework, and modified methods would perhaps need to be developed. Clearly, it would be helpful to provide a more rigorous formal treatment of this approach.

As work on summary measures gathers speed, their uses and complexities are becoming more widely appreciated. The application of simple criteria may lead to the rejection of some measures and the development of new ones. An extensive developmental agenda exists; nevertheless, the use of summary measures should not be delayed until all methodological issues have been resolved. Every effort should be made to use currently available summary measures that satisfy as many of the criteria and desirable properties as possible. The calculation of alternative summary measures should be facilitated by making the critical information on the epidemiology of non-fatal health outcomes and mortality widely available.

NOTES

1   A version of this chapter was published previously in the *Bulletin of the World Health Organization* 2000; 78(8):981-994. It is reprinted with permission from the World Health Organization.

2   Harsanyi's veil of ignorance has been described as a thin veil, in contrast to Rawls' thick veil. In Rawls' formulation (Rawls 1971), the veil excludes much more information; most importantly for this discussion, it excludes the particular circumstances of society such as the epidemiological information upon which our criteria are based.

3   Formally, the assumption that the relation "is healthier than" does not depend on the particular levels at which non-health characteristics are fixed requires separability of the health-related characteristics of a population from characteristics that are not health-related. This assumption has been questioned (Broome 1999) and several compelling examples of its violation have been presented. Nevertheless, there are reasons to believe that health is largely separable from other components of well-being. In nearly all languages and cultures there is a recognized word for health and a distinct concept of health. Common sayings to the effect that health is more important than wealth serve as a testament to the basic separability of health and non-health well-being.

In addition to the separability of health and non-health well-being, we require that individuals behind the veil of ignorance make their choice assuming that health is separable across individuals. This is required so that the statement "is healthier than" strictly reflects differences in the average level of health between populations and not the distribution of health within populations. We intend to capture distributional issues in a separate measure of inequality of health across individuals.

4   Health capital at age x, proposed as a measure of a cohort's health (Cutler and Richardson 1997; 1998), is a subjective discounted cohort health expectancy at age x. While it has not been proposed as a summary measure of population

health, it includes both prevalence and subjective expected incidence in its arguments.

REFERENCES

Anand S, Hanson K (1998) DALYs: efficiency versus equity. *World Development,* **26**(2):307–310.

Arriaga EE (1984) Measuring and explaining the change in life expectancies. *Demography,* **21**(1):83–96.

Barendregt JJ, Bonneux L (1994) Changes in incidence and survival of cardiovascular disease and their impact on disease prevalence and health expectancy. In: *Advances in health expectancies.* (Proceedings of the 7th meeting of the international network on health expectancy and the disability process REVES, February 1994, Canberra.) Mathers CD, McCallum J, Robine JM, eds. Australian Institute of Health and Welfare, AGPS, Canberra.

Barendregt JJ, Bonneux L, van der Maas PJ (1994) Health expectancy: an indicator for change? Technology assessment methods project team. *Journal of Epidemiology and Community Health,* **48**(5):482–487.

Bickenbach JE, Chatterji S, Badley EM, Üstün TB (1999) Models of disablement, universalism and the international classification of impairments, disabilities and handicaps. *Social Science and Medicine,* **48**(9):1173–1187.

Bobadilla JL (1998) *Searching for essential health services in low- and middle-income countries: a review of recent studies on health priorities.* Inter American Development Bank, Social Development Division, Washington, DC.

Bone MR (1992) International efforts to measure health expectancy. *Journal of Epidemiology and Community Health,* **46**(6):555–558.

Bowie C, Beck S, Bevan G, Raftery J, Silverton F, Stevens A (1997) Estimating the burden of disease in an English region. *Journal of Public Health Medicine,* **19**(1):87–92.

Branch LG, Guralnik JM, Foley DJ, Kohout FJ, et al. (1991) Active life expectancy for 10,000 Caucasian men and women in three communities. *Journal of Gerontology,* **46**(4):M145–M150.

Brock DW (1998) Ethical issues in the development of summary measures of population health states. In: *Summarizing population health: directions for the development and application of population metrics.* Field MJ, Gold MR, eds. National Academy Press, Washington, DC.

Bronnum-Hansen H (1998) Trends in health expectancy in Denmark. *Danish Medical Journal,* **45**:217–221.

Broome J (1999) *Ethics out of economics.* Cambridge University Press, New York.

Brown D (2000) New look at longevity offers disease insight. *Washington Post,* A9(June 12).

Brundtland GH (1998) *The global burden of disease.* World Health Organization, Geneva. (Speech delivered on 15 December).

Chiang CL (1965) *An index of health: mathematical models.* (Vital and health statistics series 2, no 5.) National Center for Health Statistics, Washington, DC.

Colvez A, Blanchet M (1983) Potential gains in life expectancy free of disability: a tool for health planning. *International Journal of Epidemiology*, **12**(2):224–229.

Concha M (1996) *Estudio carga de enfermedad. Informe final. [Chilean burden of disease study. Final report.]* Estudio Prioridades de Inversion en Salud, Ministerio de Salud, Santiago de Chile.

Crimmins EM, Saito Y, Ingeneri D (1997) Trends in disability-free life expectancy in the United States, 1970–90. *Population and Development Review*, **23**(3):555–572.

Cropper ML, Aydede SK, Portney PR (1994) Preferences for life saving programs: how the public discounts time and age. *Journal of Risk and Uncertainty*, **8**(3):243–265.

Crossette B (2000) Americans enjoy 70 healthy years, behind Europe, UN says. *New York Times*, **A10**(June 5)

Culyer AJ, Wagstaff A (1993) QALYs versus HYEs. *Journal of Health Economics*, **12**(3):311–323.

Cutler DM, Richardson E (1997) Measuring the health of the US population. *Brookings Papers on economic activity: Microeconomics*, 217–227.

Cutler DM, Richardson E (1998) The value of health: 1970–1990. *American Economic Review*, **88**(2):97–100.

Daniels N (1998) Distributive justice and the use of summary measures of population health status. In: *Summarizing population health: directions for the development and application of population metrics*. Field MJ, Gold MR, eds. National Academic Press, Washington, DC.

Deeg DJH, Kriegsman DMW, van Zonneveld RJ (1994) Trends in fatal chronic diseases and disability in the Netherlands 1956–1993 and projections 1993–1998. In: *Advances in health expectancies*. (Proceedings of the 7th meeting of the international network on health expectancy and the disability process REVES, February 1994, Canberra.) Mathers CD, McCallum J, Robine JM, eds. Australian Institute of Health and Welfare, AGPS, Canberra.

Dempsey M (1947) Decline in tuberculosis: the death rate fails to tell the entire story. *American Review of Tuberculosis*, (56):157–164.

Erickson P (1998) Evaluation of a population-based measure of quality of life: the health and activity limitation index (HALex). *Quality of Life Research*, 7(2):101–114.

Erickson P, Wilson R, Shannon I (1995) *Years of healthy life*. (CDC/NCHS, Healthy people, Statistical notes no 7.) US Department of Health and Human Services, National Center for Health Statistics, Hyattsville, MD.

EuroQol Group (1990) EuroQol: a new facility for the measurement of health-related quality of life. *Health Policy*, **16**(3):199–208.

Fanshel S, Bush JW (1970) A health-status index and its application to health services outcomes. *Operations Research*, **18**(6):1021–1065.

Field MJ, Gold MR, eds. (1998) *Summarizing population health: directions for the development and application of population metrics.* National Academy Press, Washington, DC.

Fundacion Mexicana para la Salud (1995) *Health and the economy: proposals for progress in the Mexican health system. An overview.* Fundacion Mexicana para la Salud, Mexico.

Gakidou EE, Murray CJL, Frenk J (2000) Defining and measuring health inequality: an approach based on the distribution of health expectancy. *Bulletin of the World Health Organization,* **78**(1):42–54.

Ghana Health Assessment Project Team (1981) A quantitative method of assessing the health impact of different diseases in less developed countries. *International Journal of Epidemiology,* **10**(1):72–80.

Gunning-Schepers LJ (1989) The health benefits of prevention: a simulation approach. *Health Policy,* **12**(1–2):35–48.

Gunning-Schepers LJ, Barendregt JJ (1992) Timeless epidemiology or history cannot be ignored. *Journal of Clinical Epidemiology,* **45**(4):365–372.

Gunning-Schepers LJ, Barendregt JJ, van der Maas PJ (1989) Population interventions reassessed. *Lancet,* **1**(8636):479–481.

Harsanyi JC (1953) Cardinal utility in welfare economics and in the theory of risk-taking. *Journal of Political Economy,* **61**:434–435.

Hill GB, Forbes WF, Wilkins R (1996) *The entropy of health and disease: dementia in Canada.* (Presented at the 9th meeting of the international network on health expectancy and the disability process REVES, December 1996.) Rome.

Hyder AA, Rotllant G, Morrow R (1998) Measuring the burden of disease: healthy life-years. *American Journal of Public Health,* **88**(2):196–202.

Johannesson M, Pliskin JS, Weinstein MC (1993) Are healthy-years equivalents an improvement over quality-adjusted life years? *Medical Decision Making,* **13**(4):281–286.

Katz S, Akpom CA, Papsidero JA, Weiss ST (1973) Measuring the health status of populations. In: *Health status indexes.* Berg RL, ed. Hospital Research and Educational Trust, Chicago, IL.

Katz S, Branch LG, Branson MH (1983) Active life expectancy. *New England Journal of Medicine,* **309**(20):1218–1224.

Longnecker MP (1999) The Framingham results on alcohol and breast cancer. *American Journal of Epidemiology,* **149**(2):102–104.

Lozano R, Frenk J, Gonzalez MA (1994) El peso de la enfermedad en adultos mayores, México 1994. *Salud Pública de México,* **38**:419–429.

Lozano R, Murray CJL, Frenk J, Bobadilla JL (1995) Burden of disease assessment and health system reform: results of a study in Mexico. *Journal for International Development,* **7**(3):555–563.

Mathers CD (1992) *Estimating gains in health expectancy due to elimination of specified diseases.* (Presented at the 5th meeting of the international network on health expectancy and the disability process REVES, February 1992.) Ottawa.

Mathers CD (1997) *Gains in health expectancy from the elimination of disease: a useful measure of the burden of disease.* (Presented at the 10th meeting of the international network on health expectancy and the disability process REVES, October 1997.) Tokyo.

Mathers CD (1999) Gains in health expectancy from the elimination of diseases among older people. *Disability and Rehabilitation*, 21(5–6):211–221.

Mathers CD, McCallum J, Robine JM, eds. (1994) *Advances in health expectancies.* (Proceedings of the 7th meeting of the of the international network on health expectancy and the disability process REVES, February 1994, Canberra.) Australian Institute of Welfare, AGPS, Canberra.

Mathers CD, Robine JM (1997a) How good is Sullivan's method for monitoring changes in population health expectancies. *Journal of Epidemiology and Community Health*, 51(1):80–86.

Mathers CD, Robine JM (1997b) How good is Sullivan's method for monitoring changes in population health expectancies. Reply. *Journal of Epidemiology and Community Health*, 51(5):578–579.

McDowell I, Newell C (1996) *Measuring health: a guide to rating scales and questionnaires.* 2nd edn. Oxford University Press, New York.

Mehrez A, Gafni A (1989) Quality-adjusted life-years, utility theory and healthy-years equivalents. *Medical Decision Making*, 9:142–149.

Ministry of Health, Colombia (1994) *La carga de la enfermedad en Colombia. [The burden of disease in Colombia.]* Ministry of Health, Bogota.

Murray CJL (1996) Rethinking DALYs. In: *The global burden of disease: a comprehensive assessment of mortality and disability from diseases, injuries, and risk factors in 1990 and projected to 2020.* The Global Burden of Disease and Injury, Vol. 1. Murray CJL, Lopez AD, eds. Harvard School of Public Health on behalf of WHO, Cambridge, MA.

Murray CJL, Acharya AK (1997) Understanding DALYs. *Journal of Health Economics*, 16:703–730.

Murray CJL, Chen LC (1993) In search of a contemporary theory for understanding mortality change. *Social Science and Medicine*, 36(2):143–155.

Murray CJL, Frenk JA (2000) A framework for assessing the performance of health systems. *Bulletin of the World Health Organization*, 78(6):717–731.

Murray CJL, Gakidou E, Frenk J (1999) Health inequalities and social group differences: what should we measure? *Bulletin of the World Health Organization*, 77(7):537–543.

Murray CJL, Lopez AD, eds. (1996a) *The global burden of disease: a comprehensive assessment of mortality and disability from diseases, injuries and risk factors in 1990 and projected to 2020.* Global Burden of Disease and Injury, Vol. 1. Harvard School of Public Health on behalf of WHO, Cambridge, MA.

Murray CJL, Lopez AD, eds. (1996b) *Global health statistics: a compendium of incidence, prevalence and mortality estimates for over 200 conditions.* Global Burden of Disease and Injury, Vol 2. Harvard School of Public Health on behalf of WHO, Cambridge, MA.

Murray CJL, Lopez AD (1996c) Evidence-based health policy: lessons from the global burden of disease study. *Science,* **274**(5288):740–743.

Murray CJL, Lopez AD (1997a) Alternative projections of mortality and disability by cause 1990–2020: global burden of disease study. *Lancet,* **349**(9064):1498–1504.

Murray CJL, Lopez AD (1997b) Global mortality, disability and the contribution of risk factors: global burden of disease study. *Lancet,* **349**(9063):1436–1442.

Murray CJL, Lopez AD (1997c) Mortality by cause for eight regions of the world: global burden of disease study. *Lancet,* **349**(9061):1269–1276.

Murray CJL, Lopez AD (1997d) Regional patterns of disability-free life expectany and disability-adjusted life expectancy: global burden of disease study. *Lancet,* **349**(9062):1347–1352.

Murray CJL, Lopez AD (1999) On the comparable quantification of health risks: lessons from the global burden of disease study. *Epidemiology,* **10**(5):594–605.

Murray CJL, Michaud CM, McKenna MT, Marks JS (1998) *US patterns of mortality by county and race: 1965–1994.* Harvard Center for Population and Development Studies and Centres for Disease Control, Cambridge, MA.

Mutafova M, van de Water HPA, Perenboom RJM, Boshuizen HC, Maleshkov C (1997) Health expectancy calculations: a novel approach to studying population health in Bulgaria. *Bulletin of the World Health Organization,* **75**(2):147–153.

Nord E (1995) The person-trade off approach to valuing health care programs. *Medical Decision Making,* **15**(3):201–208.

Nord EM, Pinto JL, Richardson J, Menzel P, Ubel P (1999) Incorporating societal concerns for fairness in numerical valuations of health programmes. *Health Economics,* **8**(1):25–39.

Nusselder WJ (1998) *Compression or expansion of morbidity? A life-table approach.* Doctoral dissertation. Erasmus University, Rotterdam.

Nusselder WJ, van der Velden K, van Sonsbeek JL, Lenior ME, et al. (1996) The elimination of selected chronic diseases in a population: the compression and expansion of morbidity. *American Journal of Public Health,* **86**(2):187–194.

Piot M, Sundaresan TK (1967) *A linear programme decision model for tuberculosis control. Progress report on the first test-runs. VMO/TB/Technical Information 67.55.* World Health Organization, Geneva. (Unpublished document).

Preston SH (1993) Health indices as a guide to health sector planning: a demographic critique. In: *The epidemiological transition. Policy and planning implications for developing countries.* Gribble JN, Preston SR, eds. National Academic Press, Washington, DC.

Rawls J (1971) *A theory of justice.* Harvard University Press, Cambridge, MA.

Redelmeier DA, Heller DM (1993) Time preference in medical decision making and cost-effectiveness analysis. *Medical Decision Making,* **13**(3):212–217.

Ritchie K, Jagger C, Brayne C, Letenneur L (1993) Dementia-free life expectancy: preliminary calculations for France and the United Kingdom. In: *Calculation of health expectancies: harmonization, consensus achieved and future perspectives.* REVES. Robine JM, Mathers CD, Bone MR, Romieu I, eds. John Libbey Eurotex, London.

Robine JM, Blanchet M, Dowd JE, eds. (1992) *Health expectancy.* (Proceedings of the first meeting of the international network on health expectancy and the disability process REVES, September 1989, Quebec.) HMSO, London.

Robine JM, Mathers CD, Bone MR, Romieu I, eds. (1993) *Calculation of health expectancies: harmonization, consensus achieved and future perspectives.* (Proceedings of the 6th meeting of the international network on health expectancy and the disability process REVES, October 1992, Montpellier.) John Libbey Eurotext, Paris.

Rogers A, Rogers RG, Branch LG (1989) A multistate analysis of active life expectancy. *Public Health Reports,* **104**(3):222–226.

Romeder JM, McWhinnie JR (1977) Potential years of life lost between ages 1 and 70: an indicator of premature mortality for health planning. *International Journal of Epidemiology,* **6**(2):143–151.

Ruwaard D, Kramers PGN (1998) *Public health status and forecasts. Health prevention and health care in the Netherlands until 2015.* National Institute of Public Health and Environmental Protection, Elsevier.

Sanders BS (1964) Measuring community health levels. *American Journal of Public Health,* **54**(7):1063–1070.

Sen A (1967) Isolation, assurance, and social rate of discount. *Quarterly Journal of Economics,* **81**(1):123–124.

Shryock HS, Siegel JS, et al. (1971) *The methods and materials of demography: the life table.* US Bureau of the Census, Washington, DC.

Sihvonen AP, Kunst AE, Lahelma E, Valkonen T, Mackenbach JP (1998) Socioeconomic inequalities in health expectancy in Finland and Norway in the late 1980s. *Social Science and Medicine,* **47**(3):303–315.

Sullivan DF (1966) Conceptual problems in developing an index of health. *Vital and Health Statistics,* (2):17.

Sullivan DF (1971) *A single index of mortality and morbidity. HSMHA health reports.*

Valkonen T, Sihvonen AP, Lahelma E (1997) Health expectancy by level of education in Finland. *Social Science and Medicine,* **44**:801–808.

Viscusi WK, Moore MJ (1989) Rates of time preference and valuations of the duration of life. *Journal of Public Economics,* **38**(3):297–317.

Ware JE, Sherbourne CD (1992) The MOS 36-item short form health survey (SF-36): I. Conceptual framework and item selection. *Medical Care,* **30**(6):473–483.

WHO (1996) *Investing in health research and development.* (Report of the Ad Hoc Committee on Health Research Priorities.) World Health Organization, Geneva.

WHO (1999) *The World Health Report 1999: making a difference.* World Health Organization, Geneva.

Wilkins R, Adams OB (1992) Quality-adjusted life expectancy: weighting of expected years in each state of health. In: *Health expectancy*. (Proceedings of the first workshop of the international healthy life expectancy network REVES, September 1989, Quebec.) Robine JM, Blanchet M, Dowd JE, eds. HMSO, London.

Williams A (1997) Intergenerational equity: an exploration of the "fair innings" argument. *Health Economics*, 6 (2):117–132.

Williams A (1999) Calculating the global burden of disease: time for a strategic reappraisal? *Health Economics*, 8(1):1–8.

Wolfbein S (1949) The length of working life. *Population Studies*, (3):286–294.

Wolfson MC (1996) Health-adjusted life expectancy. *Statistics Canada: Health Reports*, 8(1):41–46.

Chapter 1.3

THE INDIVIDUAL BASIS FOR SUMMARY MEASURES OF POPULATION HEALTH

CHRISTOPHER J.L. MURRAY, JOSHUA A. SALOMON
AND COLIN D. MATHERS

INTRODUCTION

In chapter 1.2, we reviewed some of the uses and conceptual debates relating to summary measures of population health (SMPH) and presented minimal criteria for evaluating SMPH. Much of the literature on SMPH has grown out of the demographic and epidemiological traditions, which take a population perspective as their starting point. For some uses such as measuring inequalities in health across individuals or measuring the health of individuals in clinical settings or intervention trials, it is important to formulate SMPH in terms of the health of some set of individuals. Many of the challenges identified in chapter 1.2 are intimately related to the linkage between population and individual health measures. Distinctions between incidence and prevalence perspectives, or period and cohort perspectives, for example, can be recast in terms of different choices as to the set of individuals (real or hypothetical) whose health is aggregated into a population measure. Recent efforts have been made to develop formal expressions of population health as aggregations of individual health measures (Cutler and Richardson 1997; 1998; Fleurbaey, forthcoming). In this paper, we attempt to set out a systematic framework for characterizing the individual basis for summary measures of population health.

To facilitate later debates in this volume, this paper addresses the question "When is one person healthier than another?" Five different answers to this question are formalized in terms of individual-level analogues to population-level health expectancies and health gaps. Precise formalization of these concepts often reveals important issues that will need to be addressed and reflected upon in future work. We end the chapter with some thoughts on the implications of this work for the development of alternative SMPH.

IS PERSON A HEALTHIER THAN PERSON B?

Imagine a casual conversation in which one participant says that John is healthier than Jack. What is the common-sense meaning of this statement? How does the use of the phrase "is healthier than" correspond to various measures of individual health? We believe that there are at least three more precise formulations of the question: "Is person A healthier than person B?"

1. Taking into account only *current* levels in various domains of health, is person A in a better state of health than person B?

2. After both person A and person B have died, will person A have lived a healthier life overall than person B?

3. For the remainder of their lives, will person A have a healthier life than person B?

We believe that the last question may be closest in meaning to the common usage of the phrase "is healthier than".

Let us illustrate the distinction between these three perspectives with a simple example. Carol and Patricia are both 35 years old, and in all domains of health (e.g., pain, mobility, cognition, affect, dexterity, vision, etc.), they have identical levels at present. Carol and Patricia have had different past health experiences: Carol was paralysed from the waist down between age 5 and age 34, at which time she underwent successful surgery that resolved her paralysis; Patricia has had full mobility all of her life. Carol and Patricia also differ in terms of current risk factors for health: Patricia has a strong family history of early onset ischaemic heart disease and smokes 2 packs of cigarettes per day, while Carol does not share either risk factor.

From the perspective of question 1, Carol and Patricia are in the same current state of health.

We do not have sufficient information to answer question 2, but Carol's experience of paralysis from ages 5 to 34 might result in Carol having a less healthy life overall than Patricia, evaluated over their entire lifespans. This depends critically on whether a family history of ischemic heart disease and tobacco consumption will eventuate in a shorter life for Patricia than Carol, and how this shortened longevity would compare to the reduction in health attributable to paralysis.

In terms of question 3, we would conclude that Carol is healthier than Patricia because of the known risks to Patricia's health that Carol does not have, all else being equal.

EX ANTE, EX INTERIM AND EX POST PERSPECTIVES

It is easy to confound the three questions asked about person A and person B with the vantage point in time when the question is asked. In fact, however, the time perspective constitutes a separate dimension along which different characterisations of individual health may be distinguished.

Question 1, which asks about individual health states, can only apply at a particular moment in time, since it refers only to the state of health of an individual at that moment in time.

Health over the entire lifespan (question 2) can be asked from three different vantage points in time:

- The *ex post* perspective reviews the lifespans of person A and person B after they have both died. The question of who had the healthier life is evaluated by adding up their experience of health at all different ages in some way.

- The *ex ante* perspective compares the expected lifespans of person A and person B at birth, before any of the health events have been realized. An *ex ante* evaluation is based on a comparison of the risks of being in different health states (including death) at different ages for person A and person B. Such an *ex ante* view of health over the lifespan is the basis of the framework for measuring health inequality presented by Gakidou et al. (2000)

- The *ex interim* perspective is located at an intermediate vantage point. For two people such as Carol and Patricia described above, the *ex interim* answer would take into account the actual health states they lived in from birth until now and their risks of being in different health states from now into the future. It is interesting to note that Williams (1997) has proposed an *ex interim* view of life expectancy as the basis for assessing inequality.

Question 3, which asks whether person A or person B will have a healthier life from now forward, is by its formulation an exclusively *ex ante* view. For two individuals evaluated at the (same) moment of birth, Question 3 is identical to the *ex ante* formulation of Question 2. At all other ages, this question differs from Question 2 by ignoring past differences in health and focusing only on the health of individuals from the present until death. This question is probably closest in spirit to the common usage of the phrase "is healthier than".

The three questions and the three time perspectives lead to five different variants of the simple question: "Is person A healthier than person B?" (Table 1). In the next sections of this paper, we present formal specifications for each of these five variants.

INDIVIDUAL HEALTH STATE

As considered in much more detail elsewhere in this volume (part 7), we assume that the health state of an individual at a particular moment in time can be characterized completely in J domains. Examples of domains include pain, affect, cognition, mobility, dexterity, vision, etc. The core set

Table 1   Different questions and time perspectives for describing
                   individual health

	Ex post	Ex ante	Ex interim
Current health		(no time dimension)	
Lifespan health	*Ex post* healthy lifespan and ex post health gap	*Ex ante* healthy lifespan and *ex ante* health gap	*Ex interim* healthy lifespan and *ex interim* health gap
Future health		Health expectancy and health gap	

of domains that should be used to describe a health state are discussed in
part 7. For each domain, we assume further that the level for an individual
may be characterized on a cardinal scale. We postulate that there is some
valuation function such that any combination of levels on the *J* domains
can be translated to a single cardinal value on a scale anchored by 1 (complete health) and 0 (a state comparable to death). The form and nature of
this function is a major subject in this volume (part 10) and in the literature (Brazier et al. 1998; Dolan 1997; Torrance et al. 1995). In this paper, our objective is to formalize comparisons of individual health
assuming that such a function is given.

More formally, we represent the valuation of a health state as follows:

$$h_i(t) = f\big(y_{1i}(t), y_{2i}(t), \dots, y_{Ji}(t)\big)$$

where $h_i(t)$ is the valuation of an individual *i*'s health state at time *t* and
$y_{ji}(t)$ is the level for individual *i* on domain *j* at time *t*. This formulation
assumes for simplicity that the valuation function $f(\cdot)$ mapping between
levels on the *J* domains is the same for all individuals.

Person A is in a better state of health than person B at time *t* if and only
if:

$$h_A(t) > h_B(t)$$

Thus, to answer the question "Is person A in a better state of health than
person B?", we need only know their levels in the *J* domains of health and
the form of the valuation function. It is possible to imagine that a valid,
reliable and cross-population-comparable survey instrument could provide sufficient information to answer this type of question for the set of
survey respondents.

EX POST LIFESPAN HEALTH

Imagine that two individuals have been observed from birth to death so
that at every age their state of health is known. To summarize their life-

time experiences of health, we need to aggregate the time spent in health states at different ages in some way. Aggregation over age presents many challenges, and many different solutions may be possible. We present four different alternatives for aggregation over the lifespan of an individual that all have SMPH analogues. Perhaps the simplest is to sum the experience of health over all ages, giving equal weight to the level of health at every age. In this formulation, we can define healthy lifespan as:

$$EPHL_i = \int_0^\infty h_i(a)da$$

where $EPHL_i$ is the *ex post* healthy lifespan for individual i, and $h_i(a)$ is the health state valuation for individual i at age a. Using this metric, person A lived a healthier life than person B if and only if:

$$EPHL_A > EPHL_B$$

The *ex post* healthy lifespan of an individual is naturally related to the health expectancy family of SMPH. In some sense, it is the realization for an individual of a health expectancy.

We can also formalize an individual health gap, which requires specification of a norm for health against which a person's experience is compared. In principle, the norm could be defined either in aggregate or age-specific terms. We define $\rho(a)$ as the normative health function that specifies a target level of health at each age for the construction of a health gap. Figure 1 illustrates a norm where individuals live in full health until age 70 years and then in somewhat less than full health until age 90.

Figure 1   Example of a norm for individual health

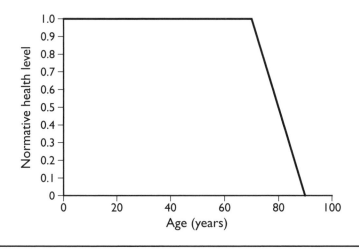

The norm illustrated in Figure 1 represents a combined norm for survivorship and health level; in this example, the implied survivorship goal is age 90, above which the normative health level is 0. A more complicated formulation of the normative health function would allow for separate specifications of a survivorship norm and a norm for health conditional on being alive at a particular age. This more flexible, two-dimensional specification may be particularly useful in accomodating complex norms that shift depending on the age that has been attained, but we use the simpler one-dimensional formulation in this paper for purposes of explication.

The healthy lifespan of an individual whose health followed the normative health curve at each age would be:

$$NHL = \int_0^\infty \rho(a)da$$

A basic health gap could be formulated simply by subtracting the *EPHL* for an individual from the total *NHL*. In this formulation, the health gap depends only on the difference between the total healthy life span in the norm and the realized lifespan, irrespective of when person *i* lived in different states of health. For all values of *EPHL* that fall below the *NHL*, this health gap formulation would produce the same ordering as *EPHL*, since each different *EPHL* is simply subtracted from a constant.

On the other hand, in defining an individual health gap, we may be concerned with the age pattern of the norm and not only with the total normative healthy lifespan. A more exacting formulation would therefore compare an individual's health to the health norm at each age, rather than simply in the aggregate. The key difference in this formulation is that any

Figure 2   Example of an individual health gap

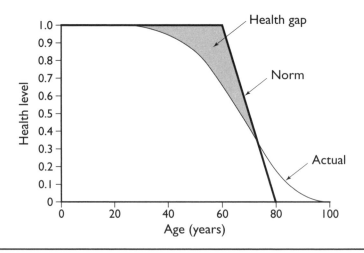

value of $h(a)$ that exceeds $\rho(a)$ counts the same as if $h(a) = \rho(a)$; in other words, when $\rho(a)$ is less than $h(a)$, the negative value is not added to the health gap. This is tantamount to saying that exceeding the norm at some ages does not make up for those other ages at which an individual falls short of the norm. Figure 2 illustrates such a case to make this distinction clearer.

Using the age-specific approach, we can formalize this type of health gap as:

$$EPHG_i = \int_0^\infty \left(\rho(a) - h_i(a) \right) \delta_i(a) da$$

where $\delta_i(a)$ is an indicator variable that equals 1 if $\rho(a) \geq h_i(a)$ and 0 otherwise. Based on this measure, we would say that person A lived a healthier life than person B if and only if

$$EPHG_A < EPHG_B$$

It is important to note that if an individual exceeds $\rho(a)$ at any age, the comparison based on $EPHG$ may produce a different ordering than the comparison based on $EPHL$.

Both the $EPHL$ and the $EPHG$ measures presented above are based on simple aggregation functions whereby any time spent in the same health state receives equal weight, irrespective of the age at which the state of health is experienced (with the exception of cases where health exceeds the normative level for a health gap). Other aggregations over different ages of an individual's lifespan are possible. A general form of aggregation incorporates a function $k(a)$ which assigns weights to time lived at different ages. A non-uniform aggregation function can be thought of as the individual analogue to age weights in SMPH. The *ex post* healthy lifespan with age-weights would be:

$$EPHL_i = \int_0^\infty h_i(a) k(a) da$$

and the *ex post* health gap with age weights would be:

$$EPHG_i = \int_0^\infty \left(\rho(a) - h_i(a) \right) \delta_i(a) k(a) da$$

In equations that follow, we include the $k(a)$ term in all formulations, as aggregation functions without age weights may be considered a special case of the general formulation, with $k(a) = 1$ for all a.

This section has presented four different types of *ex post* lifespan measures, and conclusions as to whether person A lived a healthier life than person B may be different depending on whether the metric used is *ex post* healthy lifespan, *ex post* healthy lifespan with age-weights, *ex post* health gap or *ex post* health gap with age-weights. Whether one should use the healthy lifespan or the health gap approach, and whether with or without age-weights, are themselves normative choices. These choices depend critically on whether we believe that lifespan health depends only on the total health experience over the lifetime or on the shape of the health experience. Should the loss of one year in full health from age 90 to 91 count the same in the calculus of lifespan health as two years lived in 50% health at ages 20 and 21? Many people would probably believe that living to age 90 in perfect health represents a more healthy life than living to age 91 but experiencing a 50% reduction in health during early adulthood. The construction of health gaps and/or the addition of age-weights allow some limits on the equivalence of health decrements at different ages. A health gap measure, in contrast to a healthy lifepan measure, allows for the inclusion of normative health goals that may vary by age; it may be that this notion is more consistent with the vernacular meaning of "a healthier life" than the healthy lifespan measure, which improves with increasing health levels at any age, without reference to changing normative goals.

EX ANTE LIFESPAN HEALTH

Rather than asking "*Did* person A live a healthier life than person B?" we can ask the question from birth, "*Will* person A live a healthier life than person B?" The answer to this question, *ex ante*, is a probabilistic statement, as both persons face some uncertain distribution of different lifespan paths of health. To formalize the *ex ante* view, we need to capture the probability distribution of individuals being in different health states at different ages. Because states of health at one age cannot be completely independent of states of health at other ages, we can formulate the *ex ante* view as a distribution of probabilities of different healthy lifespans under different possible states of the world:

$$EAHL_i = \sum_{s \in \Omega} r(s) \int_0^\infty h_i(s,a) k(a) da$$

where Ω is the universe of all possible states of the world and $r(s)$ is the probability of a particular state s. Gakidou et al. (2000) have used this type of formulation as the conceptual basis for the measurement of population health inequality.

It is also possible to construct an *ex ante* lifespan health gap using the same logic:

$$EAHG_i = \sum_{s \in \Omega} r(s) \int_0^\infty \big(\rho(a) - h_i(s,a) \big) \delta_i(s,a) k(a) da$$

The formalization of the *ex ante* forms of the healthy lifespan and the health gap have similarities to formulations of expected utility. Given this formal similarity, it might be natural for economists to suggest that the *ex ante* forms of these measures should be modified to include time preference and risk aversion. Time preference is defined as a pure preference for utility in the near future as opposed to the distant future. Risk aversion is defined as a preference for a particular payoff that is certain rather than the same *expected* payoff that is uncertain. In this case, however, the analogy may be inappropriate. Expected utility formulations are meant to represent how individuals choose between two uncertain options. *Ex ante* healthy lifespans and health gaps, on the other hand, are not intended to be measures of individual preferences over distributions of health pathways, but rather assessments about which distribution represents the healthier lifespan. It might be reasonable to recognize that two distributions represent the same *ex ante* levels of health over the lifespan but still to *prefer* one or the other in terms of expected utility because of discounting or risk aversion.

Since the *ex ante* question asks which person will have enjoyed the healthier lifespan once both lifespans are completed, this simply implies a prospective view of the completed life. In this case, we do not see compelling arguments in favour of time preference. Since the evaluation depends on the entire course of life over time, regardless of the point at which it is evaluated, discounting of the future does not seem relevant. Risk aversion, however, deserves more careful consideration. Imagine two individuals whose anticipated healthy lifespans are distributed with the same expected value, but different ranges of uncertainty. The question of which person will have the healthier completed lifespan is different than the question of which *ex ante* distribution may be preferred. Risk averse individuals may choose for themselves the distribution with narrower uncertainty, but the expectation of the completed healthy lifespan nevertheless is the same in both distributions. We conclude that *ex ante* healthy lifespans and *ex ante* health gaps—as characterizations of expectations of healthy life rather than of individual preferences over distributions of health prospects—should not include time preference or risk aversion.

EX INTERIM LIFESPAN HEALTH

There is a third perspective: given the past experience of health from birth until the present for person A and person B, combined with their prospects for health in the future, which person will have the healthier lifespan overall. This *ex interim* perspective combines the realization of health risks from birth to the present with an *ex ante* view of health risks from now until death. The *ex interim* healthy lifespan for an individual at age x is:

$$EIHL_i(x) = \int_0^x h_i(a)k(a)da + \sum_{s\in\Omega} r(s)\int_x^\infty h_i(s,a)k(a)da$$

The *ex interim* lifespan health gap is:

$$EIHG_i(x) = \int_0^x \big(\rho(a)-h_i(a)\big)\delta_i(a)k(a)da + \sum_{s\in\Omega} r(s)\int_x^\infty \big(\rho(a)-h_i(s,a)\big)\delta_i(s,a)k(a)da$$

FUTURE HEALTH

The fifth and final option, which asks whether person A or person B will live a healthier life from now forward, is the one that is perhaps closest to the common usage of the phrase "is healthier than". In fact, there are a number of web sites (for example, "LongToLive.com" or various "life expectancy calculators") that will provide a computation of future health prospects based on a particular risk factor profile input by an individual. Parallels to the two families of SMPH can also be formulated to answer this question for an individual. Health expectancy for an individual can be defined as:

$$HE_i(x) = \sum_{s \in \Omega} r(s) \int_x^\infty h_i(s,a) k(a) da$$

This differs from the *ex interim* healthy lifespan because it ignores previous health experience from birth until the present. The equivalent future health gap can be formalized as:

$$HG_i(x) = \sum_{s \in \Omega} r(s) \int_x^\infty \left(\rho_x(a) - h_i(s,a) \right) \delta_i(s,a) k(a) da$$

It is worth revisiting the question of risk aversion and time preference in the context of this final perspective. While we concluded that neither risk aversion nor time preference were relevant for comparisons using lifespan health measures since these measures refer to completed lifespans viewed from various time perspectives, when we are comparing current health and future prospects across individuals, particularly in thinking about the vernacular meaning of these comparisons, it may be the case that individuals exhibit risk aversion and/or time preference in making these judgments.

DISCUSSION

This chapter has presented a formal framework for constructing measures of individual health based on three different types of questions and three different time perspectives. A systematic examination of the different ways to characterize individual health will be essential in bolstering the conceptual foundation for evolving summary measures of population health. Logically, there must be some formal relationship between measures of population health and the aggregation of some measure of health across a defined set of individuals. The set of individuals may include those living, those that have died or those yet to be born, but if population health is not a function of the health of some set of individuals, then in what other way may it be interpreted?

The different ways of formulating the question "Is person A healthier than person B?" may have different applications. It can be argued that for studying inequality in health across individuals some variant of the question "Did (or will) person A have a healthier lifespan than person B?" may be the most appropriate. Gakidou et al. (2000) advocate using an *ex ante* view and Williams (1997) an *ex interim* view.

The future health formulation of the question is probably closest to the vernacular notion of individual health, which may have important implications for aggregate-level comparisons, where we ask whether population A is healthier than population B. Although some currently used population health measures account for at least part of the future stream of health consequences, none of the available measures incorporates the health prospects formulation of individual measures in a comprehensive way. Depending on the intended application, new summary measures of population health may be required in order to capture the same aspects of individual health reflected in this view.

This chapter on formalization identifies many questions that remain unanswered, such as the basis for choosing an individual normative health function, the basis for choosing age-weights and the complexity of different viewpoints. Key issues of aggregation also remain to be addressed. These aggregation issues are central to measuring average levels of population health and particularly to the problem of characterizing health inequalities. We hope that our attempts to clarify the formal basis for a range of different measures of individual health will serve as a useful starting point from which to explore different options for aggregation.

REFERENCES

Brazier J, Usherwood T, Harper R, Thomas K (1998) Deriving a preference based single index measure from the UK SF-36 health survey. *Journal of Clinical Epidemiology*, 51(11):1115–1128.

Cutler DM, Richardson E (1997) Measuring the health of the US population. *Brookings Papers on economic activity: Microeconomics*, 217–227.

Cutler DM, Richardson E (1998) The value of health: 1970–1990. *American Economic Review*, 88(2):97–100.

Dolan P (1997) Modelling valuations for EuroQol health states. *Medical Care*, 35(11):1095–1108.

Fleurbaey M (Forthcoming) On the measurement of health and of health inequalities. In: *Fairness and goodness: ethical issues in health resource allocation*. Wikler D, Murray CJL, eds. World Health Organization, Geneva.

Gakidou EE, Murray CJL, Frenk J (2000) Defining and measuring health inequality: an approach based on the distribution of health expectancy. *Bulletin of the World Health Organization*, 78(1):42–54.

Torrance GW, Furlong W, Feeny D, Boyle M (1995) Multi-attribute preference functions: Health Utilities Index. *PharmacoEconomics*, 7(6):503–520.

Williams A (1997) Intergenerational equity: an exploration of the "fair innings" argument. *Health Economics*, 6 (2):117–132.

Chapter 2.1

Applications of summary measures of population health

Paul J. van der Maas

Introduction

Population health status has so many dimensions, classifications and measurements, as well as interactions between these, that patterns and trends often cannot easily be identified. Comparisons between populations and countries are often severely hampered because different data are collected or different classifications are used. Thus the need for comprehensive population health measures and standardization of data collection is obvious and longstanding. This paper describes the possible uses of such summary measures of population health (SMPH) and some conditions that have to be met for their application. But first, summary measures in general and their composition will be discussed briefly.

Summary measures

Summary measures combine information of different types and from different sources, which together permit a rapid appraisal of a specific phenomenon. They may be used for identifying differences (e.g. between groups, countries, etc.), observed changes over time, or expected changes (e.g. as a consequence of policy measures). There are four key elements in the construction of summary measures: the selection of relevant parameters to be included, the reliable measurement/collection of these parameters, the unit in which the summary measure will be expressed, and the relative weight of each of the constituents in the total summary measure. Each of these four elements will determine how the summary measure may be applied and for what kind of applications it will be valid. Ideally a summary measure has a wide range of valid applications, but inevitably there is a trade-off between the specificity of the information that is contained in the measure and its general applicability.

The value of summary measures themselves is in producing efficient and meaningful quick-glance information, generally for non-specialists. A World Bank economist wants the information behind a GNP, and a stock exchange (e.g. the Dow Jones Industrial Average) index has very limited value for a professional investor. Nevertheless, nobody doubts the usefulness of these indicators, because of their information value and the discipline that goes into the standardized collection of the constituent data.

ELEMENTS OF SUMMARY MEASURES FOR POPULATION HEALTH

If we define population health status as the amount and the distribution of morbidity, handicap and mortality in a population, it follows that the summary measure will have to include those three aspects of ill health. Mortality can be summarized in many ways, with probably the most important distinction between expectancy measures (life expectancies) versus health gap measures (years of life lost, YLL).

The (partly related) axes for a *taxonomy of SMPH* are at least:

1. Life table population vs. real population

2. Health expectancy vs. health gap

3. Generic vs. disease-specific epidemiological input

4. Types of values/valuation procedures for expressing disability/disease in time units

5. Incidence versus prevalence measures

6. Incorporation of other values.

Together these represent a large group of SMPH, which generally will have some family resemblance or formal relationship. It should be kept in mind that, for instance, in comparing burdens of disease between countries, starting with exactly the same input, different summary measures and choices made within summary measures may yield widely different comparisons and rank orderings.

As has often been stated, SMPH inevitably have a normative character, because the choice of constituent elements represents a selection and the weights relating these elements imply a judgement about the relative importance of each constituent element. Summarizing mortality data, for instance, often implies value judgements about a reasonable or realistic life expectancy.

As mentioned already, combining a large amount of health data into one summary measure will inevitably result in information loss. This will especially occur when, owing to preventive and therapeutic interventions, the trends in incidence, duration and mortality of a certain disease evolve in different directions. These may have very different consequences for prevalence- versus incidence-based SMPH. Applications directed at estimating present health care needs would be more prevalence oriented, whereas applications directed at estimating the consequences of interventions would have to be more incidence oriented. But SMPH themselves are not intended for the detailed study of time trends in the incidence, duration and mortality of specific diseases.

DISABILITY WEIGHTS

After the publication of the Global Burden of Disease (GBD) study, the disability weights (linking mortality and disability data) and the social preference weights (age weights and discounting) have stirred much debate, which may even have obscured the paramount importance of GBD's epidemiological ambitions. Such weights may and perhaps even should be the source of a never-ending debate, and it is certainly very unlikely that there will ever be complete agreement about a universal set of disability weights for specific conditions. Fortunately, in the computation of SMPH sets of disability weights can easily be replaced. The reasons for doing so may be changes in judgements about the relative importance of specific diseases or disabilities, the amount of suffering involved, or the social consequences of specific diseases (depending on the perspective of the weighting procedure), or different policy applications of SMPH. Fortunately, all empirical research suggests that rank ordering of diseases from these perspectives is rather invariant between populations and cultures, apart from some specific types of health problems. If rank ordering is more or less stable, it is largely the size of the weight that will determine how much a specific SMPH will accentuate the importance of morbidity/disability relative to mortality.

VERSATILITY

The fact that SMPH inevitably have a limited information content and are not very sensitive to small changes in population health implies that, for many applications, continuous monitoring of SMPH may not be very informative. The frequency with which SMPH for specific applications should be reported is at least partly determined by the signal/noise ratio of that specific SMPH. It is well possible that in rich countries with high population health levels, the consequences of effective and efficient interventions will be so marginal that they will not easily be reflected in the SMPH. It is certainly possible to construct SMPH that would be sensitive to such relatively small changes due to specific interventions, but they may be less relevant for developing countries and vice versa. Thus, versatility is an important criterion in judging the usefulness of SMPH. Perhaps the most important contribution arising from the development of SMPH is that the process sets an agenda for the selection of relevant population health parameters, their uniform classification, data collection, and the consistency checking of these data.

POSSIBLE APPLICATIONS OF SUMMARY MEASURES OF POPULATION HEALTH

The reasons for developing SMPH are that diseases may vary widely in duration, severity, and lethality and that diseases may vary over time with respect to these aspects. Thus, SMPH typically combine information on morbidity, disability and mortality, generally expressed in time units (life-years, life expectancy).

The paper by Murray, Salomon and Mathers (chapter 1.2) lists eight applications.

1. Comparing the health of one population to the health of another population.

2. Comparing the health of the same population at different points in time.

3. Identifying and quantifying overall health inequalities within populations.

4. Providing appropriate and balanced attention to the effects of non-fatal health outcomes on overall population health.

5. Informing debates on priorities for health service delivery and planning.

6. Informing debates on priorities for research and development in the health sector.

7. Improving professional training curricula in public health.

8. Analysing the benefits of health interventions for use in cost-effectiveness analyses.

Applications 1 to 3 can be considered as descriptive, whereas applications 4 to 6 can be considered as intervention- or policy-directed.

DESCRIPTIVE/EXPLANATORY APPLICATIONS

The descriptive uses (comparing the health of populations, identifying time-trends, and describing the distribution of health within populations) are generally not goals in themselves, but are intended to identify differences or changes that deserve explanation and further exploration. For instance, the observation that mortality decline in the Netherlands at both young and old ages is somewhat lagging behind those of other rich countries, sparks off both scientific research on the determinants of this phenomenon and public debate about the performance of the Dutch health care system.

In order to compare health status between populations and to estimate time-trends in health status, the paramount requirement is that measurements and weights should be standardized and stable between countries and over time. Standardized information implies identical classifications, measurement and representation of collected data. For comparisons between populations, the availability of data for each constituent element would be a second requirement. For time-trends, invariance of classifications, etc. over time is obviously crucial and at the same time difficult to achieve, owing to developing knowledge and insights, as is illustrated by the successive editions of the International Classification of Diseases (ICD). Considering the required invariance of weights, their advantage is that it is a matter of consensus which set of weights will be applied, and that the sets of weights can be replaced in order to compute SMPH for specific purposes. Weights that strongly represent social value choices are less likely to be invariant over time.

POLICY APPLICATIONS

SMPH are relevant for three levels of health policy. The first level, general socioeconomic policy, is not often seen as health policy, but as long as poverty is still the major predictor of health, it should be. The systematic presentation of the distribution of health within populations and between populations should form an important input for socioeconomic policy. The second, more specific, health policy level focuses on the elimination or reduction of specific diseases or risk factors. For the planning of programmes for health protection, health promotion and immunizations and for the evaluation of such policies, the incidence- and mortality-oriented SMPH will be particularly important and helpful. The third category of health policy is specifically directed to health services. SMPH directed at informing this type of policy-making will generally focus more on prevalence measures and use weights that draw more attention to the effects of non-fatal health outcomes.

For setting agendas in biomedical research, information on the relative magnitude of health problems is very important. Obviously, other considerations, such as the intrinsic dynamics of specific research areas and the likelihood of developing breakthroughs will be at least as important. Nevertheless, the perception of a specific population health problem, either because of its present magnitude or because it may be an important threat, may often form the impetus for highly successful research, as is illustrated by many cases of especially infectious disease research.

SOCIAL VALUE CHOICES

Social value choices are meant to highlight specific elements in the health distribution within a population. Mostly this applies to age, gender, socioeconomic status or ethnicity. Social value choices may also refer to specific patient groups and specific diseases. Some brief remarks are given here.

1. Social preferences may differ between countries and change over time within countries. The use of SMPH for comparisons of burden of disease between countries or for documenting changes over time suggests that the weights relating morbidity and mortality should be as epide-

miologically oriented as possible, and that the SMPH should at least be reported without applying overall social value distributions, such as age-weights.

2. An obvious problem is that any weight to be applied to disease stages or generic health states always implies a form of interpretation (suffering, social limitations, health care use, social preferences) which may be relevant for some applications but not for others.

3. Policy-makers generally do not like the policy choices being made for them, somewhere hidden in computations. They sometimes like the consequences of different policy options to be made explicit.

4. The theoretically most universally applicable SMPH would stick as much as possible to its epidemiological basis and illustrate the consequences of different social value choices in a transparent way.

5. As health policy generally is directed at specific health problems or risk factors, the relation between these and the summary measure should remain clear.

ECONOMIC EVALUATION

Economic evaluation has traditionally used quality-adjusted life years (QALYs) as a summary measure combining mortality and disability. It is conceivable that standard evaluation techniques used in health economics may be integrated with more population health-oriented SMPH. This would require an endeavour to bridge traditional disciplinary differences, specifically the discussion of whether interventions or diseases should be the focus of study. For health policy and health care applications of economic evaluation, disease label/diagnostic information is indispensable. Allocation decisions about advanced transplantation surgery versus long-term care for mentally handicapped will (hopefully) never be decided on rank ordering of cost-effectiveness ratios.

DISEASE-SPECIFIC VERSUS GENERIC HEALTH STATUS INFORMATION

There have been many debates on whether SMPH should be based on disease-specific information, or on generic health state information, such as activities of daily living and generic quality of life measures.

Disease labels/diagnostic categories contain a wealth of information (see chapter 9.1). Although some may have limited value in establishing present and future health status in individual patients, they effectively summarize the distributions of present and future health status (including survival) in populations. They also are a shorthand for possible changes in prognosis (survival and future health status) through preventive and therapeutic interventions. Because they represent large bodies of scientific knowledge of determinants and disease processes, they are naturally at the core of both quantitative and pathophysiological biomedical research. In short, diagnostic categories are very effective heuristics for research, interventions and the understanding of suffering. On the other hand, generic health status descriptions are indispensable to put disease-specific information in perspective at the population level.

CONCLUSIONS AND RECOMMENDATIONS

1. The development of summary measures of population health is of utmost importance for many purposes. Perhaps the most important contribution in their development is not the end product, the summary measures themselves, but the fact that they force us to define exactly the required epidemiological input on mortality and disability, to stimulate the application of uniform classifications and the collection of missing information, and to systematically check the internal consistency of the epidemiological information on specific diseases. Thus, apart from setting health and research agendas they also set agendas for international comparative data collection and epidemiological research. In that respect, SMPH development will always remain work in progress, of which the periodical publication of a set of indicators is just one, albeit important and attractive, result. Another very important contribution in the development of SMPH is that it structures the debate on social preferences in health policy and that the consequences of different social preferences may be quantified in terms of population health status.

2. In the debate on SMPH, often the weights relating mortality and disability draw the most attention and generate the most discussion. This obscures the fact that the largest uncertainties surrounding SMPH stem from lack of or inconsistencies in epidemiological information. In the computation of SMPH, sets of disability weights can easily be replaced by other sets of disability weights, whereas the collection of needed epidemiological information and testing their consistency are major tasks.

3. SMPH inevitably have a normative character because their construction requires decisions on the relative weight of the epidemiological input. Nevertheless, in a taxonomy of SMPH we can include a continuum from more epidemiologically oriented SMPH to those that strongly include social preferences. For descriptive purposes the more epidemiologically oriented SMPH would be desirable, whereas for policy purposes the inclusion of social preferences may be justified.

4. Considering the previous conclusions, we must accept that there is no "one size fits all" solution for the development of SMPH. In order to keep the main purpose of the endeavour clear, to keep the discussions on the different elements focused, and to make them versatile instruments for the different purposes, a system of modular reporting is indispensable. This means that the basic epidemiological input that goes

into the construction of SMPH, including estimates to fill information gaps and corrections due to consistency checks, should always be available separate from sets of weights. Such a basic dataset should allow for the computation of a variety of SMPH for different applications. This is also important for comparisons between populations directed at specific groups of diseases or at distributions within populations, and for the future construction of time series, when different disability weights or social preferences might become relevant.

5. For all applications, SMPH based on diagnostic categories are more useful. Diagnostic categories represent a wealth of information that will direct the search for determinants and interventions and will support the setting of priorities in health care and research policy.

Chapter 2.2

On the uses of summary measures of population health

Michael C. Wolfson

Introduction

By far, the most fundamental use of summary measures of population health (SMPH) is to shift the centre of gravity of health policy discourse away from the inputs (e.g. costs, human resources, and new technologies) and throughputs (e.g. how many surgical procedures) of the health system towards health outcomes for the population.[1] This is not to imply that the resources used and activities undertaken by national or regional health systems are unimportant; quite the contrary. But our understanding of their roles and importance is more appropriate if guided by the real "bottom line", namely their influence on population health. In parallel to this applied use, SMPH can also play a fundamental role in helping to define the agenda and priorities for health research. Ideally, SMPH, and their underlying statistical systems, can be used to highlight the relative burdens experienced by a nation's or community's members attributable to various sorts of health problems or causes.

These basic roles for SMPH beg several key questions about how they ought to be constructed and presented. I shall comment briefly on these questions in turn.

SMPH and statistical systems

Any serious effort to estimate a summary measure of population health requires a substantial investment in underlying data collection and analysis. Consider what seems like a simple indicator, life expectancy (LE), as an example.

LE is derived from of a series of age-specific mortality rates. In turn, these mortality rates (ideally) presuppose a complete system of death registration, where the data collected at each death include at least age and sex. For the denominator of the mortality rate, we need a complete census of the population which, at the very least, gathers information on each individual's age and sex. However, most countries with death registration find it worthwhile, at relatively low marginal cost, also to collect items like residence geography and the principal underlying cause of death, classified according to an international standard, the WHO's International Classification of Diseases (ICD). Similarly, virtually all population censuses collect additional data such as family structure, educational attainment, geographic location, and occupation.

As a result, the underlying data system necessary to produce reliable estimates of LE by itself is very expensive. However, the death registration and population census efforts are typically multi-purpose, collecting an important range of ancillary (to LE estimates) information. At the same time, this means that LE need not be estimated in pristine isolation. It can and often is just one indicator amongst a related family—for example, age-standardized death rates by ICD-defined cause, and regional variations in mortality rates.

The fact that LE estimates can be embedded in this wider range of coherently related indicators is not just a fortuitous side-effect. It is also extremely helpful for analysts and researchers who want to do more than simply follow the evolution of overall LE as an indicator. The availability of this wider range of data allows us to "drill down" in order to better understand the patterns and trends.

Exactly parallel considerations should apply to SMPH. They should be conceived *ab initio* as the apex of a coherent structure of underlying data systems, within an explicitly designed family of indicators. One crucial set of ingredients for SMPH is exactly the same material as used for estimating LE. However, more is needed. At minimum, we also need three main ingredients (Wolfson 1999):

- a micro-level health status *descriptive system*, a carefully chosen set of structurally independent[2] health status attributes, operationalized with standardized questionnaire items, to elicit levels of functioning for representative samples of the population on a regular (e.g. annual, or quinquennial) basis;

- a micro-level *valuation function* which maps any given individual's vector of responses for these attributes into a scalar—for example, on a zero to one interval with one end-point corresponding either to death or "worst possible health state", and the other end-point corresponding to "best possible health" or "full health";[3] and

- a macro-level *aggregation formula* which rolls up the individual-level health status information, plus the mortality data, into the overall SMPH.

Let me here point out a mild disagreement with Paul van der Maas' first and fifth conclusions in this regard (chapter 2.1). As with LE, SMPH ought to be, in the first instance, descriptive. And describing the health of individuals in a population involves much more than describing diseases defined in terms of the ICD. The micro-level health status descriptive system should be more open, more vernacular, than one based only on clinical disease concepts.

As a result, the conclusions that the most important contribution of SMPH is to force "internal consistency of the epidemiological information on specific diseases", and that "for all applications, SMPH based on diagnostic categories are more useful" is far too narrow. A disease perspective or disaggregation is obviously important. But the statistical system underlying SMPH, and the family of indicators which have an SMPH at the apex, needs to be more ambitious—it needs to connect health status, since individuals are most comfortable reporting it in surveys (e.g. disabilities or functional limitations), with the more conventional clinical disease-based approaches. In turn, the SMPH should be jointly consistent with data on disease prevalence or incidence, and with corresponding data on disability or other vernacular health state descriptions.

LEVELS OF HEALTH AND INEQUALITY IN HEALTH

I argue in chapter 3.9 that it is more useful for policy purposes to develop separate measures for the average level of population health, and various aspects of the distribution of health. The SMPH is an excellent indicator for the level of health. But an SMPH, or some variant, cannot and should not be expected to bear the weight of indicating distributional features.

SMPH AND CROSS-NATIONAL COMPARISONS

The case for the usefulness of SMPH is more straightforward within a given country, because issues of cross-national comparability of data and concepts do not arise, at least not as acutely. Unfortunately, comparable international data for representative population samples, based on a common micro-level descriptive system for health status, are not available. One reason is simply inertia and priorities—many countries do not see the need to generate internationally comparable data, or do not want (reasonably) to upset important national time series. This problem is the subject of international discussions, and progress can be expected.

But there is a more fundamental problem. This is whether such comparisons can be made even in principle. There are at least two basic issues. One is whether cultural differences are so wide that even the core underlying concepts related to health, and to valuing health states, have anywhere near the same meaning in different societies. This is an open question. However, it cannot be fully avoided by eschewing international comparisons, using SMPH only within a given country. Recent levels of international migration have resulted in substantial ethnic and cultural diversity within countries like Canada, so we face this problem in any case.

The other issue is whether value systems differ too greatly between countries. It is certainly the case that SMPH embody values or norms, specifically in both the micro-level valuation function and the macro-level aggregation formula noted above. However, I do not find this concern, for example as voiced by Gavin Mooney (in chapter 12.3), that troubling. The reason is that SMPH, by virtue of the way they ought to be constructed, can be taken apart and alternatives assembled, based on different formulas or implicit normative judgements.

A simple analogy is the Consumer Price Index (CPI). This is a mixture of basic data on the prices of myriad commodities over time, and a system of weights. Prices are typically (in OECD countries) measured quarterly or monthly, and generally do not occasion much controversy (Boskin et al. 1996 is an exception). The weights come from less frequent household surveys of spending patterns. Historically, questions have been raised whether there ought to be a separate CPI for the poor or the elderly, for example. In these cases, analysts can take apart the CPI and reassemble it using different weights based on the spending patterns of those population subgroups.

Similarly, if someone objects to the weights or valuation functions embodied in a given SMPH, the raw material ought to be readily available so that analysts can, without too much difficulty, conduct a sensitivity analysis to determine if, over the relevant range of alternative weights or norms, the SMPH leads to materially different conclusions.

SMPH, ECONOMIC EVALUATION AND HEALTH CARE ADMINISTRATIVE DATA SYSTEMS

Let me come back to one of Paul van der Maas' points, this time to agree and add emphasis. While I disagree with him on the primacy of a disease perspective, I certainly do agree that SMPH must be closely linked to the evolution of epidemiological knowledge, and also to health services information. There are several practical implications, all essentially flowing from a simple observation: there are many key data collection and information creation processes unfolding in health research and health system management. The main example is the general move toward electronic patient records (EPRs). These EPR systems will routinely generate an immense wealth of longitudinal microdata on individuals' health and health care trajectories. These administrative data need to be closely connected to SMPH. The solution is the judicious and strategic construction of "Rosetta stone" data sets—data collections that include both the standard clinical or disease-based data elements, and vernacular health status as captured by the micro-level descriptive system underlying SMPH.

These Rosetta stone data sets certainly do not need to be on a census basis; they will likely only be feasible as samples. At the same time, they need to be sufficient to provide a crosswalk between the two perspectives in describing and classifying health states.

Another major example is clinical trials or studies of specific interventions in order to produce economic evaluations. These studies should include generic measures of health status, for example as recommended by the Institute of Medicine (Gold et al. 1996). And as countries upgrade or develop EPR and related information systems for the health care sector, they should include (selectively and strategically) generic measures of health status (i.e. including the micro-level descriptive system noted above).

Assigning causes to health

A final point concerns a general problem in the interpretation of SMPH. There is a widespread and reasonable feeling that SMPH are only useful if they can point to action—if movements in the SMPH can be ascribed, either historically or prospectively, to some cause, preferably one that can be influenced by an intervention of some sort. This is one of the reasons that DALYs, for example, have been based on a disease classification, and that Paul van der Maas asserts that "diagnostic categories are more useful." (The other reason presumably has to do with data availability.)

However, this is far too simplistic a reason to require SMPH to be clinically disease-based. Causal attribution is a complex question, dealt with in part 6. At this point, it is sufficient to emphasize that yes, some sort of framework for linking causes to movements in SMPH is fundamental to their usefulness; but no, that kind of causal linkage is not best approached by a mechanical insistence that the first breakdown or disaggregation of health problems ought to be from a biomedical disease perspective.

Notes

1   My general support for SMPH should not be construed as support for some specific kinds, such as DALYs. My personal preference is for the HALE (health-adjusted life expectancy) or DALE (disability-adjusted life expectancy) kind of SMPH. See chapter 6.3 for the reasons.

2   Chapter 7.2 discusses health status descriptive systems, while chapter 10.2 discusses methods for valuing health states. It should be clear, when reading these chapters together, that the descriptive system should be designed with the valuation method in mind. This imposes extra constraints over and above the usual psychometric requirements for good survey questions. In particular, given the kinds of trade-off questions required to elicit valuations, it is necessary, to avoid ambiguity, for the health states to be *structurally independent*. For example, vision and lower limb mobility are structurally independent in the sense that one can plausibly have any level of visual functioning without necessarily implying any given level of lower limb mobility. On the other hand, vision and social role function are not structurally independent in this sense, since substantial visual impairment necessarily limits an individuals' plausible range of social role function.

3   Since, empirically, a majority of a number of populations consider some living states worse than death (e.g. being completely immobile and in continuous intense pain), the numerical interval could range from some negative number

representing the worst state in the descriptive system, to 0 (zero) indicating death, to 1 indicating full health.

REFERENCES

Boskin MJ, Dulberger ER, Gordon RJ, Griliches Z, Jorgensen D (1996) Toward a more accurate measure of the cost of living. Final report to the Senate Finance Comittee (Boskin Commission). US Social Security Division, Washington, DC.

Gold MR, Siegel JE, Russel LB, Weinstein MC, eds. (1996) Cost-effectiveness in health and medicine. Oxford University Press, New York.

Wolfson MC (1999) Measuring health — visions and practicalities. Joint United Nations Economic Commission for Europe/World Health Organization meeting on health statistics, Rome.

Chapter 2.3

COMMENTARY ON THE USES OF SUMMARY MEASURES OF POPULATION HEALTH

MATTHEW McKENNA AND JAMES MARKS

INTRODUCTION

We have been asked to provide a brief commentary on the potential uses of summary health measures because we are officials from a government agency (the Centers for Disease Control and Prevention in the United States) which is involved with the application of public health interventions designed to decrease disease, disability and death. We had the opportunity to attend a World Health Organization sponsored meeting convened in Marrakech, Morocco, that dealt with the technical and ethical dimensions of these measures. Our comments have been informed and enriched by the presentations at this meeting.

The disability-adjusted life year (DALY) was first presented in the *World Development Report 1993* by the World Bank (1993). Since then, interest in summary health measures has surged. Though frequently regarded as a novel analytic tool, numerous life-year indices had been proffered prior to the DALY, starting in the 1940s with Dempsey's concept of using "years of life lost" as a metric for assessing the health burden associated with deaths occurring prior to an "ideal" life span of 65 years (Dempsey 1947). Subsequent measures incorporated non-fatal health outcomes using a life-table approach similar to the DALY methodology. In these constructs, the time lived with a disease or injury is "lost" according to the severity of the disability, pain, or distress associated with a particular malady (Erickson et al. 1989). However, even though similar summary measures such as the Years of Healthy Life have been incorporated into the overall health goals for the United States, no previous measure appears to have garnered the attention, interest, and intermittent disdain, as well as perceived usefulness, that has been directed at the DALY (Erickson et al. 1995).

Why are summary measures of population health useful?

One example of the response to the DALY's debut was from William Foege, a former Director of the Centers for Disease Control (CDC) and current senior health advisor for the Bill and Melinda Gates Foundation. He wrote in 1994:

"The DALY concept has the potential to revolutionize the way in which we measure the impact of disease, how we choose interventions, and how we track the success or failure of our intervention. Despite its potential, the DALY concept is inadequately utilized" (Foege 1994).

Besides the three applications he mentioned in this quotation (i.e. assessing overall impact of diseases, choosing interventions, and evaluating interventions), Foege also speculated in the same essay that this measure could be used to guide research priorities. This quotation suggests that the basic conceptual framework for a life-year-based index of health was novel when, in fact, the fundamental construct was several decades old. Presumably other incarnations of similar summary health measures could have prompted comparable enthusiasm and interest, but such a reception did not occur. This seems surprising since it is relatively easy to develop a set of candidate uses for any health index. Table 1 provides a set generated during meetings at the Centers for Disease Control and Prevention about the potential role of summary health measures in the planning, prioritizing, and analytic activities at that agency. Therefore, in this essay, rather than listing and describing a set of *uses*, we offer explanations as to why these set of characteristics make such measures *useful* (Table 2). We feel that the DALY, as well as other summary measures, contains many of these attributes.

Another introductory point worth noting is that our comments on summary measures arise from a population-based public health perspective. Indices designed to capture both the detailed components of individual health and the impact of clinical interventions on these components frequently require a different set of considerations than more general, population-oriented, health status measures. The methodological details and analytic implications of the distinction between these two perspectives

Table 1   Uses of summary measures of population health

Contribute to decision-making for health policy

Facilitate health planning

Supply a comprehensive reference for epidemiological estimates

Guide research priorities

Monitor population health

Provide a comprehensive assessment of interventions (clinical and community)

Guide patient care decisions (e.g. clinical trials that incorporate health-related quality-of-life measures)

Table 2   Characteristics of the usefulness of summary measures of population health

Emphasize premature mortality (not just a "body count")

Include non-fatal conditions

Require comprehensive epidemiological estimates

The estimation process emphasizes internal consistency

The measures and estimates are rigorously validated

The health outcomes are systematically given an index value

have been elegantly delineated by others (see chapter 7.2). However, it is an important distinction that is, in our opinion, too frequently overlooked.

EMPHASIS ON PREMATURE MORTALITY AND INCLUSION OF NON-FATAL HEALTH OUTCOMES

Life year-based summary measures generally attempt to combine the impact of non-fatal health outcomes as well as emphasize deaths at younger ages. This is a major step beyond the standard "body count" approach to health prioritization that inevitably results from the traditional reliance on mortality statistics (Field and Gold 1998). In developed countries, where the majority of deaths occur at ages beyond 75 years, the prioritization of research and health-care expenditures on such data tends to result in a fascination with rescue-oriented, life-saving, and technologically advanced approaches. All too often such technology-intensive procedures are implemented in frail, elderly, and frequently mentally incompetent patients without prior candid discussions about the prospects for success. This frequently results in inefficient uses of resources that accomplish little beyond denying unfortunate patients dignity at the time of death (Hamel et al. 2000). Considering measures of suffering and health-related quality of life in deliberations about priorities and interventions can help focus resources on improving function, promoting healthy life styles, and increasing vitality rather than just on lengthening life (Fries et al. 1993).

The extra weight given to premature mortality and the inclusion of the impact of non-fatal health outcomes in the computation of summary health measures are usually assumed to have obvious merit. However, the incorporation of these two attributes also has engendered substantial criticism (Williams 1999). In the formulation of and reaction to the DALY a valuable background literature has emerged that provides lucid discussions of the merits, and demerits, of these two ingredients. These works have provided compelling justifications for these choices (Murray and Lopez 1996a). For example, even though Williams has seriously questioned the age-weighting components of the DALY calculation which places greater emphasis on morbidity and mortality in younger adulthood, Nord and others have presented empirical data that these years of life are valued more than other years by persons of all ages (Nord et al. 1995). This sort of evidence prompts even Williams to suggest that the lived years in young adulthood are "the best years of our life" (Williams 1999). In our experience policy-makers generally find this emphasis intuitive and useful.

COMPREHENSIVENESS AND INTERNAL CONSISTENCY

When the DALY was introduced in the *World Development Report* in 1993, this metric was used as the primary assessment tool for delineating major health problems and identifying the most cost-effective interventions. However, undergirding all of the conclusions from this report was an enormous exercise in epidemiological analysis. Calculating summary measures like the DALY requires the estimation of age- and sex-specific incidence, prevalence and mortality rates, and the average duration for each disease or injury episode. Most of the detailed epidemiological data used in the *World Development Report* subsequently was published as part of the *Global Burden of Disease* (GBD) series (Murray and Lopez 1996b). The data from the second volume of the GBD have quickly become a standard reference for quantitative information on international health and demographics. As explained in the methods section of the first volume of the GBD by Murray and Lopez, these estimates were generated with special attention to internal consistency (Murray and Lopez 1996a). Therefore, the sum of disease-specific deaths could not exceed the overall estimate for mortality, and inconsistencies between various data sources were rigorously evaluated and resolved. In addition, the disability weights used for the more than 400 non-fatal health conditions described in the GBD also were derived with attention to internal consistency.

This attention to detail and commitment to internal consistency, as well as the encyclopaedic provision of epidemiological estimates, are welcome by-products of creating comprehensive summary measures. Indices such as the DALY or the Healthy Life Year, which was developed as part of the Ghana Health Assessment Project, become more transparent and accessible when they are accompanied by detailed epidemiological information (Hyder et al. 1998; Morrow 1984). Providing descriptive epidemiological information helps to strip summary measures of their "black box" reputation, and publication of the underlying information is important for dissemination and use of these measures for the development of health policy.

Comprehensiveness and consistency are valuable to health policy-makers and analysts beyond supplying relatively credible and detailed information. In particular, these attributes help identify important gaps in data collection and analysis. In some cases there is a paucity of high-quality, population-based data for producing widely generalizable estimates of incidence, case-fatality and morbidity rates associated with major health problems, such as ischaemic heart disease in the United States. Conversely, compilation of estimates for the calculation of summary measures also can identify "analysis gaps." For example, in attempting to execute a burden-of-disease study in the USA we have discovered that in many states there are excellent hospital discharge registries that include more detailed information about the external causes of injuries than is generally available from national data sources such as the national Hospital Discharge Survey (NCHS 1996). These state-level data can be extrapolated to the national level to provide valuable information on serious injuries. However, the state data have rarely been used to complement analyses of the descriptive epidemiology of injuries that were based on more limited national data.

ISSUES OF VALIDITY

The computation of valid summary measures requires high-quality, generalizable population-based data on all of the following: 1) the number and causes of deaths, 2) the prevalence of non-fatal conditions, 3) the incidence of non-fatal conditions, 4) the natural history of non-fatal conditions, and 5) preference-based valuations for the disability weights associated with each of these conditions. A clear tenet reiterated in the GBD is the proposition that if such quality data are not available to provide estimates for a certain condition, and as a result no estimates are generated, then that disease or injury will never be considered a significant problem. This will occur even if there is information from similar populations, or less than optimal sources of data, indicating that the condition of interest is associated with substantial disability and suffering. Therefore, studies using summary measures have an imperative to calculate estimates for all potentially important health conditions regardless of the quality of the available data. As a result, rigorous methodologists may question the validity of these estimates (Gupta et al. 1994). The accusation that these measures are not adequately "rigorous" clearly ignores the many documented inaccuracies in standard sources of health data both currently and in the past (Messite and Stellman 1996). In addition, there are many hidden details even in the construction of traditional measures, such as age-adjusted mortality rates (NCHS 1992). The implications of the choices for the estimation and interpretation of these standard measures are rarely discussed, and the ethical dimensions are usually disregarded. However, these standard measures are widely used and seem to be accepted by policy-makers and the public even when the details important to methodologists are not presented.

Summary measures grounded in the concepts of healthy-lived time and non-disabled life-expectancy help emphasize that living "long" and "well" are both important. This concept of quality-lived time seems to have an intuitive appeal which is simple to explain in the general press (Brown 2000). Therefore, many of the technical charges levied against summary measures seem potentially unwarranted because similar deficiencies in the data currently used to develop health policy are usually overlooked. When these arguments against summary measures are placed in this context, it seems that the advantages of these approaches, as long as they are grounded in analytic exactitude and are based on the best data available, clearly trump the weaknesses.

VALUATION OF NON-FATAL HEALTH OUTCOMES

A major area of concern surrounding the use of summary health measures is the validity, reproducibility, and ethics of "valuing" health outcomes. Most of the literature dealing with this issue explores methods for weighing the impact of non-fatal conditions against death and health. A critical component of this dimension is the source of the valuations. From the standpoint of usefulness for policy development, it seems inevitable that using broadly inclusive valuation methods that involve the general public, professionals, as well as other persons with an interest in the health area will be essential. There is evidence that it may be feasible to obtain scientifically defensible values that use such a broad-based approach (Essink-Bot et al. 1990).

For summary measures to achieve their full usefulness, broad-based constituencies from relevant communities should be included in the derivation of weights for non-fatal health outcomes. However, there are at least two reasons why it seems misguided to prioritize major health problems in a community simply by asking people what they want rather than by supplementing the prioritization with epidemiological information. First, in communities where conditions such as malnutrition, childhood measles mortality and similar problems have long been endemic, people may have limited awareness that these issues can be effectively addressed. People will not ask for interventions for problems that they identify as unalterable components of the "human condition". Second, the simple reality is that quantitative assessments, such as burden of disease studies, are more likely to influence the policy-makers who have the resources to effect change.

International donor organizations, elected political officials, and government agencies in developed countries that are charged with improving human welfare throughout the world are regularly beseeched for assistance by representatives from agricultural groups, business interests, educational organizations and other constituencies. These groups, usually armed with quantitative information to justify their requests for resources, are essentially competing with their counterparts in the health arena. Presentations to health officials and policy-makers using summary health measures are often more persuasive because this is the type of information they are accustomed to and believe to be scientific and credible. Therefore, even though we strongly believe that community preferences are important in bolstering the ability of summary measures to elicit interest, these preferences will be sufficiently influential only if they are bolstered by epidemiological information presented in a format that policy-makers are accustomed to using.

SUMMARY

As we stated at the outset, summary measures of health clearly are not new, but their influence on health policy deliberations seems to be growing. The surge in interest by policy-makers and the general public is augmented by the recognition that resources are not sufficient to address all health problems everywhere in the world, and that priorities must be developed for efficient use of existing health resources. Because summary measures appear to incorporate values about health, combined with more traditional, quantitative health measures, they will increase in importance as ministries of health, donor organizations, and other large institutions struggle with the prioritization of health problems, interventions, and research agendas. The discussions and debates described in this volume provide a superb opportunity to advance the structure and use of these measures. Because we are convinced that such measures will be used, such deliberations are essential for ensuring that the "revolutionary" potential of summary measures perceived by Foege in 1994 results in the most useful and positive construction of health policy.

REFERENCES

Brown D (2000) US 15th on global index of health; 1st in spending. *Washington Post*, 1:A04–A04.

Dempsey M (1947) Decline in tuberculosis: the death rate fails to tell the entire story. *American Review of Tuberculosis*, (56):157–164.

Erickson P, Kendall E, Anderson J, Kaplan R (1989) Using composite health status measures to assess the nation's health. *Medical Care*, 27(3):S66–S76.

Erickson P, Wilson R, Shannon I (1995) *Years of healthy life.* (CDC/NCHS, Healthy people, Statistical notes no 7.) US Department of Health and Human Services, National Center for Health Statistics, Hyattsville, MD.

Essink-Bot M, Bonsel G, van der Maas PJ (1990) Valuation of health states by the general public: feasibility of a standardized measurement procedure. *Social Science and Medicine*, 31(11):1201–1206.

Field MJ, Gold MR, eds. (1998) *Summarizing population health: directions for the development and application of population metrics.* National Academy Press, Washington, DC.

Foege W (1994) Preventive medicine and public health. *Journal of the American Medical Association*, 271(21):1704–1705.

Fries J, Koop C, Beadle C, et al. (1993) Reducing health care costs by reducing the need and demand for medical services. The Health Project Consortium. *New England Journal of Medicine*, 329(5):321–325.

Gupta P, Sankaranarayanan R, Ferlay J (1994) Cancer deaths in India: is the model-based approach valid? *Bulletin of the World Health Organization*, 72(6):943–944.

Hamel MB, Lynn J, Teno JM, et al. (2000) Age-related differences in care preferences, treatment decisions, and clinical outcomes of seriously ill hospitalized adults: lessons from SUPPORT. *Journal of the American Geriatrics Society,* 48(5 Suppl.):S176–S182.

Hyder AA, Rotllant G, Morrow R (1998) Measuring the burden of disease: healthy life-years. *American Journal of Public Health,* 88(2):196–202.

Messite J, Stellman SD (1996) Accuracy of death certificate completion: the need for formalized physician training. *Journal of the American Medical Association,* 275(10):794–796.

Morrow R (1984) The application of a quantitative approach to the assessment of the relative importance of vector and soil transmitted diseases in Ghana. *Social Science and Medicine,* 19(10):1039–1049.

Murray CJL, Lopez AD, eds. (1996a) *The global burden of disease: a comprehensive assessment of mortality and disability from diseases, injuries and risk factors in 1990 and projected to 2020.* Global Burden of Disease and Injury, Vol. 1. Harvard School of Public Health on behalf of WHO, Cambridge, MA.

Murray CJL, Lopez AD, eds. (1996b) *Global health statistics: a compendium of incidence, prevalence and mortality estimates for over 200 conditions.* Global Burden of Disease and Injury, Vol 2. Harvard School of Public Health on behalf of WHO, Cambridge, MA.

NCHS (1992) Reconsidering age adjustment procedures: Workshop proceedings. *Vital Health Statistics,* 4(29):3–83.

NCHS (1996) *Hospital Discharge Survey (machine-readable public-use tape).* National Center for Health Statistics, US Department of Health and Human Services, Public Health Service, CDC, Hyattsville, MD.

Nord E, Richardson J, Street A, Kuhse H, Singer P (1995) Maximizing health benefits vs. egalitarianism: an Australian survey of health issues. *Social Science and Medicine,* 41(10):1429–1437.

Williams A (1999) Calculating the global burden of disease: time for a strategic reappraisal? *Health Economics,* 8(1):1–8.

World Bank (1993) *World development report: investing in health.* Oxford University Press, New York.

Chapter 2.4

Summary measures of population health: applications and issues in the United States

Edward Sondik

Recent events

After some 30 to 40 years of research and application, summary measures of population health (SMPH) are very much on the public health agenda. The success of the Global Burden of Disease (GBD) study has prompted much of this interest, although research on measures of the health of populations has been a continuing interest for many United States researchers. Recent events have emphasized interest in exploring our understanding of the promise and limitations of SMPH. In this commentary we briefly review some of these recent events and consider several issues in the application of SMPH.

A 1998 report from a Committee of the United States Institute of Medicine (IOM) reviewed progress in developing SMPH and offered three broad recommendations (Field and Gold 1998). First, it identified the need to strengthen the understanding of the ethical and policy implications of different measurement strategies and applications. More specifically, the Committee recommended a process of analysis and public discussion to build understanding of the critical policy implications of differing designs for summary measures, their implementation approaches, and their uses. Second, the Committee recognized that different health status measures might be used for different purposes and recommended accordingly that "the Department of Health and Human Services (DHHS) create a process to establish standards for population health metrics and assess the feasibility and practicality of a compatible set of health status measures". Third, the Committee encouraged the DHHS to cooperate with other organizations, both within and outside of government, on training and education on the interpretation and use of such measures. The Committee recognized that SMPH can be important in setting policy and in leading to action but that by their very nature as summaries incorporating a variety of assumptions both analytic and ethical, their implications need to be explored. The Committee report has been influential. Prompted by it and the broad interest in the DHHS, the National Institutes of Health and the Centers for Disease Control and Prevention created the Interagency Working Group on Summary Health Measures. The purpose of this committee is to serve as a forum for research and development on summary measures. Most important, the Interagency Committee is to address the need for standards and to assure that work towards understanding the implications for SMPH use is underway.

The National Committee on Vital and Health Statistics (NCVHS), which advises the Secretary of DHHS, has also shown interest. At one of its meetings earlier in the year 2000 the NCVHS discussed the IOM report and heard from an expert panel. The panel, including a representative of Statistics Canada, discussed a number of current initiatives, and the NCVHS expressed interest in being kept abreast of these activities. The importance of an overview or index of health has also been expressed by the United States Congress, which in 1999 expressed interest in the "…development of a public health index that would serve as a benchmark for the overall progress of the nation's health status". The Congress requested that the National Center for Health Statistics (NCHS) begin "feasibility studies of the establishment of a national index…" (National Center for Health Statistics 2000).

Together, these committees, plus the variety of research and programmatic activities now underway, strongly indicate that research and applications of SMPH will be moving forward (Interagency Working Group on Summary Health Measures 2000). In fact, we can point to several examples of relatively recent work, each one different and reflecting a different use for SMPH.

- *Assessing the burden of mental health.* SMPH, specifically disability-adjusted life years (DALYs), were used in the first-ever Surgeon General's report on mental health. The report uses results from Murray and Lopez (1996) to illustrate that mental health accounts for over 15 per cent of total DALYs, ranking second in the burden of disease in established market economies, such as the United States. The burden of mental illness on health and productivity in the United States and throughout the world has long been profoundly underestimated. The use of SMPH ensures that the magnitude of health problems reflects a balance of both mortality and morbidity.

- *Estimating and quantifying disparities in health.* Researchers from the Centers for Disease Control and Prevention developed a set of state-specific measures using Years of Healthy Life (YHL). This SMPH is derived from self-assessed measures of overall health and activity limitation gathered through nationwide or state-specific surveys. In this case the data were obtained from the Behavioral Risk Factor Surveillance System, a set of state-based telephone surveys coordinated by the CDC (Morbidity and Mortality Weekly Report 1998). The original use of YHL was in the context of Healthy People 2000 (see below), based on data from the National Health Interview Survey coupled with age-specific mortality rates (Erickson et al. 1995).

• *Fostering studies of the factors causing disparities.* A recent study, "The burden of disease in Los Angeles County: A study of the patterns of morbidity and mortality in the county population" (Ho et al. 2000), uses the methodology of the GBD (Murray and Lopez 1996) coupled with Los Angeles vital statistics data. The results emphasize the differences in the rankings of health problems when morbidity data are coupled with mortality data. This paper reports the application of the DALY measure to assess racial/ethnic and gender variation in disease and injury burden in the Los Angeles County population. The age-adjusted DALY rate (per 1000 population) was higher in men than women and was highest in Blacks and lowest in Asians/Pacific Islanders. The authors note that the results are important for planning, resource allocation, and policy development.

• *Providing a framework for resource allocation.* It is appealing to consider the allocation of resources based on summary measures of population health. This may be a risky proposition since we are not guaranteed that the resources, allocated in proportion to the measure, will have an impact in like proportion. In this interesting analysis, mortality and morbidity for different diseases were combined as DALYs and used to assess the appropriateness of the distributions in the NIH research budget. This is a step very close to the use of summary measures calculated for each disease for allocating research resources across these various diseases (Gross et al. 1999). In fact, the authors show that the distribution of DALYs is a reasonable approximation to the current NIH budget distribution across diseases. The optimality of this distribution, however, can only be determined with additional analysis regarding the potential impact in each disease category.

These examples share the deficiency that the data employed on morbidity are limited. Further, the authors did not propose specific interventions as a direct part of the study. The first three examples focus on differences or disparities for populations defined by gender, race or ethnicity, or by disease. For these a next step, at least conceptually, would be to disaggregate the measures to identify the reasons for lower health status. Once identified we could move towards either developing or applying potentially cost-effective interventions and then mount these interventions in a suitable evaluation framework.

THE FUTURE

One of the most important potential applications for the use of SMPH is in the Healthy People 2010 programme, the primary prevention initiative in the United States. The programme brings together national, state, and local organizations, businesses, communities, and individuals to improve the health of all Americans (US Department of Health and Human Services 2000). Healthy People 2010 provides a set of health objectives for the United States, consisting of 28 focus areas and 467 objectives aimed at improving health status. In essence, this prevention agenda addresses risk behaviours (e.g. tobacco use, substance abuse), disease conditions (e.g. diabetes, cancer), age groups (e.g. maternal, infant, and child health), and infrastructure/system issues (e.g. public health infrastructure, food safety). The objectives provide targeted areas for improvement across these broad issues. Each objective has both a baseline and a target and, where appropriate, is broken down into various racial and ethnic groups, socioeconomic and education levels, gender, and age designations. Two over-arching goals are part of the Healthy People 2010 programme: 1) improving years and health quality of life, and 2) eliminating disparities in health.

With 467 objectives and multiple population groups involved, the summary measures may well be a useful tool for setting priorities for action. These measures may also be a help in identifying progress and problems. In addition, SMPH may well be useful to characterize health disparities across the many minority and geographically dispersed American populations. We might term the latter use identifying the "tails" of the health status distribution. For the Healthy People 2010 programme no specific summary measures have been identified, but research is underway to develop tools to summarize Healthy People 2010 for the nation and for use by states and local decision-makers in the choices they must make to implement the programme. Years of Healthy Life (YHL) was used as part of Healthy People 2000 with significant advantages and disadvantages (see below).

While summary measures can be useful, it is important that candidate measures distinguish between significant differences in health status, both the current health status and that projected on the basis of risk factor prevalence. It is also important that the measures lend themselves to application to minority populations, defined not only in terms of race or ethnicity but also in terms of the geographic region in which they live. A challenge in this task is the lack of adequate data. Healthy People 2010 has defined a set of some 20 leading health indicators to serve as a summary set of measures. A single summary of this set might prove to be very useful.

Elimination of disparities is one of the major Healthy People 2010 goals. The capability to show the relationship to national, state, and local measures and for each to identify summary measures for multiple populations—the capability to "drill down"—would be very useful. Developing this type of hierarchical set of measures would be a significant tool in helping decision-makers to grasp the impact of health disparities in specific populations.

While summary measures help to set priorities for intervention, these same measures may not be able to reflect progress in improving health status. These measures may well be relatively insensitive to interventions, especially if the impact is far in the future. Or, it might be the case that the health problem is characterized by high morbidity but relatively low mortality and that feasible interventions influence only the mortality. In this case the linkage between interventions and their ultimate impact on the summary measures needs to be developed. It seems axiomatic that a measure should complement the use for which it is to be used. This point of view was endorsed by the Institute of Medicine in its recommendation to consider a family of metrics, but testing the sensitivity of SMPH to interventions needs to be made a priority.

It is also important that we be able to calculate summary measures for each state. State public health officials are critical actors and tools for meeting the Healthy People 2010 goals, but the challenge of such extensive data gathering on a state-specific basis will require a large increase in health surveillance resources.

While Healthy People 2010 is a very broad programme, it addresses only prevention-related issues. Health status as measured by SMPH may be influenced by treatment, rehabilitation, hospice care, and other types of care. A prevention-specific measure would be desirable. Two instruments could be used, one for overall health status and another for conditions related to prevention-directed interventions. It is important that at least the prevention measure be sensitive to the changes in health status or risks to health status which the intervention programmes are designed to achieve. This may require a prevalence-oriented prevention measure that is sensitive to changes in risk factors. In engineering, systems are considered controllable if they can be brought to a desired state. This is an important concept in health as well.

One of the goals of Healthy People 2000, the forerunner to Healthy People 2010, was to increase Years of Healthy Life, a summary measure developed by the National Center for Health Statistics and its consultants. This measure is derived from self-assessed measures of overall health and activity limitation gathered through the nationwide National Health Interview Survey and coupled with age-specific mortality rates (Erickson et al. 1995). Its advantage is easy calculation from data on health status (not necessarily linked to disease or risk factors) and from vital statistics. The major disadvantage is its insensitivity over the short run to changes in the main risk factors and the fact that it is based on self-reported measures which may be unstable over short periods of time.

IMPLICATIONS FOR DATA SYSTEMS

Building data systems to develop and evaluate summary health measures is one of the principal directions outlined in the response of the National Center for Health Statistics to the Congressional directive (National Center for Health Statistics 2000). The ongoing use of measures will require a continuing availability of detailed data over time, much of which is not currently available for the required race, ethnic, and geographic detail. Other particularly important data include measures of functional status (e.g. difficulty with bathing, eating), which generally do not provide an indication of the severity of such limitations. Additionally, data are lacking on the extent to which functional limitations are mitigated by adaptations that have been made in the home or by the community.

Using such measures to maximum advantage in tracking the impact of health interventions will require detailed data at the state and local level where many public health interventions are implemented. Data on health status, functional ability, and other variables are not commonly or regularly available. Some health measures require data on the probability of making a transition from one health state to another (e.g. moving from one level of physical functioning to another). Accurately assessing these probabilities requires collecting detailed data on the same individuals over time (longitudinal studies); however, most of the United States data systems currently collect data from a given individual at only one point in time (cross-sectional studies).

The timeliness of data is also an issue. Certainly measures are most useful if they allow tracking in real time. For example, the timeliness of data on life expectancy from the nation's vital statistics system could improve markedly if states were able to invest in electronic death registration systems.

TESTING SUMMARY MEASURES

It would be helpful to understand just how sensitive various SMPH are to changes in the current health status and to changes effected to particular interventions. In the case of Healthy People 2010 one could address the sensitivity of the measures to the prevalence of tobacco use among youth, or to obesity, or to sanitary conditions, or to sexual practices, or to prenatal care. These experiments would provide a good sense of whether particular measures can be used in particular situations to identify problems (or at least lead to the identification of health problems) or be used to monitor progress in addressing the problems.

In summary, the tenor of the IOM committee report is that work needs to be done to understand the implications of SMPH in a variety of situations. Experimenting with SMPH in the context of Healthy People 2010, for example, would be a significant step forward in understanding the implications of alternative measures and in developing the necessary data sources.

REFERENCES

Centers for Disease Control and Prevention (1998) Years of healthy life - selected states, United States, 1993–1995. *Morbidity and Mortality Weekly Report,* **47**(1):5–7.

Erickson P, Wilson R, Shannon I (1995) *Years of healthy life.* (CDC/NCHS, Healthy people, Statistical notes no 7.) US Department of Health and Human Services, National Center for Health Statistics, Hyattsville, MD.

Field MJ, Gold MR, eds. (1998) *Summarizing population health: directions for the development and application of population metrics.* National Academy Press, Washington, DC.

Gross CP, Anderson GF, Powe NR (1999) The relation between funding by the National Institutes of Health and the burden of disease. *New England Journal of Medicine,* **340**(24):1881–1887.

Ho A, Simon P, et al. (2000) *The Los Angeles County burden of disease project.* Los Angeles County Department of Health Services and the UCLA Center for Health Policy Research, Los Angeles, CA.

Interagency Committee on Summary Health Measures (2000) *Department of health and human services. Summary of department activities on summary health measures.* Washington, DC.

Murray CJL, Lopez AD, eds. (1996) *The global burden of disease: a comprehensive assessment of mortality and disability from diseases, injuries and risk factors in 1990 and projected to 2020.* Global Burden of Disease and Injury, Vol. 1. Harvard School of Public Health on behalf of WHO, Cambridge, MA.

NCHS (2000) *Developing an index of health: approaches, current developmental activities, and implications.* (A report to the Senate Committee on Appropriations by the National Center for Health Statistics.) National Center for Health Statistics, Centers for Disease Control and Prevention, Washington, DC.

US Department of Health and Human Services (2000) *Healthy people 2010.* Public Health Service, Washington, DC.

Chapter 2.5

PRIORITY-SETTING IN THE HEALTH SECTOR AND SUMMARY MEASURES OF POPULATION HEALTH

PRASANTA MAHAPATRA

INTRODUCTION

This chapter is in three sections. In the first I discuss how priorities are set. I argue that macro-level priority-setting in the health sector, as in most other sectors of the economy, is a social political process which may be aided by technical inputs. I then review a few macro-level priority-setting exercises in the health sector. My emphasis in this review is to identify the technical analytical inputs usually sought for the setting of priorities. Finally I summarize the methodological characteristics that appear common to all priority-setting exercises in public health and discuss the potential uses of summary measures of population health (SMPH), particularly the health gap measures, i.e. summary measures of disease burden. I conclude that summary measures of population health are useful analytical aids to priority-setting in the health sector.

SETTING PRIORITIES IN THE HEALTH SECTOR

Real operations of a health system, on a day-to-day basis, treat certain problems, meet certain requirements, and bypass some others. Priorities are set explicitly or implicitly.[1] It is important to recognize that health sector priorities are ultimately set through social and political processes. Linkages between health policy and the social political process have been fairly well documented (for example, see Carr-Hill 1991; McKeown et al. 1994; Walt 1994). Analytical approaches to setting priorities operate within the sociopolitical environment. They modify the sociopolitical environment by changing peoples' information set. On the other hand, sociopolitical interests may engender development of specific analytical approaches. Although expressions like "priority-setting techniques" and its minor variants are used in health policy literature, they actually refer to technical and analytic aids to priority-setting. This semantic distinction is important, since a good deal of criticism of specific aids to priority-setting arises from an apprehension that they are formulist. The expression "health priority-setting" is used here to mean analytic aids to priority-setting in the health sector.

Analytical aids to priority-setting consist of processes and criteria (Goold 1996). Priority-setting criteria refer to the variables considered relevant for the ordering of alternative choices, e.g., age, sex, capacity to benefit from treatment, etc. Priority-setting processes refer to the procedures followed to arrive at certain criteria and the application of these chosen criteria to specific data. Both procedural justice and the shared criterion of fairness appear to be important for health priority-setting. Analytical aids to priority-setting can either be qualitative or quantitative. While summary measures are quantitative aids to policy analysis, the usefulness of qualitative information, such as case studies, should also be kept in perspective (Filstead 1981).

At the macro level, two distinct forms of health priority-setting can be distinguished: (a) systemic, and (b) benefit package definition or rationing. Systemic priority-setting is about health sector-wide policies. Examples are the allocation of financial and managerial resources between public health oriented interventions and clinical services, speciality profiles of outputs from education and training institutions, technology assessment, regulatory policies to discourage undesirable activities, and incentive regimes to encourage desirable services. Although systemic priorities would encourage certain services (e.g. the ones considered cost-effective) and discourage expensive services, there may still be scope for a few persons to receive the expensive services. In other words, systemic priorities act on the overall volume of services rather than on specific cases. Rationing is implicit in systemic priority-setting, although its application to individuals may vary. By definition, explicit rationing of benefit packages may be based on the same set of ethical principles and allocative criteria, but apply at an operational level.

AIDS TO PRIORITY-SETTING IN THE HEALTH SECTOR: EXPERIENCES FROM A FEW PRIORITY-SETTING EXERCISES

To understand both the process and the data requirements for health priority-setting, it will be useful to review actual priority-setting exercises in the recent past. I have reviewed four such efforts undertaken during the 1980s and early 1990s; two of them are country specific (United States and United Kingdom) and two were undertaken by international agencies. The four studies are: (a) the domestic health policy consultation in the United States undertaken by the Carter Center; (b) the interdisciplinary committee on health promotion, constituted by a group of four health care organizations in the United Kingdom; (c) a UNDP-sponsored monograph on establishing health priorities; and (d) the World Bank's *World Development Report 1993* on investing in health. All these efforts were directed towards determination of systemic priorities. A large body of literature focusing on rationing and benefit package definition exists (see, for example, Malek 1994). A well known example of a priority-setting exercise for rationing of health care is the Oregon experiment (Strosberg and et al. 1992). They are not reviewed here for two reasons: (a) the present work is concerned with a developing country perspective, and (b) the four efforts for systemic priority-setting specifically reviewed here provide enough understanding of the role of quantifying the disease burden for priority-setting, which is the focus of the present study.

Soon after its establishment in 1981, the Carter Center in the United States appointed a health policy task force to identify domestic problems in the health field. This task force identified a reduction in the size of disease burden that is preventable or treatable with current technology as a priority. In effect this was a full-scale health sector priorities review. The emphasis was on generic risk factors (also referred to as precursors in the study report) for several health problems. The study was called "Closing the gap". Methodological details and results of this consultation have been published (Amler and Dull 1987; Foege et al. 1985). Major health problems in the USA were identified in September 1983 by an expert panel using five criteria: (a) point prevalence and temporal trends; (b) severity of health impact and cost; (c) sensitivity to intervention using current scientific or operational knowledge; (d) feasibility of such interventions; and (e) generic applicability of such interventions to other health problems. Identified problem areas included: alcohol dependency, arthritis, cancer, cardiovascular diseases, dental diseases, depression, diabetes mellitus, digestive diseases, drug dependence, infectious and parasitic diseases, respiratory diseases, unintended pregnancy and infant mortality, unintended injury and violence. Definition of these problem areas are so broad that real prioritization must depend on additional criteria and data sources used to study each of them. Each problem area was assigned to a consultant, and an expert panel from different specialties, both of whom followed a common data format (Table 1) to quantify illness and its component attributable to specific risk factors. Four out of the five groups of data relate to quantification of the disease burden.

Table 1 "Closing the gap" project in the USA: common data format

Health outcome	Statistic
Mortality	Deaths, crude death rate, age-standardized death rate, age-specific mortality rates, years of potential life lost before the age of 65
Morbidity	Incidence rate, annual period prevalence, days of hospital care, hospitalizations, physician visits, days lost from work or major activity
Complications	Blindness, paralysis, amputation
Quality of life	Individual (disability, missed education opportunity, training, employment) Family (transportation to health facility, etc.) Social (greater dependency, etc.)
Direct costs	Short-stay hospital care, physician and other professional care, pharmaceuticals, special equipment and long-term institutional care

In 1985 a group consisting of four health care organizations[2] in the United Kingdom sponsored a research fellowship in health promotion and appointed an interdisciplinary committee to guide the project (Smith and Jacobson 1988). The main focus of this committee was to identify priorities for health promotion efforts. This committee listed three overall health goals and six criteria to identify health sector priorities. The three goals were: attainment of (a) longevity, (b) a good quality of life, and (c) equal opportunities for health. The six priority-setting criteria were: (i) need for action and strength of supporting evidence, (ii) feasibility or effectiveness of action and strength of evidence supporting it, (iii) public support and acceptability, (iv) professional support, (v) political support, and (vi) economic benefits. To identify the needs for action, the committee explicitly analysed the mortality patterns by broad age groups. Priorities for reduction of mortality and improvement of quality of life were identified using the mortality analysis and group consensus. Top causes of current or emerging disease burdens implicitly identified by the committee include circulatory diseases, cancers, sexually transmitted diseases, road safety, mental health, congenital abnormalities, prematurity and low birth weight, vaccine preventable diseases, and dental diseases in childhood.

Some time before 1988, the United Nations Development Programme (UNDP) commissioned the preparation of a monograph on establishing health priorities in the developing world (Walsh 1988). Walsh reviewed the literature, held discussions with scientists and programme officers in the World Health Organization (WHO), the United Nations Children's Fund (UNICEF), UNDP, the World Bank, and non-profit funding agencies, as well as faculty members from a few academic institutions. These consultations suggested that the monograph contents should be structured around the prevailing consensus on priorities in the health sector, even though no formal consensus method was used. In the monograph, Walsh first takes stock of the burden of illness, relying mainly on causes of death. About 20 disease categories were identified as leading causes of illness and death in the world. She then listed the available interventions, their cost and efficacy, and discussed the factors affecting effectiveness. Although the monograph does not give details about the manner in which estimates of mortality and intervention efficacy were gathered, it does bring out the sequence of analytical steps required for identifying priorities in health service provision and research.

The World Bank's *World Development Report 1993* (WDR) focused on the importance of investments in health and on priorities within the health sector (World Bank 1993). This report made use of two background studies: 1) the global burden of disease (GBD) study (World Bank 1993, Appendix B), and 2) the health sector priorities review (Jamison et al. 1993). The GBD study quantified the global burden of premature mortality and disability caused by about 100 diseases. Diseases cumulatively accounting for more than 90 percent of premature deaths were included in the list. A new measure of population health status, the disability-adjusted life year (DALY), was used. The health sector priorities review made use of the DALY as a common denominator to account for output from different health interventions. Each of the 25 specific diseases or disease clusters were taken up by multidisciplinary teams who studied the cost-effectiveness of available interventions.

SUMMARY AND CONCLUSION

Certain methodological characteristics appear common to all priority-setting exercises in public health, namely (a) some form of quantification of the disease burden; (b) feasibility and cost-effectiveness of the interventions; and (c) reliance on consensus among experts. The role of disease burden estimates in priority-setting needs elaboration. Evidently a disease burden estimate is only one component of a priority-setting exercise. Faced with disease burden estimates, people quickly recognize the main causes of illness and develop a motivation to reduce them. This motivation to apprehend the main causes of disease burden inevitably leads one to search for appropriate technologies and their cost-effectiveness. Considerations of technical and practical feasibility and the cost-effectiveness of interventions play a crucial role in the minds of policy-makers (along with social, political and ethical considerations) in determining which causes of the disease burden are targeted by the health care delivery system and which are the subjects for further research. Thus, the primary role of a disease burden estimate is to set the agenda by creating an environment of concern and by motivating policy-makers. In addition, disease burden estimates provide benchmarks for future evaluation of the effect of health care interventions. Specific disease burden estimates are useful for analysing the cost-effectiveness of interventions and health resource allocation modelling. Summary measures of population health are a generalization of the concept of disease burden measurement. Summary measures include measures of the health gap and measures of health expectancy. The health gap measures are nothing but measures of disease burden. Health expectancy measures, like the disability-adjusted life expectancy (DALE), can be derived from measures of disease burden, like the disability-adjusted life years and the local life table. The health expectancy measures are useful for summarizing the average health attainment of a population and for communicating this to a general audience. The health gap measures, like the DALY, allow additive disaggregation and further analysis of the causes and factors that contribute to the overall disease burden, and also help to identify the potential for enhancement of healthy life expectancy.

Limitations of disease burden information for priority-setting should also be recognized. It is sometimes believed that understanding the composition of disease burdens and identifying the main causes of illness are all that is required for priority-setting. People tend to uncritically assume that priorities are set by merely attacking the main causes of illness. This is partly true in so far as some form of "attack" on the main causes of illness is imperative. For this reason, the main causes of illness are important subjects for research. In the case of health services, disease burden information may help draw attention to the problem. However, feasibility and cost-effectiveness are additional considerations to set priorities for the organization and delivery of health care services. Health care priority-setting is distinct from research priority-setting. Health priority-setting includes both but may be used, in context, to mean priorities in service provision. Mooney and Creese (1993) discussed the role of disease burden estimates in priority-setting, while Prost and Jancloes (1993) discussed the role of epidemiology in public health priority-setting. It should be noted that disease burden estimates mostly consist of descriptive epidemiological information. Descriptive epidemiology provided traditional disease burden profiles consisting of cause-specific mortality and disease prevalence. The family of summary measures of health status do incorporate some value judgements by way of disability severity or health state preference weights, etc. (Shiell 1997). However, these measures are more sensitive to descriptive epidemiological estimates (Murray and Lopez 1996). Discussions about the role of epidemiological estimates in priority-setting would therefore apply to summary measures of disease burden estimates as well.

NOTES

1   Priorities may not be set at all and things may be allowed to drift, either due to bureaucratic habit or political corruption. The social political remedy for such a situation is to ask explicitly for set priorities and seek action conforming to those priorities. While this problem is more fundamental, the starting point for this work is that decision-makers do recognize the need for priority-setting and are willing for change.

2   The Health Education Council (name changed to the Health Education Authority from April 1987), King Edward's Hospital Fund for London, the London School of Hygiene and Tropical Medicine, and the Scottish Health Education Group

REFERENCES

Amler RW, Dull HB, eds. (1987) *Closing the gap: the burden of unnecessary illness.* Oxford University Press, New York.

Carr-Hill RA (1991) Allocating resources to health care: is the QALY a technical solution to a political problem? *International Journal of Health Services,* **21**(3):351–363.

Filstead WJ (1981) Qualitative and quantitative information in health policy decision making. *Health Policy Quarterly,* **1**(1):43–56.

Foege WH, Amler RW, White CC (1985) Closing the gap: Report of the Carter Center health policy consultation. *Journal of the American Medical Association,* **254**:1355–1358.

Goold SD (1996) Allocating health care: cost-utility analysis, informed democratic decision making, or the veil of ignorance? *Journal of Health Politics, Policy and Law,* **21**(1):69–98.

Jamison DT, Torres AM, Chen LC, Melnick JL (1993) Poliomyelitis. In: *Disease control priorities in developing countries.* Jamison DT, Mosley WH, Meashem AR, Bobadilla JL, eds. Oxford University Press for the World Bank, New York.

Malek M (1994) *Setting priorities in health care.* Wiley, New York.

Mckeown K, Whitelaw S, Hambleton D, Felicity G (1994) Setting priorities – science, art or politics. In: *Setting priorities in health care.* Malek M, ed. Wiley, New York.

Mooney G, Creese A (1993) Priority setting for health services efficiency: the role of measurement of burden of illness. In: *Disease control priorities in developing countries.* Jamison DT, Mosley WH, Meashem AR, Bobadilla JL, eds. Oxford University Press for the World Bank, New York.

Murray CJL (1996) Rethinking DALYs. In: *The global burden of disease: a comprehensive assessment of mortality and disability from diseases, injuries, and risk factors in 1990 and projected to 2020.* The Global Burden of Disease and Injury, Vol. 1. Murray CJL, Lopez AD, eds. Harvard School of Public Health on behalf of WHO, Cambridge, MA.

Murray CJL, Lopez AD, eds. (1996) *The global burden of disease: a comprehensive assessment of mortality and disability from diseases, injuries and risk factors in 1990 and projected to 2020.* Global Burden of Disease and Injury, Vol. 1. Harvard School of Public Health on behalf of WHO, Cambridge, MA.

Prost A, Jancloes M (1993) Rationales for choice in public health: the role of epidemiology. In: *Disease control priorities in developing countries.* Jamison DT, Mosley WH, Meashem AR, Bobadilla JL, eds. Oxford University Press for the World Bank, New York.

Shiell A (1997) Health outcomes are about choices and values: an economic perspective on the health outcomes movement. *Health Policy,* **39**(1):5–15.

Smith A, Jacobson B, eds. (1988) *The nation's health. A strategy for the 1990s. A report from an independent multidisciplinary committee chaired by Professor Alwyn Smith.* Kings Edward's Hospital Fund for London, London.

Strosberg MA, et al. (1992) *Rationing America's medical care.* The Brookings Institution, Washington, DC.

Walsh JA (1988) *Establishing health priorities in the developing world.* Adams Publishing Group on behalf of UNDP, Boston, MA.

Walt G (1994) *Health policy. An introduction to process and power. People, governments and international agencies – who drives policy and how it is made.* Zed Books, London.

World Bank (1993) *World development report: investing in health.* World Bank, Oxford University Press, New York.

Chapter 3.1

MEASURING THE BURDEN OF DISEASE BY AGGREGATING WELL-BEING

JOHN BROOME

DISTRIBUTIONS OF WELL-BEING

We are interested in measuring the harm that is done by disease. To look at the same question practically and positively, we are interested in measuring the good that will be done by reducing disease.

The diagram (Figure 1) illustrates very schematically the problem of measurement that concerns us. It illustrates the effects of a single epidemic. Imagine that the epidemic is expected in the future, and that it might be possible to prevent it by some public health measure. We want to measure how much harm the epidemic will do. Conversely—this comes to the same thing—we want to measure the benefit that will be achieved by preventing the epidemic.

The diagram has two halves. The right half shows what will happen if the epidemic occurs; the left what will happen if it is prevented. Each half is a multiple graph. In both, time is measured in a horizontal direction. A vertical dotted line marks the date when the epidemic occurs, if it does. Each horizontal line marks out the life of a single person; corresponding lines in the two halves of the diagram belong to the same person. Each line is the horizontal axis of a little graph that shows the course of the person's life. A person's graph begins at the time when she (or he) is born and ends when she dies. During her life, the height of the graph above the axis represents the person's *well-being*—i.e. how well her life is going. One line in the diagram has no graph on it; this indicates that one particular person will not live at all if the epidemic occurs.

The diagram shows the following effects caused by the epidemic. All of them are typical of disease.

- One person is killed at the time of the epidemic.

- One person is disabled by the epidemic, but her life is not shortened.

- One person's life is shortened by the epidemic, but she does not die immediately.

Figure 1   Well-being with and without an epidemic
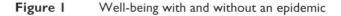

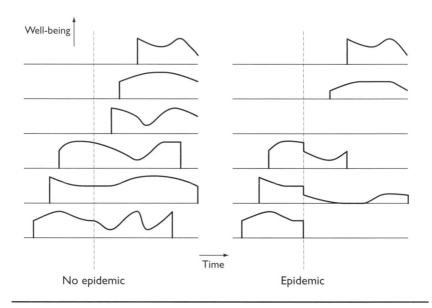

No epidemic   Epidemic

- One person who would have been born is not born as a result of the epidemic (perhaps because one of her parents is killed).

- One person born later, who would have been born healthy, is born disabled (perhaps because of genetic damage to one of her parents).

Our measure of the harm done by the epidemic must take into account events of all these sorts.

The diagram shows that, although the epidemic occurs at a single date, its effects are spread across time. This is typical of disease, and complicates our attempt to measure it. In practice, we are rarely dealing with the effects of a single epidemic. Disease is always with us, and the effort to control it always continues. Still, we shall want to know how much harm is done by the disease that occurs at a particular date, or how much benefit is achieved by a particular development in public health. This means we need to sort out the effects of events that occur at one date from the effect of events that occur at other dates. When causes act continuously, as diseases do, this is complicated. In this paper, I shall not try to sort out these causal matters. That is why I have chosen to illustrate the problem of measurement with the comparatively simple example of a single epidemic.

The vertical dimension in the diagram shows the well-being people enjoy at particular times. I shall call this *temporal* well-being whenever I need to in order to avert confusion. There are serious difficulties about measuring it, both in theory and in practice. In this paper, I shall have to skate over most of those difficulties (see chapter 5 and 6 in Broome, forth-coming). I shall simply assume temporal well-being can be measured on a cardinal scale that is comparable both between different times and between different people. The zero on the scale is also important, and I shall say something about it later in this chapter.

To measure the harm done by the epidemic, we need to compare the values of the states of affairs shown in the two halves of the diagram. The harm is the difference between their values. I assume that the value of a state of affairs is determined only by the factors that are illustrated in the diagram. That is to say, it is determined by which people exist, by the dates when those people are born and die, by their temporal well-being at all the times they are alive, and by nothing else. The value is determined only by the *distribution* of well-being, we may say. The diagram shows two alternative distributions. Our general task is to measure the value of distributions like this.

The value of a state of affairs is some sort of an *aggregate* of people's temporal well-being. Somehow, the well-being of all the people, at every time they are alive, comes together to determine the overall value of the state of affairs. This is a two-dimensional aggregation; we have to aggregate across people and also across time. When I speak of "aggregation", I do not necessarily mean simply adding up; an aggregate may be a much more complicated compound than a simple total. The main subject of this paper is to work out how this aggregation should be done. As it turns out, I shall give support to aggregation by addition.

CAN HEALTH BE MEASURED AS A COMPONENT OF WELL-BEING?

Why does my diagram show people's well-being, as opposed to their state of health? There are two answers. First, the diagram could not show just health as a component of well-being, because health cannot be separated out as a distinct component of well-being. This section argues this point. Second, even if it were possible to separate health out of well-being, it would be a mistake to do so. We should be concerned with all of well-being. The next section argues that point.

Our aim is to measure "the burden of disease". The World Health Organization (WHO) takes this to be only the reduction in *health* that people suffer as a result of disease. It takes a person's health to be part of her well-being, so the reduction in health is part of the reduction of well-being, but it may not be the whole of it. As WHO sees it, the burden of disease is not the whole reduction in people's well-being which is caused by disease, but only the part that consists in a reduction in people's health. WHO aims to measure just that part.

To suit WHO's purposes, a summary measure of health should meet two desiderata. First, it should measure health specifically, and not well-being as a whole. One place where this desideratum is expressed is in

WHO's intention to measure health as disability rather than, say, the quality of life (see Murray 1996, p. 33). WHO defines a disability as "any restriction or lack of ability (resulting from an impairment) to perform an activity in the manner or within the range considered normal for a human being". By contrast, it defines a handicap as "a disadvantage for a given individual resulting from an impairment or a disability that limits or prevents the fulfilment of a role that is normal (depending on age, sex and social and cultural factors) for that individual" (WHO 1980). These definitions indicate that a handicap is allowed to depend on factors other than health, but a disability is intended to depend on health factors only.

The second desideratum is that the measure should measure health as a component of well-being. It is to be an evaluative measure, and not merely a descriptive one; it is to measure how good a person's health is for the person, or how bad her ill-health (see Murray 1996, pp. 2–3). That is to say, it aims to measure the contribution of health to well-being.

In this section I shall argue that these desiderata cannot be simultaneously satisfied.

For the purposes of this argument, I shall set aside the problems of aggregating health across people and across time. I shall consider a single person only, and a single time in her life. A person's well-being at a time will be determined by many factors. Some are: how comfortably the person is housed, her opportunities for entertainment, how much she works and the sort of work she does, and so on. Other factors are all the ones that constitute the state of her health at the time: the quality of her eyesight, the functioning of her limbs, whether she is in pain, and so on. We could write her well-being w as a function of all these factors:

$$w = w(h_1, h_2, \ldots h_m, d_1, d_2, \ldots d_n),$$

where h_1, h_2 and so on are all the individual factors that constitute her health, and d_1, d_2 and so on are all the other factors that help to determine her level of well-being.

The two desiderata could be simultaneously satisfied to a high degree if we could write the function $w(\ )$ in the special form:

$$w(h(h_1, h_2, \ldots h_m), d_1, d_2, \ldots d_n).$$

Technically, if the function could take this form, the health factors would be said to be *separable* from the other factors. It would mean that all the health factors could be evaluated together in a separate function $h(\ )$ of their own, and then the value of this function would contribute to determining overall well-being through the function $w(\ )$. The function $h(\ )$ would be a summary measure of the person's health, and it would measure her health as a component of well-being. This measure would satisfy the first desideratum to a high degree, because it would depend only on the health factors. It would also satisfy the second desideratum to a high degree, because it would be straightforwardly a component in the person's well-being.

Actually the health factors in well-being are not separable like this. Obviously, the way in which a person's well-being is affected by the various elements of her health depends a great deal on other features of her life. For example, asthma is less bad if you are well housed, mental handicap less bad in supportive communities, blindness less bad if you have access to the internet. Conversely, features of a person's health affect the value of other things: radios are no good to the deaf, nor running shoes to the lame. The interaction between health and other features of a person's life is so intimate that health cannot be treated as separable.

Here is a simple example. Concentrate on just two health factors: the quality s of a person's sight and the quality t of her hearing. (Suppose s and t are scaled to range between 0 and 1, so that s is 0 for a completely blind person, and 1 for a person with perfect sight.) And concentrate on just two non-health contributors to the person's well-being: the number b of books she has, and the number c of CDs. Suppose her well-being is given by:

$$sb + tc.$$

Granted the stylized nature of the example, this function is plausible. The better you can see, the more benefit you get from books; and the better you can hear, the more benefit you get from CDs. Conversely, the more books you have, the more benefit you get from good sight, and the more CDs you have, the more benefit you get from hearing. In this function, the two health factors are obviously not separable. The interaction between the health factors in well-being and the non-health factors is too intimate.

To be sure, we could define some function $H(b_1, b_2, \ldots b_m)$ of the health factors alone, and use that as a summary measure of the person's health. In the example, we might choose $H(\ )$ to be $(s + t)$, say. A well-designed measure of this sort might be useful for some purposes. For instance, it might be useful in a causal investigation of the effects of a health programme. But it would be a purely descriptive measure, and it would not measure health as a component of well-being. It would satisfy the first desideratum to a high degree, but the second not at all.

Since the health factors are not separable in well-being, the two desiderata cannot both be satisfied to a high degree. This is recognized implicitly in the practice of measuring health. In practice, measures of health do not try to measure a person's health independently of other factors in her well-being. So the first desideratum is relaxed. But it need not be abandoned completely, because a measure could still count as a less perfect measure of specifically health, if the other factors in well-being were held constant during the measurement. A measure of this sort is properly called an *index* of health. An appropriate index would compare a person's actual well-being, given her state of health, with what her well-being would be if she were in good health, but if the non-health factors in her well-being were unchanged.

The commonest index is simply the former expressed as a fraction of the latter. Let H_1, H_2 and so on be the values of the health factors that represent good health. A person's actual well-being is $w = w(h_1, h_2, \ldots h_m, d_1, d_2, \ldots d_n)$, and if she were in good health her well-being would be $w_h = w(H_1, H_2, \ldots H_m, d_1, d_2, \ldots d_n)$. We can measure her health by the fraction w/w_h. This fraction is her health index; let us call it δ. The person's actual well-being is δw_h, so δ is the factor by which ill-health reduces the person's well-being, other things remaining constant. Because the health factors in well-being are not separable, we know that δ cannot depend only on the health factors.

In my simple example, the person's actual well-being is $(sb + tc)$. If she were in good health, both s and t would be 1, because they are scaled that way. So, if she were in good health but in other respects the same as she actually is, her well-being would be $(b + c)$. For her:

$$\delta = (sb + tc)/(b + c).$$

A person's state of health is fully specified by her health factors. Because δ depends also on non-health factors in well-being, δ for any particular state of health will vary from person to person according to her non-health factors. But in practice, measures of health assign each state of health a single measure; they do not let the measure vary from person to person. They use the same measure for each person in the same state of health, and they do that by taking some sort of average value for each of the non-health factors.

Ill health harms a person's well-being in various ways. Which ways are recognized in the index δ and which are not? In calculating the index, we hold constant the non-health factors in well-being. So the index takes into account only those effects that do not go through changes in the non-health factors. When a health factor affects one of the non-health factors, that effect is not included in the index. For example, if a person's poor eyesight reduces the enjoyment she gets from her books, that effect is included in the index of her ill health. On the other hand, if her poor eyesight reduces her ability to earn income, and so causes her to have fewer books, that effect is not included, because her ownership of books is a non-health factor that is held constant.

To some extent this distinction is arbitrary, because it depends on what things are included in the list of non-health factors when the index is constructed. Is the number of a person's friends included in the list? If it is, the isolation that is caused by deafness will not be included in the index for deafness; if not, it will be included.

So there is something arbitrary in an index such as δ as a measure of specifically health. It takes in other aspects of a person's well-being in a rather arbitrary fashion. Still, such a measure would satisfy the first desideratum to some extent. The real problem is that it is not practicable to hold non-health factors constant in the way the index requires. In practice, a health measure must be derived in some way from people's preferences about states of health, or from people's judgements about how bad it is to be in a particular state of health. To elicit these preferences or judgments we must ask people to exercise their imagination. They cannot be expected reliably to hold constant in their imagination factors that they know will actually not be constant.

Consequently, practical measures of health do not attempt to hold constant the non-health factors in well-being. They are not intended to. They simply take a person's well-being in her actual state of health, and compare it with the well-being she would have were she in good health. They take the former as a fraction of the latter, and use that fraction as the measure of her health.

A person's actual well-being is $w = w(h_1, h_2, \ldots h_m, d_1, d_2, \ldots d_n)$. Suppose that, if she were in good health, the values of her non-health factors would be D_1, D_2, and so on. Then if she were in good health, her well-being would be:

$$W = w(H_1, H_2, \ldots H_m, D_1, D_2, \ldots D_n).$$

One measure of her health is $\Delta = w/W$. This measure takes account of the full effect that ill health has on the person's well-being, including all the indirect effects it causes by changing her non-health factors.

Once again, for a particular state of health, the measure will in principle vary from person to person, but the practice is to take some sort of average. In WHO's studies of the burden of disease, as described by Murray, the index for a particular state of health is evaluated for "the average individual with the condition described taking into account the average social response or milieu" (see Murray 1996, p. 38). In this remark, the word "response" indicates that Murray does not think of holding non-health factors constant. Instead, he takes them to change as, on average, they actually do change as a consequence of ill health.

This is how health is measured in practice. But now, there is really nothing left in Δ to allow it to count as a measure of health specifically. It is simply a measure of well-being. It does not satisfy the first desideratum. To be sure, it measures how much well-being is reduced by ill health as a cause. But WHO's idea is to measure the reduction in health only, and health to be only a part of well-being. My own view is that we should measure the whole reduction in well-being that is caused by disease, but that is not WHO's intention.

Δ is truly a measure of well-being, rather than health. Furthermore, it is an unsatisfactory measure of well-being, because it is scaled in a peculiar way. The value of Δ for a person in good health is by definition 1, and Δ is scaled to make this so. When well-being, measured this way, is aggregated across people, the effect is to treat every healthy person as equally well off. But actually some healthy people are better off than others. So what we end up with is simply an inaccurate measure of well-being.

WE SHOULD BE CONCERNED WITH ALL OF WELL-BEING

We cannot separate out health as a component of well-being. But I think it should also be clear that we should not want to do so. We are interested in the harm done by disease, and the benefit caused by preventing disease. Disease causes harms of a great many sorts, which are often not themselves specifically changes in health. For example, some diseases prevent their victims from working, and so deprive them of income and the other benefits that accompany work: companionship, self-esteem and so on.

Indeed, the harms that *are* always treated as changes in health often consist in deprivation of goods other than health. For example, in measures of health, death is universally included as a loss of health. But death is bad—at least partly—because it deprives its victim of all the good things she would have enjoyed in the rest of her life. These are goods of all sorts, and not only elements of health. So the badness of death consists in the loss of many things that are not themselves elements of health. Similarly, much of the harm caused by disabilities is not particularly a matter of health. For instance, if you are paralysed, you do not have access to many of the ordinary goods that other people enjoy. That is a major part of your loss.

So we ought not to be trying to measure the harm done by disease in terms of health only, but in terms of the whole of well-being. The measure we shall emerge with may accurately be called a measure of the burden of disease, but it would be inaccurate to call it a measure of health. If it is not a measure of health, why should the World Health Organization take any particular interest in it? Because it measures the harm caused by disease, or the benefit caused by controlling disease. The *cause* is specifically to do with health. The *effect* is harm or benefit in general.

In practice we need a measure now, and we cannot wait till someone has developed a way to measure well-being. We will not soon have a good theory of well-being, let alone a practical way of measuring it. Yet we do already have sensible measures of a person's health. More accurately, we have measures of the badness of particular sorts of ill-health (see Murray 1996, pp. 22–33). I think it is sensible to start using these measures immediately, but recognize that they are only approximations.

All the measures we have are scaled in such a way that a year of healthy life always has the value of 1. Years in less good health have a value less than 1. So a year of healthy life always makes the same contribution to the aggregate measure, however good or bad that year is in respects other than health. This too may be defensible as an approximation. As a rough approximation, when we are working on a very large scale, it may be defensible to assume that all healthy people are equally well off. But it is defensible as an approximation only. If we could find ways to be more accurate, we should use them.

However, many authors think it is a matter of principle that we should count each healthy year equally. It is not merely an acceptable approximation. They think there is actually a moral reason why the measurement of health should be scaled in this way. They believe fairness demands it (Culyer 1990, pp. 9–27; Murray 1996, p. 7). In this respect, they think our measurement of health should be guided by the consideration of fairness.

Murray explains this view using the example of two patients who are each in a coma caused by meningitis (see Murray 1996, p. 7). Only one can be treated, and the other will die. One is richer than the other. Suppose that, because she is richer, her well-being will be higher if she is saved. Then more good would be done by saving her. Should she be chosen for the treatment on that account? Murray thinks not. He evidently believes that would be unfair to the poorer patient. For this reason he thinks our measurement of the benefit of treatment should be blind to the person's wealth. This can be achieved by assigning the same value to a year of good health, regardless of other aspects of a person's well-being such as her wealth.

I agree with Murray that we ought not to give priority to the richer patient. But I do not agree that this should lead us to distort our measurement of goodness. The truth is that, if one patient will live a better life than the other, as we are assuming, then more good would be done by saving her than by saving the other. We should not hide this truth. Instead, we should learn something different from the example: doing the most good should not be our only criterion in making decisions of this sort. We also need to take account of fairness. In this case fairness requires us to be impartial between the patients, even though maximizing good would lead us to discriminate between them. Furthermore, fairness is a very important consideration, and in this case outweighs the extra benefit that would be achieved by saving the rich patient. We ought to choose in a non-discriminatory way, perhaps by holding a lottery (see chapter 14.4). Once we see that fairness is a distinct consideration from goodness, we will not need to try and incorporate considerations of fairness into our measure of goodness.

In any case, Murray's attempt to incorporate fairness into goodness fails. Let us modify his example. Suppose neither of the coma patients is richer than the other, but one is disabled and the other is not. Say that one has lost an arm. Should the other be saved on that account? Murray appears to be ambivalent about a case of this sort (see Murray 1996, pp. 22–33), but I do not think we need be ambivalent. If it is unfair to discriminate between patients on grounds of their wealth, it is certainly unfair to discriminate on grounds of this disability. It would plainly be unfair to let the disabled person die because she has already lost an arm. But we cannot make our measurement of health blind to disability, because disability is one of the main things we aim to measure. Our measure is bound to show that more good is done by saving the person who is not disabled. Yet this is unfair. So we have to recognize fairness as a separate consideration, which cannot be incorporated into our measure of goodness.

I have been oversimplifying. I think fairness is itself a sort of good. The separation I am really making is between fairness on the one hand and other sorts of good on the other. But for convenience I shall continue to use the terms "goodness" and "well-being" to contrast with fairness. Strictly, these terms include all sorts of good *apart from fairness*. Why separate out fairness from other sorts of good? Because it works differently. Fairness is essentially a matter of how people fare in comparison with each other. Consequently, the arithmetic of fairness is different from the arithmetic of other goods; a simple example appears in my "All goods are relevant" (chapter 14.4). Fairness therefore needs separate accounting.

Figure 1 shows people's well-being apart from fairness. Fairness does not appear in the diagram.

AGGREGATION AND SEPARABILITY OF PEOPLE

We have to aggregate temporal well-being across people and across time. How should we do it? Here is a simple possibility. First aggregate each person's well-being, to determine an aggregate value for each person. We may call this personal aggregate the person's *lifetime* well-being. Then aggregate together people's lifetime well-beings to determine the overall value of the distribution. This simple route to aggregation takes the two dimensions separately. First we aggregate across time for each person. Then we aggregate across people. The two questions of *how* to aggregate across times and across people remain open. I shall come to them in due course: I will discuss (see below) aggregation across people, and aggregation across times in a person's life.

This is a comparatively simple way to aggregate, but is it correct? At the first stage of aggregation, it requires us to assess each person's lifetime well-being on the basis of her temporal well-being at all the times in her life. We can only do this if each person's life can be correctly evaluated independently of how things go for other people. The assumption that this is possible I call *"separability of people"*. Is it a correct assumption?

At first, you might well think not. You might well think we should attach value to equality between people and, at first sight, this concern seems inconsistent with separability between people. If we are interested in equality, we are interested in how some people fare in comparison with other people. Are some much better off than others, or are most people at about the same level? If one person has a good life, say, we might assign her life more value if most other people are at about the same level than we would if she were much better off than most other people. In the latter case, her good life contributes to inequality in the society; in the former case it does not. This suggests we cannot value one person's life separately from other people's, so the assumption of separability is false.

Various replies may be made to this objection to separability on grounds of equality. In my book *Weighing Goods* I gave one that I favour on theoretical grounds (Broome 1991, chapter 9), but here I shall give a more pragmatic one. I have already stated the basis of it above. If equality is indeed valuable, that can only be because inequality is unfair. It is unfair that some people are worse off than others are, if they do not deserve to be. But I have just argued that fairness must be accounted for separately from goodness; it should not be incorporated into our measure of goodness. The assumption that people are separable is about the aggregation of goodness. Consequently, this matter of fairness cannot be an objection to it.

If fairness is to be accounted for separately, we cannot determine how we should act simply on grounds of goodness. Suppose we are wondering where to concentrate our resources on promoting health. Suppose it turns out that more good will be done by concentrating them on the cities rather than the country; suppose the resources will promote people's well-being more effectively in the cities. This is not enough to determine that the cities are where they should be used. Separately, we also need to consider fairness. If city-dwellers are already well off compared with people in the country, it might turn out unfair to give the city-dwellers still more. If so, the extra benefit of using the resources in the cities will need to be weighed against the extra fairness of using them in the country.

That deals with one possible doubt about separability of people. You might have a different doubt. We have to bear in mind that our decisions about health will affect the numbers of people who exist. A person exists in one half of my diagram who does not exist in the other half. In comparing the values of the two halves, we cannot ignore this difference. This means, in effect, that we shall have to attach a value (positive or negative) to the person's existence. I know that many people find it intuitively difficult to accept the idea that existence has value, and I shall say more about it below. Here I shall only point out a consequence of assuming separability of people. It implies not only that we can evaluate a person's life independently of how things go for other people, but also that the value of a person's existence is independent of how many other people exist and of how things go for them.

This conflicts with an assumption that people very commonly make when they think about population. They think that we should aim for the greatest well-being, on average, for the people who live. For example, when China chose to limit the number of Chinese, I presume its motive was to try and achieve the greatest average well-being for the Chinese people. It assumed that increasing population tends to decrease average well-being, and for this reason it decided to control the increase in population.

If your objective is the average well-being of the people, you will be in favour of adding a person to the population if her existence will increase the average. This will be so if her well-being will be above the average of the people who already exist, and if her existence will not harm other people. You will be against adding a person if her well-being will be below the average, and if her existence will not benefit other people. So the value of adding a person depends on how her well-being will compare with the well-being of the people who already exist. This conflicts with separability of people, which requires the value of her existence to be independent of the well-being of other people.

As it happens, I think separability wins this particular conflict. The average principle is mistaken, precisely because it conflicts with separability. But I shall not try to justify this claim in this paper. In this paper, I cannot go deeply into the value of population. I needed to mention the second doubt about separability, but having mentioned it I shall pass on.

ADDITION ACROSS PEOPLE

Separability of people permits the two-stage route to aggregation I mentioned: first aggregating temporal well-being across times to determine each person's lifetime well-being, and then aggregating lifetime well-beings across people. But separability does much more than this. It also allows us to derive remarkable conclusions about how the second step of aggregation is to be done. Consequently, I shall discuss this second step first, and come to the first step afterwards.

Separability of people turns out to be a remarkably powerful assumption. If it can be justified, a very strong conclusion can be drawn from it by mathematical means. It implies that aggregation across people must take an *additively separable form*. This means that a distribution's value takes the form:

$$f_1(g_1) + f_2(g_2) + \ldots + f_P(g_P). \tag{1}$$

In this formula, g_1, g_2 and so on stand for the lifetime well-beings of each person. The functions $f_1(\ )$, $f_2(\ )$ and so on are *transformations* that are applied to the well-beings before they are added up. The addition runs over all the people who exist. Missing people, like the one missing on the right of the diagram, are ignored.

The spectacular conclusion expressed in formula (1)—more precisely its derivation from separability of people—stems originally from a mathematical theorem first established by Harsanyi (1955), and subsequently developed and interpreted by many other authors (see Broome 1991, chapter 10). There is a lot of background to it which I have not mentioned and do not propose to mention. It makes several other assumptions besides separability of people, and several of them are controversial. I do not pretend that formula (1) is established truth. However, with some qualifications, I believe it can be soundly defended. I shall take it for granted in this paper.

The presence of the transformations $f_1(\ )$, $f_2(\ )$ and so on allows formula (1) to accommodate the so-called *priority view*. This is the view that we should be more concerned about the well-being of less well-off people than about the well-being of better-off people (Atkinson and Stiglitz 1980; Parfit 2000).[1] We should attach more value to increasing the well-being of the less well-off; we should give priority to the worse-off. If the transformation functions in (1) are all the same, so $f_1(\ ) = f_2(\ ) = \ldots = f_P(\ )$, and if they are strictly concave, they will have the effect of giving priority to the worse-off. This is how the priority view can be accommodated.

The priority view does not value equality directly, but it gives a derivative value to equality. For any given total of well-being, it prefers this well-being to be more equally distributed rather than less equally. That is one of its attractions.

I think the priority view is mistaken. The argument that leads me to this conclusion is long and arduous, and I do not need to rehearse it here (see Broome 1991, chapters 9 and 10). Only the result matters here. But for anyone who is interested, here is a brief sketch. For the priority view even to make sense, we must have an arithmetical (more precisely, *cardinal*) scale of people's lifetime well-being, which is defined before we come to aggregating well-being across people. Well-being measured on this independent scale is transformed by the transformations $f_1(\ )$, $f_2(\ )$ and so on. But I do not believe we have a clearly defined arithmetical scale. I believe our quantitative notion of well-being is actually formed by the process of aggregating across people. Implicitly, we define the scale of well-being for ourselves in such a way that we can aggregate well-being simply by adding, without transformation:

$$g_1 + g_2 + \ldots + g_P. \tag{2}$$

Part of the attraction of the priority view is the indirect value it assigns to equality. But it is not the only way of assigning value to equality. I explained above that the value of equality is best understood as the value of fairness, and I explained that I am not treating fairness as a part of goodness in this paper. It needs to be accounted for separately. So if we adopt formula (2) as our account of goodness, we need not repudiate a concern for fairness and equality.

POPULATION

Formula (2) is more or less correct, but not quite. It is slightly oversimplified; it is correct only if we are evaluating distributions that all contain the same number of people. For most of this paper I shall ignore changes in population, so formula (2) will be adequate. But the diagram (Figure 1) shows that when we concern ourselves with health, we really ought to allow for different numbers of people. In that case, the correct formula is:

$$(g_1 - v) + (g_2 - v) + \ldots + (g_P - v). \tag{3}$$

Here, v stands for a particular level of lifetime well-being that I call the *neutral* level. Imagine a person is added to the population, and her well-being is neutral. Then formula (3) tells us that adding her is neither good nor bad; the distribution that contains this extra person is equally as good as the distribution that does not. In this sense, adding this person is ethically neutral; hence the name "the neutral level". Formula (3) says that to evaluate a distribution of well-being, we first calculate how much each person's lifetime well-being exceeds the neutral level. (This will be a negative amount if it falls below the neutral level.) Then we add these amounts across people.

Once again, I shall not argue for formula (3), but simply mention sources. This formula was first defended by Blackorby and Donaldson (1984), and there is a further defence in my *Weighing Lives*.

Although it can be derived by reasonably secure arguments, formula (3) is very contentious. It is much more contentious even than the simple additive formula (2), used to compare distributions that have the same population. Formula (3) implies there is only a single neutral level of well-being. It implies it is a good thing to add a person to the population if her well-being is above the neutral level, and a bad thing to add a person if her well-being is below the neutral level. Only if her well-being is exactly at the neutral level is her addition ethically neutral. This is strongly in conflict with many people's intuitions. Many people believe that adding a person to the world is *generally* neutral. That is to say, increasing the world's population is not in itself either good or bad. Adding a person no doubt has effects on other people. For example, the existence of a new person may be harmful because of the demands the person makes on the earth's resources. But apart from such external effects, the addition of a person is neutral in itself. Call this the "intuition of neutrality". It says there is not just one neutral level, as formula (3) implies, but that most levels of well-being are neutral. (I say "most" because adding a person whose life will be bad is intuitively not neutral, but bad.)

The intuition of neutrality must be wrong. Consider three options. Option A is to add a person whose lifetime well-being would be high. Option B is not to add this person at all. Option C is to add her (the same person), but in such a way that her well-being would be less than it is in A. Everyone apart from the added person is equally as well off in A as she is in B and in C. According to the intuition, A is equally as good as B. The difference between A and B is simply that the person is added in A, and that is neutral. Similarly B is equally as good as C, according to the intuition of neutrality. "Equally as good as" is a transitive relation, so it follows that A is equally as good as C. But this is false. A and C have the same population; the difference between them is only that our added person is better off in A than she is in C. Everyone else is equally well off in A and C. So A must be better than C.

Given that the intuition of neutrality is false, we have to face up to the question of the value of adding people to the population. This is particularly inevitable when it comes to measuring health. One of the greatest effects of disease is that it restricts the world's population. One of the greatest effects of reducing disease is that it expands the world's population. The amazing explosion of population that has occurred in the last two centuries is primarily due to improvements in public health, and this population explosion is perhaps the most important thing that has ever happened to humanity. It cannot be ignored. Up to now, I suspect it has been ignored in measures of health because of the presumption that it has no value in itself. This is the intuition of neutrality, and it is not sustainable.

On a small scale, Figure 1 shows how odd it would be to ignore the addition of a person to the population. The epidemic illustrated in the diagram kills one person, and we count the years of life that person loses as a harm done by the epidemic. It causes one person, not yet born, to live a disabled rather than a healthy life, and we count the disability as a harm caused by the epidemic. It causes one person, not yet born, never to be born at all. Suppose we were to count that as neutral, as the intuition of neutrality suggests; in comparison to our treatment of the other two cases, that would be odd.

In this chapter I shall not try to pursue the question of how to value population. Nor shall I insist very firmly that formula (3) is the right one. I chiefly want to emphasize that the problem of valuing population cannot be ignored. Having said that, I shall from here on ignore it.

IS LIFE INCOMMENSURABLE?

Separability of people has brought us to a simple formula for aggregating people's lifetime well-beings. For the most part, we simply add up. That solves one part of the aggregation problem; we know how to aggregate across people. Our other problem is to aggregate across time in each person's life, to determine her lifetime well-being as an aggregate of her temporal well-being.

Before coming to the details of aggregation across time, I should take up a preliminary topic. In setting up the problem of aggregation, I have taken it for granted that a person's lifetime well-being depends both on the length of her life and on her temporal well-being while she is alive. Both factors contribute to her lifetime well-being, and that makes them implicitly comparable in value. As a general rule, I assume that a decline in temporal well-being at some time could be made up for by an increased length of life. This assumption is certainly implicit in any summary measure of health: a summary measure is a single measure that is supposed to incorporate both the length of people's lives and the quality of their lives.

Yet some people think there is something wrong with this assumption. They think of life as a special sort of good, which cannot properly be put on the same scale as the mundane goods that make up the quality of life.

One version of this view gives absolute priority to prolonging life over other sorts of good; any extension of life is worth any sacrifice to achieve. A more moderate version is that prolonging life is incommensurable with other sorts of good; they cannot be measured on the same scale. If this is so, it means we cannot put length of life and quality of life together in a single measure of health. Either version threatens summary measures. So I need to say something about this view.

First, it is very plausible that the value of living is nothing more than the value of receiving other sorts of good. The only benefit of staying alive is to gain the opportunity of enjoying all the ordinary goods that life brings. If this is right, there can be no problem about weighing the value of life against ordinary goods. The value of life is just the same thing as those ordinary goods.

True, there may be problems of incommensurability among the ordinary goods themselves. Perhaps the value of love cannot be precisely weighed against the value of good health, for example. But I have already ignored that problem when I assumed there is such a thing as a unified notion of temporal well-being. Implicitly, I set aside any problems there might be about weighing one sort of ordinary good against another. I am not suggesting that love and health can be precisely weighed against each other, but implicitly I assumed they can be roughly weighed—well enough to let us make sense of a scale of temporal well-being. My present suggestion is that there is no further problem about weighing life against these goods.

That may not be a sufficient answer to the idea that life is incommensurable with other goods, because some people believe life has a value of its own, quite apart from the good things it contains. That may be so. But even if it is so, it does not follow that its value cannot be weighed against other goods. No doubt we cannot expect to weigh it precisely, but it might be weighed against health, say, as much as love can be weighed against health.

Some evidence that life can be weighed against other goods is that in our own lives we regularly do this sort of weighing, and feel it right to do so. We sometimes pursue other goods even at the risk of shortening our lives. For example, mothers sometimes sacrifice their health, and so shorten their lives, in the course of bringing up their children. We do weigh life against other goods, and it does not seem absurd to do so. It seems no more absurd than, say, weighing honour against money.

So I think the onus of proof is on those who doubt that life can be weighed against other goods. We need at least a special argument why this sort of weighing, in particular, should be impossible.

ADDITIVITY ACROSS TIMES: THE DEFAULT

Now to temporal aggregation itself. It is much less clear-cut than aggregation across people. I believe there are solid arguments for the interpersonal additive formula (3). But for aggregation across time, I can offer nothing more than a "default" theory. I do not insist it is correct. I see it more as a convenient basis for organizing the discussion. Still, it is simple and attractive, and I do not think we should depart from it without a good reason. I shall mention some putative reasons that have been offered for doing so, but I find none of them very convincing. They are mostly mere intuitions, without the backing of argument. I would rather stick with the default.

As it happens, there are some formal arguments that could be used in support of this default. Aggregating well-being across time is roughly analogous to aggregating well-being across people. Consequently, the default theory may be defended by formal arguments that are roughly analogous to the arguments for formula (2). However, these arguments depend on an assumption that I have no faith in: separability of times in a life. I have no need to spell out exactly what this amounts to, but it is analogous to separability of people. Whereas I think separability of people is correct, I have no faith in separability of times. Consequently, I do not put my trust in the formal arguments for the default theory.

The default theory is simply that a person's lifetime well-being is the total of the temporal well-being in her life:

$$g_p = g_p^1 + g_p^2 + \ldots + g_p^T \qquad (4)$$

This is a formula for the well-being of a person who is identified by the index p. g_p is this person's lifetime well-being, and g_p^1, g_p^2 and so on are her temporal well-beings at the times she is alive. For convenience in writing this formula, I have divided time into discrete periods.

This additive formula only makes sense once we have an arithmetical (strictly, cardinal) scale for temporal well-being. I have already said that in this chapter I shall not try to deal with the construction of this scale. But I need to say something about the zero. If we were comparing only lives of equal length using formula (4), the zero would make no difference; a cardinal scale of temporal well-being would be enough. However, for lives of different length, the zero matters.

The formula shows us how we must interpret the zero of temporal well-being. Suppose a person's life is made longer by one period, and her well-being in that period is zero. Then according to the formula, her lifetime well-being is unaffected. Extending a person's life at level zero is equally as good for the person as not extending it. This means we must interpret the zero of well-being as the level of well-being such that living a period of life at that level is equally as good as not living it. I call this the "neutral level of temporal well-being" (to distinguish it from the neutral level of lifetime well-being I mentioned above). We might say it is the level that lies on the borderline between periods of life that are worth living and periods that are not worth living.

If this neutral level is to serve as our zero of well-being, it must be a constant. It must not depend on how the rest of the person's life has gone. Its constancy is questionable. Some intuitions are against it. For example, we might think a life that has been lived at a high level would be spoiled by having a merely mediocre period at the end. At the end of this high-level life, then, the neutral level of well-being would be high. On the other hand, if a life has been generally mediocre, an extra period that is slightly less mediocre might improve the life as a whole. If so, the neutral level of well-being at the end of a mediocre life is low. So the neutral level will depend on how the rest of the life has gone.

If the neutral level is not constant, the default theory shown in formula (4) is not correct. I have no strong reason for rejecting the intuition I described in the previous paragraph. Nor do I have a strong reason for accepting it. So I shall stick to the default in this respect.

OTHER PATTERNS OF AGGREGATION ACROSS TIME

Let us continue to review the reasons we might have for doubting the default theory. One is the thought that perhaps we should give some priority to worse times in a life. This would be analogous to giving priority to the worse-off people, when aggregating across people. It could be achieved by applying a strictly concave transformation $f(\ )$ to temporal well-being before adding up. It would give us the formula:

$$g_p = f(g_p^1) + f(g_p^2) + \dots + f(g_p^T).$$

However, I see no particular reason why we should give priority to worse times. There is a case for giving priority to the worse-off, but this case depends on the separateness of persons, to use Rawls' phrase. The better-off are separate people from the worse-off. Consequently, the higher well-being of the better-off does not compensate the worse-off for their lower well-being. That is a precondition for the idea that we should give priority to the worse-off people. But the good times in a life can indeed compensate for the bad times: they compensate the single person whose life it is. So the corresponding precondition for giving priority to the worse times is not satisfied.

A second thought that conflicts with the simple formula (4) is that "inclines" may be better than "declines" (see Velleman 1991). Take two lives that have the same total of temporal well-being, and suppose they last for the same length of time. But suppose one goes uphill—it gets progressively better and ends well—whereas the other goes downhill. It is plausible that the former is a better life than the latter. Yet the default theory implies the two lives are equally good.

The view that inclines are better than declines might be formalized in various ways. The simplest way is to say that the later periods of life count for more in lifetime well-being than the earlier periods. This means modifying formula (4) by adding weighting factors to different periods in life:

$$g_p = a^1 g_p^1 + a^2 g_p^2 + \ldots + a^T g_p^T,$$

where a^1, a^2 and so on are weights. Later periods have bigger weights.

This formulation can join forces with the slightly different thought that the end of a person's life is particularly important in determining how good the life is. Suppose we are evaluating a person's life once it has ended. I think we are inclined to put much more weight on the closing years than on the person's childhood. An unhappy childhood is unfortunate, but for someone who has lived a long time it may count for very little. But an unhappy old age will always be significant. Again, this suggests that later years should have greater weight.

The idea that the later times in life count for more than the earlier times is intuitively attractive. However, measures of health in practice are much more often influenced by the opposite view, that well-being in later years should be discounted compared with earlier years. Later times are often discounted in two ways. First, the temporal well-being that comes in the later years of a person's life is counted for less than the temporal well-being that comes in earlier years. Second, the lifetime well-being of people who are born later is counted for less than the lifetime well-being of people who are born earlier.

Why should we discount later well-being? There are various sources for the idea of discounting, and I cannot possibly examine them all in the detail they require. I can only mention some and assess them very briefly.

One is the supposition that people typically discount their own later well-being in their decision-making. Let us grant this as a fact, and ask whether it licenses us to apply discounting in forming measures of health or other measures of well-being. When a person makes a decision, she does so at a particular time, and makes it from the perspective of that time, looking forward at the future. From the perspective of that time, later future times are more distant than earlier future times. It may well be a feature of our person's psychology that she counts later times for less because they are more distant. Distant objects look smaller, even though in fact they are not.

Later times will not always be more distant. When the person looks back over the same period, the later times will be closer than the earlier times. Will she still count them for less? I do not think so. When we evaluate past stretches of our life, I do not think we give extra weight to times in the more distant past. The later times are nearer, and for that reason, I think we tend to count them for more.

Decision-making is special in that it is inevitably forward-looking. This is because we can only affect the future. Decision-making takes the perspective of a particular time, and looks forward from then. Later times are therefore more distant than earlier ones. This explains psychologically why later times may seem less important in our decision-making. When we draw up measures of health, should we similarly take the perspective of a particular time? We should not. We should look at the world impartially, and give each time its proper weight. It is surely incorrect to count a period for less just because, at the moment, it happens to be more distant. That is a distortion.

A second source of discounting is that some sorts of good are genuinely less valuable in later years than in earlier years. Money is an example. $1 in December 2001 is less valuable than $1 in December 2000. This is because $1 in December 2000 can actually be exchanged for *more* than $1 in 2001, by leaving it in a bank at interest. Most economic commodities are like that. You can exchange beer in December 2000 for more beer in December 2001 by selling it now, banking the proceeds at interest, and using the money plus accrued interest to buy beer in December 2001. Provided the price of beer has not gone up by more than the rate of interest, you will end up with more beer. The ultimate explanation of why this is possible is that we have a productive economy. The economy is able to turn economic commodities used as inputs into a greater quantity of economic commodities as outputs at a later date. It is therefore correct practice in economics and accounting to value later commodities less than earlier ones. More precisely, this is correct for produced commodities. But for scarce resources, which are not produced, it is not normally correct, and normally these goods ought not to be discounted.

Like scarce resources, people's well-being does not participate directly in the economy's productive process. True, we can exchange well-being at one time for well-being at a later time. Suppose you save some of your present wealth instead of spending it. Suppose you invest it, and use the proceeds for spending in the future. You sacrifice some of the well-being you might have derived from your wealth in the present, and instead gain some well-being in the future. This is exchanging present well-being for future well-being. But there is no guarantee you will get more well-being in the future than you sacrifice in the present. With most economic commodities, there is a good reason why you will normally end up with more of them if you choose to exchange present ones for future ones. This is because they directly participate in the productive process. But well-being does not directly participate, and there is no reason why you should end up with more of it.

I state all this boldly. It takes some detailed economic analysis to support it[2] and I would be misleading you if I did not admit that the economic analysis leads to some debate. Still, the outcome is as I say. There is good reason for discounting most economic commodities. This has created a habit of discounting. But the reasons for discounting commodities cannot legitimately be transferred to well-being.

I conclude that the grounds for discounting temporal well-being are weak. If we discounted, we would attach greater weight to earlier years than to later ones. I see no reason for departing from the default in that direction. On the other hand, I mentioned some intuitions that attach greater weight to later years than earlier ones. These are attractive, but they are merely intuitions, and I think they are not enough reason for departing from the default in that direction either.

In the calculation of DALYs, a different pattern of weights has been used (see Murray 1996 pp. 54–61). More weight is given to the middle periods of life, and less to early and late periods. However, the reason given by Murray for this system of weights is not that he thinks well-being in the middle period of life is actually more valuable than well-being at other periods. The reason is to do with the benefits that people bestow on each other. People in the middle years of life support the young and the old economically, and they give benefits to the young and the old in other ways too. For that reason they are more valuable. In economists' terms, this value is an *externality*.

In a diagram like mine in the first section, showing a distribution of benefit, the benefit that one person, p, gives to another, q, will show up within q's life. It will automatically be incorporated in the value we assign to the distribution when we aggregate well-being across it. There is no need to allow for it by a further system of weights like Murray's.

Murray accounts for externalities differently, by attaching weights to the quality of p's life. He is forced to this expedient because he restricts his attention to states of people's health. The external benefits that p bestows on q will not normally take the form of improvements in q's health. So they will not normally appear directly in any measure that is based on states of health only. Murray's weights are the only way he has of taking them into account, given the restricted nature of his measure.

As I said above, our measure of the harm done by disease ought not to be based on states of health only. The harm done takes many forms, and ill-health is only one of them. This is an example. If a disease kills people in the middle years of life, one harmful consequence is that the old and young are deprived of support and other benefits that they would otherwise have received. This is a harm caused by disease that is not a change in their state of health. Consequently, it can only be incorporated in Murray's measure by distorting the aggregation of states of health. That is the effect of his weights. The correct way to take the harm into account is to use a measure that is based more generally on well-being.

In sum, it gives no reason to depart from the default theory of aggregation.

CONCLUSIONS

I believe that existing measures of the burden of disease are all additive, except that they sometimes discount later well-being and sometimes apply age-weighting. I have supported additivity. Additivity across people can be supported by fairly solid argument. Additivity across time has less argument behind it, but it is a reasonable default position. I have argued that there is no good reason to apply different weights to well-being that comes at different dates. For instance, there is no good reason to discount, or to apply age-related weights.

I have argued that measures of the burden of disease should be based on people's well-being rather than on the state of their health only. This is because the bad effects of disease are multifarious, and not confined to health. Measures of the burden of disease usually ignore the effect of disease on the world's population. I have argued that this is a very large effect, and it cannot be assumed to be neutral in value. It therefore must not be ignored.

Notes

1 I believe the name comes from Parfit, 2000, but the idea was well-established in economics long before then. For instance, see textbook by Atkinson and Stiglitz, 1980, p. 340.

2 The argument is in Broome (1994). There is also an excellent analysis in Murray (1996) pp. 44–54, which I agree with to a large extent.

References

Atkinson AB, Stiglitz JE (1980) *Lectures on public economics.* McGraw-Hill, London.

Blackorby C, Donaldson D (1984) Social criteria for evaluating population change. *Journal of Public Economics,* **25**(1-2):13–33.

Broome J (Forthcoming) *Weighing lives.* Oxford University Press, Oxford.

Broome J (1991) *Weighing goods.* Blackwell, Cambridge, MA.

Broome J (1994) Discounting the future. *Philosophy and Public Affairs,* **23**(2):128–156.

Culyer AJ (1990) Commodities, characteristics of commodities, characteristics of people, utilities, and the quality of life. In: *Quality of life, perspectives and policies.* Baldwin S, Godfrey C, Propper C, eds. Routledge, London.

Harsanyi JC (1955) Cardinal welfare, individualistic ethics, and interpersonal comparisons of utility. *Journal of Political Economy,* **63**:309–321. (Reprinted in Essays on ethics, social behavior, and scientific explanation, Reidel, 1976, pp 6–23)

Murray CJL (1996) Rethinking DALYs. In: *The global burden of disease: a comprehensive assessment of mortality and disability from diseases, injuries, and risk factors in 1990 and projected to 2020.* The Global Burden of Disease and Injury, Vol. 1. Murray CJL, Lopez AD, eds. Harvard School of Public Health on behalf of WHO, Cambridge, MA.

Parfit D (2000) Equality or priority? In: *The ideal of equality.* Clayton M, Williams A, eds. Macmillan, Hampshire.

Velleman D (1991) Well-being and time. *Pacific Philosophical Quarterly,* **72**:48–77.

WHO (1980) *International classification of impairments, disabilities, and handicaps: a manual of classification relating to the consequences of disease.* World Health Organization, Geneva. (Reprint 1993)

Chapter 3.2

THE SEPARABILITY OF HEALTH AND WELL-BEING

DAN W. BROCK

INTRODUCTION

A host of measures, both general and disease specific, have been developed to measure the impact of disease and its treatment on people's health. The Global Programme on Evidence for Health Policy at the World Health Organization (WHO) employs summary measures of population health (SMPH) to measure those impacts. We are interested in people's health because of how it affects their overall well-being. Well-being is a moral or normative notion which I shall take here to refer to how well off a person is overall, how good the person's life is. Ordinary thinking considers health to be one aspect or contributor to people's overall well-being, along with their education, work, social relationships, etc. If the contribution of health to people's well-being can be determined without reference to their other conditions or circumstances besides their health, or other aspects of their well-being, then health and well-being are separable.

John Broome argues in this volume that health is not separable from well-being or from other aspects of a person's condition or well-being (chapter 3.1). As a theoretical matter I believe there is no question that he is correct. For example, loss of fine motor control in one's fingers from disease is an impairment of one's health, but its effect on one's well-being will be very different if one is a concert pianist or, instead, a writer who can dictate her work. If one loses the ability to do physical labour from a back injury, the impact on one's well-being will vary greatly depending on whether one has sufficient education to obtain non-physical work and on whether one's society has retraining programmes to enable one to obtain other employment. Even assuming that health can in principle be fully distinguished conceptually from other aspects of well-being, the value of different health states for a person is not separable from the non-health states of the person or from other aspects of the person's well-being. As

Broome correctly notes, even if health does have intrinsic value, its value is surely largely instrumental; health is necessary to pursue most of what else we value in life, and disease and disability are bad for us because they prevent our doing so.

As I have said, these theoretical claims about health's non-separability from well-being seem to me unquestionably correct and should not be controversial. Broome draws from them (though with occasional qualifications) the implication that we should measure the burdens of disease on overall well-being, not health. Yet the health research literature is replete with measures of health and health-related quality of life, and monitoring the health of populations with a variety of SMPH occupies enormous manpower and resources worldwide. As Murray noted in discussion at the Marrakech conference, the WHO, which sponsored this volume and the conference from which it grew, is the World *Health* (not Well-Being) Organization. If health and well-being are in theory not separable, is current practice that apparently assumes their separability fundamentally misguided or incoherent? Must we give up SMPH in favour of SMPWB? I shall sketch one line of reasoning that may justify the standard practice of apparently ignoring the non-separability of health and well-being and focusing only on health. I shall then comment more briefly on Broome's analogous claims that a measure of the burdens of disease should measure all the burdens, not just the health burdens; if some burdens should be ignored in resource prioritization on grounds of fairness, Broome argues that we should take account of the concern for fairness separately and not do so in a way that distorts the measure of the burdens of disease. But I believe this ignores important pragmatic considerations.

QUANTITATIVE VERSUS EVALUATIVE ASPECTS

One issue dividing those who assume the separability of health and well-being and those who reject it may lie in Broome's distinction between the natural and evaluative facets of health, or what he has called elsewhere the quantity versus the goodness of health (Broome 1991; Broome, forthcoming). Broome grants that health in its natural facet, the quantity of health, is separable from well-being and denies separability only for the goodness of health. However, he argues that our concern should be with the goodness of health and the harm of disease, and with the contribution of health to people's well-being. We want to know the harm that is done to people by disease so that we can prioritize interventions to prevent or reduce that harm. Simple measures of population health like life expectancy or infant mortality rates, however, appear to be measures of the quantity of health in a society, not the goodness of health, as do frequency measures in a population of a disability such as deafness. And I believe that many who develop and use SMPH implicitly assume it is the natural facet or quantity of health that they are measuring. Oversimplifying greatly, suppose that disease is a condition causing an adverse deviation in normal species function, and that health in turn is the absence of disease. Suppose also that normal species function, and so health, for organisms such as human beings can be determined by biological science. Health in its natural, non-evaluative facet is normal species function and decline in or loss of a normal function like sight or the ability to move one's limbs are reductions in health. While we might ask how good a person's health is, and be told "not too good" or "getting worse" because the person is losing his sight, this question and reply seem to call only on the natural or quantitative sense of health, not the evaluative sense concerning the extent to which health contributes to a person's well-being.

Summary measures of individual or population health, however, require overall judgments about the levels of health of persons in the face of different combinations of functional limitations caused by disease. A quantitative SMPH requires the assignment of quantitative values to decrements in health resulting from different specific levels of different functional limitations. Most SMPH determine these values, typically on a scale of 0 for death and 1 for full health, by asking people their preferences, using for example standard gambles or time tradeoffs, for living with the different functional limitations. When people make these judgments, they cannot still be employing only the natural, non-evaluative conception of health; they must be making judgments about the goodness of health, the degree to which different functional limitations reduce overall well-being. It is not even clear how to make sense of an overall measure of the quantity of health that assigns relative weights to different functional limitations or disabilities in purely naturalistic, non-evaluative terms.

If people are asked how bad their health would be on a 0 to 1 scale when, for example, they have lost the ability to move their legs or have lost their sight, they might try to make sense of and answer the question in at least two different ways. First, they might consider how much the particular impairment would limit their ability to pursue their own particular life plan—that is, roughly, how much it would reduce their overall well-being. Second, they might consider the question from a more general perspective asking how much the particular impairment would limit the pursuit of normal human activities, taking account of the typical relative importance of the different activities and the degrees to which they would be limited. From either perspective they must also make assumptions about the nature of their society, such as whether wheelchairs and access ramps to buildings and transportation are widely available. These two perspectives may not differ much in practice in their results for disability weights, since in the first a sufficiently large and diverse sample of individuals should be used to wash out the impact of unusual life plans and values.

Measuring the value or goodness of health

Each of these ways of thinking about the relative importance of different impairments of health illustrate the lack of separability between health and well-being that Broome argues for, since each asks how a particular functional impairment affects a specific or typical individual's overall lifeplan or well-being. But while they support the non-separability of health and well-being, they also suggest that in practice it may be less of a problem both for SMPH and for health policy than Broome's examples imply. SMPH are used to provide a summary measure of the health of a population such as a country. In that context, differences between individuals will largely wash out and not be important. As SMPH are applied across increasingly diverse social, cultural, economic and historical contexts, the dependence of the value or goodness of health, and in particular of specific aspects of health, on other aspects of well-being can become more important; this suggests caution in using a summary measure of population health across very diverse international contexts. Despite such important cautions, either of the two approaches I have suggested may permit the practical use of SMPH as a measure of the goodness of health; this does not deny the theoretical non-separability of health and well-being, but only questions its importance for some practical and policy purposes.

A different approach locates the moral importance of health in its impact on people's opportunity, not well-being. In Norman Daniels' influential account of justice in health care, health is understood in terms of normal species function and disease as impairment of normal function. The moral importance of health care and health is their role in preserving or restoring fair equality of opportunity from being undermined or threatened by disease and disability (Daniels 1985). Fair equality of opportunity requires that individuals have a fair share of the normal opportunity range in their society. Differences in the importance of a particular impairment of health or disability will generally be greater for a particular person's well-being from specific features of that person and her life plan than for her access to a fair share of the opportunity range for her society; in Broome's example, the effect on a music lover's well-being will be very different depending on whether she loses her hearing or sight, but the effect on her opportunity range will be much less closely tied to her specific life plan. If the moral importance of health is its effect on opportunity, not well-being, the separability issue may be less worrisome for our normative use of SMPH.

Pragmatic considerations

I shall now illustrate briefly the relevance of pragmatic policy considerations to separability. In the WHO work on measuring the burden of disease the only differences between persons that are taken account of in the summary measure are age and gender. My concern is not whether both these differences are relevant to the measure, but rather with other differences that were ignored. Broome discusses the case of whether to save a rich man with a good life or a poor man with a less good life in an emergency room; he argues that we do more good by saving the rich man and our measure of goodness should reflect that fact. Analogously, it would seem that our summary measure of goodness should assign more value to saving lives in wealthy developed countries than in very poor developing countries. Not to do so assumes that the burdens of a disease and the benefits of a health intervention in a population measured with SMPH are separable from how good that population's lives are in other respects, including their wealth. I believe Broome would argue that an accurate measure of the burden of disease and of the good done by health interventions should not ignore real differences in wealth between countries and its effects on the goodness of individuals' lives in them. For reasons of fairness he agrees that we should not prefer to save the rich man, and so should not prefer to save lives in rich developed countries rather than in very poor developing countries.

But fairness and goodness are distinct moral concerns and Broome argues it distorts our measure of goodness and of disease burden to introduce considerations of fairness into it; simple analytic clarity supports separating measures of disease burden from fairness. Nevertheless, there are some obvious pragmatic and policy concerns that I believe point in the other direction that are relevant to an ultimately practical project like the Global Burden of Disease (GBD) study. A measure that seems to have the evident and straightforward implication that saving lives and, for example, preventing AIDS in developing countries does less good and has less value than doing so in developed countries—that the lives of the rich are of more value than those of the poor—would obviously be subject to and would no doubt receive serious attack in political and policy contexts. Insisting that although the good produced by saving a life in the developing world is indeed less than in the developed world, on grounds of fairness we do not want to give priority to the latter over the former, might do little to deflect that attack in a world marked by deep sensitivity and suspicion by many in the developing countries about inadequate concern in the developed countries for them and their problems. If there are good reasons of fairness, and perhaps other reasons as well, for ignoring other non-health differences in the goodness of lives across countries, pragmatic policy or political considerations may support not strictly separating all fairness concerns from the burden of disease measure. Here, fairness supports ignoring the non-separability of the values of health, specifically preserving life, and other conditions of persons, specifically differences in the goodness of their lives from differences in wealth. Where the balance of theoretical, moral and pragmatic reasons falls for how to treat particular aspects of the separability issue is, of course, complex and controversial; my point here is only that pragmatic concerns are not irrelevant to these choices in WHO's work.

REFERENCES

Broome J (Forthcoming) *Weighing lives*. Oxford University Press, Oxford.

Broome J (1991) *Weighing goods*. Blackwell, Cambridge, MA.

Daniels N (1985) *Just health care*. Cambridge University Press, Cambridge, MA.

THE LIMITED MORAL ARITHMETIC
OF HEALTH AND WELL-BEING

Daniel M. Hausman

INTRODUCTION

In attempting to quantify the global burden of disease, the World Health Organization (WHO) seeks to define summary measures of the health of the world's population. This choice is not inevitable, because disease diminishes well-being and people's capacities to achieve what they value; and one might measure the global burden of disease by measuring the impact of disease in terms of wider consequences than the impact on health.

John Broome argues for such a proposal. He suggests measuring the burden of disease in terms of its consequences for well-being. In his view, the consequences for the population should be calculated by summing the total consequences for each individual person, and the life-time consequences for each individual should be determined by summing the consequences for each year with no discounting and every age counting equally.

FOCUS ON CONSEQUENCES

Why should one examine the consequences for well-being rather than the narrower consequences for health or the wider set of consequences with respect to everything that matters to the individuals who are affected by disease? Broome argues that WHO should not focus only on health consequences because health is not separable from well-being and because health measures will be misleading for evaluative purposes. He maintains that in focusing only on health consequences, one will arrive at misleading estimates of the relative significance of different diseases.

Broome is right that health is not separable from well-being and that the significance of a disease for well-being may differ from its significance for health, but how serious is this objection to WHO's proposed summary measures? How large will the mistakes be if one takes health to be separable and focuses only on health consequences? Philosophers can point out that there is a question here, but they do not have the expertise to answer it. No one imagines that a summary measure of population health could be perfect.

In arguing that WHO should focus on the consequences of disease for well-being rather than health, Broome also needs to consider why WHO should confine its concern to the consequences of disease for well-being rather than to a wider set of consequences consisting of all those things that matter to people? Although this last point may seem very abstract, I think that it points to a serious objection to focusing on the consequences of disease for well-being rather than for health. Measuring the burden of disease by its consequences for well-being commits WHO to the view that health and disease matter only insofar as they affect well-being. Perhaps this is correct—though I personally dispute it—but it is a controversial philosophical position. Its content depends on what counts as "well-being". On a theory of well-being as some sort of mental state, the burden of disease depends entirely on the effects of disease on mental states. On a theory of well-being as the satisfaction of preferences, one would have to measure the burden of disease by determining the strength of people's preferences for the consequences. Of course, there are broader theories of well-being, but it would be better if WHO did not commit itself to any theory of well-being and if it could leave open the possibility that the burden of disease on human capacities cannot be measured in terms of well-being, regardless of how well-being is understood. Indeed, the conceptualization of disability-adjusted life years (DALYs) in fact emphasizes the links between health states and functioning more than the links between health states and well-being (Murray 1994, p. 438). In focusing on health consequences, WHO should leave open the question of their ultimate significance.

PROBLEMS OF EQUALITY

An additional, though less serious problem with attending to consequences for well-being,[1] is that it may be questioned whether the well-being of a group is the sum of the well-being of its members. Broome makes a technical argument for the additivity of well-being, which rests on the premise that well-being is separable across people. What this means is that whether *P* is better off than *Q* does not depend on the unchanging level of well-being of others. Broome takes the objections to the separability of well-being across persons to derive from the importance of equality. In his book, *Weighing Goods* (Broome 1991), he addresses these difficulties by arguing that equality matters only when it affects the good of individuals and that the influence of inequalities is already incorporated into the measures of individual good. In his essay in this volume, in contrast, he argues that one should separate concerns about fairness sharply from concerns about goodness and that equality is relevant to fairness not to goodness.

There are other telling objections to the separability of well-being across people. When there are interdependencies among the good of different individuals, how well off P is compared to Q may depend on the level of well-being enjoyed by others. For example, measures that improve the well-being of children also improve the well-being of adults who love them both absolutely and relative to those who are indifferent to children. Although there may be other arguments why overall well-being should be the sum of individual well-being, one cannot argue for additivity on the grounds of separability. On the other hand, one can use Broome's argument to argue for the additivity of health, which is, unlike well-being, separable across people to a high degree of approximation. So the average health of a population is the average health of its members.

Unfortunately, this is about the only substantial conclusion concerning the measurement of average health that can be established without controversy. Although health is probably not more difficult to measure than well-being, it is not much easier to measure either. Even the definition of health (or disease) is controversial. The controversy only grows when one attempts to make comparisons between the health of different individuals and different populations.

PROBLEMS OF MAKING COMPARISONS

How can health states—either of one individual at different times or of different individuals—be compared? Comparisons along particular dimensions of health may be straightforward. For example, someone who is bedridden is less mobile than someone in a wheel-chair and in this way in a worse health state. But how are health states that differ across different dimensions to be compared? Is someone who is bedridden but in the full possession of their faculties in a better or worse health state than someone with dementia who is capable of moving in a wheel-chair? It seems that the comparison between the health states of particular individuals must rest on a theory of the impact of the diminished health states on these people's lives.

In this way, one might be led directly back to considerations of well-being. It might appear that the comparison involves asking which health state most diminishes the well-being of individuals, given their specific circumstances and ideals. But the measurement of health need not be tied this closely to well-being. One might, for example, also compare health states in terms of their impact on the "functionings" discussed by Sen (1992, chapter 3) and Nussbaum (2000) (see also Nussbaum and Sen 1993).

Even if in some such way one is able to judge whether A is healthier than B or vice versa at every instant during some time interval, one would not necessarily know whether on average over the interval A is healthier than B. To compare A's health to B's over some period during which A was sometimes healthier than B and B was sometimes healthier than A, one needs to know how much healthier A was when A was healthier and how much healthier B was when B was healthier. One needs a cardinal or interval measure of health, and one will only have one if one can say, quantitatively, how much being bedridden diminishes *A*'s quality of life and how much dementia diminishes *B*'s quality of life. One also needs a cardinal measure in order to "add up" health states, which one must do in order to compare the health of populations. In addition, to compare population health one needs a very substantial theory of well-being or of human functionings in order to be able to say how much, on average, health states diminish the quality of life. Devices such as the standard gamble, time trade-offs and person trade-offs are ways of attempting to elicit the quantitative comparisons that are needed.

To compare *A*'s and *B*'s health over some period, it is also necessary to take into account the amount of *time* that *A* was healthier than *B*. The obvious thought is that one should graph *A*'s and *B*'s health—or the difference between their health—on the vertical axis and time on the horizontal axis and derive the comparison between their health over the whole period by integrating. But what justification is there for this "obvious thought?" If health were separable across times as well as across individuals, then one would be justified in adding up health across time. But health—like well-being or functionings—is not separable over time. The effect of health states on average health during a period depends on how the states are distributed during the period. One minute of a severe five-hour migraine is not $\frac{1}{300}$th as bad as the whole migraine. A period of confinement to a wheel-chair has a very different impact if it is episodic than if it is concentrated.

Furthermore, the average impact of a health state may vary considerably depending on the stage of the life of the individual. Mobility restrictions that would be devastating to teenagers might be of little importance to those who are middle-aged. This second difficulty could be addressed by taking the mobility restriction of a teenager to be a different health state than the mobility restriction of someone who is middle-aged. It is not specifically a problem about the additivity of health states at different times. Both of these problems should be distinguished from questions about whether health states should be age-weighted. Age-weighting counts health states of *all* kinds—pain, perceptual failures, and so forth—differently depending on a person's age.

We can compare the health of particular individuals over an extended period by thinking about how their physical and mental states impinge on their specific capacities and on the overall quality of their lives. But there is no way to specify how a variety of health states over an extended period impinges on average on people's general capacities and well-being. The treatment of time is consequently bound to be a rather unsatisfactory compromise. That compromise need not be simple unweighted addition or integration of momentary health states, but no simple formula taking severity of health states as more or less than proportional to the time that they last will be satisfactory either. Though, as we have seen, the effect of a period of pain may be more than proportional to its length, the burden of twenty years of blindness might be much less than twenty times the impairment and distress caused by one year of blindness.

Recognizing connections between health, well-being, and human functioning might not appear very fruitful, because there is no generally accepted theory of well-being or functioning. Indeed, it seems that there is more consensus in untutored judgments about whether one individual is healthier than another and what it means to make such a judgement than in beliefs concerning whether one individual is better off than another and concerning the basis for making such comparisons. Economists are famous for maintaining that interpersonal comparisons of welfare are impossible, but nobody asserts that interpersonal health comparisons are impossible.

The sense that health comparisons are more tractable than welfare comparisons or comparisons of functioning may, however, be deceptive. Since there are a few fixed points upon which there is general agreement, and since those fixed points in fact permit many of the comparisons health professionals have typically made, it seems much easier to make health comparisons among populations than it actually is. Consider some of these fixed points: Greater longevity indicates better health—at least if it is not too strongly correlated with increasing disabilities. Lower rates of infant mortality and lower rates of debilitating infectious diseases reflect better health. Since such indicators are often strongly correlated with one another and since they have permitted intuitively plausible comparisons of health in different nations, in different classes within nations, and in consequence of different policies, it seems as if health comparisons are not that difficult. But analogous comparisons of well-being or functioning can be made just as easily! It is just as uncontroversial to claim that longevity contributes to well-being and functioning and that infant mortality and infectious diseases diminish them.

EXPLORING THE NATURE OF WELL-BEING

One possible moral to be drawn is that significant philosophical work needs to be done to answer controversial questions concerning human well-being and functioning and so to construct conceptions that are both more broadly accepted and more precise. A better theory of health and better measures of population health could then be built on this philosophical foundation. I doubt, however, that such a foundation can be provided. Questions concerning the nature of well-being and the significance of human capacities have been unresolved for millenia, and there are no indications that moral philosophers are on the verge of a revolutionary breakthrough.

Furthermore, it is doubtful whether all of the important open questions have answers. It is hard to see how to answer questions such as whether a particular cognitive disability diminishes well-being or functioning more than some physical disability. The answer might vary from person to person and culture to culture. Even relativizing the question to a detailed specification of the circumstances, why believe that there is some single "correct" notion of functioning or well-being that would permit such comparisons?

Moreover, even if such questions had objective answers and even if philosophers could find them, there are cultural and political barriers to employing this knowledge. Although some distance from the notions of functioning and well-being accepted in particular societies is needed in order to correct for biases resulting from injustices and manipulative socialization, comparisons of health cannot be just the comparisons of some group of experts. They must be comparisons that the populations involved can come to accept. So while there is, of course, no reason not to continue to explore notions of well-being and functioning and to seek more refined notions and measures of health, I do not think one should expect too much of these efforts.

One might instead conclude that refined health comparisons are simply not possible. For example, can one say whether middle-aged women who live in wealthy countries are healthier than middle-aged men, let alone do so with quantitative precision? Women are less likely to die, but they must cope with many symptoms related to menopause, and losing the ability to reproduce is itself arguably a loss of health. Rather than supposing that there must be some answer to the question "Who is healthier?", perhaps what is needed is some thought about what to do when such comparisons cannot be made.

Not only should one think about the logic of incomparability, but one also needs to think about how the inability to make fine comparisons ought to affect policy. Should one treat populations whose health cannot be compared in the same way as one treats populations whose health is equally good? Suppose, for example, that it were impossible to make an overall comparison between the health of two populations and that their health differed in some regard that affected their relative status, political rights, or material prospects? How much should one be influenced by the overall incomparability of the health of the populations, and how much should policies be influenced by specific differences?

Conclusions

One might attempt to base health policy on measures of particular dimensions and aspects of health rather than on measures of overall health. After measuring particular dimensions of health such as age-specific mortality rates, rates of specific classes of disabilities, and so forth, perhaps those concerned with health policy should conceive of the task of determining how to cope with the differences along many dimensions as a normative problem concerning how justly to take people's interests into account rather than as a technical problem concerning how to construct an overall measure of health.

In this way, pressing questions about how to measure health may ultimately lead one *beyond* questions about what is good for individuals to questions concerning justice, both in circumstances in which health comparisons can be made and especially in the cases where health comparisons cannot be made.

NOTES

1   I am avoiding talking here of quality of life, which I shall, like others, use as a blanket term that includes well-being as well as relatively objective matters of functioning.

REFERENCES

Broome J (1991) *Weighing goods*. Blackwell, Cambridge, MA.

Murray CJL (1994) Quantifying the burden of disease: the technical basis for disability-adjusted life years. *Bulletin of the World Health Organization*, 72(3):429–445.

Nussbaum M (2000) *Women and human development: the capabilities approach*. Cambridge University Press, Cambridge.

Nussbaum M, Sen A (1993) *The quality of life*. Clarendon Press, Oxford.

Sen A (1992) *Inequality re-examined*. Russel Sage, New York.

Chapter 3.4

A NOTE ON MEASURING WELL-BEING

JAMES GRIFFIN

DO WE ADD IN REACHING OVERALL JUDGEMENTS ABOUT WELL-BEING?

Most of us, perhaps all of us, think that we can, in some way, aggregate well-being. By "aggregating" I mean merely that we can rationally move from judgements about how good certain components of a person's life are to a judgement about how good the life is overall, and perhaps also that we can move from how well-off various individuals are to how well-off the group they form is. But to aggregate in these ways is not necessarily to add. The difference I have in mind between addition and aggregation will become clearer as the discussion proceeds, though one difference just stipulated is that adding is only one form of aggregating.

Some people think that we do indeed aggregate a person's well-being by adding—for instance, adding one's levels of well-being at various times to get one's well-being over a long stretch of time. But I doubt it. What is more, many of them hold this independently of holding any view about what human well-being actually is. But can one decide the form of a measure of well-being without knowing the substance of well-being? Can one, for instance, hold that the form of aggregation for well-being is addition, while we are agnostic about substantive accounts of well-being? I doubt that too.

A SUBSTANTIVE ACCOUNT OF WELL-BEING

Let me take one particular substantive account. It is, to my mind, the most plausible one (Griffin 1986; 1996); it is also, I believe, the one most widely held among philosophers. It says that what makes a life good is the presence, not of a single substantive super-value (pleasure or happiness, say), but of one (or more) of several irreducibly different substantive values, which can be listed. For instance:

1. *Accomplishment*: doing in the course of one's life the sort of things (for example, finding a cure for AIDS, raising one's children well) that give it weight or point, i.e. the sort of thing which means that one's life is not wasted.

2. *Deep personal relations*: when personal relations become deep, reciprocal relations of friendship and love, they have a value distinct from the pleasure and profit they bring.

3. *Enjoyment*.

4. *Understanding*: knowing about oneself and one's place in the universe, including how to take account of the value represented by other people, is a good in itself.

5. *The components of human dignity*: living as a rational agent, being able to pursue a course through life chosen by oneself, is valuable over and above the happiness it might bring.

This sort of substantive account of well-being is now often called an "objective list" account (Parfit 1984, appendix I) though I should prefer calling it simply a "list" account because I have reservations about the objective-subjective distinction as it is used here (Griffin 1996, chapter II, section 6).

Now, it does not especially matter for present purposes whether the particular list I have given is quite right. What matters is that the right list may contain prudential values of a long-term, life-structuring nature. It usually takes a fairly long while for a "deep" personal relation to be a good-making feature of life (overcoming the natural distance between persons, even those supposedly "close" to one another); what we value is having a life containing personal relations of that sort. It characteristically takes the major part of one's productive life to "accomplish" certain things that have the sort of weight that ensures that one's life is not wasted. And living autonomously and at liberty is a way of living that one hopes will characterize one's whole life. Unlike pleasures, which can come in short doses, the realization of deep personal relations and of accomplishment and of rational agency are very long-term, often lifetime, projects.

Consequences for measurement

Let us see how these prudential values Figure in our aggregating judgements. It seems to me that there are pairs of values such that *no* amount of one can equal a certain amount of another (Griffin 1986, pp. 83–89). For example, suppose that I am the sort of person for whom living autonomously causes stress and strain—more than the average amount. Just having to decide for myself causes me above average stress, and I am a rather bad practical reasoner and so take a lot of false turns in my life, which cause me more than average strain to straighten out. You, let us say, are prudentially shrewd and offer to take over the general management of my life. Well, even if I thought you would do a considerably better job than I in reducing my stress and strain, I would not accept. So long as my autonomy caused me only common (though, as I have said, above average) stress and strain, not crippling anxiety, and so long as my false turns produced only common discomfort and embarrassment, not catastrophe, I should prefer remaining autonomous. And rightly so; autonomy is a major part of rational agency, and rational agency constitutes what moral philosophers have often called, with unnecessary obscurity, the "dignity" of the person. It is rational of me to think that *no* amount of stresses and strains, so long as they remained below the threshold just roughly indicated, could outweigh the value of my autonomy. Stresses and strains below that threshold still have a negative value, but still no amount of them would add up to the value of living life autonomously. I have elsewhere called this feature of certain pairs of values "discontinuity" (Griffin 1986, pp. 85–89). Addition is here defeated; one cannot add certain negative values, no matter how many, so that they become equal to a certain finite positive value.

There is something more here. Perhaps one can see how to add up "stresses and strains". Perhaps all "stresses" have intensity and duration, and the calibration of those two dimensions would be at least a start on getting what we need for addition. Similarly for "strains". But can one form any idea of adding up the component values of living autonomously? What would the components be? Each autonomous decision or action? Surely not. What we value is something already highly inclusive: we value living as an autonomous agent. It is a way of life that we value.

Take another example. Let us say that, having devoted virtually the whole of your productive life to finding a cure for AIDS, you finally succeed. It is an immense accomplishment, in the technical sense of that term introduced earlier. But this ambitious, striving life also involved its stresses and strains for you (though still, let us say, within the limits described a moment ago). Looking back, you ask yourself: would my life have been better, in terms of my own well-being, lived the way I lived it, or lived less ambitiously with no stress and strain but no accomplishment to speak of either? To answer your question, would you have to add up some components or other? I am not saying that one cannot point to a single place in the thought processes that go into aggregating values (that is, that go into reaching an all-values-considered judgement) in which we *might* be doing what could reasonably be called "addition". My point is that we do much more than add. The most important part of aggregation is aggregating features or dimensions of life, not periods of it. In this particular aggregation we have to compare the value of this particular accomplishment and the disvalue of this particular sort of life of stress and strain. And here the crucial judgement, I should say, is that the value of this accomplishment is greater than (perhaps even discontinuously greater than) avoiding these stresses and strains. That final judgement is not a matter of adding up time-slices, or indeed anything else. And it is not led up to by prior addition. There might be, as I conceded, some episodes of deliberation that can properly be considered addition, but the final valuing of this accomplishment is not arrived at by adding up anything. For example, pleasure can come in short doses. But even if one were comparing a life full of short-term pleasures with a sterner life of fewer pleasures but considerable accomplishment, one would not first add the values attached to the individual pleasures and then compare the sum to the value of the life of accomplishment. One would compare the two lives as wholes: how good is such a life of short-term pleasures measured against this life of accomplishment?

In the process of understanding *that* accomplishment is prudentially valuable, one also understands *how* valuable various tokens of it are. These are not independent pieces of knowledge. And in understanding how valuable a certain token is we understand how valuable it is *compared to* tokens of other things that one similarly understands to be prudentially valuable. One does not have to sum anything to arrive at these overall judgements; they are part of the initial judgement that such-and-such is valuable.

This point is related to a gap in the conception of adding levels of well-being at periods of time. How do we determine which periods of time to take? A minute? A day? A year? The answer depends upon what in particular one thinks one should look at, and a substantive account will tell one. If we know that pains and strains are bad, then we can identify episodes of pains and strains and weigh them. But what about accomplishing something with one's life? One cannot calculate the level of accomplishment between eleven and twelve o'clock and then between four and five o'clock, or today and then tomorrow, and so on. The appropriate time period seems to be a whole life, or something close to it, and the overall (aggregative) value of what someone has accomplished in life is not arrived at by adding time-slices.

The crucial judgment that I imagined one is having to make is how valuable what one has accomplished in the course of one's productive life, against the sort of stressful life one has had to lead. We do not arrive at that judgement by adding up value components of each and seeing which sum turns out greater. An example of "discontinuity", which this example may anyway be, simply makes this point especially starkly: a judgement of discontinuity is a judgement that no amount of, say, stress and strain (within the limits indicated) can add up to, say, accomplishment at the level one has reached. Of course, stresses and strains could come so thick and fast in a life that some other evil were present, but I am limiting the example simply to the ordinary stresses and strains that commonly come with a striving life. The way we seem to arrive at the crucial judgement is, rather, by comparing items that are already highly aggregated, namely something on the order of ways of life, what life deals one, what sort of person one is, and so on.

I do not want to deny that we aggregate. For instance, I should have to consider what I have accomplished in my life, how much I have enjoyed life, what frustration and pain I have suffered in the course of it, how rich my personal relations have been, and so on. It is not surprising that I should have to consider these various things, because the list account tells us that they are precisely what make up the quality of life. Having come to reflect on these things, then I should be in a position to estimate the value of my life as a whole. And I should do that by making the sorts of comparisons I sketched above—by comparing items that are already highly aggregated. I would not add.[1]

NOTES

1   Some of the points in this short piece are elaborated in Griffin J, *Well-being*, pp. 34 ff., ch. V, pp. 243 ff.

REFERENCES

Griffin J (1986) Well-being: its meaning, measurement, and moral importance. Clarendon Press, Oxford.

Griffin J (1996) Value judgement. Clarendon Press, Oxford.

Parfit D (1984) Reasons and persons. Clarendon Press, Oxford.

Chapter 3.5

FAIRNESS, GOODNESS AND
LEVELLING DOWN

JOHN BROOME

In chapter 3.1, "Measuring the burden of disease by aggregating well-being", I argued that a measure of the burden of disease should not be influenced by considerations of fairness. The burden of disease is a matter of goodness—of the harm done by disease. Fairness should be accounted for separately; we shall need a distinct measure of fairness. So we need a goodness measure G and a fairness measure F. The value of equality is a consideration of fairness, and will need to be included in F.

When a decision has to be made, both fairness and goodness need to be taken into account. Usually, some of the options available will be fairer, and others will do more good. To compare the values of these options, fairness and goodness will need to be weighed against each other. Consequently, we shall need a combined objective, which puts fairness and goodness together. This will be some combination of G and F, making a combined measure. A simple example is just the weighed sum $G + aF$, where a is some weight. The size of a in this example reflects the relative importance of fairness compared with goodness.

Since the value of equality is a consideration of fairness, this combined measure will include the value of equality. It has sometimes been argued that treating the value of equality as a separate consideration from goodness will inevitably run up against a problem.[1]

Imagine some change damages the health of the best-off people in the society, and does no good to anyone; this is called a "levelling down". The change improves the society's degree of equality, so it must increase F. It will also decrease G. But—the argument goes—F and G are independent. So there must be a possibility that, in the combined measure, the increase in F outweighs the decrease in G. Our accounting would then say the change is a good thing.

At least—the argument goes—we have no principled way of ruling out this possibility. Take the additive formula $G + aF$ as an example. Perhaps some suitable choice of the weight a will prevent the decrease in F from outweighing the increase in G. But such a choice would be arbitrary. Once we have set up a distinct fairness measure to capture the value of equality, in principle it might outweigh the goodness measure when a levelling down takes place. So the argument goes.

Yet—the argument goes—levelling down cannot possibly be a good thing, because it is good for no one. So this way of accounting for the value of equality must be incorrect.

I agree that a levelling down cannot possibly be a good thing. I believe that no change can be good unless it is good for someone—I call this "the principle of personal good". But I think this argument based on levelling down is mistaken. It is easy to construct measures G and F, and form a combined measure from them, in such a way that levelling down can never be accounted a good thing. Here is a very simple example.

Suppose there are only two people, with well-being w_1 and w_2 respectively. Let the goodness measure be the sum of well-being:

$$G = (w_1 + w_2).$$

Let the fairness measure be minus the absolute value of the difference in well-being:

$$F = -|w_1 - w_2|.$$

F measures the degree of equality in well-being. It is scaled in such a way as to be a negative number unless there is perfect equality, and in that case it is zero. Let us combine G and F in the additive fashion as $G + aF$, and choose a to be 2. We get

$$(w_1 + w_2) - 2|w_1 - w_2|.$$

This formula is strictly increasing in w_1 and w_2. That is to say, a decrease in w_1 or in w_2 always decreases the value of the formula. This is very easy to check. So this formula implies that levelling down is always a bad thing.

According to the argument I described, my choice of a as 2 must have been arbitrary and unprincipled. However, I chose a to ensure that my formula would conform to the principle of personal good. I take this principle to constrain our evaluation of distributions of well-being. No formula can be correct unless it satisfies this principle. So my choice was not arbitrary; it was constrained by principle.

CORRIGENDUM

Summary measures of population health: concepts, ethics, measurement and applications.

Edited by: Murray CJL, Salomon JA, Mathers CD, Lopez AD: Geneva: WHO; 2002.

Page 136.

11th last line:	Replace 'choose a to be 2' by 'choose a to be '½'
10th last line:	Replace '2' by '½' in formula
6th last line:	Replace 'choice of a as 2' by 'choice of a as ½'

NOTES

1   The argument is one version of the "levelling-down objection". The levelling-down objection appears in Derek Parfit's article on "Equality or priority", but Parfit's version of it is not the one I present here. In fact, on pp. 112–115 of "Equality or priority", Parfit himself gives an argument that could serve as a response to the version I present here. It is close to my own response.

REFERENCES

Parfit D (2000) Equality or priority? In: *The ideal of equality*. Clayton M, Williams A, eds. Macmillan, Hampshire.

Chapter 3.6

MY GOODNESS — AND YOURS: A HISTORY, AND SOME POSSIBLE FUTURES, OF DALY MEANINGS AND VALUATION PROCEDURES

ERIK NORD

INTRODUCTION

In the Global Burden of Disease (GBD) project the question has been raised whether disability-adjusted life years (DALYs) should measure average health only, or also capture concerns for fairness and equity. The following is a brief comment on this issue. I first distinguish between goodness in health care in terms of objective health gain, individual utility, and societal value. I then show the role of these concepts and their operationalization in the history of DALYs. I proceed to discussing the latest proposal for defining health in the GBD project (Murray et al. 2000), and its possible implications for procedures for determining disability weights. I finally discuss the pros and cons of different candidate weighting procedures.

GOODNESS

Goodness can be discussed with respect to a given state of affairs in population health or with respect to improvements in population health. For simplicity I focus on the latter in the following.

It is common to distinguish between three kinds of good or goodness in health care:

1. *Objective health gains*. Gains in functioning or life expectancy.

2. *Individual utility*. Individuals' valuations of health improvements for themselves (determined by their subjective perceptions of quality of life and personal valuations of gained life years).

3. *Societal value*. Judgements by representatives of society at large of the relative goodness of different health programmes (determined by ob-

jective health gains, gains in subjectively perceived quality of life, and concerns for fairness and equity across individuals).

There is also a fourth concept: *Individuals' valuations of health programmes from behind a so-called "veil of ignorance" about the consequences for themselves.* This may be seen as a mixture of individual utility judgement and societal value judgement. For a thorough discussion, see Menzel (1999). I return to this below.

QUANTITIES AND VALUES

Some objective health gains may be compared in terms of *size*. For instance, ten gained life years is twice as much as five gained life years, and ten life years gained in a healthy person may be said to be a bigger health gain—meaning a bigger production of "well-life"—than ten life years gained in a disabled person.

On the other hand, far from all objective health gains can be compared in terms of *size*. One cannot, for instance, say that getting one's eyesight back is a "bigger" or "smaller" gain than getting one's hearing back, or "bigger" or "smaller" than getting to live five extra years. To make such comparisons, one has to look at the *value* of the gains—to the individuals concerned (= individual utility) or to society (= societal value)—by means of techniques like the standard gamble, the time trade-off, the person trade-off and willingness to pay.

There is no simple linear relationship between "quantifiable" objective health gains and individual utility. Ten extra years may be valued less than twice as much as five added years (in terms of willingness to sacrifice to obtain them), and disabled people may value avoided premature death (= gained life years) as much as able people do.

There is also no simple linear relationship between individual utility and societal value. For instance, for given gains in health and utility, the general public tends to value programmes more, the more severe the initial state of illness is (Callahan 1994; Nord 1993; Richardson 1997; Ubel 1999).

These observations suggest that summary measures of population health (somewhat paradoxically) cannot be based on the measurement of health as "objective functioning". They must be based either on the concept of individual utility or on the concept of societal value (or as we shall see later, a mixture of these), and it makes a difference which of them is chosen.

In the history of DALYs, views on this choice have changed over time.

THE GBD VALUATION HISTORY

In the original DALY work, it seems that disability weights were meant to express the "badness" of different states of illness (i.e. the loss of quality of life) to the individuals concerned (= individual disutility). The weights were then obtained by asking panels of people to locate selected states of illness on a rating scale from zero to unity (Murray 1994).

Since one of the purposes of DALYs was to inform resource allocation decisions, it was later felt that disability weights should encapsulate not only individual (personal) quality of life considerations, but also a broader set of societal distributive values (Murray 1996). For this reason (as I understand it), the valuation protocol was changed entirely in 1995, and the rating scale was replaced by the person trade-off (PTO) technique. Preliminary PTO-valuations for 22 indicator conditions were subsequently published by Murray and Lopez (1996), and the 1995 protocol has since been used in various settings in the GBD enterprise.

European experiences

The 1995 GBD protocol includes two different ways of asking person trade-off questions—PTO1 and PTO2. PTO1 basically asks: If programme A can extend the life of 1000 healthy people, and programme B can extend the life of N people with a given disability (e.g. blindness), how big must N be for you to be indifferent between the two programmes? If, for instance, average N for blindness is 1250, then the value for blindness will be 0.8 (1000/1250) and the disability weight for blindness will be 0.2. *Only responses higher than "1000" are accepted*. There is, in other words, an underlying assumption that the value of extending the life of disabled or chronically ill people is less than the value of extending the life of healthy people. Researchers in an ongoing European DALY project rejected this idea as unethical (Arnesen and Nord 1999). PTO2, on the other hand, compares health-improving programmes with life-saving ones. There is nothing unethical about PTO2, but the European researchers found it difficult to understand. They therefore developed an alternative version of the PTO (PTO3) which essentially goes as follows:

> Imagine that you are a decision-maker. You have a choice between two programmes that will reduce the incidence of disease in a few years from now.
>
> Programme A will prevent the occurrence of a rapidly fatal disease in 100 people in your country.
>
> Programme B will prevent the occurrence of disease X (chronic state described in detail) in N people in your country.
>
> The programmes are in all other respects equal. Choose the value for N that would make you indifferent between the two programmes.

If, for instance, $N = 1000$, then the disability weight for disease X will be 0.1 (100/1000). The phrasing raises no ethical problems. At the same time, it is easy to understand and maintains the societal value perspective.

The current proposal from the GBD-project

Following the strong reactions to PTO1 and PTO2 in the European project, Murray et al. (2000) argue that the change in 1995 in the construction and perspective of DALYs may have turned it into a too complex concept, with a less clear, common sense meaning. They suggest that perhaps it is better after all to keep the DALY as a summary measure of health only and to "distance the development of this measure from the complex value that must be considered in the allocation of scarce resources" (p. 986). They tentatively propose a specific way of defining health that arguably would allow disability weights to be estimated without societal distributive concerns being invoked. The proposition is that population A should be deemed healthier than population B if and only if (most) individuals behind a veil of ignorance personally would prefer to be in population A rather than in population B, when all non-health characteristics of A and B are the same.

Operationalization

The proposal of Murray et al. is an interesting one, and I can see a fairly straightforward way of operationalizing it. Suppose one wants to obtain a disability weight for *severe asthma*, subjects can then be faced with two hypothetical cohorts, A and B, of 100 people each (Table 1):

Table I   Two hypothetical cohorts for valuing a health state

Cohort	Healthy	Asthma at 40 with detailed description	Fatal disease at 40	Sum
A	80	20	0	100
B	95	0	5	100

Each subject can then be asked: Behind a veil of ignorance, to which cohort would you rather belong? One can then change the number of asthma cases until the subject is indifferent. If the median indifference number in an appropriate sample of subjects is in fact 20, the disability weight for asthma will be $5:20 = 0.25$.

This operationalization may be seen either as a variant of the person trade-off technique or as a probability trade-off resembling the standard gamble technique (Menzel 1990; 1999; Nord 1999). Whether it should be seen as the former or the latter depends on the considerations that people take into account when they respond.

Murray et al. are assuming that by using the veil of ignorance construct in their definition of health they exclude societal concerns for fairness and thus capture individual utility only. But the veil of ignorance construct does not necessarily work that way. Suppose, in the asthma example above, that a subject is indifferent between A and B. This *could* be because he is a maximizer of expected utility and thinks the disutility to him personally of severe asthma is one fourth of that of fatal disease. He would then be thinking in terms of personal risk, and the measurement would in effect capture a probability trade-off. But his indifference could also be the net result of two considerations: Personally he thinks the disutility of fatal disease Y is less than four times that of severe asthma but, on the other hand, being a person with a social conscience, he prefers to belong to the cohort where the distribution of health is more equitable. In the example, he might feel that that is cohort A. Both aspects considered, he is indifferent. The judgement of personal value (utility) then mixes with concerns for equity, and the response resembles more a person trade-off.

This example is more than a theoretical speculation. In an Australian study, preferences for belonging to a fair system seemed to override interests in utility maximization when people were asked what role treatment costs should have in priority-setting across patient groups (Nord et al. 1995). Similarly, preferences for letting severity of illness strongly influence priority-setting (as opposed to setting priorities on the basis of expected benefit only) seem to be strong even when people are asked behind a veil of ignorance (Nord 1994; Richardson and Nord 1997; Ubel 1999).

The point is that in many, perhaps most countries, people are inclined not to think only about themselves when they think about health policy or "which population they would prefer to belong to". To avoid ambiguities and difficulties of interpretation, the veil of ignorance approach therefore needs some further specification. To achieve the goal of Murray et al. the instructions to the valuation procedure outlined above could for instance say that "in this thought experiment we ask you to think only of your own self-interest and to have in mind how different kinds of health problems would affect quality of life for you personally". This seems quite feasible. Alternatively, subjects could be instructed to think of both self-interest and concerns they might have for fairness and equity. The operationalization above could then be seen as an alternative to PTO3 in asking about societal value. For a more detailed discussion, see Menzel (1999).

Comparison of methods

With the above operationalizations there seem to be (at least) three interesting candidate procedures for establishing disability weights in future Global Burden of Disease statistics: a revised person trade-off with an explicit societal perspective (PTO3 above); a veil of ignorance approach as described above with an individual, self-interest perspective; and a veil of ignorance approach as described above with a broader ethical perspective. The following are some points to consider in a choice between these three.

1. I cannot see any ethical problems with any of the approaches.

2. All three valuation tasks seem quite easy for subjects to understand.

3. I agree that a summary measure of population health should as much as possible accord with ordinary people's use (= common sense) of the word "health". It is possible that the introduction of societal concerns for fairness in a summary measure may run counter to this goal. On the other hand, it is not clear that ordinary people will immediately nod their heads understandingly when they see health defined as above by means of the veil of ignorance construct.

4. One might argue that ordinary people will never understand summary measures of health, and that these are primarily aids for reasonably well educated and informed policy-makers. If this is true, it is the common sense of the latter that is of interest. Murray et al. are then in effect suggesting that population health understood as "average population health" is more in keeping with the policy-makers' common sense than "average health adjusted for skewedness in distribution". I am not so convinced that this is true in most countries. Are we dealing with culture-specific values and a myth of objectivity here?

5. The previous point highlights the value side of DALYs. Murray et al. argue that "we can quite reasonably choose to measure population health in one way and conclude that scarce resources should not be allocated simply to maximize population as so measured" (p. 986). On the other hand, they previously stress that "summary measures should be considered to be normative" and that "great care must be taken in the construction of summary measures precisely because they may have far-reaching effects" (p. 982). So perhaps the former point is more a theoretical than a real one. It will be tempting to use DALYs as a measure of benefit in cost-effectiveness analysis. Perhaps they should then not fail to incorporate concerns for fairness.

FINAL REMARK

There is a somewhat disturbing lack of continuity in the thinking about valuation in the Global Burden of Disease project. The change from a rating scale to the person trade-off in 1995 seemed to be based on very careful reflection at the *conceptual* level: What are DALYs supposed to measure, given their purported use in health policy-making? Later events showed that the specific operationalization that was then chosen (PTO1 and PTO2) was unfortunate. This, however, does not in itself give reason for changing the underlying concept or aim of the measure from societal value back to individual utility. PTO3 was developed to cover what PTO1 and PTO2 were meant to cover, and thus to be in keeping with the idea of the 1995 DALY. A veil of ignorance approach that draws attention to distributive concerns in addition to self-interest would also be in keeping with this idea. One would perhaps expect that the feasibility of these approaches will be carefully examined before a more fundamental conceptual change in burden of disease measurement is proposed.

ACKNOWLEDGEMENT

I am very grateful to Paul Menzel for helping me clarify concepts in this paper.

REFERENCES

Arnesen T, Nord E (1999) The value of DALY life: problems with ethics and validity of disability adjusted life years. *British Medical Journal,* 319(7222):1423–1425.

Callahan D (1994) Setting mental health priorities: problems and possibilities. *Milbank Quarterly,* 72(4):451–470.

Menzel P (1990) *Strong medicine: the ethical rationing of health care.* Oxford University Press, New York.

Menzel P (1999) How should what economists call "social values" be measured? *Journal of Ethics,* 3(3):249–273.

Murray CJL (1994) Quantifying the burden of disease: the technical basis for disability-adjusted life years. *Bulletin of the World Health Organization,* 72(3):429–445.

Murray CJL (1996) Rethinking DALYs. In: *The global burden of disease: a comprehensive assessment of mortality and disability from diseases, injuries, and risk factors in 1990 and projected to 2020.* The Global Burden of Disease and Injury, Vol. 1. Murray CJL, Lopez AD, eds. Harvard School of Public Health on behalf of WHO, Cambridge, MA.

Murray CJL, Lopez AD, eds. (1996) *The global burden of disease: a comprehensive assessment of mortality and disability from diseases, injuries and risk factors in 1990 and projected to 2020.* Global Burden of Disease and Injury, Vol. 1. Harvard School of Public Health on behalf of WHO, Cambridge, MA.

Murray CJL, Salomon JA, Mathers CD (2000) A critical examination of summary measures of population health. *Bulletin of the World Health Organization,* 78(8):981–994.

Nord E (1993) The trade-off between severity of illness and treatment effect in cost-value analysis of health care. *Health Policy,* 24:227–238.

Nord E (1994) *Workshops on a value table for prioritizing in health care.* (In Norwegian.) (Working paper no 1/1994.) National Institute of Public Health, Oslo.

Nord E (1999) *Cost value analysis in health care: making sense out of QALYs.* Cambridge University Press, Cambridge.

Nord E, Richardson J, Street A, Kuhse H, Singer P (1995) Who cares about cost? Does economic analysis impose or reflect social values? *Health Policy,* 34(2):79–94.

Richardson J (1997) *Critique and some recent contributions to the theory of cost-utility analysis.* (CHPE working paper no 77.) Monash University, Centre for Health Program Evaluation, Melbourne.

Richardson J, Nord E (1997) The importance of perspective in the measurement of quality adjusted life years. *Medical Decision Making,* **17**(1):33–41.

Ubel P (1999) How stable are people's preferences for giving priority to severely ill patients? *Social Science and Medicine,* **49**(7):895–903.

Chapter 3.7

EVALUATING SUMMARY MEASURES
OF POPULATION HEALTH

JEFF RICHARDSON

INTRODUCTION

To select the most appropriate summary measures of population health (SMPH) from the large number of candidate statistical measures it is necessary to have selection criteria. This chapter addresses the issue of how to choose these selection criteria. It then discusses the implications of a set of proposed criteria for the choice of SMPH.

In summary, it is argued that SMPH should be selected from those measures that best answer the questions which are of interest to us; the selection criteria should therefore fully describe the attributes of an SMPH which will provide a complete, reliable and valid answer to these questions.[1] The argument is not trite. It is not uncommon to reverse the methodology: to commence with an intuitively appealing concept, and then to search for the many questions which, it is felt, the concept must help to answer. "Utility" and "health" are two such appealing concepts.

It is also commonplace to ask for the "conceptual basis" of a metric. This somewhat ambiguous phrase seems to suggest that SMPH must be the outcome of an established theory. For example, it has been argued that the standard gamble is the "theoretically correct" instrument to measure health-related quality of life (HRQoL) as it is the instrument implied by the von Neumann Morgenstern axioms of Expected Utility Theory. This approach is explicitly rejected here. The conceptual basis of the metric should be a statement of what it is that the metric seeks to measure and why the metric fulfils the purpose of interest. This may or may not involve reference to a theory other than the "theory" that the metric truly measures what it purports to measure (validity). There is, for example, no complex conceptual basis associated with the use of "death" as an indicator of interest. Mortality statistics are of importance because life is an endpoint in itself and because we wish to quantify our success in achieving this objective.

Focusing upon the purpose of an SMPH—the question it has to answer—clarifies two of the themes of this chapter. First, if there is more than one purpose, then it is likely that there will need to be more than one SMPH. Analogously, if there is more than one economic policy objective, then the theory of economic policy suggests that, except fortuitously, there will need to be more than one policy instrument. Secondly, as the questions to be answered relate directly or indirectly to social objectives, the choice of SMPH must reflect social–ethical values. This adds a significant dimension of complexity as such values are hard to elicit and may vary with the context and between population groups.

These more general issues of purpose and context are amplified below. In the following section a set of criteria are proposed for selecting SMPH which are relevant to economic evaluation and the measurement of the Burden of Disease (BoD). These are used to discuss two questions in the section that follows; viz, the choice of a scaling instrument (time trade-off, standard gamble, etc.) and the perspective—patient or social—to be embodied in an SMPH.

QUESTIONS, CONCEPTS AND CONTENT

The possible aims of SMPH include:

1. describing life expectancy (for both individual and social planning and, self evidently, for individual interest);

2. making cross national comparisons of health to be used either as a benchmark for national performance or to parenthesize particular national problems;

3. making cross national comparisons to determine the priority for health-related aid;

4. measuring the BoD by disease category (to highlight the need for health-related action within a country);

5. quantifying changes in the quality of life (QoL) across a country or through time (to determine the success of social policy and to formulate subsequent policy);

6. measuring the individual benefits arising from a health programme or service (for orthodox economic evaluation); and

7. measuring the "social value" of these benefits (for less orthodox economic evaluation!).

The distinction between individual and social benefits alluded to above has only recently been explicitly identified. Factors included in the latter but not the former include: age weights, indices of the severity of the initial health state, health potential, the maintenance of hope, the achievement of a "fair innings" (life expectancy), and the distribution of benefits

(Menzel et al. 1999; Nord et al. 1999; Williams 1998 and Tsuchiya, chapter 13.1).

Numerous SMPH already exist which, to a greater or lesser extent, may satisfy these objectives. They include a variety of mortality-related indices (life expectancy, years of life lost, etc.), lives, life years, quality-adjusted life years (QALYs) and its many variants[2] which result from the choice of scaling instrument (time trade-off, standard gamble, etc.), perspective (patients or public), the group from whom values are elicited (patient, provider or public); reference time (anticipated versus realized health state), and time from the commencement of an episode of illness (year, full episode, full life). Finally there has been increasing attention given to the inclusion of indicators of social–ethical preferences with respect to age, disease severity, fair innings, etc. Some of these SMPH may have multiple uses. However, a satisfactory answer to each of the earlier questions is likely to require the adoption of several SMPH.

For example, while mortality statistics describe life expectancy they do not indicate the QoL. The years of life lost (YLL) plus HRQoL help describe the BoD but may not represent a comprehensive measure of the social value of life-years gained from a health programme. Developing countries may be primarily concerned with mortality, but international aid agencies may wish to take other factors into account and these factors may reflect the willingness to pay and the values of the donor, not the recipient, nations.

The following section is concerned with the criteria for selecting SMPH for two purposes: to measure the BoD and to measure social preferences in the context of an economic evaluation. Before turning to this task there is a final general point. Each of the questions and each of the potential SMPH is value laden. Mortality is used as an indicator because of the self-evident importance placed upon life by society. The use of QALYs similarly reflects the social importance of HRQoL. More generally, the selection of the questions to be answered by SMPH and the choice of SMPH implicitly or explicitly represents an ethical judgement concerning the importance of the issue and how it is to be answered.

Incorporating social values is complicated by the fact that the values—health related or otherwise—are often context specific. The value of water to a person dying of thirst differs from the value to an individual in normal circumstances. As noted by Allais in 1953, an incremental increase in the probability of a favourable outcome is valued differently in the context of near certainty and in the context of a low probability of a favourable outcome. Incremental income is of greater value in the context of poverty. A second complicating factor is that the criteria of value may also be context specific. Clothing may be judged primarily by elegance in temperate climates. In colder climates the most important criterion may be warmth.

The importance of context for the relevance of an SMPH is nicely illustrated by the debate over "double jeopardy", i.e. the assertion that

QALYs imply discrimination against the permanently disabled because restoration of the disabled to their best possible health state (disability) results in a smaller health gain and a lower priority for treatments than the restoration to best possible health of normal patients. Ubel et al. (1999) found, however, that survey respondents clearly discriminated between the treatment of long-term quadriplegics and the treatment of previously healthy patients who would become quadriplegics after treatment. Specifically, the respondents did not consider that saving the life of a long-term quadriplegic was of less value than saving the life of a normally healthy person. While the utility gain by the quadriplegic would clearly be less, respondents considered that the context was morally relevant to their social decision. The social value of a possible subsequent cure for quadriplegia would be unaffected by this conclusion as the context of the cure would be quite different from the context of a life-saving treatment.

CRITERIA FOR ASSESSING SOCIAL VALUE

Since economists regularly offer advice which purports to assist with the achievement of social objectives, it is surprising that there is so little critical discussion of the criteria for determining social objectives. At a high level of abstraction, economic theory acknowledges the existence of a "social welfare function" (SWF) which, in principle, can incorporate any social arrangement that contributes to (undefined) social well-being. The term "function" is presumably used to add gravitas to an otherwise vacuous acknowledgment that society may have a variety of objectives. The SWF becomes an ethical theory with ethical content when it postulates that social welfare is a function of individual utilities: it becomes the orthodox theory of welfarism.

If the assumptions of welfarism and economic orthodoxy were correct, they would largely eliminate the need for an independent enquiry into the criteria for selecting an SMPH to measure social value. With the exception of the distribution of initial wealth, social values are assumed. However, for the reasons discussed in chapter 12.1, the use of these assumptions in the health sector is not warranted and consequently there is a need for explicit criteria. These will necessarily be ad hoc, in the sense that they are not derived from an orthodox and established theory. But, as noted earlier, they should be judged by their capacity to answer questions of interest and not by their adherence to an orthodoxy which itself is necessarily based upon once-ad hoc assumptions.[3]

Murray et al. (2000) are among the few who recognize both that multiple objectives may imply the need for multiple SMPH and that an explicit procedure is needed to choose between alternative SMPH. They propose that Rawls' veil of ignorance be used for this latter purpose. Five criteria are derived. While these are shown to eliminate some SMPH, it is questionable whether they justify the use of a Rawlsian veil. The criteria could almost certainly be justified without a veil: it is unlikely that anyone would disagree that a useful definition of "healthiness" would identify populations with lower mortality, age- and sex-specific incidence, prevalence of poor health, etc.

It is also unlikely that the veil of ignorance will produce an unambiguous criterion for "Healthiness". Consider the two populations in Table 1. There is no obvious way of determining the "healthier" population. From behind a veil of ignorance the individual's choice will depend very largely upon their risk behaviour. A risk plunger or someone adopting a maximum-minimum criterion would prefer membership of population 1. Someone who was risk averse or maximized the expected value of health would select population 2. In sum, it is unclear what people will think behind a veil of ignorance, and the inclusion of irrelevant risk or uncertainty in the decision process only casts doubt upon its validity.

Previously (Richardson 1994) I proposed four criteria for evaluating the units of an SMPH to be used for measuring benefits in the context of an economic evaluation and, more specifically, to be used for assessing the scaling techniques that have been used in cost-utility analysis to convert life-years into "utility" or units of social value (TTO, SG, PTO, RS, ME[4]). I believe these four criteria are still appropriate. They are that:

1. More units are considered to be of greater social value.

2. The units should have a clear and unambiguous meaning.

3. (a) The units should have a "weak" interval property, i.e. that incremental units should, in some *easily understood sense*, mean the same irrespective of the number of units already obtained.

   (b) The units should have a "strong" interval property, i.e. that an x per cent increase in measured quality of life at any point along the QoL spectrum should have, *in an easily understood sense*, the same value as an x per cent increase in the length of life.

4. The scaling techniques should be sensitive to a change in a health state and be reliable and valid.

Table 1   Frequency distribution of population utility

QoL (Utility score)	Population 1 (%)	Population 2 (%)
1.0	50	
0.8	—	90
0.4	50	—
0.0 (Dead)	—	10
Total	100	100
E(U)	0.70	0.72

The reasons for these criterion are fairly self evident. However, I now believe that Criterion 1 requires supplementation as follows:

1. (a) The SMPH should embody relevant ethical values, which are consistent with stable population values and which reflect any relevant context-dependent values.

   (b) Units should fully measure all dimensions of the subject of measurement and be sensitive to changes in health status.

   (c) The numerical value of the units should not be influenced by extraneous factors.

The case of double jeopardy discussed earlier illustrates the need for criterion 1(a). Benefits from the treatment of quadriplegia may be measured in a way that satisfied criterion 1 but still permits unwanted discrimination. Criterion 1(a) implies that, with the usual social values, saving the life of a quadriplegic and a normally healthy person would receive equal priority. Criterion 1(b) is introduced to eliminate instruments which, while satisfying other criteria, are insensitive and fail to fully measure some dimensions of health improvement.

Criterion 1(c) is less benign than it may first appear. Especially in the psychometrics discipline, there is a legitimate tradition of seeking underlying—latent—variables implied by, and correlated with, observed or manifest variables (IQ is an example of this). There is an attraction to the argument that the latent variable represents the "true quantity" and that observations are only manifestations of this. The argument is treacherous. If the TTO (hypothetically) provided an exact measure of the SMPH required for economic evaluation (it met all criteria, or even defined the desired concept), its combination with other imperfect indices (RS, PTO, SG) would permit the creation of a latent variable capable of explaining variation in the observed data and capable of creating functional relationships with each of the manifest variables. In this contrived example, the latent variable is not a gold standard but a deviation from it. The conclusion illustrated by this example is that statistical composites are beguiling but difficult to interpret, evaluate and validate.

The importance of criterion 2 should also be parenthesized. SMPH and especially those measuring HRQoL and social value will be used by policymakers who must trade off competing objectives. Their capacity to do this is impaired if they do not truly understand what different indices mean and imply. Even more importantly, there is no method, at present, for ensuring that scales have the strong interval property (criterion 3b). The only basis for believing it exists arises from the nature of the question asked to survey respondents and the validity of their answers. Thus, a correctly answered TTO question will ensure that a person will truly trade life for quality of life and in the proportions indicated by the instrument's score. Units derived from more complex procedures are less likely to retain this defining property of the QALY. The existence of extraneous information violating criterion 1(c) would be hard to detect or interpret by policy-makers.

CHOICE OF SCALING INSTRUMENT

It was suggested above that different SMPH might be required for the measurement of the BoD and the social benefits of economic evaluation. The need for this depends upon the precise question of interest. If the BoD was intended to measure the present social value of disease, then it could borrow the SMPH used for economic evaluation. If, however, it is intended to measure the quantum of suffering associated with current disease, then the appropriate SMPH would include the duration and intensity of the suffering but not the indicators of the social value of the suffering. This implies that life-years and the utility value of the health state—duration and the quality of the sensations associated with it—would be included in the metric for the BoD; the intellectualized value of these which lead to age, time or other value weights would only be included in the SMPH used for quantifying social value in economic analyses (see chapter 13.2).

In an earlier paper (Richardson 1994) I used the first four criteria above to assess the relative merits of the available scaling instruments for this latter purpose. It was argued (i) that the RS and ME did not have a clear meaning and that there was no possible link between them and the (all-important) strong interval property defined in criterion 3b; (ii) that, by contrast, the three trade-off instruments all required a comparison of the quantity and quality of life; (iii) that the meaning and the interval property of units derived from the SG were seriously confounded by the (irrelevant) risk context of the instrument; and (iv) that the choice between the PTO and TTO should be determined largely by the perspective—personal or societal—that was wanted in an analysis.

While still supporting the framework for assessing the instruments, i.e. the application of explicit criteria, I would now modify this conclusion. All three trade-off instruments are confounded and for the same reason. The technique used to elicit a numerical score, i.e. varying the risk of death, length of life, and distribution of benefits, introduces a (normally) extraneous factor into the assessment. Thus all three violate criterion 1(c). The risk embodied in the SG will normally be quite different to the risk facing a patient who may be receiving a service which does not affect the likelihood of death. The TTO is confounded by time preference and the different life expectancies in the contrived TTO question. The PTO introduces a distributional consideration which will normally be quite dissimilar to the distributional implications, if any, of the programme under review.

Supporters of each scaling instrument may seek to defend its integrity by arguing that what is called an "extraneous element" here—risk, time or distribution—is, in fact, a part of what is to be measured. In the case of the standard gamble, advocates have gone one step further and argued that the introduction of risk is necessary for the measurement of "utility."

Values calculated in the shadowy world of "Under-Risk" are mutated in some way due to their contact with risk—not the risk associated with the real world context of the decision, but with any risk—and magnitudes emerge as "utility" which, because of the connotations of the word, is presumed to be an accurate reflection of the intensity of a person's preferences and the appropriate object of measurement. The world of "Under-Risk" is described as "shadowy" because the way in which the risk of instant death captures the intensity of a person's preferences with respect to the relief of, for example, pain—and the risk that the mild analgesic taken will not relieve the pain—has not been explained in the literature, and the relationship implied appears to be more mystical than empirical.

In all three cases the argument that the extraneous factor is justified is demonstrably wrong. Each of the instruments varies a contrived health state scenario and in each case the measured utility will be determined by two elements; viz, the true utility score but also the direct effect upon utility of the instrumental variable, i.e. risk per se (SG), time horizon and the rate of time preference (TTO), and the distribution of benefits (PTO). Varying one element of an instrument permits the unique identification of only one (not two) elements of the reported utility, and the stated purpose of each instrument is that this element should be the health-related quality of life—not the effect upon utility of the instrumental variable. In sum, a single instrument cannot (except by chance[5]) simultaneously measure two unrelated values. This may be demonstrated formally[6] and the truth of the proposition is made self-evident by the fact that the second element (the real world risk, time or distributional dimensions of the health state being assessed) are not normally included in the health state description presented to patients.

The final choice of scaling instruments should depend, *inter alia*, upon the magnitude of the contamination—the size of the second, extraneous, element. If, for example, TTO values did not change significantly with the length of time described by the instrument[7] (something reported by Dolan et al. 1996) and if the contamination of the PTO and SG arising from distribution and risk per se was significant, then the TTO might be the preferred instrument. This issue, however, is empirical not conceptual.

There are other sources of potential bias in these instruments. For example, it has been noted in the literature on adaptation that the utility score assigned to poor health states by those who have experienced them is generally greater than the score assigned by the public. Evidence suggests that a contributory factor to this discrepancy is that those contemplating the state will be influenced by the sadness of entering the state. To the extent that this is generally true and to the extent that we wish to measure the utility of a state per se, then the person trade-off instrument is subject to a second confounding effect if it is implemented in a way that suggests that previously healthy patients will be returned to a health state (the state being evaluated) less than full health[8] (Kahneman 1999). That is, there is a conflation of the health state disutility and the sadness—disutility—of the process of entering the state.

A further and similarly empirical issue is the extent to which survey respondents understand and respond accurately to the three types of question. Economics, as a discipline, has a tradition of assuming rationality and good information and this is reflected in the implicit assumption that the answer received from a respondent will literally and precisely reflect a considered opinion. Studies which have encouraged deliberation have not found empirical support for this assumption (Murray and Lopez 1996; Dolan 2000; Shiell et al. 2000). However, there is no good evidence about the techniques which best promote deliberation. The methods in the studies cited above may or may not improve deliberation. A recent search by the Monash Health Economics Unit failed to identify a substantive literature discussing and validating alternative procedures for encouraging deliberation. Perversely, some doubt was cast upon the intuitively plausible use of focus groups.

Finally, there is significant literature on whose perspective and values should be incorporated into an SMPH. This has been reviewed by Brazier et al. (1999). While there is a broad consensus that a patient perspective should be adopted, it is commonly argued that the values incorporated should be those of a cross-section of the population because it is the community, as taxpayers, who must pay for health programmes. This argument is not compelling. Taxpayers do not specify how their funds should be spent in other contexts. We do not vote on the composition of the armed forces, the location of roads, etc. and we do not specify how recipients of social service payments should spend their money. It is perfectly reasonable (and universal practice) for taxpayers to fund health services which are prioritized by others.

In a recent contribution, Nord et al. (1999) combined elements from both sides of this argument and proposed a two-stage procedure in which the patients' perspective and values are used to produce utility scores, and societal representatives are then used to convert these into units of social value. It should be recognized, however, that decisions concerning perspectives and values are ethical, not technical, and economists have no particular expertise in this area.

The relevance of this final issue—the authority of economic analyses—is that it illustrates the methodological weakness of the economics discipline once orthodox theory is inapplicable or is rejected. Arguments are largely ad hoc. Nord et al. may correctly argue that patient values lead to a more coherent concept of the Burden of Disease which may subsequently be valued. Others might wish to defend the hybrid concept of a publicly evaluated burden. Resolution of this debate requires prior agreement upon criteria. Those suggested here include criterion 1(a)—that an SMPH should embody relevant ethical values *which are consistent with stable population values*. In the present context, this implies consistency with the populations' preferred approach to decision-making and choice of decision-makers, i.e. the public, patients, or both, as required by Nord et al. (1999). Resolution of this issue implies structured communication with the population. The process is described in chapter 12.1 as "empirical ethics" and requires deliberation, systematic ethical criticism, and empirical re-examination of population values after clarification of the consequences. The choice of perspective is an obvious subject for empirical ethics.

Conclusions

There has been surprisingly little discussion about the choice and application of criteria for selecting SMPH. Within the economics discipline this is, in part, attributable to the fact that orthodox economic theory bypasses the need for such an analysis by assuming objectives and axioms of behaviour which dictate conclusions. The first of the two major themes of this chapter has been that explicit criteria should be adopted for the evaluation of SMPH. As the objective of different SMPH is to quantify concepts of interest, candidate criteria should themselves be judged by how well they promote this objective. The criteria proposed here explicitly sought to describe the properties needed in a reliable and valid SMPH for use in the context of economic evaluation and the measurement of the Burden of Disease.

When the proposed criteria are employed to discriminate between the scaling instruments used to quantify the HRQoL, the outcome is inconclusive. The criteria eliminate the Rating Scale and Magnitude Estimation. They do not discriminate between the time trade-off, person trade-off and standard gamble. This reflects the fact that in each case the measurement of HRQoL is contaminated by the "instrument variable"—time, distribution and risk—used to quantify the HRQoL, and the extent of the contamination is an empirical issue. There is, consequently, a need to investigate the properties of these scaling instruments more thoroughly than has occurred to date.

For the reasons given by Richardson (1994) and by Dolan et al. (1996) the TTO may well be the most appropriate scaling instrument for estimating utility scores. If the desired concept of social value was simply individual utility, then this would imply that the TTO might also be the scaling instrument of choice. As the preferences for other elements of social value—age, severity, etc.—are not experienced solely by patients, then the use of the PTO and the values of the general population may be preferred or employed in a second-stage analysis to convert individual "utility" into "social value". These are not issues, however, which may be resolved by *a priori* theory alone. Instrument reliability and validity also depend upon the empirical questions associated with instrument bias, respondent comprehension and deliberation, and also upon the perspective which society or its representatives wish to have embodied in health state valuations.

None of these are "technical issues" to be resolved by *a priori* "economic theory".

The second main theme of the chapter has been that multiple questions imply the need for multiple concepts which, in turn, implies the need for multiple SMPH. As an example, it was argued that there are separate, useful and coherent concepts of the Burden of Disease, and of individual and social value associated with disease cure. The suggested concept of the BoD corresponds with quantities which are time based and which determine a flow of sensations, i.e. duration-based suffering (lowered HRQoL) and loss of life years (the loss of any time-based sensations). The social value of these quantities depends upon intellectualized preferences including a preference for benefits to particular groups of the community, at particular points in time and, probably, in particular contexts. Except for time preference, there has been little investigation of these and almost no research which employs the melding of empirical and ethical analyses as described and advocated in chapter 12.1.

There is still a large research agenda!

NOTES

1　Secondary criteria might include the cost of obtaining the required data and, related to this, the possibility of an indicator serving more than one purpose.

2　These variants include healthy year equivalents (HYEs) and disability-adjusted life years (DALYs).

3　The axioms of neoclassical economic theory are ad hoc in the sense that they are not created from a prior theory. Any attempt to base all theories and assumptions upon prior theories and assumptions encounters an infinite logical regress (See chapter 12.1).

4　TTO = time trade-off;　SG = standard gamble;　PTO = person trade-off; RS = rating scale; ME = magnitude estimation.

5　It is possible that a particular procedure might expose a person to a real risk of death of, for example, 0.4 and that the utility value of the health state before the procedure was 0.6. Then and only then would it be possible to argue that the standard gamble captured the relevant attitude towards risk. An analogous argument applies with respect to the TTO and duration; the PTO and distribution.

6　In the theory of policy it is known that, except by coincidence, the simultaneous achievement of n objectives requires n policy instruments. More formally, a system of n simultaneous equations—one determining the value of each policy objective—can only be solved if there are at least n independent variables whose values may be adjusted as policy instruments. In the present case, $n = 2$: we wish to set both QoL and the other variable—risk, time or distribution—at their real world values and "solve" for the numeraire or instrument variable. But with only one instrument we can only "solve" for (determine the equivalent value of) one—not two—of the real world variables and the existence of two variables confounds the relationship—there is no unique solution.

7   For example survey respondents might be asked to consider scenarios with either a 20-year or a 10-year period of poor health and then be asked to select the (shorter) period of good health which would be of equivalent value. A positive rate of time preference (RTP) would affect the 20-year scenario more than the 10-year scenario. If the RTP was zero, both scenarios would produce the same response.

8   The PTO technique asks survey respondents to compare the value of a programme which returns x patients to full health and a programme which returns y patients to health state S. The value of y is varied until the two programmes are of equal value to the respondent. The procedure thus envisages x patients entering the health state S.

References

Brazier JE, Deverill M, Green C, Harper R, Booth A (1999) A review of the use of health status measures in economic evaluation. *Health Technology Assessment,* 3(9):1–164.

Dolan P (2000) The measurement of health-related quality-of-life for use in resource allocation decisions in health care. In: *Handbook of health economics. Vol. 1B.* Culyer AJ, Newhouse J, eds. Elsevier, Amsterdam.

Dolan P, Gudex C, Kind P, Williams A (1996) Valuing health states: a comparison of methods. *Journal of Health Economics,* 15(2):209–231.

Kahneman D (1999) How can we know who is happy: conceptual and methodological issues. In: *Well-being: the foundations of hedonic psychology.* Kahneman D, Diener E, Schwarz N, eds. Russell Sage Foundation, New York.

Menzel P, Gold MR, Nord E, Pinto JL, Richardson J, Ubel P (1999) Toward a broader view of values in cost-effectiveness analysis of health. *Hastings Center Report,* 29(3):7–15.

Murray CJL, Lopez AD, eds. (1996) *The global burden of disease: a comprehensive assessment of mortality and disability from diseases, injuries and risk factors in 1990 and projected to 2020.* Global Burden of Disease and Injury, Vol. 1. Harvard School of Public Health on behalf of WHO, Cambridge, MA.

Murray CJL, Salomon JA, Mathers CD (2000) A critical examination of summary measures of population health. *Bulletin of the World Health Organization,* 78(8):981–994.

Nord EM, Pinto JL, Richardson J, Menzel P, Ubel P (1999) Incorporating societal concerns for fairness in numerical valuations of health programmes. *Health Economics,* 8(1):25–39.

Richardson J (1994) Cost-utility analysis: what should be measured? *Social Science and Medicine,* 39(1):7–21.

Shiell A, Seymour J, Hawe P, et al. (2000) Are preferences over health states complete? *Health Economics,* 9(1):47–55.

Ubel P, Richardson J, Pinto-Prades JL (1999) Lifesaving treatments and disabilities: are all QALYs created equal? *International Journal of Technology Assessment in Health Care,* 15(4):738–748.

Williams A (1998) If we are going to get a fair innings, someone will need to keep the score! In: *Health, health care and health economics*. Barer M, Getzen TE, Stoddart GL, eds. Wiley, Chichester.

Chapter 3.8

An equity motivated indicator of population health

Norberto Dachs

Introduction

Not withstanding all the work done recently on summary measures of population health,[1] the area is still open for new research and the development of new proposals for more satisfactory ways of accomplishing the task at hand, which is to be able to present in one value (or a few values) enough useful information for meaningful comparisons between countries and subpopulations, in such a way that both the levels (averages) and the inequalities (dispersions) are also taken into account. In relation to the measurement of inequalities in health in particular, there are several proposals but they generally come from adaptations of previous works in epidemiology and economics.[2] However, there has been controversy and discussion on whether these measurements should be done for subgroups of populations or at the individual level (Braveman et al. 2000; Murray et al. 1999).

The aim in this chapter is to show that it is possible to develop useful and meaningful ways of measuring both the levels and inequalities using measures which have "decomposability" properties, making it possible to use them both at the "individual level" and in "subgroups" of a given population and, at the same time, taking into account equity considerations.

There are two general ways of approaching the problem of measuring population health. The first one is to suppose that the population has n individuals, and that to each one of them it is possible to associate a value x_i that would be a measure of "health" of the ith individual. The second way is to adopt a distributional approach and suppose that health in the population has a (probability) distribution F that belongs to a family F of possible distributions. Both approaches present advantages and disadvantages. Many times it is difficult or impossible to associate a value of health to an individual member of the population, and in others it is not immediately clear for what class of distributions F should be used. The two approaches are reconcilable, and in effect are alternative simplifying representations of this inherently complex problem.[3] They are called individual and distributional approaches, respectively.[4] With either of these two broad approaches it is then possible to develop measures for inequality either informally (ad hoc) or axiomatically.[5] The family of summary measures to be presented here is obtained by an axiomatic approach.

NOTATION

Let A be a population of n individuals, represented by a vector $a = (a_1, a_2, \ldots, a_n)$. To the ith individual in this population it is possible to associate (or to think of) a number x_i which is a measure of his/her health status. The health of the population is thus represented by the vector $x = (x_1, x_2, \ldots, x_n)$. In the alternative distributional approach the "health" of an individual in the population would be a random variable X with distribution $F \in F$ for some appropriate family of (probability) distribution functions.

It is necessary that this be a positive health measure, in other words, $x_i > x_j$ means that a_i has better health than a_j. One example of such a measure is a survival probability, for example the survival probability to age one. Another example is a health-adjusted life expectancy (HALE). One type of HALE is the measure used in the *World Health Report 2000* of WHO.[6] It will be further supposed that the support of F is [0,1], in other words, that the health measure for an individual lies between zero and one. This is true for survival probabilities and can be obtained normatively for HALEs and in many other cases by dividing the values by a reasonably attainable (or already attained) upper limit.

A summary measure of population health H is then a function from X to R^θ, where R is the set of real numbers, and (the positive integer) θ should preferably have a (very) small value. In this work the study is restricted to the particular case of $\theta = 1$. This function will be further restricted to have values in [0,1]. Again, in most cases, this can be obtained either by appropriate transformations or by restricting to functions already in [0,1]. If the distributional approach is to be used, H would be a functional $H(F) \rightarrow [0,1]$.

A CLASS OF MEASURES

The axioms used here are specific to health status. Several of them, but not all, are similar to the axioms used to derive measures of economic inequality. As is always the case, the choice of the axioms is a matter of personal preference and choice. A short argument will be presented for each axiom to justify its inclusion, as well as brief justifications of why some of the ones used in economic studies have to be dropped when considering health status.

The axioms will be presented for the individual approach. They can also be formulated for the distributional approach, but it is easier to understand their intuitive appeal in the individual formulation. They are the following:

A1—Weak equity. Given two persons, i and j, with unequal health status $x_i < x_j$, the impact on the value of a summary measure of the health status of a population that includes these two individuals will be higher for a (health) improvement $\Delta x > 0$ in x_i than an equal improvement in x_j. In other words, if $x_i < x_j$, then $H(x_1,..., x_i + \Delta x,..., x_j,..., x_n) > H(x_1,..., x_i,..., x_j + \Delta x,..., x_n)$.[7]

A2—Replication invariance. If the population x is obtained from y by a replication of any length so that $x = (y, y, ..., y)$, then $H(x) = H(y)$. This ensures that the measure H reflects health status in a "per capita" basis.

A3—Symmetry. If x is obtained from y by a permutation, then $H(x) = H(y)$. This is also known as the assumption of anonymity. It requires the summary measure to use only the information contained in the values of the x's themselves and not some other characteristics like sex, educational status, etc. of the individuals (the a's) themselves. This will not prevent the possibility of partitioning the population according to these (and other) characteristics to understand or explain differences in the health status of population subgroups. Taking this property into consideration it is then possible to simplify the notation and to identify a and x, in other words, the population itself and the vector of the health status of its individuals, as will be done from now onwards.

A4—Weak additive decomposability. If the population x is constituted by the aggregation of two subpopulations y and z of sizes n_1 and n_2, respectively, with $n = n_1 + n_2$, then $H(x) = H(H(y),..., H(y), H(z),..., H(z))$, with $H(y)$ repeated n_1 times and $H(z)$ repeated n_2 times. This property can easily be extended to the case of k subpopulations. This is the property that will make it possible to try to understand and eventually explain variations of health status between subgroups of x. The only requirement is that the subgroups are not overlapping, in other words it is necessary to partition the population x into a collection of mutually exclusive and collectively exhaustive subsets $x(1),..., x(k)$. For example, if y is the population of one province and z of another province, of a country constituted by these two provinces, then the measure of health status for the whole country is the combination of the measures of the health status of the two provinces.

This could be also applied to the study of other subgroups of the population (ethnic groups, urban/rural populations, etc.).

A5—Monotonicity. A gain in health for any individual in the population will be reflected by an increase in the summary measure H. In other words, $1 \le i \le n$, and $\Delta x > 0$, then $H(x_1,..., x_i + \Delta x,..., x_n) > H(x_1,..., x_i, ..., x_n)$.

In distributional terms this property gains a new light. It is equivalent to saying that if F_Δ is obtained from F by translating a mass Δ rightwards (irrespective from where it is taken) in the distribution, then $H(F_\Delta) > H(F)$.[8]

Now for properties that should not be required for summary measures in the special case of health.

The most evident of them is the principle of transfers (or Pigou-Dalton condition). This property states that for $0 < \Delta x < x_i \leq x_j$, then $H(x_1, \ldots, x_i + \Delta x, \ldots, x_j - \Delta x, \ldots, x_n) > H(x_1, \ldots, x_i, \ldots, x_j, \ldots, x_n)$ or, in other words, that if one "transfers" Δx from x_j to x_i when x_j is better off than x_i (but by an "amount" such that the worse off does not get better than the other), then the summary measure increases. It seems evident that this should not be required in the case of health status since it is difficult (impossible?) to conceive a meaningful way of transferring "health status units" from one individual to another. It does not seem possible in general to improve the health status of one individual by taking health status units from another. An interesting discussion would result if instead of health status the measure were to be for health care (either access or utilization or financing.)

Scale invariance and translation invariance are two other properties that are many times required of measures of inequality derived through the construction arising from welfare functions. The rigorous statement of these properties and the discussion of their implications in the case of health status measures exceed the scope of this work. Stating loosely, scale invariance would be equivalent to saying that given two populations $x = (x_1, x_2, \ldots, x_n)$ and $y = (y_1, y_2, \ldots, y_m)$, with $H(x) - H(y) = \Delta H$, and then, if the values of all x's and all y's are multiplied by the same constant α, representing by $\alpha x = (\alpha x_1, \alpha x_2, \ldots, \alpha x_n)$ and αy the new populations, then $H(\alpha x) - H(\alpha y) = \alpha \Delta H$. Similarly for a translation, which would be an addition of the same constant value to all individuals in both populations. They are not explicitly required from the summary measure H in the forms above, although the measure to be presented below satisfies weaker versions of both properties.[9]

The family of Atkinson's welfare functions:

$$W(x) = \frac{1}{n_x} \sum_{i=1}^{n} u(x_i) \tag{1}$$

where u is a continuous function with positive first derivative and negative second derivative and, in particular, the functions of the form presented in (2) satisfy all the axioms and properties A1 through A5. Instead of presenting formal demonstration which can be found in many books of economics, the five properties will be illustrated in very simple cases of populations with two to four individuals.

$$H(x) = \left(\frac{1}{n} \sum_{i=1}^{n} x^{(1-\varepsilon)} \right)^{\frac{1}{1-\varepsilon}} \tag{2}$$

For example, if $x_1 = 0.6$ and $x_2 = 0.8$ and $\varepsilon = 1.5$, then $H(x_1,x_2) = 0.689$. If there is a health status gain of $\Delta x = 0.1$ for x_1 from 0.6 to 0.7, then the new value is $H(0.7,0.8) = 0.747$ whereas if the gain had been of the same amount, but for x_2 from 0.8 to 0.9, then the new value is $H(0.6,0.9) = 0.727$. The increase in H is 0.058 $(0.747 - 0.689)$ in the first case and 0.0038 $(0.727 - 0.689)$ in the second case. If we chose $\varepsilon = 2$, then $H(0.6,0.8) = 0.686$, $H(0.7,0.8) = 0.747$ and $H(0.6,0.9) = 0.720$ and the increases in H are 0.061 and 0.034, respectively.

The other important property to investigate in more detail is the weak decomposability. Let us consider an example with two subpopulations, each of size two, as shown in Table 1. The first, y, with individuals with health status 0.6 and 0.7. The value of H for y is 0.647, smaller than the average of health status of the two constituent individuals in the population. The second population is z with individuals with health status 0.8 and 0.9 and the value of H for z is 0.848. The value of H for a population of two individuals with health status 0.647 and 0.848 is 0.737 which is equal to H for $x = (y,z)$ or $H(0.6,0.7,0.8,0.9) = 0.737$. According to the property of replication invariance, the value of $H(0.647,0.848) = H(0.647,0.647,0.848,0.848)$.

The choice of the parameter ε will be dictated by how much importance is to be assigned to the weak equity axiom. The choice of ε depends on the relative importance we wish to place on dispersion of the values in relation to level of the values. The larger the value of ε the greater the so called aversion to inequality. The final choice of ε must be the result of a social and political decision, as in Lindholm and Rosén (1998).

A DISTRIBUTIONAL EXAMPLE

Many of the distributions of health status in populations can be well approximated by Beta distributions (compare Figures 1 and 2, as well as the distributions of DALEs in Figure 2.3 of WHO' s *World Health Report 2000*, p.30).

The expected value and the variance of a Beta(a,b) random variable are:

$$u = \frac{a}{a+b} \qquad v = \frac{ab}{(a+b)^2 (a+b+1)} \qquad (3)$$

Table 1   Example (for $\varepsilon = 1.5$) of weak decomposability of the measure H

Subpopulation **y**	= (0.6,0.7)	H(**y**) = 0.647
Subpopulation **z**	= (0.8,0.9)	H(**z**) = 0.848
Population **x** = (**y**,**z**)	= (0.6,0.7,0.8,0.9)	H(**x**) = 0.737

According to the weak decomposability of **H** we have:

H(x) = **H(H(y),H(z))** = **H**(0.647,0.647,0.848,0.848) = 0.737, as expected.

To explore the possibility of obtaining values for $H(x)$ under this assumption, simulations were performed for different values of u and v, and for values of e equal to 1.5, 2, 3, 5 and 9. It is possible to express H as a function of u and v in the form:

$$H = u + d\left|(1-v)^{(1-\varepsilon)} - 1\right| \tag{4}$$

Figure 1   Densities of three different Beta[0,1] distributions wih parameters (100,10), (30,10) and (100,6), respectively

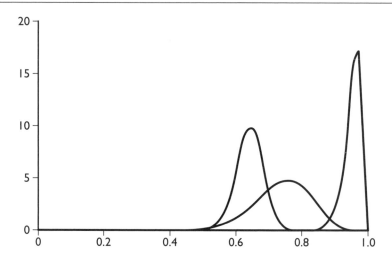

Figure 2   Distributions of survival probabilities below one year of age in four regions of Brazil, 1998

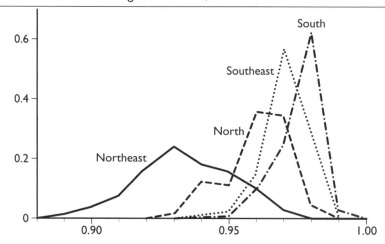

where d is a function of u and ε. The graph in Figure 3 presents d for values of $\varepsilon = 1.5, 2, 3, 5$ and 9 for u ranging between 0.8 and 0.99.

With data for the survival probabilities in the micro regions of Brazil (Simões 2000), it is possible to compute the values of H for each region[10] and for the whole country. It is also possible to assume that the distributions in each region have approximately a Beta distribution and use formula (4) to do the computations.

The values obtained by application of the expression for H, formula (2) are:

North: $H = 0.9597$ Neast: $H = 0.9340$

Seast: $H = 0.9708$ South: $H = 0.9763$

Using the approximation from formula (4) the values are:

North: $H = 0.9567$ Neast: $H = 0.9270$

Seast: $H = 0.9695$ South: $H = 0.9744$

The value of H for the whole country is 0.9579. This would correspond to a mortality rate below age one of 0.0421 for 1998, or 42.1 per thousand. The estimated value for this year is approximately 33.7 per thousand. The 25% larger value obtained from H is due to the great dispersion of the values. The difference between the observed (average) value and H can be used in itself as an inequality measure.[11]

The differences for the values obtained by direct computation and by supposing a Beta distribution for the values in each region are all fairly small.[12]

Figure 3   Values of d of formula (4) for u ranging between 0.8 and 0.99 and for $\varepsilon = 1.5, 2, 3, 5$ and 9

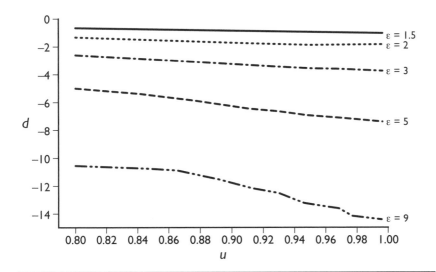

In other situations it is possible to model survival probabilities using socioeconomic (and other types of) covariates. For measures like H it may then be possible to express the health status of populations taking into account level and dispersion as a function of these covariates. This is a promising area for searching for meaningful interventions related to these covariates, which will (in a hopefully known way) affect the value of H in a given population.[13]

Notes

1 For example, Murray and Lopez (1996) and Field and Gold (1998).

2 Wagstaff et al. (1991) as well as Mackenbach and Kunst (1997).

3 For a mathematically rigorous treatment of these two approaches, see Cowell (1998).

4 Cowell (1998), pp. 1–4, refers to these as the Irene-Janet and the parade approaches.

5 A third way of devising meaningful measures should be mentioned, the "welfare-theoretic", Cowell (1998).

6 The measure there is called DALE: Disability Adjusted Life Expectancy.

7 This is not the same as a "Rawlsian" or minimax approach. See Rawls (1971), Lindholm et al. (1996) and Sen (1997).

8 Some people might not feel comfortable with this axiom since it postulates that the population health measure would increase even if only the largest x_i increases, and they would probably prefer to consider a much weaker property, which could be called *property of population gain*. In the case of health status, this is equivalent to requiring that the summary health measure in the population increases only if there is a gain for all individuals. This, jointly with *A1*, could perhaps be called a *strong equity property*.

9 There are also weaker versions of scale and translation invariance that require only that the order of the H's be preserved under the respective transformations.

10 See Figure 2. The micro regions of the states of Mato Grosso, Goiás and the Federal District were included in the Southeastern region, and those of the state of Tocantins in the Northern region.

11 Deaton (1997), page 136ff., for example.

12 All the values computed from the Beta distribution are slightly smaller. They would be closer to the actual values if the sizes of each micro region had been taken into account for the computations. This would make the variances smaller since each value is repeated several times. With smaller variances the values from formula (4) would be bigger and the differences between the two methods smaller.

13 This would be the case for child survival functions that could be modelled using survival analysis models. See for example the work of Wagstaff (1999).

REFERENCES

Braveman P, Krieger N, Lynch J (2000) Health inequalities and social inequalities in health. *Bulletin of the World Health Organization,* 78(2):232–233.

Cowell FA (1998) Measurement of inequality. DARP discussion paper no 36. In: *Handbook of income distribution.* Atkinson AB, Bourguignon F, eds. London School of Public Health, Distributional Analysis Research Programme, London.

Deaton A (1997) *The analysis of household surveys: a microeconomic approach to development policy.* The Johns Hopkins University Press, Baltimore, MD.

Field MJ, Gold MR, eds. (1998) *Summarizing population health: directions for the development and application of population metrics.* National Academy Press, Washington, DC.

Lindholm L, Rosén M (1998) On the measurement of the nation's equity adjusted health. *Health Economics,* 7(7):621–628.

Lindholm L, Rosén M, Emmelin M (1996) An epidemiological approach towards measuring the trade-off between equity and efficiency in health policy. *Health Policy,* 35(3):205–216.

Mackenbach JP, Kunst AE (1997) Measuring the magnitude of socio-economic inequalities in health: an overview of available measures illustrated with two examples from Europe. *Social Science and Medicine,* 44(6):757–771.

Murray CJL, Gakidou E, Frenk J (1999) Health inequalities and social group differences: what should we measure? *Bulletin of the World Health Organization,* 77(7):537–543.

Murray CJL, Lopez AD, eds. (1996) *The global burden of disease: a comprehensive assessment of mortality and disability from diseases, injuries and risk factors in 1990 and projected to 2020.* Global Burden of Disease and Injury, Vol. 1. Harvard School of Public Health on behalf of WHO, Cambridge, MA.

Rawls J (1971) *A theory of justice.* Harvard University Press, Cambridge, MA.

Sen A (1997) *On economic inequality. (Expanded edition with substantial annex by JE Foster and A Sen).* Clarendon Press, Oxford.

Simões CC (2000) *Estimativas da mortalidade infantil por microregiõs e municipios. [In Portugese].* Ministério da Saúde, Brasilia.

Wagstaff A (1999) *Inequalities in child mortality in the developing world. How large are they? How can they be reduced?* (April, 19–23. Ninth Annual Public Health Forum.) London School of Hygiene and Tropical Medicine, London.

Wagstaff A, Paci P, van Doorslaer E (1991) On the measurement of inequalities in health. *Social Science and Medicine,* 33(5):545–557.

Chapter 3.9

LEVELS OF HEALTH AND INEQUALITY IN HEALTH

MICHAEL C. WOLFSON

As I noted in chapter 2.2, by far, the most fundamental use of summary measures of population health (SMPH) is to shift the centre of gravity of health policy discourse towards the basic objective of health policy, namely improving the health of the population. Without valid and broadly accepted measures of health, it is much more difficult to focus resources and activities in ways that have the most beneficial impact in improving health. And analogously with the economy and incomes, there are always concerns about both the average levels of health in the population and the pattern or distribution of health among individual members of the population. A fundamental question of indicator design is how to measure not only levels, but also dispersion or inequalities in health.

As part of the discussion at the conference that gave rise to this volume, objections were raised that this question had already been answered. SMPH, it was claimed, by their very nature, already embodied—indeed even obfuscated—strong normative judgements about the distribution of health.

As a matter of arithmetic, it is absolutely correct that any given SMPH defines an "equivalence class" where distributional changes have no effect. For example, given all the specific details of the micro-level descriptive system, the micro-level valuation function, and the macro-level aggregation formula (see chapter 2.2), an infinite range of examples can be constructed in accord with the following: reducing person i's health by x, and increasing person j's health by y, leaves the arithmetical value of the SMPH unchanged.

However, this criticism can equally be levelled at many other widely used measures such as GDP per capita, average family income, or the increase in government revenue associated with a particular tax change. The overwhelming response, both by statistical systems and by policy analysts, is not to throw out these measures. Rather, it is to complement them with other measures, such as regional differences in GDP per capita, or decile shares for family income, or average tax changes by age group and family type. There is a long history in economics, for example, of distinguishing the "size of the pie" from the way it is divided.

In an exactly analogous fashion, concerns about the distribution of health are far better handled by producing a complementary range of indicators, not by abandoning SMPH as hopelessly value laden or confounded with implicit distributional assessments.

It is very important to reinforce, in this connection, the idea of conceiving SMPH in conjunction with their requisite underlying data systems. We know right from the beginning that discussion of the trends or patterns for any given SMPH will quickly and legitimately also raise distributional questions. As a result, the underlying data systems should be designed not only to support the construction of the SMPH in question, but also to enable a range of analyses of distributional matters. This should not be too difficult if the underlying population survey data on health status, for example, are available as (appropriately non-identifiable) micro data sets to researchers and policy analysts.

Still, it is important to recognize that SMPH are much more complex indicators than, say, average family income. As noted in chapter 2.2, SMPH require three major components: a micro-level descriptive system, a micro-level valuation function, and a macro-level aggregation formula. Some of the concerns raised during the conference about the value judgements implicit in any given SMPH relate primarily to the micro-level valuation function, for example whether it is based on an individual perspective (e.g. time trade-off) or on social choice-based questions (e.g. person trade-off). My sense is that for the purposes for which we wish to use SMPH, it would be best if a process of internationally coordinated research and consensus building could arrive at an agreed approach. Nevertheless, it would still be important, from time to time, to estimate individuals' summary health status (i.e. the result of applying the micro-level valuation function to the micro-level descriptive system for a representative sample of the population) using several reasonable alternative methods or valuation frameworks, and then to conduct sensitivity analyses to assess the implications for overall SMPH results.

Such sensitivity analyses would address concerns of the following form: "I do not agree that raising person i's health status (HS) level from 0.6 to 0.8 is equivalent to raising person j's HS from 0.3 to 0.5." These concerns, while possibly well founded, are not concerns about equity or the measurement of inequality. They are more basic concerns about the reasonableness of the underlying micro-level valuation function itself.

On the other hand, assuming agreement on the micro-level descriptive system and valuation function, there is considerable room for a wide range of health inequality indicators. As a first pass at a taxonomy, we can divide inequality measures into a univariate or marginal group on the one hand, and a bivariate or conditional group on the other. The first group conceives of health inequality like income inequality—some people are healthier than others, and the key question is how dispersed are individuals along a (uni-dimensional) spectrum of health status.

The bivariate or conditional approach, on the other hand, focuses on the more widely held view that inequalities in health involve at least two variables, health status plus some other characteristic like income. The most common expression of this view is the observation that high income individuals tend to be healthier than lower income individuals. Indeed, there is overwhelming evidence that there is a socioeconomic gradient in health status—whether socioeconomic status (SES) is measured in terms of income, education, or occupation, and health is measured in terms of self-report, clinical disease incidence or prevalence, or mortality—that every step up the socioeconomic spectrum is accompanied by an improvement in health, with strong evidence of causality running from SES to HS, though not exclusively so.

For convenience, let me refer to this latter conception of health inequality as the bivariate view. In this case, indicators of inequality turn not so much on the marginal distribution of health (i.e. the univariate view), irrespective of socioeconomic status, but rather on the extent of correlation between SES and health.

Another way to split health inequality indicators is between (direct) cross-sectional and (synthetic) cohort approaches. Cross-sectional indicators are based directly on survey results and/or mortality rates, and are not in the same class as SMPH. Examples would include the dispersion of age-standardized mortality rates across sub-national geographic areas for a univariate measure, and graphs of the "gradient" showing the pattern of average health status by income range based on results from a health survey for a bivariate measure.

Cohort indicators, in contrast, are in the same class as SMPH. These could be univariate, for example based on a set of life expectancies estimated from mortality rate quantiles, which in turn were based on small area variations in age-specific mortality rates (Rowe 1988). Or they could be bivariate, for example based on disability-free or health-adjusted life expectancies (DFLEs or HALEs) for income or educational quartiles (e.g. Nault et al. 1996; Wilkins and Adams 1983). Note that at the moment, we are leaving aside the question of which summary measure or statistic, like the Gini coefficient, would be used. Rather, we are focusing on the quantities over which such a summary statistic would be computed. Indeed, in many cases, it is more useful not to bother computing a statistic like the Gini coefficient, and instead to inform the discussion of inequality using something like a graphical display of quintile shares (univariate or marginal approach), or a histogram of DFLEs or HALEs by SES group (bivariate or conditional approach).

In turn, the cohort approach can be broken down by the manner in which the results are estimated, and the kinds of data on which they draw. This variety of cohort methods also pertains to the macro-level aggregation formula used for the SMPH itself. There is a range of possibilities here:

- The Sullivan method based on mortality rates and health state prevalences, versus a method drawing on longitudinal data which allow direct estimation of health state dynamics.

- Among the latter, methods using first order versus higher order (i.e. more lags) in the transition dynamics.

- Methods using unconditional (e.g. mortality as a function of age and sex only), or conditional transition dynamics (e.g. mortality as a function not only of age and sex, but also prior health status, and possibly SES).

- Methods focusing directly on outcomes (e.g. deaths, a given health state), versus those focusing on the *risks* or predispositions of outcomes.

Essentially, a univariate approach to health inequality would be based on a sample of life table results representing the observed variability in the underlying prevalences or transition rates in a population in a given time period, while a bivariate approach would condition the sample of life tables on another important factor like SES. Gakidou et al. (2000), for example, argue for and develop the concepts for a univariate version of the latter most challenging kind of cohort measure, focusing on heterogeneities in health risks over the life course. They propose a specific method for doing so. We have elsewhere criticized this approach and proposed an alternative (Wolfson and Rowe 2001).

At the least, this variety of views on the basic concepts of health, the methods for constructing cohort measures, and the form of health inequality (univariate versus bivariate), plus the fundamental importance of the core question of health inequality, means that a range of indicators should be conceived, articulated, and estimated. To be coherent and meaningful, these inequality indicators can and should build on the same underlying data systems and framework as SMPH, especially the micro level descriptive system and valuation function. But they are necessarily complementary to, and not subsumed in, the SMPH.

References

Gakidou EE, Murray CJL, Frenk J (2000) Defining and measuring health inequality: an approach based on the distribution of health expectancy. *Bulletin of the World Health Organization,* **78**(1):42–54.

Nault F, Roberge R, Berthelot JM (1996) Espérance de vie et espérance en santé selon le sexe, l'état matrimonial et le statut socio-économique au Canada. *Cahiers Québécois de Démographie,* **25**(2):241–259.

Rowe G (1988) *Mortality risk distributions: a life table analysis.* (Research paper series no 19.) Statistics Canada, Analytical Studies Branch, Ottawa, Ontario.

Wilkins R, Adams O (1983) Health expectancy in Canada, late 1970's: demographic, regional and social dimensions. *American Journal of Public Health,* **73**(9):1073–1080.

Wolfson MC, Rowe G (2001) On measuring inequalities in health. *Bulletin of the World Health Organization,* **79**(6):553–560.

Chapter 4.1

HEALTH EXPECTANCIES: AN OVERVIEW AND CRITICAL APPRAISAL

COLIN D. MATHERS

INTRODUCTION

In the last two decades, there has been a considerable international effort to develop summary measures of population health that integrate both mortality and non-fatal health outcomes, and international policy interest in such indicators is increasing. As a result, two major classes of summary measures have been developed: health expectancies, such as disability-free life expectancy; and health gaps, such as disability-adjusted life year (DALY). This chapter describes the concept of health expectancy, a taxonomy of the types of health expectancy and an overview of methods of calculation.

Health expectancy is a generic term for all population indicators that estimate the average time (in years) that a person could expect to live in various states of health. Health expectancies may relate to defined states of health (breaking up the continuum of health into dichotomous or polychotomous states), or to equivalent years of good health (using health state valuations to calculate health-adjusted life expectancies, or disability-adjusted life expectancies). The best known example of a dichotomous health expectancy is the disability-free life expectancy at birth. This measure estimates the average expected years of life "free of disability" for a newborn in a population, if current disability and mortality conditions continue to apply. The best known example of a health-adjusted life expectancy is healthy life expectancy (HALE) calculated for 191 countries by the World Health Organization for 1999 (WHO 2000) and 2000 (WHO 2001a). This measure estimates the average equivalent "healthy" expected years of life for a newborn in a population, if current disability and mortality conditions continue to apply.

This chapter also examines issues in the conceptualization, measurement and valuation of health status that must be addressed before using health expectancies as summary measures of population health. Some major methodological and empirical issues are identified that must be considered before developing a standard approach to estimating health expectancies for populations.

Finally, the chapter includes a critical comparison of health expectancy indicators against the desirable criteria for summary measures of population health proposed by Murray et al. (2000) and proposes a health expectancy indicator that meets all these criteria.

BACKGROUND

The concept of combining population health state prevalence data with mortality data in a lifetable to generate estimates of expected years of life in various health states was first proposed in the 1960s (Sanders 1964) and developed in the 1970s (Sullivan 1966; 1971). The disability-free life expectancy (DFLE) was calculated for a number of countries during the 1980s and an international research network, the Network on Health Expectancy (Réseau Espérance de Vie en Santé, or REVES), was established in 1989 (Mathers and Robine 1993). The objectives of REVES are to promote the use of health expectancy as an indicator of population health and as a tool for health planning. REVES has focused its efforts on harmonizing calculation methods and identifying conditions necessary for comparing health expectancy estimates, both across populations and over time (Bone 1992; Mathers and Robine 1993).

Since the late 1980s, there has been a dramatic increase in the number of health expectancy calculations carried out, almost all using the Sullivan method (Robine et al. 1999). Proceedings of several REVES meetings have been published (Robine et al. 1992; 1993; Mathers et al. 1994) and REVES has also produced bibliographies and statistical yearbooks summarizing the available health expectancy calculations (Robine et al. 1999). In 1993, Organisation of Economic Co-operation and Development (OECD) included disability-free life expectancy among the health indicators reported in its health database (OECD 1993) and by 1999 the number of OECD countries for which some estimates of disability-free life expectancy were available had grown to 12 (OECD 1999). Overall, estimates of dichotomous health expectancies (disability-free life expectancy or life expectancy in good health) are now available for 49 countries (Robine et al. 1999). In the year 2000, the World Health Organization published first estimates of disability-adjusted life expectancy (DALE) for 191 countries in 1999 (WHO 2000) and has recently updated these estimates for the year 2000 using information from the Global Burden of Disease Study and from health surveys carried out in 63 countries (WHO 2001a).

The recent growth in interest in health expectancy indicators at national and international level reflects the fact that health expectancies are easily comprehensible indicators that combine both mortality and morbidity into a single composite indicator. They are thus a very attractive tool for summarizing and comparing levels of population health, for monitoring long-term trends in the evolution of population health and, in particular, for addressing the issue of compression or expansion of morbidity.

Three major hypotheses have been advanced for the evolution of population health in countries where birth and death rates are low and death rates continue to fall, particularly at older ages, with consequent increasing life expectancies. The first hypothesis, compression of morbidity, was proposed by Fries (1989) who suggested that adult life expectancy is approaching its biological limit. As a result, if the incidence of incapacitating disease can be postponed to later ages, then morbidity will be compressed into a shorter period of life. The second hypothesis, expansion of morbidity (Gruenberg 1977; Kramer 1980), postulates that the decline in mortality is due to decreasing case-fatality rates for diseases and not to a reduction in their incidence or progression. Consequently, the decline in mortality is accompanied by an increase in chronic illness and disability. Further arguments have been developed from evolutionary biology that support this second hypothesis (Olshansky et al. 1991). The third hypothesis was proposed by Manton (1982; 1987), who suggested that the decline in mortality may be partly due to decreased fatality rates, but at the same time the incidence and progression of chronic diseases may be decreasing, leading to a dynamic equilibrium.

Attempts have been made to use time series measures of health expectancy to test these hypotheses (Robine et al. 1996; 1999). Despite the growth in dichotomous health expectancy calculations, there are only 8 countries for which time series data are available (Robine et al. 1996), and the lack of comparability of definitions and measurements across countries limits the conclusions which can be drawn. These data reinforce the importance of ensuring that summary measures of population health are sensitive to severity levels of disability and are measured consistently across countries and over time.

Health expectancy indicators are also potentially useful for comparing the health of groups within populations, or for examining health inequality, although again care must be taken to ensure the indicators are comparable. Available comparisons suggest that health expectancies show larger inequalities for disadvantaged population subgroups (e.g. minorities, people with low income or low levels of education) than do mortality or morbidity indicators. Mortality inequalities are compounded by disability and handicap inequalities for such groups (Robine et al. 1996; Valkonen et al. 1994). Recently, Gakidou et al. (1999) proposed a framework for measuring health inequality in populations, based on the health-adjusted life expectancy.

A TYPOLOGY OF HEALTH EXPECTANCIES

HEALTH EXPECTANCIES AND HEALTH GAPS

A wide array of summary measures of population health has been proposed (Murray et al. 2000). On the basis of a simple survivorship curve, these measures can be divided broadly into two families: health expectancies and health gaps. The bold curve in Figure 1 is an example of a survivorship curve $S(x)$ for a hypothetical population. The survivorship curve indicates the proportion of an initial birth cohort that will remain alive at a given age, x. Life expectancy at any age x, (e_x), is given by the area under the curve from x onwards:

$$e_x = \int_x^\infty S(a)\,da \qquad (1)$$

The area A under the survivorship curve represents life expectancy at birth. Health expectancies are measures of this area that weight the area A differentially according to the health states of the survivors. More formally, if we use the same notation as in Murray, Salomon and Mathers (chapter 1.3) for $h_i(a)$, the valuation of the health of an individual i at age a, then we can define a health expectancy for this population as:

$$HE_x = \int_x^\infty \left[\int_0^1 w(h(a))\, h(a)\, S(a)\,dh \right] da \qquad (2)$$

where $w(h(a))$ is the the prevalence density of health state valuation h at age a, normalized so that for each a

$$\int_0^1 w(h(a))\, dh = 1$$

Figure 1   Survivorship functions for a population

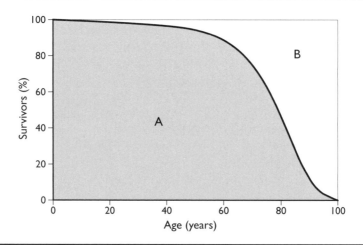

In the most general case, the health state valuation h may be a function of age a as well as the health state defined by levels on a set of health domains.

In contrast to health expectancies, health gaps quantify the difference between the actual health of a population and some stated norm or goal for population health. The health goal implied by Figure 1 is for every-one in the entire population to live in ideal health until the age indicated by the vertical line enclosing area B at the right.[1] The health gap, there-fore, is area B plus some function of area A.

TERMINOLOGY

In the mid-1990s, REVES developed a set of recommendations for termi-nology that has been widely adopted (Mathers et al. 1994):

- *Health expectancy* (HE): Generic term for any expectation of life lived in a defined state of health, whether that is a state of good health (e.g. disability-free) or poor health (e.g. disabled, dependent).

- *Health-adjusted life expectancy* (HALE): Summary measures which use explicit weights to combine health expectancies for a set of discrete health states into a single indicator, indicating the expectation of equiva-lent years of good health.

With the development of health gaps measures in the 1990s, there has been some shift in the use of these terms, and health expectancy is now used to denote the general class of summary measures that relate to the area under the survival curve. It is thus timely to propose a revision of the terminology as follows:

- *Health expectancy* (HE): Generic term for summary measures of popu-lation health that estimate the expectation of years of life lived in vari-ous health states. This includes expectations for specific health states (e.g. disability-free life expectancy) and for "equivalent good health" (e.g. disability-adjusted life expectancy). Health expectancies are mea-sures of the area under the survivorship curve that take into account differential weights for years lived in different health states.

- *Health-adjusted life expectancy* (HALE): General term for health ex-pectancies which estimate the expectation of equivalent years of good health. HALE is calculated for an exhaustive set of health states defined in terms of disability severity. HALEs give a weight of 1 to years of good health, and non-zero weights to at least some other states of less than good health. Healthy life expectancy is used as a synonym for HALE, rather than its previous usage for a health state expectancy for perceived (self-reported) good health.

- *Disability-adjusted life expectancy* (DALE): Synonym for HALE.

Using this terminology, we can categorize health expectancies into two main classes: those that use dichotomous health state weights and those that use health state valuations for an exhaustive set of health states.

Examples of the first class include:

- *Disability-free life expectancy*: This health expectancy gives a weight of 1 to states of health with no disability (above an explicit or implicit threshold) and a weight of 0 to states of health with any level of disability above the threshold. Other examples of this type of health expectancy include active life expectancy and independent life expectancy.

- *Life expectancy with disability*: This is an example of a health expectancy which gives 0 weight to all states of health, apart from one specified state of less than full health (in this case, disability above a certain threshold of severity). If health state 3 in Figure 2 is "moderate disability", then the area under the survival curve corresponding to health state 3 represents life expectancy with moderate disability. Other examples of this type of health expectancy include handicap expectancy and severe handicap expectancy.

Examples of the second class include:

- *Health-adjusted life expectancies*: These have been calculated for Canada and Australia using population survey data on the prevalence of disability at four levels of severity, together with more or less arbitrary severity weights (Mathers 1999; Wilkins et al. 1994; Wilkins and Adams 1992). More recently, Canada has produced the first estimates of health-adjusted life expectancy, based on population prevalence data for health states and measured utility weights (Wolfson 1996). The World Health Report 2000 and the World Health Report 2001 (WHO 2000; 2001a) have published estimates of healthy life expectancy (HALE) for 191 Member States.

- *Disability-adjusted life expectancy*: This was calculated for the Global Burden of Disease Study for seven severity levels of disability, using disability weights that reflected social preferences (Murray and Lopez 1996). Mathers et al. (1999) calculated DALE for Australia, using prevalence data and preference weights from the Global Burden of Disease Study and from a Dutch study using similar valuation methods (Stouthard et al. 1997).

HEALTH-ADJUSTED AND DISABILITY-ADJUSTED LIFE EXPECTANCY

Although health states form a continuum, in practice they are generally conceptualized and measured as a set of mutually exclusive and exhaustive discrete states, ordered on one or more dimensions. If we enumerate health states using a discrete index, k, then we can calculate disability- or health-adjusted life expectancy as:

$$HALE_x = \int_x^\infty \left[\sum_k w_{k,a} h_{k,a} \right] S(a) da \qquad (3)$$

If the weight, h_k, for state k is independent of age a, then

$$HALE_x = \sum_k \left(h_k \times \int_x^\infty w_{k,a} \times S(a) da \right) = \sum_k w_k \times HE_{kx} \qquad (4)$$

where HE_{kx} is the health expectancy at age x for years lived in state k.

In terms of the four health states illustrated in Figure 2, if $HE_{1,0}$ to $HE_{4,0}$ are the health expectancies at birth for each of the four states, and we give age-independent weights w_2, w_3, w_4 (less than 1) to the three states of less than full health, then the health-adjusted life expectancy at birth and total life expectancy at birth are given by:

$$HALE_0 = HE_{1,0} + w_2 \times HE_{2,0} + w_3 \times HE_{3,0} + w_4 \times HE_{4,0} \qquad (5)$$

$$LE_0 = HE_{1,0} + HE_{2,0} + HE_{3,0} + HE_{4,0} \qquad (6)$$

Murray and Lopez (1996) presented estimates of DFLE and DALE for each region of the world using Sullivan's method and the severity-weighted prevalence of disability derived from the YLD estimates in the Global Burden of Disease Study. For these calculations, severity-weighted disability estimates were not discounted or age weighted. Murray and Lopez calculated disability prevalences for seven disability classes with an adjustment to allow for independent co-disability between different disability classes. The expected years of healthy life lost ranged from 8% in the Established Market Economies (life expectancy at birth of approximately

Figure 2   Survivorship functions for four health states

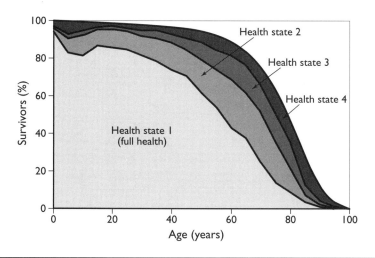

77 years) to 15% in sub-Saharan Africa (life expectancy at birth of about 50 years).

The Australian Burden of Disease Study (Mathers et al. 1999) also estimated the DALE for Australia using Sullivan's method. Total DALE at birth was 68.7 years for males and 73.6 years for females, similar to the values for the EME estimated in the Global Burden of Disease study. Approximately 9% of total life expectancy at birth is lost due to disability for both males and females in Australia, again similar to the 8% lost in the EME. Figure 3 shows DALE (years of healthy life) and years lost due to disability (total life expectancy minus DALE) for males and females at ages 0, 15, 40 and 65 years.

The World Health Organization has published estimates of healthy life expectancy for 191 Member States in 1999 (WHO 2000) and 2000 (WHO 2001a). Healthy life expectancy (DALE) estimates for 1999 were based on analysis of mortality rates, life expectancies and cause of death distributions for 191 countries, together with internally consistent estimates of the incidence, prevalence and disability distributions for 109 disease and injury causes by age group, sex and region of the world, and an analysis of 60 representative health surveys across the world (Mathers et al. 2001, see also Sadana et al., chapter 8.1). Sullivan's method was used to compute healthy life expectancy for males and females in each WHO member country (see Figure 4). After the publication of the World Health Report 2000, a substantial effort was invested in improving the methods and in developing and refining data sources used for estimating healthy life expectancy. WHO has developed a standardized description of health

Figure 3   Expected years of healthy life and expected years lost due to disability at birth, 15, 40 and 65 years of age, by sex, Australia 1996

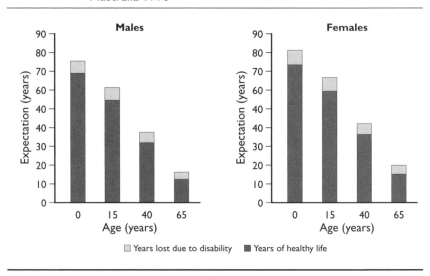

☐ Years lost due to disability   ■ Years of healthy life

states for use in population surveys and health state valuation, together with calibration methods that can be used in household and postal surveys, to improve the cross-population comparability of self-report data (see Murray et al., chapter 8.3). Estimates of healthy life expectancy for WHO Member States in the year 2000 were published in the World Health Report 2001 (WHO 2001a).

A TAXONOMY OF HEALTH EXPECTANCIES

Murray et al. (2000) classified health expectancies in terms of five key aspects:

1. *Cohort versus period measures*: Almost all health expectancy calculations to date have used current population health data to calculate period health expectancies. Long time series of population health data are rarely available and those cohort health expectancies that have been calculated were based on models or projection scenarios (see Murray et al. 2000 for details).

2. *Prevalence versus incidence measures*: There are two main methods of calculation, described below in section 4. The Sullivan method uses current prevalence data for health states; other methods use current transition rates (incidence, remission, case fatality). It has been argued

Figure 4   Disability-adjusted life expectancy (DALE) by total life expectancy at birth, by sex, 191 countries, 1999 (Mathers et al. 2001)

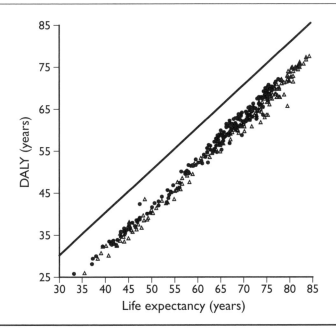

that prevalence is a stock variable reflecting past flows, rather than current health risks (Robine et al. 1992). This issue is discussed in more detail in section 6.

3. *Definition and measurement of health states*: Health expectancies have been calculated for health states defined in different ways. These have included single dimensions of health, such as disease, impairment, disability, handicap, multidimensional health state descriptions such as the Health Utilities Index, and global measures of health, such as self-reported health. Issues relating the definition and measurement of health states are discussed below in section 5.

4. *Health state valuations used*: As discussed above, health expectancies can be distinguished by the type of health state weights used. Dichotomous weights have been widely used for measures such as disability-free life expectancy. Polychotomous or continuous weights are used to produce health-adjusted life expectancies. These weights can be further distinguished according to whether they are "arbitrary" severity weights, or measured preference or utility weights.

5. *Other values*: As noted above, HALEs could be calculated with health state valuations that are age dependent, by allowing health states to be valued differently according to the age they are lived at. Similarly, it would be possible to discount years of life lived at ages further into the future. The Global Burden of Disease study used age weights and time discounting in its health gap measure, the DALY. Lindholm et al. and Lindholm and Rosen (1998; 1998) have calculated a form of health expectancy with equity weights.

METHODS OF CALCULATION

Three methods for calculating health expectancies have been used: Sullivan's method, the double decrement life table method, and the multistate life table method. Sullivan's method uses the observed prevalence of disability at each age in the current population (at a given point of time), to divide the hypothetical years of life lived by a period life table cohort at different ages into years, with and without disability.

SULLIVAN'S METHOD FOR DICHOTOMOUS HEALTH STATE WEIGHTS

Sullivan's method requires only a population life table (which can be constructed for a population using the observed mortality rates at each age for a given time period) and prevalence data for the health state or health states of interest. Such prevalence rates can be obtained readily from cross-sectional health or disability surveys carried out for a population at a point in time. Surveys of this type are carried out regularly in most developed countries. As a result, Sullivan's method has been widely used during the

1980s and 1990s to estimate disability-free life expectancy and other forms of health expectancy.

Sullivan's method uses the life table functions:

l_x the number of survivors at age x in the hypothetical life table cohort

L_x the number of years of life lived by the life table cohort between ages x and $x + 5$

$prev_x$ the prevalence of health state D (e.g. disability) between ages x and $x + 5$ in the population

to calculate:

$YD_x = L_x \times prev_x$ Years lived in state D between ages x and $x + 5$

$YWD_x = L_x \times (1 - prev_x)$ Years lived without state D between ages x and $x + 5$

Health expectancy free of state D is the sum of YWD_i from age $i = x$ to w (the last open-ended age interval in the life table) divided by l_x (survivors at age x):

$$DFLE_x = \frac{\sum_{i=x}^{w} YWD_i}{l_x} \tag{7}$$

Health expectancy for state D is the sum of YD_i from $i = x$ to w, divided by l_x (survivors at age x):

$$DLE_x = \frac{\sum_{i=x}^{w} YD_i}{l_x} = LE_x - DFLE_x \tag{8}$$

Sullivan's method for disability-adjusted life expectancy (DALE)

Suppose we have classified the entire population into a set of $S + 1$ health states as shown in Table 1. These $S + 1$ health states include all people from

Table 1   Classification of population into $S + 1$ health states

	State				
	0	1	2	...	S
Prevalence	D_0	D_1	D_2		D_S
Description	No disability	Disability level 1	Disability level 2		Disability level S

these in good health to those in the most severe levels of disability. Thus, the sum of the prevalences across all states 0 to S is equal to 1.0.

If we have weights w_0, w_1, w_2, etc., measured on a scale where 1 = good health (state 0), then the years lived in good health between age x and $x+5$ are given by:

$$YLH_x = L_x \times \sum_{s=0}^{S} w_s \times D_{si} = L_x \times \left(1 - \sum_{s=1}^{S} dw_s \times D_{si}\right) \qquad (9)$$

Note that if disability weights dw_s are given in the DALY form (0 = good health and 1 = death), then the weight $w_s = 1 - dw_s$ and YLH can be calculated using the second form of the formula. Note that the second formula does not include the disability-free state $s = 0$.

Disability-adjusted life expectancy is:

$$DALE_x = \frac{\sum_{i=x}^{w} YLH_i}{l_x} \qquad (10)$$

This is the same formula as for *DFLE*, except that YLH_x is replaced by the weighted sum of the years lived across all health states.

MULTISTATE LIFE TABLE METHOD

Multistate life table methods for calculating health expectancies were proposed by Rogers et al. (1989a; 1990) to take into account reversible transitions between good health and one or more disability (or other health) states. Their data for persons aged 70 years or more from the US Longitudinal Survey on Aging showed that transition rates from dependence to independence can be surprisingly high, even for the very old. In addition, the multistate life table method allows one to calculate health expectancies for population subgroups in a specific health state at a given age, such as those not disabled at age 65, whereas the Sullivan method gives only the average health expectancy for the entire population at a given age.

The multistate life table generalizes the single state life table, which analyzes the transition from a single "alive" state to the "absorbing" death state, to include reversible transitions between two or more non-absorbing "alive" states. It is theoretically attractive because it is based on transition rates that represent current health conditions (like the mortality-based period life table); it allows transitions in both directions between all states except death; it allows death rates to differ by health state; and it allows conditional health expectancies to be calculated for people in a specified state at a given age.

Figure 5 illustrates the possible transitions in a two-state life table with a non-disabled state (denoted by subscript 1) and a disabled state (subscript 2). The number of survivors in state k ($k = 1, 2$) and age x is denoted by l_{xk}. The transition probability q_x of the single-state life table becomes a transition matrix giving the probabilities of transition between states j

Figure 5   Transitions in a 2-state multistate life table

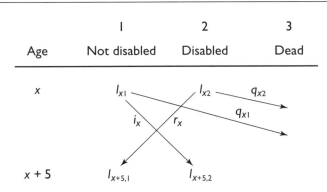

and k in the age interval $(x, x+5)$. The transition probability, i_x, is the probability that a person not disabled at exact age x will become disabled at exact age $x + 5$, and is closely related to the incidence rate of disability for the age interval $(x, x + 5)$. The transition probability, r_x, is the probability that a person disabled at exact age x will be free of disability at exact age $x + 5$, and is closely related to the recovery rate from disability for the age interval $(x, x + 5)$. Once the transition probability matrix has been specified, it is possible to calculate the survivorship functions, l_{xk}, for all ages x, given assumptions about the initial distribution of the lifetable population in the two health states.

Multistate life tables can be either population-based, which assume that the initial distribution of survivors is that seen at the relevant age in the population (Crimmins et al. 1994; 1996), or status-based, which assume that everyone enters the lifetable in a given state (Rogers et al. 1989b; 1990). For a more detailed review of multistate methods see Saito et al. 1999.

DOUBLE DECREMENT METHOD

Double decrement life table methods are based on the incidences of disability or death during the study period (Katz et al. 1983). This method assumes that both the disability and death states are irreversible, so there can only be a transition from disability to death. Thus the disability state used with this method must either be irreversible (e.g. senile dementia), or one where the probabilities of recovery can be assumed negligible. The double decrement method is a special case of the multistate life table method, where the remission rate for the state of less than full health is assumed to be zero.

MICROSIMULATION METHODS

Laditka and Wolf (1998) have applied a microsimulation technique to estimate health expectancies from transition probabilities between health states. The microsimulation approach has similar properties to the multistate method: it is based on transition rates rather than prevalences; it allows transitions from all health states except the "absorbing" state of death; and it allows conditional health expectancies to be calculated. For HALEs based on more than two health states, the multistate life table becomes increasingly complex, and microsimulation methods may be preferable for calculating incidence-based HALEs, or the population-averaged HALE proposed in section 5.

UNDERLYING ASSUMPTIONS AND VALIDITY OF SULLIVAN'S METHOD

A pure cross-sectional indicator is one that summarizes the health experience of a population at a given point in time, in terms of the transition rates or probabilities of changing health state, or of dying. An example is the standard form of period life expectancy, such as the life expectancy at birth for French males in 1996. This indicator gives the expectation of life for a person at each age of their life, based on the risk of dying for that age. Sullivan's method, unlike the standard life table method for calculating period life expectancy, does not produce a "pure" cross-sectional indicator derived from the current health transition rates in the population (Bebbington 1992; Brouard and Robine 1992).

Sullivan's method does not give a pure period indicator because the prevalence rates are partly dependent on earlier health conditions of each age cohort (i.e. the incidence, recovery and state-specific mortality rates applying at earlier times or ages). The prevalence of disability is a stock that is dependent on past history, whereas the incidence of disability is a flow (Brouard and Robine 1992). To construct a purely cross-sectional indicator using Sullivan's method, one would have to use the equilibrium prevalences observed in a fictitious cohort which had always been exposed to the observed cross-sectional transition rates between health states. In an equilibrium or stationary population, where all transition rates are constant over time, Sullivan's method gives the same health expectancies as the multistate methods. The problems with Sullivan's method arise, not because it uses prevalence and mortality data averaged over all health states, but because the data it uses are dependent on past conditions in the population (Mathers 1991).

As Sullivan's method is the only method for which data are widely available, there is considerable concern about potential biases and limitations of the method for tracking changes over time (Barendregt et al. 1994; Bebbington 1992). Mathers and Robine (1997) developed a simulation model using data for France, which allowed them to compare the Sullivan estimate with the pure period estimate from the multistate life table, for a population which has experienced realistic changes in transition rates over time. They concluded that the difference between the estimates produced by the two methods is small when transition rates are changing relatively slowly over time, as postulated by the principal scenarios for evolution of population health; and that Sullivan's method is acceptable for monitoring long-term trends in health expectancies for populations.

Barendregt et al. (1994) also carried out a simulation comparing Sullivan's method with the multistate method. Their hypothetical example was based on a sudden and very large change in survival rates, stable incidence rates and varying prevalence rates, and showed that the Sullivan method was not capable of monitoring the resulting changes in health expectancy. This confirms the conclusion that Sullivan's method is not appropriate for detecting sudden changes in population health. Barendregt et al. (1994) generalized their conclusion to state that Sullivan's method is not appropriate for the analysis of changes in health expectancy over time under any circumstances. However, simulations undertaken by Mathers and Robine (1997) showed that Sullivan's method provides acceptable estimates of the true period value of health expectancy, if there are smooth and relatively regular changes in transition rates over a reasonably long-term period, and in particular, provides good estimates of trends in health expectancy.

DEFINING AND MEASURING HEALTH STATUS

Health expectancies were originally conceived as measures of the expectation of life without disability, handicap, dependency or disease. The most common measures, disability-free life expectancy, active life expectancy and independent life expectancy have all been framed in terms of dichotomous health states, defined in terms of disability (functional limitations) or handicap (role limitations, dependence, restrictions in participation). During its first round of meetings, the Network on Health Expectancy agreed that the WHO International Classification of Impairments, Disabilities, and Handicaps (ICIDH) (WHO 1980) should provide the conceptual framework for the development of health expectancy indicators based on impairment, disability and handicap states. Robine and Jagger (1999) reviewed the ICIDH and other models of the disablement process and noted that there is considerable confusion and disagreement over the boundaries between impairment and disability, and disability and handicap, particularly in relation to where functional limitations and complex activity restrictions fall.

The second revision of the ICIDH, renamed the International Classification of Functioning, Disability and Health or ICF (WHO 2001b) replaces the concepts of disability and handicap by the concepts of capacity and performance and applies these constructs to a single list of activity and participation domains (see Üstün, chapter 7.3). The ICF has been used to design a WHO health status measurement module, which measures performance in six core domains and, in its long form, 16 additional domains (see Sadana, chapter 7.1).

Classification of individuals into health states based on capacity or performance limitations requires a standard classification of limitation severity (including the threshold for any limitation) and a parsimonious set of domains of functioning for which limitations are measured (see chapters 7.1, 7.3 and 8.3). Some surveys use a single global question about performance limitations due to illness or injury (Verbrugge and van den Bos 1996), others use a set of activities of daily living (ADLs), typically including around 6–10 domains. The so-called OECD instrument (de Bruin et al. 1996) provides an example of an instrument which measures disability in relation to specific functions or ADLs.

As well as ADL instruments, some surveys also ask about more complex activities such as housework, shopping, managing money, etc. Such activities are referred to as instrumental activities of daily living (IADL). The Euro-REVES II group (Robine and Jagger 1999) reviewed 16 recent European health interview surveys and found 10 had used an ADL scale to measure functional health. Of the 7 instruments reviewed to date, it was found that not all items were comparable across the surveys, and that the wording of items had been changed beyond changes due to translation. Even with identical survey instruments, self-report data suffers from severe problems of cross-population comparability (see Sadana et al., chapter 8.1) and, apart from the WHO healthy life expectancy calculations, no health expectancies to date have been cross-population comparable.

Mathers (1996a), Nord (1997) and Wolfson (1998) have argued that summary population health measures should relate to a narrower definition of health than total wellbeing. These authors also argued that the conceptualization of health should be restricted to domains, such as impairments and activity limitations that are intrinsic to the person or "within the skin", rather than use dimensions of broader well-being that are determined substantially by the interaction between the individual (and their health) and the social and environmental contexts. Here, "within the skin" includes mental health and function as well as physical health and refers to functioning at the level of the body and of the individual (in the terms used by the ICF).

Any health state measurement instrument that will be used to estimate SMPH should be designed to take the following issues into account:

- *Scope:* the instrument should clearly specify the health domains that are encompassed.

- *Duration:* the duration of disability may be short-term (transient) or long-term (chronic). Most DFLE calculations have been based on prevalence data for long-term disability only. Mathers (1996a) has argued that health status instruments for use with SMPH should not exclude short-term health states.

- *Severity:* measuring the degree of limitation is important, not only for more precisely specifying the health state, but also for defining the threshold for classifying a person as disabled (or in less than ideal health). Much of the lack of comparability of disability prevalence data arises from differences in the threshold level of severity of disability included. Additionally, many ADL and IADL instruments define severity in terms of numerical scoring systems which give arbitrary weightings to the different items and levels.

Threshold issues are of much less importance for severity-adjusted measures of disability that use preference weights. Disability around the threshold will make a much smaller contribution, since the preference weights for mild disability states are extremely close to that for no disability. In addition, most of the variation in self-reported disability associated with changing perceptions and standards arises at the very mild end of the disability spectrum, and the prevalence of severe disability is much less subject to social or temporal variations in perceptions and reporting of disability. Thus, severity-weighted disability measures will be much less subject to the problems of self-reported measures discussed below.

Measured prevalence of disability is also sensitive to the precise wording of the disability instrument and the means of administration (self-completion, personal interview or telephone interview), and it will be important to improve the comparability of population survey data by working towards consistent collection instruments. It will also be necessary to use appropriate calibration tools to deal with the problem of cross-population comparability (see Murray et al., chapter 8.3).

The immediate causes of disability in terms of disease, injury and impairment (and the broader determinants, such as risk factors and environmental conditions) are also of great relevance for policy makers and ideally should be measured in combination with disability and handicap in population surveys or other population health datasets. Population data on the severity distribution of disability associated with specific health conditions would also assist in the consistent calculation of DALYs and health expectancies. It would also avoid the need to include this aspect in the estimation of health state valuations.

One common approach to standardizing health state descriptions is to use a health status instrument that describes health as a profile of levels on a series of domains (Patrick and Erickson 1993). The SF-36 is an example of such an instrument, with eight domains covering self-perceived health, vitality, bodily pain, mental health, physical functioning (mobility and self-care activity limitations), social functioning (participation), role-physical (participation) and role-emotional (participation). The SF-36 domains are scored on a continuous scale from 0 to 100, which results in a very large number of health states. Health state profiles intended for use with health state valuations tend to use a more limited number of levels in each domain.

WHO is developing a standardized description of health states for use in population surveys and health state valuation (see chapters 7.1 and 7.3). The challenge in seeking a standardized description involves trade-offs between completeness of description and parsimony. Other desirable properties include cross-cultural validity, and usability by younger and older adults with widely varying education levels and cultural backgrounds.

To date, few health expectancy calculations have been carried out based on health state profiles. The Health Utilities Index has been used to estimate health-adjusted life expectancy for Canada (Wolfson 1996), and data from 63 countries collected using the WHO health status and valuation modules has been used in the calculation of healthy life expectancy for WHO Member States (WHO 2000; 2001a).

CRITICAL APPRAISAL OF HEALTH EXPECTANCIES

Murray et al. (2000) proposed a set of desirable properties for evaluating SMPH based on common sense notions of population health of the following type:

> If two populations are identical in every way except that infant mortality is higher in one, then we expect that everybody would agree that the population with the lower infant mortality is healthier.

They suggested a minimal set of desirable properties for summary measures that will be used to compare the health of populations:

- *Criterion 1*: If age-specific mortality is lower in any age group, *everything else being the same*, then a summary measure should be better (i.e. a health gap should be smaller and a health expectancy should be larger).[2]

- *Criterion 2*: If the age-specific prevalence of some health state worse than ideal health is higher, *everything else being the same*, a summary measure should be worse.

- *Criterion 3*: If the age-specific incidence of some health state worse than ideal health is higher, *everything else being the same*, a summary measure should be worse.

- *Criterion 4*: If the age-specific remission for some health state worse than ideal health is higher, *everything else being the same*, a summary measure should be better.

- *Criterion 5*: If the severity of a given health state is worse, *everything else being the same*, then a summary measure should be worse.

We briefly assess health expectancies against these five criteria. Health expectancies based on prevalence data (for example, those calculated using Sullivan's method) meet criteria 1 and 2, but fail criteria 3 and 4 (until prevalence rates change to reflect the change in transition rates). Health expectancies based on transition rates (for example, those calculated using the multistate life table method) meet criteria 1, 3 and 4, but fail criterion 2.

Health-adjusted life expectancies (HALE) meet criterion 5, whereas health expectancies using dichotomous health state weights (e.g. disability-free life expectancy) do not. Table 2 summarizes these conclusions.

Table 2   SMPH criteria met by various forms of health expectancies

	Dichotomous weights (e.g. DFLE)	Polychotomous weights (e.g. HALE)
Prevalence-based measures	1, 2	1, 2, 5
Transition-rate based measures	1, 3, 4	1, 3, 4, 5
Population averaged health expectancies (see text)	1, 2, 3, 4	1, 2, 3, 4, 5

Most health expectancies have been characterized by the use of dichotomous health states (e.g. disability-free, with disability). Years of life lived with disability are given an implicit value of zero (equivalent to the valuation of death) for disability above a certain threshold; below this threshold the valuation is 1. This means that the summary indicator is not sensitive to changes in the severity distribution of disability within a population (criterion 5). The overall DFLE value for a population is largely determined by the prevalence of the milder levels of disability, and comparability between populations or over time is highly sensitive to the performance of the disability instrument in classifying people around the threshold.

These problems are illustrated in Figure 6 by Australian estimates of handicap-free life expectancy for 1981, 1988, 1993 and 1998, based on disability prevalence data from the Australian population surveys of disability. The prevalence of handicap increased substantially between 1981–1988, from 9.4–13.7% for males and from 8.7–12.2% for females. It is highly likely that a substantial part of these increases is due to changes in

Figure 6   Trends in disability-free life expectancy (DFLE), handicap-free life expectancy (HFLE), severe handicap-free life expectancy (SHFLE) and total life expectancy (LE), by sex, Australia 1981–1998

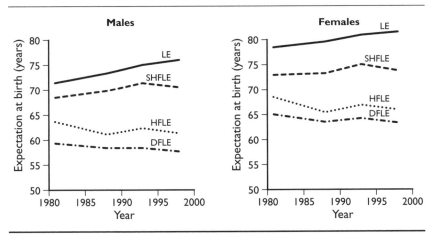

community awareness and perceptions of handicaps, changes in income support programmes, availability of aids, and increasing levels of diagnosis of some health problems (Mathers 1996b). In contrast, the prevalence of severe handicap remained largely unchanged over the period 1981–1993, then jumped substantially between 1993–1998. The latter change is thought to be at least partly due to changes in survey methodology, although the actual questions used were largely unchanged (AIHW 1999).

Murray et al. (2000) have pointed out that no existing health expectancy measure fulfils criteria 2 and 3 together. Prevalence measures are widely recognized as important for planning current curative and rehabilitative services, while incidence-based measures are more relevant to planning prevention activities. While these long-standing arguments have their merits, they do not overturn the conclusion that a summary measure should be sensitive to both incidence and prevalence. Most people would consider a population with lower incidence (but not prevalence) of states worse than full health at a point in time to be more healthy than a comparison population. Similarly, most people would also consider a population with lower prevalence (but the same incidence) of states worse than full health to be more healthy than the comparison population.

Murray and co-authors (chapter 1.2) proposed that some aggregate of cohort or period health expectancies could be constructed that would satisfy all five criteria. In chapter 1.3, they outlined a formalization of individual health, which provides a basis for constructing aggregate health expectancies for populations. In principle, the population health expectancy defined as the average of all the *ex interim* individual health expectancies for the people comprising the population at a given point of time satisfies all five criteria of Murray et al. (chapter 1.2). Ex interim individual health expectancies require assumptions about future incidence, remission and mortality rates that the individuals will face, whereas currently computed period health expectancies provide a measure based only on currently measurable aspects of health. For this reason, we may choose to define and estimate individual health expectancies by assuming that future incidence, remission and mortality rates that the individuals will face reflect current health conditions only. We can then calculate a population-based aggregate health expectancy which satisfies the five criteria.

Suppose that the current prevalence of each health state h in the population aged x is $prev_{hx}$. The period health-adjusted life expectancy $HALE_{hx}$ for an individual in health state h at age x can be calculated from the current transition rates observed in the population in the usual way (this assumes that the individual faces the transition risks at each future age observed for that age group in the current population). Note that $HALE_{hx}$ here is not the same as the dichotomous measure HE_{hx} referred to in equation 4. $HALE_{hx}$ is a measure of the conditional expectation of equivalent years of good health for an individual specified to be in health state h at age x. HE_{hx} is the expected years lived in health state h averaged across all individuals aged x (whatever health state they are in at age x).

The average health-adjusted life expectancy at age x for the actual prevalence distribution of individuals in the population is thus:

$$HALE_x = \sum_h prev_{hx} \times HALE_{hx} \tag{11}$$

where the prevalences are defined so that at each age x,

$$\sum_h prev_{hx} = 1 \tag{12}$$

A summary measure for the population could then be based on some aggregation of the average health-adjusted life expectancies at each age, such as a simple average across all individuals in the population:

$$\overline{HALE} = \frac{\sum_x \left(n_x \times \sum_h prev_{hx} \times HALE_{hx} \right)}{\sum_x n_x} \tag{13}$$

where n_x is the number of individuals aged x. This aggregate measure would reflect both incidence and prevalence and would be age-structure dependent. This summary measure would satisfy all five criteria and would also be easily interpretable as the average expected years of good health (averaged across all people in the actual population) assuming current transition rates remain unchanged.

A summary measure independent of age structure could also be constructed by age-standardizing the age-specific health expectancies. If p_x is the proportion of people aged x in the standard reference population, then the standardized summary measure is:

$$\overline{\overline{HALE}} = \sum_x \left(p_x \times \sum_h prev_{hx} \times HALE_{hx} \right) \tag{14}$$

This measure reflects current prevalence rates in a population, as well as current incidence, remission and mortality transmission rates. Its calculation would require substantially more information than currently available for most populations. It does not, however, require substantially more information than is already required to calculate $HALE$ using the multistate lifetable method or microsimulation techniques.

OTHER DESIRABLE PROPERTIES OF SUMMARY MEASURES

Murray et al. (2000) proposed two other desirable attributes of summary measures if they are to be used to inform policy discussions. These are not attributes based on arguments about whether a population is healthier than another, but rather on practical considerations:

- Summary measures should be comprehensible and feasible to calculate for many populations. Comprehensibility and complexity are different. Life expectancy at birth is a complex abstract measure, but is easy to understand. Health expectancies are popular because they are also easily understood.

- Summary measures should be linear aggregates of the summary measures calculated for any arbitrary partitioning of subgroups. Many decision-makers, and very often the public, desire information that is characterized by this type of additive decomposition. In other words, they would like to be able to answer what fraction of the summary measure is related to health events in the poor, in the uninsured, in the elderly, in children and so on. Additive decomposition is also often appealing for cause attribution.

Most health expectancies satisfy the first attribute. Even the population-averaged health expectancy, HALE, is relatively easily understood as the average expected healthy years of life across all individuals alive in an actual population at a point in time. No health expectancy meets the second additive decomposition attribute in relation to cause attribution. Most health expectancies do not have additive decomposition in relation to population sub-groups either. The population-averaged health expectancy is an exception, as it is explicitly constructed by addition across individuals in the population.

Health-adjusted life expectancies are additively decomposable into health expectancies for specified levels of disability severity (refer to equation 4). This form of decomposition may be useful in understanding whether changes in population health are occurring predominantly at mild levels of disability. Health expectancies for particular health states may be better conceptualized in terms of health state decomposition of a HALE summary measure, rather than as SMPH in themselves. The latter interpretation requires that we accept very unusual dichotomous health state valuations, whereas the former interpretation is closer to the usual ways in which families of health expectancies are presented (e.g. as DFLE together with a set of health expectancies for various levels of disability severity). This interpretation would lead us to exclude health expectancies based on dichotomous valuations from the family of SMPH and see them as components of a health state decomposition of an SMPH.

Health-adjusted life expectancy remains very appealing as a candidate for a single summary measure of population health, even though it cannot be additively decomposed with respect to causes. Wolfson (1998) has outlined a vision of a coherent and integrated statistical framework, with a summary measure of population health status at the apex of a hierarchy of related measures, rather than a piecemeal set of unconnected measures. The macro measures at the apex of the system, such as health-adjusted life expectancies and DALYs, would provide a broad population-based overview of trends and patterns (HALE) and cause-specific summary measures of population health that are additive (DALYs). The health gap measures would be used for quantifying the causes of health losses, for identifying the potential for health gain and for linking health interventions to changes in population health. Such a system should include the capability to "drill down" below the summary measure to component parts such as incidence rates, prevalence rates, severity distributions, case fatality rates, etc. It should also allow us to drill down below the whole of the population level to examine inequalities in health and to estimate the impacts of a given intervention on various subgroups.

CONCLUSIONS

There is rising interest in summary measures of population health among national and international policy makers and health planners. The US Institute of Medicine recently released a report on summary measures, which concluded that "all measures of population health involve choices and value judgements in both their construction and their application" (Field and Gold 1998). Because of their potential influence on international and national resource allocation decisions, summary measures must be considered as normative measures. Great care must be taken in the construction of such summary measures precisely because they may have far-reaching effects.

Health expectancies are very attractive summary measures of population health as they are readily understandable and measured in units (years of life expectancy) that are intuitively meaningful to the average person. To date, the only health expectancies which can be compared across countries are the healthy life expectancies (HALE) published by WHO (2000; 2001).

Most health expectancies are also characterized by the use of dichotomous health states (e.g. disability-free, with disability). This means that the summary indicator is not sensitive to changes in the severity distribution of disability within a population. The overall DFLE value for a population is largely determined by the prevalence of the milder levels of disability, and comparability between populations or over time is highly sensitive to the performance of the disability instrument in classifying people around the threshold. For these reasons, health-adjusted life expectancies are to be preferred as SMPH, and it is probably more appropriate to view health expectancies based on dichotomous weights as components of an additive severity decomposition, rather than SMPH in their own right.

WHO has commenced a major research programme to develop cross-population comparable measures of health status. Further development of this instrument to provide estimates of the average distribution of disability severity for entire episodes of specific diseases or injury (either through longitudinal surveys or through modelling based on cross-sectional data) will enable HALE and DALYs to be calculated in a manner consistent with each other and appropriately used to complement each other in describing the health of a population and the contribution of specific conditions to loss of health.

Notes

1   Figure 1 is only a correct representation of a health gap in absolute terms in a stable population with zero growth.

2   This criterion could be weakened to say that if age-specific mortality is lower in any age-group, *everything else being the same*, then a summary measure should be same or better. The weaker version would allow for deaths beyond some critical age to leave a summary measure unchanged. Measures such as potential years of life lost would then fulfil the weak criterion.

References

AIHW (1999) *Australia's welfare 1999*. Australian Institute of Health and Welfare, Canberra.

Barendregt JJ, Bonneux L, van der Maas PJ (1994) Health expectancy: an indicator for change? Technology assessment methods project team. *Journal of Epidemiology and Community Health*, **48**(5):482–487.

Bebbington AC (1992) Expectation of life without disability measured from the OPCS disability surveys. In: *Health expectancy*. (Proceedings of the first meeting of the international network on health expectancy and the disability process REVES, September 1989, Quebec.) Robine JM, Blanchet M, Dowd JE, eds. HMSO, London.

Bone MR (1992) International efforts to measure health expectancy. *Journal of Epidemiology and Community Health*, **46**(6):555–558.

Brouard N, Robine JM (1992) A method for calculation of health expectancy applied to longitudinal surveys of the elderly in France. In: *Health expectancy*. (Proceedings of the first meeting of the international network on health expectancy and the disability process REVES, September 1989, Quebec.) Robine JM, Blanchet M, Dowd JE, eds. HMSO, London.

Crimmins EM, Hayward MD, Saito Y (1994) Changing mortality and morbidity rates and the health status and life expectancy of the older population. *Demography*, **31**(1):159–175.

Crimmins EM, Hayward MD, Saito Y (1996) Differentials in active life expectancy in the older population of the United States. *Journals of Gerontology. Series B, Psychological and Social Sciences*, **51B**:S111–S120.

de Bruin A, Picavet HSJ, Nossikov A (1996) *Health interview surveys: towards international harmonization of methods and instruments. European series no 58*. WHO Regional Publications, European Series No. 58. World Health Organization, Regional Office for Europe, Copenhagen.

Field MJ, Gold MR, eds. (1998) *Summarizing population health: directions for the development and application of population metrics*. National Academy Press, Washington, DC.

Fries JF (1989) The compression of morbidity: near or far? *Milbank Quarterly*, **67**(2):208–232.

Gakidou EE, Murray CJL, Frenk J (1999) *A framework for measuring health inequality.* (GPE discussion paper no 5.) World Health Organization/Global Programme on Evidence for Health Policy, Geneva.

Gruenberg EM (1977) The failures of success. *Milbank Memorial Fund Quarterly — Health and Society,* 55(1):3–24.

Katz S, Branch LG, Branson MH (1983) Active life expectancy. *New England Journal of Medicine,* 309(20):1218–1224.

Kramer M (1980) The rising pandemic of mental disorders and associated chronic diseases and disabilities. *Acta Psychiatrica Scandinavica,* 62(285):282–297.

Laditka SB, Wolf DA (1998) New methods for analyzing active life expectancy. *Journal of Aging and Health,* 10(2):214–241.

Lindholm L, Rosen M, Emmelin M (1998) How many lives is equity worth? A Proposal for equity adjusted years of life saved. *Journal of Epidemiology and Community Health,* 52(12):808–11.

Lindholm L, Rosen M (1998) On the measurement of the nation's equity adjusted health. *Health Economics,* 7(7):621–8.

Manton KG (1982) Changing concepts of morbidity and mortality in the elderly population. *Milbank Memorial Fund Quarterly – Health and Society,* 60(2):183–244.

Manton KG (1987) Response to "an introduction to the compression of morbidity" by James Fries. *Gerontologica Perspecta,* 1:23–30.

Mathers CD (1991) *Disability-free and handicap-free life expectancy in Australia 1981 and 1988. AIHW health differentials series no 1.* AGPS, Australian Institute of Health, Canberra.

Mathers CD (1996a) *Issues in the measurement of health status.* (Invited paper: 9th REVES work-group meeting of the international network on health expectancy and the disability process, December 1996.) Rome.

Mathers CD (1996b) Trends in health expectancies in Australia 1981–1983. *Journal of the Australian Population Association,* 13(1):1–16.

Mathers CD (1999) Gains in health expectancy from the elimination of diseases among older people. *Disability and Rehabilitation,* 21(5–6):211–221.

Mathers CD, Robine JM (1993) Health expectancy indicators: a review of the work of REVES to date. In: *Calculation of health expectancies, harmonization, consensus achieved and future perspectives.* (Proceedings of the 6th meeting of the international network on health expectancy and the disability process REVES, October 1992, Montpellier.) Robine JM, Mathers CD, Bone MR, Romieu I, eds. John Libbey Eurotext, Paris.

Mathers CD, Robine JM (1997) How good is Sullivan's method for monitoring changes in population health expectancies. *Journal of Epidemiology and Community Health,* 51(1):80–86.

Mathers CD, Robine JM, Wilkins R (1994) Health expectancy indicators: recommendations for terminology. In: *Advances in health expectancies.* (Proceedings of the 7th meeting of the international network on health expectancy and the disability process REVES, February 1994, Canberra.) Mathers CD, McCallum J, Robine JM, eds. Australian Institute of Health and Welfare, AGPS, Canberra.

Mathers CD, Sadana R, Salomon JA, Murray CJL, Lopez AD (2001) Healthy life expectancy in 191 countries, 1999. *Lancet,* 357(9269):1685–1691.

Mathers CD, Vos T, Stevenson C (1999) *The burden of disease and injury in Australia.* Australian Institute of Health and Welfare, Canberra. *www.aihw.gov.au/publications/health/bdia.html.*

Murray CJL, Lopez AD, eds. (1996) *The global burden of disease: a comprehensive assessment of mortality and disability from diseases, injuries and risk factors in 1990 and projected to 2020.* Global Burden of Disease and Injury, Vol. 1. Harvard School of Public Health on behalf of WHO, Cambridge, MA.

Murray CJL, Salomon JA, Mathers CD (2000) A critical examination of summary measures of population health. *Bulletin of the World Health Organization,* 78(8):981–994.

Nord E (1997) *A review of synthetic health indicators.* (Background paper prepared for the OECD Directorate for Education, Employment, Labour, and Social Affairs.) National Institute for Public Health, Oslo.

OECD (1993) *OECD health systems: facts and trends 1960–1991.* Organisation for Economic Co-operation and Development, Paris.

OECD (1999) *Eco-santé. OECD health database 1999.* Organisation for Economic Co-operation and Development, Paris.

Olshansky SJ, Rudberg MA, Carnes BA, Cassel CK, Brody JA (1991) Trading off longer life for worsening health. The expansion of morbidity hypothesis. *Journal of Aging and Health,* 3(2):194–216.

Patrick DL, Erickson P (1993) *Health status and health policy: quality of life in health care evaluation and resource allocation.* Oxford University Press, New York. Robine JM, Blanchet M, Dowd JE, eds. (1992) *Health expectancy.* (Proceedings of the first meeting of the international network on health expectancy and the disability process REVES, September 1989, Quebec.) HMSO, London.

Robine JM, Jagger C (1999) *Developing consistent disability measures and surveys for older populations.* (Background paper prepared for OECD meeting on implications of disability for ageing populations: monitoring social policy challenges.) Organisation for Economic Co-operation and Development, Paris.

Robine JM, Mathers CD, Bone MR, Romieu I, eds. (1993) *Calculation of health expectancies: harmonization, consensus achieved and future perspectives.* (Proceedings of the 6th meeting of the international network on health expectancy and the disability process REVES, October 1992, Montpellier.) John Libbey Eurotext, Paris.

Robine JM, Mathers CD, Brouard N (1996) Trends and differentials in disability-free life expectancy: concepts, methods and findings. In: *Health and mortality among elderly populations.* Caselli G, Lopez AD, eds. Clarendon Press, Oxford.

Robine JM, Romieu I, Cambois E (1999) Health expectancy indicators. *Bulletin of the World Health Organization*, 72(2):181–185.

Rogers A, Rogers R.G., Belanger A (1990) Longer life but worse health? Measurement and dynamics. *Gerontologist*, 30(5):640–649.

Rogers A, Rogers R.G., Branch LG (1989) A multistate analysis of active life expectancy. *Public Health Reports*, 104(3):222–226.

Rogers RG, Rogers A, Belanger A (1989) Active life among the elderly in the United States: multistate life-table estimates and population projections. *Milbank Quarterly*, 67(3–4):370–411.

Saito Y, Crimmins EM, Hayward MD (1999) *Health expectancy: an overview.* (NUPRI research paper series no 67.) Nihon University, Population Research Institute, Tokyo.

Sanders BS (1964) Measuring community health levels. *American Journal of Public Health*, 54(7):1063–1070.

Stouthard MEA, Essink-Bot ML, Bonsel GJ, et al. (1997) *Disability weights for diseases in the Netherlands.* Erasmus University, Department of Public Health, Rotterdam.

Sullivan DF (1966) Conceptual problems in developing an index of health. *Vital and Health Statistics*, (2):17.

Sullivan DF (1971) *A single index of mortality and morbidity. HSMHA health reports.*

Valkonen T, Sihvonen AP, Lahelma E (1994) Disability-free life expctancy by level of education in Finland. In: *Advances in health expectancies.* Proceedings of the 7th meeting of the international network on health expectancy and the disability process REVES, February 1994, Canberra. Mathers CD, McCallum J, Robine JM, eds. Australian Institute of Health and Welfare, AGPS, Canberra.

Verbrugge L, van den Bos T (1996) *A REVES Enterprise: developing a global disability indicator.* (Presented at the 9th meeting of the international network on health expectancy and the disability process REVES, December 1996.) Rome.

WHO (1980) *International classification of impairments, disabilities, and handicaps: a manual of classification relating to the consequences of disease.* World Health Organization, Geneva. (Reprint 1993)

WHO (2000) *The World Health Report 2000. Health systems: improving performance.* World Health Organization, Geneva.

WHO (2001) *The World Health Report 2001. Mental health: new understanding, new hope.* World Health Organization, Geneva.

Wilkins R, Adams OB (1992) Quality-adjusted life expectancy: weighting of expected years in each state of health. In: *Health expectancy.* (Proceedings of the first workshop of the international healthy life expectancy network REVES, September 1989, Quebec.) Robine JM, Blanchet M, Dowd JE, eds. HMSO, London.

Wilkins R, Chen J, Ng E (1994) Changes in health expectancy in Canada from 1986 to 1991. In: *Advances in health expectancies.* (Proceedings of the 7th meeting of the international network on health expectancy and the disability process REVES, February 1994, Canberra.) Mathers CD, McCallum J, Robine JM, eds. Australian Institute of Health and Welfare, AGPS, Canberra.

Wolfson MC (1996) Health-adjusted life expectancy. *Statistics Canada: Health Reports,* 8(1):41–46.

Wolfson MC (1999) Measuring health – visions and practicalities. Joint United Nations Economic Commission for Europe/World Health Organization meeting on health statistics, Rome.

Chapter 4.2

A NEW HEALTH EXPECTANCY CLASSIFICATION SYSTEM

JEAN-MARIE ROBINE

The idea of a health expectancy indicator was first suggested 35 years ago by Sanders, who proposed modifying the life table to produce a new analysis of population health status:

> In such an analysis we would not only determine for each age the probability of survival, but also the subsidiary probabilities of those surviving on the basis of their functional effectiveness. This would range from individuals who are completely dependent on others, even for carrying on their daily living activities, to those fully equipped to carry on with no apparent handicaps all the functions characteristic of their age and sex (Sanders 1964).

In 1971, Sullivan proposed the first method for calculating health expectancies, and in 1989 an international research network (REVES) was set up to promote the use of health expectancy indicators and improve their comparability. Today, indicators such as the disability-adjusted life expectancy (DALE) are widely used sociological tools (Mathers et al. 2000; WHO 2001).

Ten years later, the outcomes from REVES are modest: a first estimation of health expectancy is available for only 49 countries, mostly for developed countries; a chronological series of health expectancies have been produced for only 15 countries; and the health expectancies are not directly comparable from one country to another, because they were calculated using national health surveys with different study designs. This was also a weakness of previous health expectancy estimates (Robine et al. 1999). Only the European Union has estimates that can be compared across countries, based on the European Community Household Panel (Robine et al. 2001).

Even though the WHO mortality database contains vital registration system data for only about 70 countries (Wilmoth 2000), the Global Programme on Evidence for Health Policy, recently established at the

WHO, has used a wider set of data on mortality and comparable disability data for almost 200 countries, allowing

> for the first time, the WHO to calculate healthy life expectancy for the children born in 1999 with the help of an indicator designed by the scientists of the WHO, the DALE (Disability Adjusted Life Expectancy) (WHO 2001).

The new indicator, the DALE, belongs to the class of health-adjusted life expectancy indicators (HALEs), in a previous classification system for health expectancies (HEs) established by REVES for the WHO (Robine et al. 1995; WHO 1995).

This classification system was based on previous work by TNO Prevention and Health (Boshuizen, van de Water 1994), and by REVES (Mathers et al. 1994), whose work distinguished between HEs and HALEs at the same level:

- *Health expectancy* is defined as: "The general term referring to the entire class of indicators expressed in terms of life expectancy in a given state of health (however defined). Health expectancies are hypothetical measures and indicators of current health and mortality conditions. Health expectancies include both 'positive' and 'negative' health states, which may be defined in terms of impairment, disability, handicap, self-rated health, or other concepts. The sum of health expectancies in a complete set of health states should always equal total life expectancy."

- *Health-Adjusted Life Expectancy* is defined as: "A generic term for weighted expectation of life summed over a complete set of health states (however defined). Weights for health states typically range from zero (dead) to unity (optimum health). It is a statistical abstraction based on health expectancies in a number of discrete health states and explicit weights for each of those health states. The weights may be empirically derived, based on expert opinion, or arbitrarily chosen" (Mathers et al. 1994; Robine et al. 1995).

Today, WHO seems to use "healthy life expectancy", "health expectancy", "disability-adjusted life expectancy", and "life expectancy in good health" interchangeably (WHO 2001). Under these conditions, the best means of promoting the use of a common and consistent terminology is to modify the REVES classification system and incorporate health-adjusted life expectancies, especially the DALE, as proposed by Mathers (see preceding chapter). The REVES classification system distinguished between four classes of indicators according to four broad concepts: (1) disease, as defined by the International Classification of Diseases, leading to disease-free life expectancies; (2) disability, as broadly defined by the International Classification of Impairments, Disabilities and Handicaps, leading to impairment-free, functional limitation-free, activity restriction-free and handicap-free life expectancies; (3) the perceived health approach, leading to life expectancies in good perceived health or in bad perceived health; and finally (4) health-adjustment by weighting, leading to HALEs (Robine et al. 1995).

Mathers has proposed that HE be used as a generic term to refer to all four indicators and to subdivide these into two main classes, *health state expectancy* (HSE) and HALE, to distinguish the indicators previously gathered as HEs on the one hand, and HALEs on the other (see preceding chapter). Thus disease-free life expectancies, disability-free life expectancies, and life expectancies in perceived health would be subclasses of the HSE class. The use of the term HSE clarifies the specificity of the indicators previously gathered by REVES as health expectancies.

On the other hand, the inclusion of DALE among the health expectancy classification system would encourage the WHO to use a common language with researchers in the field of health indicators. The new classification system will ensure that WHO scientists realize that the term "healthy life expectancy" (or "life expectancy in good health") clearly refers to a specific health state, "healthy" (or "in good health"), and that it should not be used as a synonym for DALE, or even for HE. The new classification system would also highlight the main difference between HSEs and HALEs. No weighting is involved in the calculation of HSEs, these being simply a decomposition of the life expectancy (LE) into a minimum of two HSEs. Thus, this calculation leads to a family of indicators expressed in years. In contrast, there is an explicit set of weighting in the calculation of HALEs leading to a summary measure of population health, through a transformation of the life expectancy. Thus the health-adjusted life expectancies are expressed in "transformed years" depending on the transformation made. It could be, for example, the "equivalent years of full health" or the "equivalent years without disability".

Rearranging the equations proposed by Mathers in the preceding chapter, we have:

$$LE = HSE_1 + HSE_2 + HSE_3 + \dots + HSE_n \qquad (1)$$

$$HALE = HSE_1 + w_2 \times HSE_2 + w_3 \times HSE_3 + \dots + w_n \times HSE_n \qquad (2)$$

where $w_2, w_3, \dots w_n$ are weights below 1 for the states, HSE_2, HSE_3,... HSE_n, of less than full health.

The equations clearly show that a HSE is an additive decomposition of LE, leading to a family of indicators expressed in years; and that HALE is a transformation of LE that produces a new indicator expressed in "weighted years", and which summarizes the different HSEs.

HEALTH STATE EXPECTANCIES

The use of current health state prevalences allows the number of years lived at different ages by the population of the period life table to be decomposed into the numbers of years lived in the different health states, from which health state expectancies can be calculated. In the same way that a specific weighting does not need to be given to men and women to count how many men or women are in a population, no weighting needs be given to the health state to compute health state expectancies.

To obtain a health state expectancy, the period life expectancy in a minimum of two health state expectancies needs to be decomposed, leading to a family of at least three indicators: the life expectancy and its two components. Examples of simple decomposition are disability-free life expectancy (DFLE) and life expectancy with disability (LEWD), or life expectancy in good perceived health (LEGPH) and life expectancy in bad perceived health (LEBPH). Thus:

$$\text{DFLE} + \text{LEWD} = \text{LE} \text{ and } \text{LEGPH} + \text{LEBPH} = \text{LE} \qquad (3)$$

In fact, life expectancy is often decomposed into more than two components by the use of severity levels. For example, LEWD may be broken down into life expectancy with severe disability (LEWsD) and life expectancy with light or moderate disability (LEWlmD):

$$\text{DFLE} + \text{LEWlmD} + \text{LEWsD} = \text{LE} \qquad (4)$$

Most of the time, ratios of health state expectancy to life expectancy are computed in addition to calculating health state expectancies themselves. These ratios give the proportion of life expectancy lived in the studied health states. For example, DFLE/LE gives the proportion of life expectancy lived free of disability.

Lastly, life expectancy is often decomposed according to different sets of health states illustrating different approaches to health or different concepts, leading to a large family of indicators.

This family of indicators aims to answer practical questions. Is the increase of life expectancy accompanied by an increase of the time lived with disability? Is the DFLE increasing faster than LE, leading to a compression of the time lived with disability? Is the time lived in the different disability states (light, moderate or severe) evolving in the same way, leading to a redistribution of the time lived with disability between the different severity levels. Answering these three questions would allow us to differentiate between the main hypotheses concerning the evolution of the population health, while mortality continues to decline, particularly at old ages. The hypotheses are the "pandemic of mental disorders and disabilities" (Gruenberg 1977; Kramer 1980); the "compression of morbidity" (Fries 1980); and the "dynamic equilibrium" (Manton 1982).

Health state expectancies aim also to assess differentials in the evolution of LE, DFLE and life expectancy without chronic disease (WHO 1984), and also in the evolution of life expectancy without functional limitation, and life expectancy without activity restriction (Robine et al.

2000b). The disablement process, from accidents or chronic diseases to activity restrictions and social participation limitations, is quite complex. Interventions to stop it can take place at different levels. Thus an increase in the time lived with functional limitation is not necessarily followed by an increase in the time lived with activity restriction or social participation limitation. Another question is whether or not an increase in the time lived without disability is accompanied by an increase in the time lived in good perceived health, a closer indication of individual satisfaction. Thus, the goal of health state expectancies is clearly to monitor health transitions at work through its different components: mortality/longevity, measured or reported morbidity, functional limitation at the body level, activity restriction in daily life (i.e. in the daily environment), and perceived health.

The period life table offers a strong conceptual and statistical framework allowing the design of a complete family of integrated indicators. Thus, health state expectancies, together with life expectancy make a coherent set of health indicators to monitor health transitions currently at work in different countries. All the indicators are expressed in years; thus basic combinations, like summation or ratios, are easy to calculate and immediately meaningful.

In the calculation of health state expectancies, the years lived at different ages have the same value and there is no discount for "years of life lived at ages further into the future" (Murray et al. 2000), because the aim of these indicators is to summarize the health and mortality conditions of a period of time. This period characteristic is the essential condition allowing the monitoring of change over time by repetition of the calculations.

In the preceding chapter, Mathers comments on DALE, estimated for Australia, with these words: "Approximately 9% of total life expectancy at birth is lost due to disability for both males and females in Australia..." The estimation commented upon is not a DFLE and cannot be expressed in years, or as a proportion of the life expectancy. It should be understood that: "Approximately the equivalent in full health of 9% of the duration of life expectancy at birth is lost due to disability..." (Mathers, chapter 4.1). In fact, if the mean value of a year lived with disability is half the value of a year of full heath, 18% of life expectancy is lived with disability to get this 9% Figure; and if the mean value of a year with disability is one-third of the value of a year of full heath, which is more probable, 27% of the life expectancy is lived with disability.[1]

Mathers also refers and discusses criteria for evaluating summary measures of population health proposed by Murray et al. (2000). In doing this, it is important to remember that population statistics combine flows and stocks and that the condition *ceteris paribus* cannot apply at the same time for the flows and the depending stocks. In demography, for instance, the population depends on births, migrations and deaths and if age-specific mortality rates decrease (criterion 1 of Murray), *ceteris paribus*, (i.e. no change for migrations and births), the population will change: bigger size, more elderly, or more sick people, for example. In the same way in epidemiology, the prevalence depends on incidence, recovery and lethality, and if the prevalence of some state of health changes (criteria 2 of Murray), at least one flow must change. These remarks equally apply to the other criteria.

Lastly, Mathers computes an "average health-adjusted life expectancy", taking into account the age structure of the population and leading to a Figure corresponding to an average person in a population which satisfies all the criteria. This proposal may be somewhat provocative and needs to be carefully assessed since the main advantage of LE over any other population mortality indicator is that it is independent of any age structure. This allows a direct comparison of the mortality conditions from one country to another. On the other hand, other population mortality indicators have to be standardized on a common age structure standard to be comparable.

Despite these criticisms, the inclusion of HALEs, such as DALE, in the REVES health expectancy classification system is welcome and it should promote the use of a more consistent terminology among the WHO scientists and other researchers working in the field of health indicators.

NOTES

1   The World Health Organization makes the same confusion when commenting its new DALE estimates for all countries of the world: "These lost healthy years range from 20% of total life expectancy at birth in sub-Saharan Africa down to 10% for the low mortality countries in the Western Pacific region, primarily Japan, Australia, New Zealand and Singapore" (WHO 2001). The "equivalent healthy years" are first called "healthy years" and then years of life.

REFERENCES

Boshuizen HC, van de Water HPA (1994) *An international comparison of health expectancies.TNO report.* TNO Health Research, Leiden.

Fries J (1980) Aging, natural death, and the compression of morbidity. *New England Journal of Medicine,* 303(3):130–135.

Gruenberg EM (1977) The failures of success. *Milbank Memorial Fund Quarterly – Health and Society,* 55(1):3–24.

Kramer M (1980) The rising pandemic of mental disorders and associated chronic diseases and disabilities. *Acta Psychiatrica Scandinavica,* 62(285):282–297.

Manton KG (1982) Changing concepts of morbidity and mortality in the elderly population. *Milbank Memorial Fund Quarterly – Health and Society,* 60(2):183–244.

Mathers CD, Robine JM, Wilkins R (1994) Health expectancy indicators: recommendations for terminology. In: *Advances in health expectancies.* (Proceedings of the 7th meeting of the international network on health expectancy and the disability process REVES, February 1994, Canberra.) Mathers CD, McCallum J, Robine JM, eds. Australian Institute of Health and Welfare, AGPS, Canberra.

Mathers CD, Sadana R, Salomon JA, Murray CJL, Lopez AD (2000) *Estimates of DALE for 191 countries: methods and results.* (GPE discussion paper no 16.) World Health Organization/Global Programme on Evidence for Health Policy, Geneva.

Murray CJL, Salomon JA, Mathers CD (2000) A critical examination of summary measures of population health. *Bulletin of the World Health Organization,* 78(8):981–994.

Robine JM, Jagger C, Egidi V, eds. (2000) *Selection of a coherent set of health indicators: a first step towards a user's guide to health expectancies for the European Union.* Euro-REVES, Montpellier.

Robine JM, Jagger C, Romieu I (2001) Disability-free life expectancies in the European Union countries. *Genus,* 57(2):89–101.

Robine JM, Romieu I, Cambois E (1999) Health expectancy indicators. *Bulletin of the World Health Organization,* 72(2):181–185.

Robine JM, Romieu I, Cambois E, van de Water HPA, Boshuizen HC, Jagger C (1995) *Global assessment in positive health.* (Contribution of the network on health expectancy and the disability process to the World Health Report 1995: bridging the gaps. REVES paper no 196.) INSERM.

Sanders BS (1964) Measuring community health levels. *American Journal of Public Health,* 54(7):1063–1070.

WHO (1984) *The uses of epidemiology in the study of elderly. Technical report series no 706.* World Health Organization, Geneva.

WHO (1995) *The World Health Report 1995: bridging the gaps.* World Health Organization, Geneva.

WHO (2001) *Health adjusted life expectancy indicators: estimates for 2000.* World Health Organization, Geneva.

Wilmoth JR (2000) *Berkeley mortality database: overview and future directions.* Max Planck Institute for Demography, University of California, Berkeley, CA.

Chapter 4.3

Health expectancies: what can we expect from summary indicators of population health?

Eileen M. Crimmins

Introduction

Summary measures of population health have been proposed and developed as useful tools for health policy-makers and analysts. The questions policy-makers would like to be able to address include: Is health improving or deteriorating? Do some groups have better health than others? Where can resources be most effectively spent to improve health and to reduce differentials? Has the expenditure of resources resulted in an improvement in health?

The term "summary measures" of population health now appears to encompass all measures that link schedules of age specific mortality and morbidity. The categorization of summary measures into two classes, health expectancies and health gaps, has been a valuable contribution of the WHO work. In chapter 4.1, Mathers provides a clear formulation of the differences between these two classes of measures. Health expectancies attempt to measure the current length of healthy life; while health gaps measure the difference between what is and what the length of healthy life should or could be.

Mathers also provides an insightful summary of the work on health expectancies over the past three decades (chapter 4.1). He highlights the issues that have captured the attention of researchers and policy-makers in the field: how to measure health states, how to value health states, and what methods are appropriate to use in developing summary measures (Bone et al. 1995; Saito et al. 1999). His review clarifies not only the extent of the discussion but the lack of closure on any of these topics.

Mathers ends his summarization of the state of work in this area by proposing another summary measure, after subjecting existing indicators to evaluation using a questionable set of criteria. Certainly, new indicators are potentially valuable additions to existing measures, but no one indicator is going to be useful in addressing all of the questions posed by policy-makers and researchers. In the following sections, I review the health process that we are trying to capture using summary measures of population health and provide examples of the wealth of information that can be developed from a family of summary measures. I argue that a variety of summary measures will provide the most useful set of indicators for both researchers and policy-makers. Summary measures need to be chosen in light of the health problems that are of interest and the potential policies that are being evaluated.

DIMENSIONS OF POPULATION HEALTH

As Mathers makes clear, measurement of health remains a major differentiating factor among measures of health expectancy. Health expectancies have been based on one dimension of health or on many dimensions of health, singularly or combined. There are no strong proponents of the idea that only one dimension of health is appropriate for inclusion in a summary measure of health. There is general agreement that multiple dimensions of health should be included in summary measures, although there is some disagreement as to how multiple measures should be included. Most existing empirical estimates of healthy life expectancy reflect disability-free life simply because of data availability, rather than because of a strong belief that disability is the most important dimension of health. The issue of which dimensions of health are appropriate for summary measures and how they should be combined relates to the questions being addressed, as well as the availability of data.

Classification schemes of the dimensions of health have helped clarify thinking about the process of health change. There is acceptance of the general approach laid out in the ICIDH even though intense discussion of the categories and vocabulary continue. For populations, we generally see health change as progressing from diseases, conditions and impairments to functioning loss, disability or handicap, and then death. This is a loose scheme and does not need to apply at the individual level where some functioning loss occurs without any specific underlying condition, some disability is unrelated to mortality, and death sometimes occurring with no forewarning of disease or disability. Using the words employed both by the ICIDH and North American researchers the dimensions of health could be loosely classified as in Figure 1. All of these dimensions of health might be usefully approached using summary measures.

Figure I

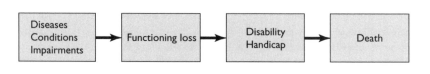

SUMMARY MEASURES

It is possible to develop summary measures by combining all or some of the dimensions in Figure 1 (and other aspects of health) into one index, as has been done in the United States and in Canada (Erickson et al. 1995; Wolfson 1996). It is also possible to develop a family of summary indicators based on the different dimensions of health. These would indicate the length of life with and without disease and with and without disability or functioning loss. Such indicators have been suggested for health monitoring by the European Union (Robine et al. 2000) and a similar series of indicators has been developed for the United States as part of an approach to setting goals for health policy. In this paper I provide examples of the indicators being developed in the US for monitoring health trends and health gaps. These indicators include years with and without diseases (Table 1) and years with and without disability of various types (Table 2).

Table 1　Expected length of life at birth with and without disease: 1994, United States

Expected length of life	Total	Males	Females
Total	75.7	72.6	78.8
Without heart disease	69.0	66.3	72.0
Without arthritis	63.5	63.8	63.6
Without diabetes	72.5	69.9	75.4
Without hypertension	64.8	63.4	66.6
Without asthma	71.5	69.4	74.0
Without bronchitis/emphysema	70.7	68.6	73.1
With heart disease	6.7	6.3	6.8
With arthritis	12.2	8.8	15.2
With diabetes	3.2	2.7	3.4
With hypertension	10.9	9.2	12.2
With asthma	4.2	3.2	4.8
With bronchitis/emphysema	5.0	4.0	5.7

Table 2　Expected years of life at birth free of and with specified types of disability: 1994, United States

Expected length of life	Total	Males	Females
Total	75.7	72.6	78.8
Free of any limitation	62.1	60.3	64.0
Free of major disability	71.5	68.4	74.5
Able to perform personal care	74.3	71.5	77.1
With some limitation not major	9.4	8.1	10.5
With major disability but can PPC	2.8	3.1	2.6
Unable to perform personal care	1.4	1.1	1.7

These examples are offered simply to show the value of a family of measures and the potential for many summary measures to be used in health policy. They are not necessarily seen as the best or most appropriate measures. They are measures which could be developed with available data. As Mathers notes, there is still a strong need for evaluation of the basic health data collected by national and international bodies.

LIFE WITHOUT DISEASE

Measures of the length of life with and without disease are very useful for health planners because most health treatment is disease-based. Major chronic diseases increasingly are treated pharmaceutically from the time of diagnosis until the time of death. Knowing how many years of treatment are likely to be related to diagnosis, and being able to estimate how this would change with changes in mortality rates or treatment and prevention, provides a valuable tool to health planners. In the table below information is provided for both men and women to indicate the size of the gender gap. Based on the population prevalence in 1994 in the United States, the average age at onset of heart disease is 69 and the average number of years lived with heart disease is 6.7 (Table 1). Women and men both experience about 6.5 years of heart disease because women's heart disease has an age of onset almost 6 years later than that of men. The average length of time a person would be treated for hypertension would be about 11 years. Females would require 12 years of treatment for hypertension and men only 9, because the difference in age at onset is only about 3 years. Arthritis is a disease for which both men and women have an average age of onset of about 64; however, because women spend the rest of their longer lifespan with arthritis, the years lived with arthritis for women are almost double those of men.

LIFE WITHOUT DISABILITY

Examination of expected life at birth with and without three levels of disability for the United States in 1994 is shown in Table 2. Disability ranges from mild—having any difficulty in performing any activity because of health—to very severe—being unable to provide personal care such as eating, dressing or bathing. The length of life with these various types of disability ranges from 9 years for the most moderate to 1.4 years with the most severe. Dividing disability into a number of meaningful levels produces a series of measures that can be used to estimate the average length of life with a certain type of care or accommodation needed and the length of life when such care would not be needed.

Some have argued against the use of single disability state-based summary measures because of the sensitivity of the measures to the definition of disability. Certainly all measures reflect only the health levels measured, but a set of disability measures clarifies the length of life in the set of disability states. This may actually be more useful than weighting years of life according to the severity of disability, because the weighting approach does not provide information on the number of years lived in each state which is often useful in estimating needed services or care.

It is also possible to limit disability summary measures to specific life stages and specific types of disability. An example relevant to working life is shown in Table 3. The expected length of life between ages 20–69 with and without disability, divided into years unable to work, and into years when one can work but with some limitation, is calculated for the US in 1994. There is very little gender difference in the length of life unable to work, or in the length of life able to work with limitation during the working years. For both men and women, there are about 4 years when they would be unable to work because of health and about 6 years when they are able to work as long as there is some accommodation in the amount or type of work. Such summary measures for the working years can provide useful indicators for evaluating labour force potential, as well as for evaluating the need for employer and pension plan accommodation.

LIFE WITH HEALTH RISKS

In another approach to summarizing population health, a set of indicators can be built to represent health behaviours or risk factors for the onset of poor health outcomes. Expected years with a doctor visit and without a doctor visit are shown, together with years with and without obesity for the U.S. population in 1994 (Table 3). Both lack of medical care and obesity are risk factors for poor health outcomes, including disease onset,

Table 3   Expected years of life at birth with and without at least one doctor visit; expected life at age 20 obese and not obese[a]

Expected length of life	Total	Males	Females
Total expected life 20–69	42.8	41.2	44.6
Unable to work	3.8	3.6	3.9
Limitation in work ability	6.3	6.1	6.4
Able to work with no limitation	32.7	31.5	34.3
Total expected life at birth	75.7	72.6	78.8
With a doctor visit	58.8	52.4	65.2
Without a doctor visit	16.9	20.2	13.6
Total expected life at age 20	56.9	53.9	59.7
With BMI $\geq$ 25	29.1	32.2	25.8
With BMI < 25	27.8	21.7	33.9

a. Obesity is defined in terms of body mass index (BMI), weight (kg) divided by height squared (m^2), as BMI $\geq$ 25 (kg/m^2).

disability, and death. Summary indicators show that even though men live an average of about 6 years less than women, they average 20 years during their lives with no doctor visit, while for women only 14 years are without a doctor visit (Table 3). If an annual doctor visit is a health goal, this measure clearly indicates the gap between the current state and the goal.

Men spend a greater number of years and proportion of their lives obese than women. On average American men spend 32 years after age 20 with a body mass index higher than 25, a marker for obesity. Women, by contrast, spend an average of only 26 years obese. The public health goal is to eliminate obesity and this summary indicator shows how far the current situation is from this ideal.

The measures above are offered as example of summary measures of health based on a variety of indicators representing a number of health dimensions. Each one provides information about the levels and gaps in population health. All of these measures are based on cross-sectional prevalence of health states and current mortality. As such, they are indicators of the current health state of the population that have been developed for a life table population so that they are comparable across time and place.

POPULATION HEALTH STOCK VERSUS POPULATION HEALTH FLOWS

Population health at any one point in time is defined by the stock of health states among people. This stock of population health, however, is determined by the processes or flows leading to the onset and recovery from diseases, functioning loss, disability, and death. Thus current population health is a stock that is determined by a large number of flows that have occurred over the lifetime of the population. Summary measures of population health reflect the current stock of health if they are based on prevalence estimates. The use of incidence-based approaches to estimating summary measures results in estimates of the implications of the continuation of current flow rates. Like conventional life tables they reflect the life expectancy and the life table population that would result from continued flows into and out of health states. It is unlikely that any actual population will have the health distribution implied for the life table population, just as it is unlikely that any real cohort will experience the period life table experience. This is one reason governments and international agencies have relied on cross-sectional data to provide summary measures of population health. No country currently has adequate data for routinely estimating summary measures of population health with incidence-based data across the life span.

When incidence-based life-tables have been developed, they are often highly parameterized and based on a variety of methodological assumptions. In addition, the inherent instability of estimates based on small numbers of incident events, even with very large samples, makes these methods virtually impossible to use for monitoring population health even if data existed. However, incidence-based life tables are theoretically valuable for indicating the long-term effect of current conditions on population health. They are also valuable as a basis for models that can be developed to examine the process of health change, because they clarify the effect of changes in different aspects of the process of health change. Cross-sectional approaches are of little use in determining explanations for change in population health. Incidence–based models are needed to effectively address health policy by determining the process by which interventions are likely to influence population. This leads to the conclusion that not only are several dimensions of health usefully included in measures of population health, but multiple methods and multiple types of data are also needed for full understanding of the process of health change.

ACKNOWLEDGEMENTS

Support for the work has been provided by the U.S. National Institute on Aging and the AARP Andrus Foundation.

REFERENCES

Bone MR, Bebbington AC, Jagger C, Morgan K, Nicolaas G (1995) *Health expectancy and its uses*. HMSO, London.

Erickson P, Wilson R, Shannon I (1995) *Years of healthy life*. (CDC/NCHS, Healthy people, Statistical notes no 7.) US Department of Health and Human Services, National Center for Health Statistics, Hyattsville, MD.

Robine JM, Jagger C, Egidi V, eds. (2000) *Selection of a coherent set of health indicators: a first step towards a user's guide to health expectancies for the European Union*. Euro-REVES, Montpellier.

Saito Y, Crimmins EM, Hayward MD (1999) *Health expectancy: an overview*. (NUPRI research paper series no 67.) Nihon University, Population Research Institute, Tokyo.

Wolfson MC (1996) Health-adjusted life expectancy. *Statistics Canada: Health Reports*, 8(1):41–46.

Chapter 4.4

INCIDENCE- AND PREVALENCE-BASED SMPH: MAKING THE TWAIN MEET

JAN J. BARENDREGT

INTRODUCTION

Summary measures of population health (SMPH), by definition, combine morbidity and mortality in a single indicator of population health status. Based on this definition a large variety of indicators has been constructed: there are health expectancies and health gap indicators, disability-free and disability-adjusted indicators, for example. Additional variety is caused by the use of weighting schemes for age and/or time (see chapter 1.2).

The resulting SMPH can be classified into incidence- and prevalence-based indicators, and the relative merits of prevalence-based indicators for detecting and monitoring trends in population health status have been the subject of much debate (Barendregt et al. 1994; 1995; 1997a; Mathers and Robine 1997; Rogers et al. 1990; van de Water et al. 1995). However, the issue of incidence- versus prevalence-based indicators has wider implications than just the appropriateness of the indicator for trend monitoring. Incidence- and prevalence-based indicators measure different things (Crimmins et al. 1993). When used for policy-making an incidence-based indicator will, under certain circumstances, induce a different policy than a prevalence-based one. The question is whether this peculiarity is desirable, and if not, avoidable.

In this chapter we examine the difference between incidence- and prevalence-based SMPH, and investigate under what circumstances they produce different results. We argue that the divide between incidence- and prevalence-based approaches forces policy-makers to choose between a current and a future perspective on population health, and that this choice is unfortunate, because both aspects should count and need to be balanced. Investigation of the causes of the difference between incidence- and prevalence-based indicators suggests that a dynamic method is needed to unite both approaches. We conclude by discussing implications of this finding.

Because we use health expectancy for the detailed examples, this chapter is in the Health Expectancies section, but we would like to stress that the arguments equally apply to health gaps.

INCIDENCE VERSUS PREVALENCE

Incidence- and prevalence-based health expectancy (HE) indicators are both calculated using a life table, but of a different kind. Incidence-based indicators use a multi-state life table and data on the transition probabilities between the states. States to be distinguished are at least "healthy", "diseased" and "dead", and the respective transition probabilities are "incidence", "remission" and "case fatality". The multi-state life table is in fact a model of the disease process, and, depending on purpose and data, a more complex model with additional states and transitions may be specified. With the transition probabilities, the multi-state life table calculates the prevalence of the diseased state, which in turn is used to calculate the number of diseased years lived by the life table cohort, from which the HE is derived (see appendix for details).

Ideally, the transition probabilities are estimated on a longitudinal study. But even when such data are available additional assumptions are needed, such as the number of transitions from the healthy to the diseased state and back, that occurs between the waves of the longitudinal study. Lacking longitudinal data it is also possible to estimate the transition probabilities from cross-sectional data, but then assumption of steady state is needed (see below).

Prevalence-based HE indicators start out with a normal life table, which has only two states: "alive" and "dead". Years in the "alive" state are then divided into healthy and diseased years using the observed prevalence of the diseased state. The direct use of observed prevalence in the calculation of the HE is often called the "Sullivan method". The prevalence data are typically measured in a cross-sectional survey.

The incidence-based indicator is more complex and has more demanding data requirements. Either registries with record linkage, or longitudinal studies with a long follow-up period and a sufficient number of waves are needed, while for the prevalence-based indicator a quick (and cheap) cross-sectional survey will do. Despite these disadvantages, researchers often prefer incidence-based indicators because of their specific properties.

STOCKS VERSUS FLOWS

Incidence- and prevalence-based indicators will frequently differ, even when measured on the same population, because different variables are used as inputs. Incidence-based indicators use *flow* variables: the transition probabilities determine the flow from one state to another. Prevalence is a *stock* variable: it is the result of past flows into and out of the diseased state.

The bath tub offers an appropriate analogue. The level of the water, a stock variable, is determined by the flows into and out of the tub (from the tap and drain, respectively). The level of the water at any given moment, however, is determined by the flows of the past: it takes a long time for a bath tub to fill and to empty. A stock variable is therefore in part a historical variable, in that it describes the current situation, but this situation reflects the circumstances of the past. How large the historical part is depends on the relative size of the flow variables to the stock variable: a big drain empties a small bath tub quickly.

The historical part in observed prevalence is what makes a prevalence-based indicator different from an incidence-based one. For an incidence-based indicator a prevalence is calculated in the multi-state life table, based on current flow variables. The resulting prevalence can be called a *synthetic* prevalence, as an analogue to the synthetic cohort that is calculated in a life table from current cross-sectional mortality.

When the past and present conditions are sufficiently the same, incidence- and prevalence-based indicators will produce the same result. In theory, "sufficient" is when the past transition probabilities have been the same as the present for a period of time equal to the difference between the highest age considered in the life table and the lowest age at incidence of the disease (see appendix for derivation). Depending on the kind of morbidity, that may be a long time.

In practice, much depends on the probability of leaving the diseased state. A diseased state with high remission and/or case fatality probabilities will have a relatively small historical part, and will be mostly determined by current flows, and vice versa.

PRESENT VERSUS FUTURE

The synthetic prevalence of the incidence-based method is often interpreted as the future prevalence—the "prevalence expectancy". This interpretation is correct to the same extent as life expectancy predicts the expected age at death of a newborn: life expectancy is a good estimator of expected age at death, if mortality remains constant in the future. But since we expect mortality to decline in the future, life expectancy underestimates the expected age at death.

In the case of disease prevalence we do not have such unequivocal expectations. In many cases, case fatality is expected to decline, with increased prevalence as a consequence. But if incidence declines too, the prevalence may well remain the same or even decrease. When interpreting the synthetic prevalence as the "prevalence expectancy"—the prevalence as it will be in the future—all the uncertainty about the future of disease epidemiology should be kept in mind.

Whether and when this future will arrive depends on disease characteristics. In particular, the trends in the transition probabilities in the recent past (and hence the degree of discrepancy between currently observed prevalence and the synthetic one), and the probability of leaving the diseased state (determining prevalence inertia), are both important. A problem is that the life table method gives no clue whatsoever as to when the future will arrive: it may be anything from tomorrow to many decades from now.

Given this interpretation of the incidence-based indicator as an estimator of things to come, the question arises as to which indicator to use: the incidence-based or the prevalence-based? The consensus is that it depends. Prevalence-based indicators are best for studying the current population health status, because they measure the current burden of disease. In contrast, incidence-based indicators are preferred for assessing which way the population health status is heading, because they measure what the burden of disease will eventually be, even if they do not say how long it will take to get there.

Suppose, for example, that you want to measure the burden of disease of poliomyelitis in a country that introduced comprehensive vaccination 40 years ago. The incidence-based indicator will show that this burden is zero: nobody gets infected anymore. The prevalence-based indicator, on the other hand, will show a burden of disease: there will still be people paralyzed as a consequence of infection among those older than 40 years. The obvious conclusion is that, while poliomyelitis is still affecting population health, as a health problem it is on its way out as long as vaccination is maintained.

In this example, it is relatively easy to see how long it will take before incidence- and prevalence-based indicators are in agreement. Because remission is zero and excess mortality is not very high, the prevalence-based indicator will gradually decline to zero as the exposed cohorts go extinct, which will take several decades.

PRESENT AND FUTURE

While the consensus on when to use which indicator makes a lot of sense, it is still unfortunate that the division into either present or future exists. People care about their current health, but also about their future health. Many forego short-term pleasures in the hope of improving their long-term health. Many treatments involve a short-term deterioration of health, but this decline is offset by the prospect of a future improvement. Assuming people do not care about their future health is saying that we are all like the man who jumps off the 40th floor, and when asked at the 20th floor how things are, answers that he is suffering no ill effects.

On the other hand, the future is not all-determining. Many people do engage in short-term pleasures and ignore the long-term consequences. Painful surgery to prevent a future health problem will be postponed, or even forgone, depending on how distant the future health problem is.

People's health-related behaviour clearly shows that they care about both current and future health, and when the present and the future are in conflict they balance the two. There is empirical evidence that people care more about their health in the near term, than in a far off future, but how much more is determined by a person's degree of time preference. And from the diversity in their behavior it can be concluded that people differ in their degree of time preference.

If people are indeed concerned about current and future health, this should have consequences for SMPH. The goal of such composite health indicators is to summarize population health status in a single indicator that can be used as a gauge for policy-making. An indicator used to steer health policy should reflect people's preferences about health, because such an indicator becomes normative.

In practice policy-making is not just concerned with current population health and health care needs, but also with their development in the near and not-so-near future. For example, when confronted with the prospect of a major new epidemic 15 years ago, many governments mounted big public awareness campaigns against HIV. At that time, the burden of disease of HIV was negligible, as measured by a prevalence-based indicator. It was the expected future burden of disease, calculated with disease models, that prompted governments into action.

On the population level, too, current and future health concerns may be in conflict. For example, preventing HIV from becoming a major epidemic requires expenditures now, which will compete with current health care needs, while the benefits of prevention are many years into the future. When health research is drawn into the equation, the conflict between current and future needs becomes even larger.

In summary, there is a strong case for SMPH that bridge the divide between incidence- and prevalence-based indicators. The health-related behaviour of people shows that they care about their current and future health. The public health policies of at least some governments properly reflect these concerns, but these policies cannot be based on a single SMPH and at least two indicators are needed: an incidence-based one and a prevalence-based one. Moreover, since the incidence-based indicators do not tell how far away in time the expected burden of disease is, it is not possible to explicitly balance current and future population health status.

It is therefore desirable to construct an indicator which includes both the incidence and prevalence perspectives, such that both present and future population health count, and can be balanced against one another using an appropriate rate of social time preference. In the remainder of this chapter we will investigate what such an indicator should look like.

AGE AND TIME

The different results produced by incidence- and prevalence-based indicators originate from the way age and time are handled in the methods. Time and age are often considered synonymous: we grow older in step with the passage of time. Describing a population through time, however, requires separate age and time dimensions. This is best illustrated by the life table method for calculating HE. Life tables can be classified as either "period" or "cohort" tables (Shryock et al. 1976). Cohort tables reconstruct the mortality of a cohort using historical data. For example, the cohort life table of the 1900 birth cohort uses mortality of 0-year olds from 1900, of 1-year olds from 1901, etc. The life expectancy from such a life table is of course not a good indicator of current population health status, because mortality has declined dramatically since 1900. It is possible to use a cohort life table to estimate the life expectancy of the current birth cohort, but then assumptions about mortality up to 100 years into the future have to be made. Most researchers are not prepared to make such assumptions.

To obtain current estimates of mortality, the period life table uses currently observed, cross-sectional mortality. With this current mortality a synthetic cohort is created, synthetic because no real cohort has ever experienced or will experience such a mortality (unless mortality remains unchanged for 100 years, for example). The life expectancy calculated with such a period life table is a better indicator for current population health status, although it probably underestimates the life expectancy of the current birth cohort. As a result the period life table is usually employed for HE indicators.

The period life table has two interpretations (Shryock et al. 1976): the cohort interpretation of the period life table; and the stationary population interpretation. In the first interpretation, the period life table describes a single birth cohort through time as it ages, and the age axis of the life table describes age and time simultaneously. In contrast, the stationary population interpretation considers the life table to describe a complete population at one point in time, and the age axis measures age only. There is no time component in this interpretation. The stationary population method is more appropriate for calculating the HE, because the indicator is intended to reflect the current population health status.

The stationary population interpretation of a life table as a description of the current population fits well with the prevalence-based indicator since the prevalence is currently observed. For the incidence-based indicator things are less clear. As we stated above, the incidence-based indicator is interpreted as saying something about the future, but does not specify how far away this future is. So for the incidence-based indicator the stationary population interpretation of the life table is of a population at some, but not specified, point in the future.

Given that people show time preference in their evaluation of future health, it is important to know how far away this future is. Is it next year, or 50 years from now? If the future is still some time off, the intermediate years become important too. Will current health status gradually evolve into future health status, or will it remain constant and then change suddenly? To evaluate current and future health simultaneously we need an indicator that starts with current health status and then describes health status as it evolves over time. This requires a method that describes a population over time and uses separate age and time axes. In other words, the indicator needs a dynamic population method.

A DYNAMIC METHOD

A dynamic population method can be depicted as a series of linked life tables, one for each point in time. The life tables are linked such that the population at age a and time t depends on the population at age $a-1$ and time $t-1$, and on incidence and mortality between $t-1$ and t.

At $t = 0$ the current population health status is used as starting point. Input is cross-sectional mortality and prevalence of the diseased state. For each $t > 0$ prevalence and mortality are calculated from the previous population, using as input the transition probabilities as they are currently observed (or as we expect them to be in the future).

The result is a stream of future mortality schedules and disease prevalences, from which the HE is calculated for each time point. To evaluate the stream of the current and future health expectancies and allow for time preference, a weighted average is calculated, with weights for future HEs determined by an appropriate discount rate.

This solves the problem of the divide between incidence- and prevalence-based indicators. The dynamic method combines both approaches and adds an explicit way to include time preference. Of course, this latter point introduces the problems of dealing with time preference, such as which discount rate to use and how long the evaluation period should be (Barendregt et al. 1997b; Barendregt and Bonneux 1999). But these are problems shared by all methods that try to deal with time preference, and we shall not attempt to solve them here.

DISCUSSION

The argument above has been restricted to HE indicators as examples of SMPH. The question is whether the conclusions generalize to other SMPH, such as disability adjusted life years (DALY). DALYs are not measures of health expectancies, but instead measure health gaps, the difference between an ideal number of healthy years and reality, see chapter 1.2 and Murray (1994). However, the DALY uses both age and time inputs to described population health, similar to the health expectancy indicator, and the dynamic method described above is also applicable to DALYs.

Using the dynamic method it is possible to merge the incidence- and prevalence-based approaches to a single indicator, that reflects both current and future population health status, balanced against one another using a rate of social time preference. The dilemma of having to choose between a current and a future perspective on population health can thus be avoided, but this comes at the cost of increased complexity and data requirements. The dynamic method needs input data from both the incidence and the prevalence methods, although this is a relatively small increase over the data needed for the incidence method. The increased complexity of the dynamic method is a more serious impediment. It is more difficult to explain and requires far more calculations. The calculations can still be done in a spreadsheet, but it will be a big one. On the other hand, the simplicity of the life table method is rather deceptive. While the calculations may be simple, the problems discussed in this chapter illustrate that the interpretation is not.

We have already noted that the dynamic method has to deal with the problems of time preference, such as which discount rate to use and how long the evaluation period should be. Solutions to these problems are severely needed, but unfortunately these are not in sight.

Is it worthwhile to merge incidence- and prevalence-based indicators? The answer is that it depends. It may be worthwhile when there have been trends in the past, or when there are trends expected in the future. These trends may be such that the incidence- and prevalence-based indicators produce substantially different results. Under these circumstances the dynamic method is able to solve the artificial dilemma produced by the limitations of the life table.

Appendix

A: Life expectancy

Life expectancy is calculated by assigning age-specific mortality probabilities to a "synthetic" birth cohort of (usually) 100 000. The birth cohort is called synthetic because the mortality probabilities used are current probabilities. A real birth cohort would have been subjected to past mortality probabilities that were generally higher than current ones; and a cohort of newborns will face future probabilities that we expect to be lower yet. Because of these changes in mortality, current life expectancy at age 0 will not be equal to the average number of years of life expected for a cohort of newborns.

If we denote the synthetic cohort with l_a, with a the age index and a_{max} the highest age considered, and the mortality probabilities with q_a, then the life expectancy e_a is given by the total number of years to be lived by the cohort at age a divided by the number alive at that age:

$$e_a = \frac{\sum_{a}^{a_{max}-1} 0.5(l_a + l_{a+1}) + l_{a_{max}} e_{a_{max}}}{l_a} \tag{1}$$

Using $l_{a+1} = l_a(1 - q_a)$ we can rewrite (1) to:

$$e_a = \frac{\sum_a^{a_{max}-1} l_a(1 - 0.5q_a) + l_{a_{max}} e_{a_{max}}}{l_a} \qquad (2)$$

Life expectancy is a static estimator: because $l_{a+1} = l_a(1-q_a)$ for all a any change in the current mortality q_a is instantly reflected in the total number of years lived to its full effect. In fact, the life expectancy estimator assumes that the mortality probabilities have been unchanged for at least a_{max} years.

B: HEALTH EXPECTANCY

Health expectancy is calculated by not letting years defined as "unhealthy" count towards the total number of years to be lived. When P_a is the age specific prevalence of unhealthiness (expressed as a proportion) then the health expectancy h_a can be calculated by:

$$h_a = \frac{\sum_a^{a_{max}-1} l_a(1 - 0.5q_a)(1 - P_a) + l_{a_{max}} e_{a_{max}} (1 - P_{a_{max}})}{l_a} \qquad (3)$$

Equation (3) can be used for both the prevalence as the incidence method, the difference is where the prevalence P_a comes from.

C: EMPIRICAL VERSUS SYNTHETIC PREVALENCE

The prevalence method uses empirical prevalence data obtained through a survey or some similar method, while the incidence method uses the prevalence calculated in the life table itself from current transition probabilities. The cross-sectional prevalence for a very simple disease process with incidence I_a and mortality M_a and no cure the prevalence at time t is given by:

$$P_a^t = (P_{a-1}^{t-1} + I_{a-1}^{t-1})(1 - M_{a-1}^{t-1}) \qquad (4)$$

Applying (4) recursively to itself and assuming that prevalence at birth equals zero, we can rewrite (4) to:

$$P_a^t = \sum_{j=0}^{a-1} (I_j^{t-a+j} \prod_{k=j}^{a-1} (1 - M_k^{t-a+k})) \qquad (5)$$

The prevalence as given by (5) is used by the prevalence method. For the incidence method in the multi-state life table the following equations apply:

$$P_a^t = (P_{a-1}^t + I_{a-1}^t)(1 - M_{a-1}^t) \tag{6}$$

$$P_a^t = \sum_{j=0}^{a-1} (I_j^t \prod_{k=j}^{a-1} (1 - M_k^t)) \tag{7}$$

This multi-state disease prevalence might be referred to as a "synthetic prevalence", as an analogue to the life table cohort. Unlike cross-sectional prevalence, synthetic prevalence is not a stock variable, because it is a function of current transition probabilities only and does not depend on past values.

D: Steady state

From (5) and (7) it can be deduced under which conditions the cross-sectional and multi-state disease prevalences at age a and time t will be equal:

$$I_j^{t-a+j} = I_j^t \forall j \in [0 \dots a-1] \tag{8}$$

$$M_j^{t-a+j} = M_j^t \forall j \in [0 \dots a-1] \tag{9}$$

To put it another way: past age-specific transition probabilities must have been equal to the current transition probabilities for, depending on age, up to a years. When a_{min} stands for the lowest age at which incidence occurs this requirement relaxes to $a - a_{min}$ years. Because the calculation of the health expectancy always uses the prevalence of the highest age a_{max} (see Equation 3) this implies that the prevalence-based health expectancy equals the incidence-based health expectancy when age specific transition probabilities have been constant for up to $a_{max} - a_{min}$ years.

E. Dynamic method

The dynamic method uses Equation 4 to calculate disease prevalences for $t = 1, 2 \dots$. At $t = 0$ the observed prevalence is used. Equation 3 then allows to calculate *HE* for $t = 0, 1, 2 \dots$. Then a weighted average $\overline{HE}$ over the stream of *HE*s is calculated using:

$$\overline{HE} = \frac{\sum_t \dfrac{HE_t}{(1+r)^t}}{\sum_t \dfrac{1}{(1+r)^t}} \tag{10}$$

with r the discount rate. Note that this equation requires a time horizon.

REFERENCES

Barendregt JJ, Bonneux L (1999) The trouble with health economics. *The European Journal of Public Health*, 9(4):309–312.

Barendregt JJ, Bonneux L, van der Maas PJ (1994) Health expectancy: an indicator for change? Technology assessment methods project team. *Journal of Epidemiology and Community Health*, 48(5):482–487.

Barendregt JJ, Bonneux L, van der Maas PJ (1995) Reply to van de Water et al. *Journal of Epidemiology and Community Health*, 49(3):330–331.

Barendregt JJ, Bonneux L, van der Maas PJ (1997a) How good is Sullivan's method for monitoring changes in population health expectancies? Letter. *Journal of Epidemiology and Community Health*, 51:578

Barendregt JJ, Bonneux L, van der Maas PJ (1997b) The health care costs of smoking. *New England Journal of Medicine*, 337(5):1052–1057.

Crimmins EM, Saito Y, Hayward MD (1993) Sullivan and multistate methods of estimating active life expectancy: two methods, two answers. In: *Calculation of health expectancies: harmonization, consensus achieved and future perspectives.* (Proceedings of the 6th meeting of the international network on health expectancy and the disability process REVES, October 1992, Montpellier.) Robine JM, Mathers CD, Bone MR, Romieu I, eds. John Libbey Eurotext, Paris.

Mathers CD, Robine JM (1997) How good is Sullivan's method for monitoring changes in population health expectancies. *Journal of Epidemiology and Community Health*, 51(1):80–86.

Murray CJL (1994) Quantifying the burden of disease: the technical basis for disability-adjusted life years. *Bulletin of the World Health Organization*, 72(3):429–445.

Rogers A, Rogers R.G., Belanger A (1990) Longer life but worse health? Measurement and dynamics. *Gerontologist*, 30(5):640–649.

Shryock HS, Siegel JS, et al. (1976) *The methods and materials of demography.* Condensed Edition by Edward G.Stockwell, ed. Academic Press, Orlando, FL.

van de Water HPA, Boshuizen HC, Perenboom RJM, Mathers CD, Robine JM (1995) Health expectancy: an indicator for change? *Journal of Epidemiology and Community Health*, 49(3):330–331.

Chapter 5.1

HEALTH GAPS: AN OVERVIEW AND CRITICAL APPRAISAL

CHRISTOPHER J.L. MURRAY, COLIN D. MATHERS, JOSHUA A. SALOMON AND ALAN D. LOPEZ

INTRODUCTION

Chapter 1.2 defined two major families of summary measures of population health (SMPH): health expectancies and health gaps. In this chapter, we review the concept of health gaps, present an overview of the key conceptual and methodological issues around the construction of health gaps, and compare different types of health gaps against the desirable criteria for summary measures of population health proposed by Murray et al. in chapter 1.2.

HEALTH EXPECTANCIES AND HEALTH GAPS

Different summary measures of population health may be divided broadly into two families: health expectancies and health gaps. The distinction between these two families may be illustrated using a survivorship curve (Figure 1), which indicates, for each age x, the proportion of an initial birth cohort that will survive to that age. In Figure 1, life expectancy at birth is computed as the area under the survivorship curve (area A), while a health expectancy measure extends the notion of life expectancy by weighting the time lived at each age according to the health states of the surviving cohort members (see chapter 4.1 for a detailed examination of health expectancies).

Health gaps quantify the difference between the actual health of a population and some stated norm or goal for population health. As with health expectancies, health gaps include weights that account for time lived in health states worse than ideal health. A variety of health gaps have been proposed and measured, for example disability-adjusted life years (DALYs) (Murray and Lopez 1996) and healthy life-years (HeaLYs) (Hyder et al. 1998; Hyder and Morrow 2000), and many others can be derived. Although health gaps are usually presented in absolute terms (e.g. representing the total number of healthy years "lost" in a population), a life table health gap measure, such as that presented in Figure 1, may also

Figure I   Survivorship function for a population

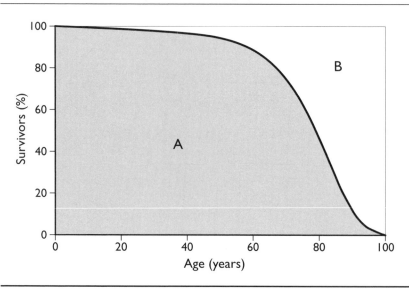

be used as a simple heuristic: this example illustrates a health goal of full survivorship in perfect health through age 100. In mathematical terms, the life table health gap is computed as area B plus some function of area A:

$$\text{Health Gap} = B + g(A)$$

where $g(\cdot)$ is a function that assigns weights to health states less than full health.

More formally, the life table health gap (HG) can be defined in terms of a loss function, $L(a)$, which specifies the normative goal for survivorship at age a:

$$HG_x = \int_x^\infty \left\{ \int_0^1 w(h(a)) \cdot [1 - h(a)] \cdot S(a)dh \right\} da + \int_x^\infty d(a)L(a)da$$

where $w(h(a))$ is the prevalence density of health state valuation h at age a, normalized so that

$$\int_0^1 w(h(a)) \cdot dh = 1$$

The health state valuation h is measured on a scale ranging from 0 (states equivalent to death) to 1 (ideal health), and $d(a)$ is the number of deaths occurring at each age a (given by the derivative of the survival function, S). In the most general case, the weights may also be functions of age a.

Various types of health gaps can be defined, according to the standards chosen for:

- the selected normative target used to measure the difference (health gap) from current health conditions in a population.

- the method used to value time spent in health states less than ideal health.

- the inclusion of other social values, such as age-weights, time preference and equity weights.

DEFINING THE NORMATIVE HEALTH FUNCTION

The most important conceptual issue relating to health gaps is the choice of the normative goal for health against which the health of the current population is compared. There are several important elements that may distinguish different classes of normative functions, including the level of definition (i.e. individual or population), the use of multi-dimensional vs. combined norms, and the use of unconditional vs. conditional norms.

1. Individual vs. population norms

One simple type of norm would be a reference population-level health expectancy, which could be compared to the health expectancy in a particular population to compute a life table health gap measure, as illustrated in Figure 1. While this type of norm allows for simple graphical heuristics, it adds little information to what is already conveyed by the health expectancy in most cases, and may be less easily interpreted.

Norms specified at the individual level are more useful for computing health gaps in absolute terms and allow for a more intuitive appreciation of the way that population health measures relate to the health of the individuals who comprise the population. As described in chapter 1.3, clarification of the individual basis for SMPH is helpful in understanding distinctions between period and cohort viewpoints, or between incidence and prevalence perspectives, and in specifying the particular set of health outcomes that will be included in different SMPH.

Points 2 and 3 below focus on additional conceptual choices that are particularly relevant for individual-level norms.

2. Combined vs. two-dimensional norms

The normative health function includes both a normative survivorship function and a normative function for the health states of survivors. These may be combined in a single norm or defined separately. An example of a combined norm might be a simple curve for target health levels at each age, with the normative survivorship limit implied by the point at which the health goal declines to zero.

More flexibility in defining the normative health function is possible with a two-dimensional norm that separates the survivorship target from the health goals for survivors. A two-dimensional norm allows health gaps to be decomposed easily into separate components for mortality and non-fatal health outcomes. For example, DALYs represent the combination of years of life lost due to premature mortality (YLLs) and years lived with disability (YLDs). The two-part norm simplifies causal attribution, as YLLs may be computed directly from age-specific death numbers, and YLDs from either incidence or prevalence of relevant health states (which are defined in YLDs in reference to disease and injury sequelae).

3. Unconditional vs. conditional norms

A further distinction may be made between unconditional and conditional norms. An unconditional norm defines a set of age-specific target levels for health and/or mortality that do not change depending on the age an individual has attained, while a conditional individual norm may vary as individuals advance in age. For example, an unconditional (combined) norm may be defined as survivorship in full health up to age 100. An individual who lives to 101 in full health thus exceeds this norm and contributes nothing to the health gap measure. In contrast, a conditional norm, such as the two-part norm implemented in the DALY, may set a survivorship goal that is specific to the age that has already been attained. In this case, an individual who lives to age 101 in full health may still contribute to the health gap, given a norm for healthy life expectancy at age 101 that is greater than 0. The conditional norm allows for all individuals in the population to contribute to the total health gap, no matter what age they attain.

In addition to the distinctions introduced here, we may further characterize different types of survivorship norms based on the specific nature of the loss function applied to deaths at different ages. In the following section, we review different categories of survivorship norms that have been introduced in the extensive literature on mortality gaps.

Classes of survivorship norms

The concept of mortality gaps was proposed first by Dempsey (1947), who argued that all deaths are not equivalent: a death at a younger age represents a greater loss of life than a death at an older age. She proposed a class of indicators, years of life lost, that use time rather than death counts as the unit of measure. In the past 50 years, a variety of measures have been developed that attempt to assess the stream of life lost due to deaths at different ages (Haenszel 1950; Kohn 1951; Perloff et al. 1984; Romeder and McWhinnie 1977). These measures can be divided into four families: potential years of life lost (PYLL); period expected years of life lost (PEYLL); cohort expected years of life lost (CEYLL); and standard expected years of life lost (SEYLL). We describe these four families of measures briefly here and refer readers to more detailed discussions in Murray (1996).

When used as measures of the population burden of premature mortality, all these families of indicators measure the gap between the current mortality pattern of a population and a reference norm for survivorship.

POTENTIAL YEARS OF LIFE LOST

The general notion behind PYLL is that a death at age 5 years, for example, represents a greater loss of potential life than a death at age 70 years. The normative survival goal for PYLL takes the simplest possible form of a constant value such as 65 years, and would be represented in Figure 1 by a vertical line at the normative survival age. For the potential limit to life specified in PYLL, different groups have suggested ages ranging from 60 to 85 years (e.g. Centers for Disease Control 1986). The major criticism of PYLL has been that deaths averted for people older than the arbitrarily-chosen potential limit of life do not contribute to the burden of premature mortality. If such a measure were to be used to influence the allocation of health resources, it implies that there is no benefit to health interventions that reduce mortality over the potential limit to life. This is at odds with clinical practice and with the values of most societies.

PERIOD EXPECTED YEARS OF LIFE LOST AND COHORT EXPECTED YEARS OF LIFE LOST

In a period life table, life expectancy at each age is the estimated duration of life expected at each age if the current age-specific mortality patterns were to hold in the future. To calculate PEYLL, deaths at each age can be weighted by the expected years of life lost at each age, based on a current life table.

Given past secular trends in mortality, the average individual alive today at any given age is likely to live substantially longer than period life expectancy at that age. As distinct from period life expectancy, cohort life expectancy is the estimated average duration of life a cohort would actually experience. Cohort life expectancy is usually substantially higher than period life expectancy.

Using a measure such as expected years of life lost, deaths at every age contribute to the estimated burden of disease, in contrast to PYLL where deaths over the potential limit do not. Expected years of life lost (whether period or cohort), however, are a strange way to define the gap between a population's current mortality rates and some idealized norm. It is confusing to define a population's present mortality rates as the norm against which current achievement is being assessed. If expected years of life lost are used as a measure of the burden of disease, a death in a rich country where life expectancy at each age is higher would be considered a greater burden than a death in a poor country with a lower life expectancy. This violates one of the basic principles of comparative analyses of population health, namely that like events should be counted identically in all populations.

Standard expected years of life lost

The advantages of an expectation approach, where every death contributes to the burden of disease, and the equitable approach of PYLL, where every death of a given age contributes equally to the calculation of the burden of disease irrespective of the population in which it occurs, can be combined by using a standard expectation of life at each age as the reference norm. One example of such an approach is the DALY, which uses the Coale & Demeny West Model Level 26 life table (Coale and Guo 1989) to provide a global standard for the definition of the expected years of life lived at each age for females.

There are a number of considerations in choosing the standard life table. Among the most important of these is whether a different expectation of life at each age should be used for males and females. As these measures of years of life lost can be used to measure the gap between present conditions and some ideal, one can argue that the same standard should be used for the two sexes. Alternatively, one might argue that there is a biological difference between male and female survival potential (Verbrugge 1989; Waldron 1983). One could argue that this absolute difference in potential expectation of life should be incorporated into the calculation of SEYLL by using separate male and female standards.

Murray and Lopez (1996) in the 1990 Global Burden of Disease Study argued that, while the gap between male and female life expectancy in developed countries is still high (7 years or more), in the wealthier groups the gap is much smaller. Modeling exercises (Manton 1986; Pressat 1973) have also suggested that the biological difference in survival is likely to be on the order of 2 to 3 years.

The choice of a standard life expectancy schedule need not be based on model life tables. In the United States Burden of Disease and Injury (USBODI) Study (Murray et al. 1998) variations in life expectancy at birth at the county level were examined, ranging from 56.5 years for American Indians and Alaskan Natives in Bennett, Jackson, Mellette, Shannon and Todd counties (South Dakota), to 97.7 for Asians and Pacific Islander females in Bergen (New Jersey).

Following an extensive preliminary exploration of how best to capture differences among the health status of different population groups in the United States, the USBODI study defined eight different "Americas" according to a ranking of life expectancy values at birth for race/sex units at the county level. Cut-off points for each of the eight Americas were defined following a percentile distribution. America 1, with the highest life expectancy, was then chosen as the standard against which to measure the size of the current health gap in the United States.

Years of life lost (YLL) values were calculated for approximately 100 major causes of diseases and injuries for each of the eight Americas. The YLL gap was measured between each of the lower seven Americas and America 1 for each specific cause. The total YLL was computed by adding YLL values for each of the seven Americas. This approach identifies which are the major contributing diseases and health conditions to the current gap in population health in the United States.

More generally, there is a vast literature on what the probable length of the human lifespan is, given what is currently known or knowable about measures and technologies to reduce disease impact and extend life. Among the most commonly used limits to life expectancy (as opposed to lifespan) is the estimate of 85 years by Fries (1980), using arguments about the compression of morbidity.

The standard DALY uses a loss function based on standard model life tables for males and females with life expectancies at birth of 80.0 and 82.5 years respectively. It should be noted that even for populations, such as the Japanese, where current period life expectancies exceed these standards, there is still a health gap for every death, since the model life table is being used to define the loss function (lost years of life for a death at each age) rather than the normative population survival.

WHICH INDIVIDUALS AND EVENTS?

The calculation of health gaps requires explicit choices about the time perspective adopted for defining event rates for the various input parameters, along with the precise set of individuals and events that are incorporated. Chapter 1.3 described three different time perspectives for computing individual health assessments, including the "snapshot" characterisation of health at an instant, the holistic view of health over the entire lifespan, and the assessment of current and future health. Of the currently used health gaps, none are computed purely as aggregates of any of these perspectives over a defined population. Rather, the primary focus of health gaps has been at the level of health events such as deaths or the incidence of defined conditions. Alternative health gaps could be computed based on the current and future health prospects for all of the individuals living in a population. Such a "current and future" health gap would be the analogue of the current and future health expectancy discussed in chapter 4.1.

For gaps based on counts of health events, important choices must be made as to the time perspectives for each of the critical inputs, namely incidence, remission, case-fatality and general mortality. Thus, for example, one could calculate health gaps as a pure *cohort* measure, where all parameters are based on observed events in a cohort. This would require tracing a birth cohort until every member had died. Alternatively, cohort event rates by age could be estimated. Health gaps could also be pure *period* measures, where all events rates are calculated for a hypothetical cohort assumed to experience current age-specific event rates throughout life.

A series of hybrid gap measures based on a mixture of period and cohort perspectives can also be imagined. For example, the following combinations of types of input measures might be defined:

	Incidence	Remission	Case-fatality	Mortality
Type I	Past	Past	Past	Past
Type II	Current	Future	Future	Future
Type III	Past	Past	Past	Current

Thus, a Type I gap would be based entirely on event rates estimated to have occurred in the past, at different ages, and at different times. Type II, on the other hand, is a gap measure which uses current incidence, but applies the estimated future event rates for all other parameters.

Pure cohort health gaps are conceptually the most appropriate framework for calculating health gaps in that they would utilize real or observed event rates for a cohort. The issue of waiting time for event rates could be circumvented by projecting rates based on current and past experience. In fact, this process is implicit in the definition of pure period gaps which assume current rates will remain constant.

CAUSAL ATTRIBUTION

A key concern in the construction of SMPH is the identification of the relative importance of different diseases, injuries or risk factors to the summary measure. In the case of health gaps, the total gap can be uniquely and exhaustively decomposed into a non-overlapping set of contributions attributed to various diseases and injuries (see chapter 6.1 for a more detailed discussion). This list of diseases and injuries is based on the latest version of the International Classification of Diseases, Injuries and Causes of Deaths. The main advantage of categorical attribution is that all disease/injury contributions sum to the total health gap (additive decomposition property). Additive decomposition is also readily understood by policy-makers and the public.

Additive decomposition for risk factors is not possible, however, since there is no known (or knowable) set of mutually exclusive and exhaustive exposures which collectively sum to any population health gap. If additive decomposition is a critical property, then the contribution of diseases and injuries to a SMPH can only be assessed if that measure is a health gap. This contribution can be assessed in absolute terms, or perhaps more meaningfully, relative to the size of the current health gap.

Counterfactual analysis is an alternative method of causal attribution for identifying the relative importance of diseases, injuries or risk factors to a health gap. This method assumes some alternative hypothetical scenario for the levels of a disease, injury or risk factor. For example, one might ask how much a health gap would be reduced if motor vehicle accidents could be eliminated, or reduced to some feasible or plausible level. In the case of health gaps, adopting a counterfactual scenario will produce results that reflect the age and sex composition of the population. This is clear from the example of motor vehicle accidents which disproportionately affect young males. This may well be appropriate for policy since the results would identify those causes which contribute most in terms of lost health years for the population as a whole.

CRITERIA FOR HEALTH GAPS

Murray, Salomon and Mathers (2000) proposed a set of desirable properties for evaluating SMPH based on common sense notions of population health:

Criterion 1. If age-specific mortality is lower in any age-group, *everything else being the same*, then a summary measure should be better (i.e. a health gap should be smaller and a health expectancy should be larger).

Criterion 2. If age-specific prevalence of some health state worse than ideal health is higher, *everything else being the same*, a summary measure should be worse.

Criterion 3. If age-specific incidence of some health state worse than ideal health is higher, *everything else being the same*, a summary measure should be worse.

Criterion 4. If age-specific remission for some health state worse than ideal health is higher, *everything else being the same*, a summary measure should be better.

Criterion 5. If the severity of a given health state is worse, *everything else being the same*, then a summary measure should be worse.

It is useful to assess health gaps against these criteria. Some measures of health gaps such as potential years of life lost do not meet Criterion 1. This criterion could be weakened to say that if age-specific mortality is lower in any age-group, *everything else being the same*, then a summary measure should be the same or better. The weaker version would allow for deaths beyond some critical age to leave a summary measure unchanged. Measures such as potential years of life lost would then fulfil the weak criterion. Measures which define the gap based on local life expectancy, however, do not meet even the weak version of Criterion 1.

Health gaps based on health state incidence and remission data meet Criteria 1, 3 and 4 but fail Criterion 2. It would be possible to construct a health gap using methods analogous to Sullivan's method for health expectancies, which meets Criterion 2 but fails to meet Criteria 3 and 4.

Returning to the question of the defined normative health function in gap measures, we may consider two potential additional criteria for health gaps, relating to the different interpretations of the normative health function at the individual and population levels. For an individual, the target health function may be conceptualized in terms of a *loss function* that indicates the number of years of life lost due to a health event (e.g. a death) at each age. In some cases, it may also be appealing to examine the implied population normative function associated with a specified loss function. Thus two potential criteria for health gaps, additional to the five general criteria proposed by Murray et al. (2000), might be as follows:

A. *The loss function for any event at age a should be invariant across different populations.*

B. *The normative survivorship goal should be constant across populations.*

From an individual perspective, we argue that the loss of life for an individual at a given age should be constant, regardless of which population he or she belongs to. This has compelling ethical support, but is also essential if health gaps are to be compared across populations. One possible deviation from this principle is to recognize the biological difference in survival between males and females which arguably is not subject to policy intervention and therefore is not of interest or concern for calculating health gaps. We argued that this biological differential should be factored into the derivation of different loss functions for males and females.

Criterion B seems intuitively appealing at first, because it allows for the simple heuristic representation of the life table health gap in terms of an implied target health expectancy. If both criteria A and B are to be fulfilled, however, then it can be demonstrated that the only possible functional form of the normative survivorship curve is an age-invariant normative survival (i.e. a vertical line in the life table space of Figure 1). If this is accepted, the issue arises as to what age should be chosen as the normative standard. One requirement might be that all events should contribute to the calculation of a health gap, in which case the normative age would need to be set at, or beyond, the human lifespan (i.e. 125 years). The disadvantage of such a choice is that the relative contribution of YLLs by age will alter as the standard is moved to progressively higher ages. Another disadvantage is that the relative YLL to YLD contribution is highly sensitive to the choice of a normative age, with the YLD component declining with an increasing standard age. Equity considerations demand that criterion A will be satisfied. However, there is no consensus on whether criterion B is acceptable. Because the key interest in summary measures of population health is to provide information on the health of a set of individuals, we conclude that the loss function (i.e. individual-level) interpretation of the normative health function is the appropriate viewpoint, so that only criterion A provides a compelling addition to the core criteria described by Murray et al. (2000).

CONCLUSIONS

This chapter has provided a general overview of the development and evaluation of different health gap measures. As indicators of the difference between the health in a current population and some target for population health, health gaps provide a useful way to compare populations and to monitor progress. Health gaps are particularly valuable for comparing the contributions of different diseases, injuries and risk factors to the overall health of a population, as they allow quantification of the burden of disease and injury in terms of absolute numbers of life years, and provide comprehensive assessments that exhibit additive decomposition across population groups or health conditions.

The most fundamental conceptual question for developing health gap measures is the definition of the normative health function. We have considered a variety of different issues relating to the specification of this normative function and highlighted some of the advantages and disadvantages of alternative approaches. We conclude that health gaps are most usefully defined in terms of individual norms (e.g. loss functions) rather than in terms of normative population survival curves. That said, it may be desirable to choose individually-based norms that result in an appropriately meaningful normative population survival curve.

The conditional two-part norm used in the standard DALY has a number of appealing features. In particular, deaths at any age contribute to the health gap, and the normative level of health is always assumed to be full health at each age. The use of a standard life table rather than a population-based period or cohort life table to define the norm ensures that the additional criterion A (that the loss function for an event at age a should be invariant across populations) is met. Most importantly, criterion A implies that loss functions based on national survival curves should not be used for international comparative health gap analyses, although such loss functions may be used for various other types of national studies.

A number of challenges remain in resolving ongoing debates relating to currently used health gap measures (such as the definition of the most appropriate survival standard), and there is considerable scope for developing new health gap indicators that allow for different types of comparisons (for example, a measure of current and future health gaps in a population). As interest in comparative assessments of health problems rises, the continuing evolution of health gap measures will provide a valuable set of tools for analysts and policy-makers.

REFERENCES

Centers for Disease Control (1986) Premature mortality in the United States: public health issues in the use of years of potential life lost. *Morbidity and Mortality Weekly Report,* 35(2S):1–11.

Coale AJ, Guo G (1989) Revised model life tables at very low levels of mortality. *Population Index,* 55(4):613–643.

Dempsey M (1947) Decline in tuberculosis: the death rate fails to tell the entire story. *American Review of Tuberculosis,* (56):157–164.

Fries J (1980) Aging, natural death, and the compression of morbidity. *New England Journal of Medicine,* 303(3):130–135.

Haenszel W (1950) A standardized rate for mortality defined in units of lost years of life. *American Journal of Public Health,* 40:17–26.

Hyder AA, Morrow RH (2000) Applying burden of disease methods in developing countries: a case study from Pakistan. *American Journal of Public Health,* 90(8):1235–1240.

Hyder AA, Rotllant G, Morrow R (1998) Measuring the burden of disease: healthy life-years. *American Journal of Public Health,* 88(2):196–202.

Kohn R (1951) An objective mortality indicator. *Canadian Journal of Public Health,* 42:375–379.

Manton KG (1986) Past and future life expectancy increases at later ages: their implications for the linkage of chronic morbidity, disability and mortality. *Journal of Gerontology,* 41(5):672–681.

Murray CJL (1996) Rethinking DALYs. In: *The global burden of disease: a comprehensive assessment of mortality and disability from diseases, injuries, and risk factors in 1990 and projected to 2020.* The Global Burden of Disease and Injury, Vol. 1. Murray CJL, Lopez AD, eds. Harvard School of Public Health on behalf of WHO, Cambridge, MA.

Murray CJL, Lopez AD, eds. (1996) *The global burden of disease: a comprehensive assessment of mortality and disability from diseases, injuries and risk factors in 1990 and projected to 2020.* Global Burden of Disease and Injury, Vol. 1. Harvard School of Public Health on behalf of WHO, Cambridge, MA.

Murray CJL, Michaud CM, McKenna MT, Marks JS (1998) *US patterns of mortality by county and race: 1965–1994.* Harvard Center for Population and Development Studies and Centres for Disease Control, Cambridge, MA.

Murray CJL, Salomon JA, Mathers CD (2000) A critical examination of summary measures of population health. *Bulletin of the World Health Organization,* 78(8):981–994.

Perloff JD, LeBailly SA, Kletke PR, Budetti PP, Connelly JP (1984) Premature death in the United States: years of life lost and health priorities. *Journal of Public Health Policy,* 5(2):167–184.

Pressat R (1973) Surmortalité biologique et surmortalité sociale. *Revue Française de Sociologie,* 14:103–110.

Romeder JM, McWhinnie JR (1977) Potential years of life lost between ages 1 and 70: an indicator of premature mortality for health planning. *International Journal of Epidemiology,* 6(2):143–151.

Verbrugge LM (1989) The twain meet: empirical explanations of sex differences in health and mortality. *Journal of Health and Social Behavior,* 30(3):282–304.

Waldron I (1983) The role of genetic and biological factors in sex differences in mortality. In: *Sex differentials in mortality.* Lopez AD, Ruzicka LT, eds. ANU Press, Canberra.

Chapter 5.2

Healthy life years (HeaLYs)

Adnan A. Hyder and Richard Morrow

Introduction

The healthy life year (HeaLY) is a composite measure that combines the amount of healthy life lost due to morbidity, plus that attributed to premature mortality (Hyder 1998). It is an evolution of the seminal work on days of life lost by the Ghana Health Assessment Team several years ago (GHAPT 1981). The HeaLY can be applied to population groups to determine the impact of a particular disease or disease group, to work out the effects of an intervention or package of interventions, or to compare areas, populations, or socioeconomic groups (Hyder and Morrow 2000; Last 1995).

The need to weigh the benefits of health interventions against their costs is the principle reason for attempting to describe the consequences of disease as a single number. The HeaLY approach focuses on the pathogenesis and natural history of disease as the conceptual framework for assessing morbidity and mortality and for interpreting the effects of interventions (Figure 1). For the purpose of estimating healthy life lost or gained, disease has been defined as anything an individual experiences that causes, literally, 'dis-ease,' anything that leads to discomfort, pain, distress, disability or death from whatever cause including injuries and psychiatric disabilities.

With some exceptions, those with infection or some biological characteristic such as AS-haemoglobin are considered healthy unless they have specific identifiable symptoms or signs. Pre-clinical or sub-clinical disease is not generally counted. However, the diagnostic criteria for some conditions such as hypertension, human immunodeficiency virus (HIV) infection, or Onchocerciasis (diagnosed by skin snip) include individuals without signs or symptoms. Such criteria (e.g. indicators of infection, high blood pressure, or genetic markers) are appropriate when they serve as the basis for intervention programmes. Interventions may also be directed at reducing identifiable risk factors, such as tobacco smoking or risky sexual

Figure 1   Conceptual basis of the HeaLY method: the disability-death
                  model

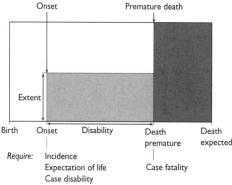

behaviour. To the extent that risk reduction can be translated into disease reduction, the approach to measuring the benefits and costs of a risk reduction intervention programme remains the same.

The onset of disease will usually be dated from the start of symptoms or signs, as determined by the individual afflicted, a family member, medical practitioner or a lab test. There are several different patterns of disease evolution depending on the specific condition. Healthy life lost from disability and from premature death due to typical cases of cirrhosis, polio and multiple sclerosis will differ in terms of onset, extent and duration of disability, as well as termination (Figure 2).

The conclusion of the disease process depends on a host of factors, from correct diagnosis to appropriate treatment. Possible outcomes include clinical recovery (the complete disappearance of clinical signs and symptoms) and premature death, death as a result of the disease, or progression to what is considered a different disease entity. The latter includes death directly caused by the disease and death that is indirectly brought upon by the disease as a result of disability. Termination of a disease state may also be marked by recovery followed by progression to another disease.

COMPUTING HEALYS

The variables and formula for calculating HeaLYs are described below and summarized in Table 1. Each disease will have a distribution of ages at which onset or death may occur, but for most diseases the *average age* will provide a satisfactory approximation. In view of data limitations, this is the starting assumption for applying the HeaLY method. However, if data or sensitivity testing indicate that the average age is not satisfactory, then estimates may be based on age distributions. Similarly, if the natural his-

Figure 2 Patterns of healthy life lost

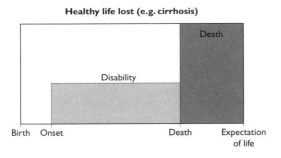

Healthy life lost (e.g. cirrhosis)

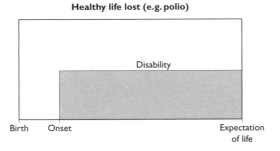

Healthy life lost (e.g. polio)

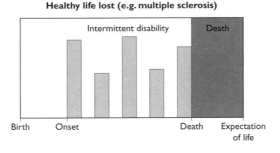

Healthy life lost (e.g. multiple sclerosis)

tory of a disease is different in different age groups, the disease can be specifically classified by age. Diseases in the under-5 years old age group may be considered different from the same disease in adults (e.g. neonatal tetanus as compared to adult tetanus and childhood pneumonia compared to adult pneumonia) and may have different interventions.

In recurrent diseases or diseases with multiple episodes (e.g. diarrhoea), age at onset denotes the average age at first episode. For some diseases, such as malaria, which is characterized by recurrent episodes, and schistosomiasis, in which reinfection occurs at frequent intervals, it may be useful to view them as single lifetime diseases. For example, malaria in Africa may be considered for each individual as a single, lifelong disease

Table I   Variables for estimating healthy life years (HeaLY)

Sign	Explanation	Expression
I	Incidence rate per 1000 population per year	/1000/year
Ao	Average age at onset	Years
Af	Average age at death	Years
E(Ao)	Expectation of life at age of onset	Years
CFR	Case fatality ratio: proportion of those developing the disease who die from the disease	0.00–1.00
CDR	Case disability ratio: proportion of those developing the disease who have disability from the disease	0.00–1.00
De	Extent of disability (from none to complete disability equivalent to death)	0.00–1.00
Dt	Average duration of disability for those disabled by the disease; a composite of temporary and permanent disability based on the proportion of cases in each category.	Years
HeaLY	Healthy life years lost per 1000 population per year: = I × {[CFR × {E(Ao) – [Af – Ao]}] + [CDR × De × Dt]}	HeaLYs per 1000 per year

with chronic, usually asymptomatic parasitemia. Malaria has intermittent severe clinical attacks with high mortality in late infancy and early childhood while immunity is being acquired. This can be followed by recurring, mild clinical episodes with virtually no mortality after age 10 years.

The expectation of life in HeaLYs has been based upon normative expectations of what should be achieved under optimal circumstances. This is approximated by women in Japan, who have the highest global expectation of life. The expectation has been taken from female estimates of regional, low mortality model life tables (Coale et al. 1983). The west model represents the most general mortality pattern, with an expectation of life at birth of 82.5 years for females (level 26), and it has been used for the HeaLY method (Coale and Guo 1989; Hyder and Morrow 2000). However, mortality pattern is a variable and different standards can be used for specific national or regional applications of the HeaLY method.

The value of the case disability ratio is normally 1.00 by definition, since all cases are disabled (to varying degrees and duration) if they have been labelled as diseased. However, there are some diseases, such as sickle cell anaemia and genetic diseases, where cases may not be considered diseased by definition, and these need to be noted. The average duration of disability in years is important since disability can be either temporary or permanent. If the disability is temporary, the duration of that disability until recovery is Dt (Table 1).

If the disability is permanent and the disease does not affect life expectation, then Dt is the expectation of life at age of onset of disease [Dt = E(Ao)]. On the other hand, if the disability is permanent and the disease does reduce life expectation, then Dt is the expectation of life at age of onset, reduced by the difference between ages of fatality and onset

$[Dt = E(Ao) - (Af - Ao)]$. For permanent disability therefore, $Dt = \{CFR \times [E(Ao) - [Af - Ao]]\} + \{[1 - CFR] \times E(Ao)\}$, which marks the onset of disease as the point of reference stated above and includes periods of disability prior to death.

The Ghana Health Assessment Team, in collaboration with the Ministry of Health, community members, and clinicians from the University of Ghana Medical School, developed a disability severity scale, largely using expert opinion and group consensus (Table 2). The severity of disability caused by specific diseases or injuries was scored into four equal classes between 0.01–0.99; two additional classes indicated no disability (0.00), and disability equivalent to death (1.00). For example, the loss of one limb is ranked as 0.25 disabled; and the loss of two limbs as 0.50 disabled. These scores represent an estimate of the *average* disability suffered by typical cases of the specific disease or injury over its course. The Ghana scale is simple and has been used in published work on HeaLYs. Similar types of scales may be developed in countries interested in burden of disease studies.

The healthy life years lost from premature death and from disability are added and expressed as the total years of life lost due to death and disability from a specific disease per 1 000 population per year. These effects are cumulated for all the new cases from the time of onset and include events that may happen many years later. These are all attributed to the year in which disease onset occurred. This is analogous to a "prospective" view of the event (disease onset) and its consequences, as cases are "followed" over time.

UNDERSTANDING HEALYS

The healthy life lost that is attributable to the incident cases in a given year includes the stream of life lost due to premature death and disability in future years, as well as that in the current year. The health status of a population is determined by the amount of healthy life it achieves, expressed as a proportion of the healthy life it could achieve under optimum

Table 2   Disability classification systems[a]

Class	Severity	Examples
1	0	Normal health
2	0.01–0.25	Loss of one limb
3	0.26–0.50	Loss of two limbs
4	0.51–0.75	Loss of three limbs
5	0.76–0.99	Loss of four limbs
6	1.00	Equivalent to death

a. Source: Ghana Health Assessment Team (1981)

conditions. A cohort of 1 000 newborns with an expectation of life of 82.5 years has the potential of 82 500 years of healthy life. In a steady state, a random sample of 1 000 from such a population has the potential of 41 250 years of healthy life (Hyder 1998; Morrow and Bryant 1995). Each year this population would lose 1 000 years of healthy life to mortality, with a distribution of age at death equivalent to that which leads to a life expectation of 82.5 years. Any disease that leads to disability or to death earlier than that set by this age-at-death distribution would increase the amount of healthy life lost beyond this *minimum*. Discounting future life or adding productivity, dependency, or age weighting would affect these denominator numbers.

HeaLYs measure the *gap* between the current situation in a country and that in an ideal country or standard, as defined by the selected expectation of life. In recent work the standard has been based on the life expectation approximated in Japan. Thus, if exactly the same method was used to estimate the HeaLY losses for females in Japan, they would amount to zero per 1 000 people for loss due to mortality; only those due to disability would be counted. For an ideal population where there was also no disability, there would be no gap to measure. This does not mean that the ideal population is not losing years of healthy life, but it is only losing the minimum defined by the structure of the population and the expectation of life, as described above. Any country that experiences losses greater than this minimum, either as a result of excess mortality or disability, will have a measurable gap and that is what the HeaLYs register.

COMPARING HEALYS

HeaLYs can be compared to other health gap measures using criteria proposed by WHO:

HEALYS AND DALYS

HeaLYs are very much like DALYs and the data requirements, input variables, value choices and estimation procedures are comparable. The HeaLY may be considered a simplified health gap and was created with the intention of:

- Allowing Health Ministry decision-makers in developing countries to readily estimate a summary measure of health.

- De-linking some value choices from the calculations *per se*.

- Making estimates of healthy life lost from premature mortality and disability consistent with each other and with the natural history of disease concept (see below) (Hyder and Morrow 1999).

HeaLYs clearly define a population health target and then measure the gap between current conditions and the target. Age weighting, discounting and valuing of life (except for placing mortality and morbidity at par) are not part of the calculations, but are left as additional manipulations for national and regional decisions. We have chosen to use a 3% discount rate when comparing results with DALYs. It is important to note that HeaLYs do not reduce the data demands for health gaps in any way, but present a simplified way to construct a composite indicator.

AGE WEIGHTING

Age weighting, as proposed by the DALY approach, is a value choice. According to the age curve (World Bank 1993), higher weights are given to years lived in young adult ages—that is, a year of life at age 25 is valued more than a year lived at age 5 years or 65 years. This results in a higher weighting for younger ages between 5 and 15 years and a lower weighting for the older ages, when compared with measures of the stream of healthy life lost that do not use age weighting (Barendregt et al. 1996; Hyder et al. 1998). Thus, regardless of ethical and equity arguments, age weights further emphasise losses of healthy life at youngest ages—a fact that may not be easily recognized.

ATTRIBUTION OF DEATHS

The DALY comprises two components: i) the loss from premature mortality (years of life lost, YLL) is based on deaths occurring in a defined base year; ii) the loss from disability is based on morbidity that will occur throughout a lifetime in those with onset of disease in the base year. Losses from deaths in the base year could also be attributed to the year of onset of disease for each death. This would be consistent with the natural history of disease concept and would focus both components—losses from premature mortality and disability—to the year of onset of disease. This is the basis of the HeaLY (Hyder and Morrow 1999).

For diseases which are at steady state or approximating it, the difference in attributing deaths to either base year or year of onset will not be marked. However, for conditions that are in a dynamic state and changing, such as with the HIV/AIDS epidemic, a working hypothesis was that these differences would be marked and important to note. To test this, data for the HIV/AIDS epidemic from the 1990 Global Burden of Disease study was used to construct both scenarios (Table 3).

Data from the *Global Health Statistics* volume (Murray and Lopez 1996a) were used to construct premature mortality losses from HIV infection for three regions of the world. Since the DALY/YLL attributes all deaths in the base year to the base year only, losses measured by this method are much lower. If the incidence of HIV infection is used to estimate losses and all deaths occurring in the cohort are attributed to the base year (regardless of current deaths), then the losses are far greater, as demonstrated by the healthy life years for premature mortality only (HeaLYpm) indicator. The differences peak in areas such as sub-Saharan Africa with a several-fold difference in estimates.

Table 3   Impact of HIV on premature mortality: attribution of deaths in DALY/HeaLY[a]

Parameter	Middle Eastern Crescent	India	Sub-Saharan Africa
Incidence (1000/yr)	0.05	0.21	2.10
Case fatality ratio	1.00	1.00	1.00
Age of onset (yr)	31.60	31.00	27.50
Duration (yr)	7.00	7.00	6.50
Age of death (yr)	38.60	38.00	34.00
No. deaths (000)	1.00	1.00	239.00
DALY/YLL (000)	16.00	17.00	7 020.00
DALY/YLL rate (/1000)[b]	0.03	0.02	13.80
HeaLYpm (000)	642.00	4 554.00	28 493.00
HeaLYpm rate (/1000)[b]	1.30	5.40	55.80

a. Source: Murray and Lopez (1996a; 1996b).

b. DALY/YLL and HeaLYpm reflect loss of healthy life from premature mortality only, inclusive of expectation of life (West, level 26) and discounting (3%/year). DALY/YLL also include age weighting.

This difference in perspective is important, both for measurement and decision-making. If the incidence of a disease remains relatively constant, and there are no interventions and populations remain relatively stable, then steady states would be approximated and these differences would not matter. However, with situations such as the HIV/AIDS epidemic, the numbers provide a different perspective to decisions that need to be taken today, if the stream of healthy life loss from HIV onset in the base year is to be prevented. Indeed, the perspective used in the HeaLYs is a better focus for interventions that aim to reduce incidence, which would be primarily preventative in nature. It also adds consistency to the two components of the summary measure.

HeaLYs and the criteria

WHO has proposed a set of criteria for summary measures of population health. The criteria are based on a minimal set of desirable properties for these measures, such that two populations may be distinguished with respect to their health status alone. The philosophical perspective used to develop the criteria has been that of individual choice from behind a "veil of ignorance". The Rawlsian veil of ignorance is a useful philosophical construct for setting initial conditions, particularly for establishing a rational basis for social contracts; however, the application of a modified version of such a construct for the development of criteria for measures is new.

The criteria proposed by WHO obviously do not reflect the entire spectrum of purposes for which a summary measure may be developed and used. At the same time, the five criteria are neither mutually exclusive nor independent. The criteria are not stated in a parallel fashion; criteria 1 and 4 posit improvements in the summary measure, while criteria 2, 3 and 5 reflect the summary measure getting worse. The interdependence of prevalence, incidence and duration of disease means criteria 2 and 3 are not independent. It should be remembered that other properties, such as clarity, transparency and ease of use, are also as important as the five criteria described.

A comparison of HeaLYs with the proposed five criteria for summary measures yields the following conclusions:

- HeaLYs fulfil criterion 1 (age-specific mortality changes), since any reduction of age-specific mortality will lead to a lower HeaLY loss in a population. For comparative purposes HeaLYs have used a fixed normative goal for population survivorship.

- HeaLYs fulfil criterion 2 (age-specific prevalence higher), since an increase in prevalence would be the result of increased duration (at constant incidence) and that would increase the HeaLY losses from disability. HeaLYs do not use the prevalence perspective *per se* in any component of the calculation (see sections above).

- HeaLYs fulfil criterion 3 (incidence of health state worse than full health changes), since any increase in incidence of a health state worse than full health would increase the HeaLY losses for a population. HeaLYs count the loss of healthy life from disability, based on the incidence of that disability.

- HeaLYs fulfil criterion 4 (remission of health state worse than full health higher), since if remission from disability is higher then there would be fewer HeaLYs lost from disability.

- HeaLYs would fulfil criterion 5 (effect of one worse-off individual), if they were meant to measure the impact of each individual in the population. As currently developed, HeaLYs evaluate the average levels in a population and unless that changes, HeaLY losses would not be affected by individual variation. (When the individual is in a worse health state and affects population estimates of the disability weight for a specific disease, however, this would cause more loss of HeaLYs in the population).

- HeaLYs were developed with easy comprehension and feasibility of calculation in mind, especially for the developing world.

- HeaLYs, like other health gaps such as DALYs, have the property of additive decomposition.

In addition to the criteria for summary measures, WHO is also exploring criteria for health gaps (Murray et al. 2000). Evaluation of the two proposed criteria indicate that:

- For criterion 1, the loss function from premature mortality for an individual at any age is invariant in HeaLYs, since a standard survivorship function is used. For all individuals at that age, the loss would be determined by the number of people at that age in the population, which in turn is dependent on the age structure of the population. For loss of healthy life from disability, this criterion is not relevant, as the incidence, duration, extent and prevalence of disability in populations would have to be the same for it to apply.

- For criterion 2, HeaLYs already use a normative survivorship goal, which is constant across populations, when they are used for comparative purposes. In other words, when the objective of using HeaLYs is cross-national comparisons a fixed survivorship standard is used. If HeaLYs are used for other purposes a different survivorship standard may be applied—the objective determines the standard.

The criteria proposed by WHO may be useful in thinking through summary measures of population health. However, the development of new measures, and innovative applications of current ones, should largely be determined by the purpose of the measure. It is also relevant that the allocation of scarce resources will be the leading issue in stimulating the development of appropriate measures. Thus, efforts at de-linking the measurement of the burden with allocation issues, although theoretically useful, are less important in practice.

USING HeaLYs AND HEALTH GAPS

If the goal of developing health gaps is to influence policy, especially international and national resource allocation decisions, then a set of criteria may be developed for using health gaps in decision-making. First, health gaps would serve decisions within the health sector and not issues between the health and other sectors. Second, decisions within the health sector are made not on diseases or disabilities *per se*, but on health interventions for them. A large part of such decisions are to do with the allocation of resources for interventions and estimating the effects of interventions. Although there are decisions that pertain to policy development, legislation, standard setting, enforcement, manpower development and deployment, resource distributions underlie many of these as well.

From a decision-making perspective, a set of questions may be posed to stimulate the development of criteria for using health gaps.

WHAT IS THE TIME FRAME FOR DECISION-MAKING?

Ministries of Health, Planning and Finance, especially in the developing world, often work with 3–5 year development plans. This would be the time frame for major decisions within the health sector and data that supports this process needs to be made available. Health measures generated within the country by nationals also need to be available to affect this process. How can health gaps aid in this process, especially if their generation requires time and effort that may not be currently available in these countries?

WHAT TYPES OF INFORMATION WILL ASSIST IN DECISION-MAKING?

It has been argued that incremental changes as a result of policies are more central to decisions than the pre- and post-decision levels of any factor (Williams 1999). Under this premise, for example, it is more important to know how policy y would decrease the current infant mortality rate compared to policy x, rather than know the current level of the infant mortality rate. Clearly, there is merit to knowing both options and the artificial scenarios of having one versus the other information is largely academic. What is more important is that many statistical data routinely collected in the developing world is irrelevant to health planning or health care evaluation. Attention needs to focus on the key information that should be collected (as a normative function) by ministries of health. Can the process of estimating health gaps be a mechanism for achieving this objective?

WHAT PRECISION IS REQUIRED FOR DECISION-MAKING?

Decisions within the health sector may change if there is significant evidence to support a change (dependent on the political process of decision making). "Significance" here does not refer to statistical significance, but to policy importance (i.e. in terms of the orders of magnitude of health gains achievable). Is the data currently available for the generation of health gaps sufficient for this level of precision, even if it is not for epidemiological purposes?

DO HEALTH GAPS CHANGE DECISIONS?

In the final analysis, the impact of health gaps will be felt if decisions based on them are substantially different than those based on traditional indicators. Health gaps need to inform these policy- and priority-setting processes in countries and regions, and such cases will form the evidence for using health gaps. Proponents of health gaps need to collect, demonstrate and disseminate such scenarios effectively.

CONCLUSION

Health gaps define a group of composite indicators (SMPH) that assess the health status of populations based on a defined standard. The central challenge to the construction and use of health gaps, especially in the developing world, remains the data that will serve as input, since it is either not available, not valid or unreliable. This is the essential need for developing countries—to know how many people are dying and from what cause. The challenge then becomes to use the data effectively to improve the health status of the population.

Our intention in raising these issues is not to offer a solution to a specific summarization problem. Rather, we want to point out that candidate measures need not (we would argue should not) be limited to unidimensional measures. While our ability to think in several dimensions is limited, it can be improved with practice. That practice has proven crucial in attacking problems in physical engineering systems, and there is no reason to suppose it will be less important in tackling more complex social policy issues. In instances where many people must make informed choices based on the same scientific data but with different values, multidimensional measures are essential for providing sufficient information for rational choice.

REFERENCES

Barendregt JJ, Bonneux L, van der Maas PJ (1996) DALYs: the age-weights on balance. *Bulletin of the World Health Organization*, 74(4):439–443.

Coale AJ, Demeney P, Vaughan B (1983) *Regional model life tables and stable populations*. Academic Press, Inc., New York.

Coale AJ, Guo G (1989) Revised model life tables at very low levels of mortality. *Population Index*, 55(4):613–643.

Ghana Health Assessment Project Team (1981) A quantitative method of assessing the health impact of different diseases in less developed countries. *International Journal of Epidemiology*, 10(1):72–80.

Hyder AA (1998) *Measuring the burden of disease: introducing health life years*. Doctoral dissertation. Johns Hopkins University, Baltimore, MD.

Hyder AA, Morrow RH (1999) Steady state assumptions in DALYs: effects on estimates of HIV impact. *Journal of Epidemiology and Community Health*, 53(1):43–45.

Hyder AA, Morrow RH (2000) Applying burden of disease methods in developing countries: a case study from Pakistan. *American Journal of Public Health*, 90(8):1235–1240.

Hyder AA, Rotllant G, Morrow R (1998) Measuring the burden of disease: healthy life-years. *American Journal of Public Health*, 88(2):196–202.

Last JM (1995) *A dictionary of epidemiology*. 3rd edn. Oxford University Press, New York.

Morrow RH, Bryant JH (1995) Health policy approaches to measuring and valuing human life: conceptual and ethical issues. *American Journal of Public Health*, 85(10):1356–1360.

Murray CJL, Lopez AD, eds. (1996a) *Global health statistics: a compendium of incidence, prevalence and mortality estimates for over 200 conditions*. Global Burden of Disease and Injury, Vol 2. Harvard School of Public Health on behalf of WHO, Cambridge, MA.

Murray CJL, Lopez AD, eds. (1996b) *The global burden of disease: a comprehensive assessment of mortality and disability from diseases, injuries and risk factors in 1990 and projected to 2020.* Global Burden of Disease and Injury, Vol. 1. Harvard School of Public Health on behalf of WHO, Cambridge, MA.

Murray CJL, Salomon JA, Mathers CD (2000) A critical examination of summary measures of population health. *Bulletin of the World Health Organization,* 78(8):981–994.

Williams A (1999) Calculating the global burden of disease: time for a strategic reappraisal? *Health Economics,* 8(1):1–8.

World Bank (1993) *World development report: investing in health.* Oxford University Press, New York.

Chapter 5.3

Using achievable mortality reductions to define a survivorship standard for calculating mortality gaps

Kiyotaka Segami

Introduction

The recent national health plan, Healthy Japan 21, establishes various health goals such as a reduction in potential years of life lost (PYLL) and an improvement in health expectancy. It also has concrete targets, such as decreasing the prevalence of overweight and obesity (Body Mass Index of 24.2 kg/m^2 or more) from 32.8% to 25.0% in males and from 27.1% to 20.0% in females; and increasing the number of daily walking steps by 1 000 steps on average, from 8 202 steps to 9 200 steps in males and from 7 282 steps to 8 300 steps in females as an indicator of physical exercise.

The plan also mentions the importance of setting graduated realistic targets to enable goals to be achieved gradually. This is especially relevant for prefectural governments planning specific interventions in these areas in the near future. The national health plan also proposes that prefectural governments use health target indices such as the Systematically Attainable Longevity Target (SALT) mortality index (Segami 1999; 2000). This article illustrates the use of the SALT method to set a realistically attainable mortality standard for calculating mortality gaps.

The global burden of disease in Japan

Fukuda et al. (1999) have estimated the total burden of disease in Japan for 1993 to be 12.76 million disability-adjusted life years (DALYs) (Table 1). When mortality rates are ranked by disease and cause of injury, and compared with the ranking of burden of disease in DALYs for Japan, the greatest difference is for mental disorders and traffic accidents (Ikeda 1998), Figure 1.

The DALY is an excellent index for assessing health problems internationally. But for Japan, which has the best life expectancy in the world, the use of the Global Burden of Disease (GBD) standard life expectancy

Table 1   National burden of disease in Japan in 1993[a]

	Total DALYs	Males		Females	
		YLL	YLD	YLL	YLD
All causes[a]	12 759 400	4 233 400	3 008 700	2 845 500	2 671 800
I. Communicable	929 100	378 400	88 300	270 000	192 400
II. Non-communicable	10 535 800	3 145 200	2 820 600	2 305 700	2 264 300
Malignant neoplasms	2 577 300	1 329 900	210 500	909 600	127 300
Depression	1 021 100	100	349 100	200	671 700
Cerebrovascular disease	1 078 000	388 200	185 200	358 200	146 400
III. Injuries	1 440 000	709 800	295 900	269 700	164 600

a. Source: Fukuda et al. (1999).

b. Calculated using the number of deaths due to all causes.

Figure 1   Comparison of ranking of disease groups according to
DALYs and mortality rate, Japan 1993

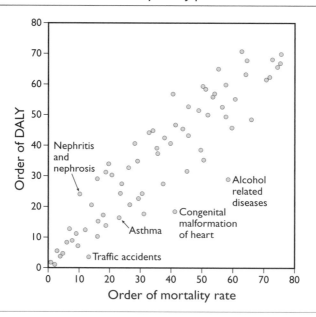

Source: Ikeda (1998).

for calculating mortality gaps implies an unrealistically large normative
standard for life expectancy, particularly when examining regional mortality gaps within Japan. This paper examines the use of an alternative,
more realistic standard for calculating regional mortality gaps.

THE USE OF MORTALITY GAPS IN JAPAN

PERIOD EXPECTED YEARS OF LIFE LOST (PEYLL) IN JAPAN, 1998

Murray and Lopez (1996) defined a variety of mortality gaps, based on various implied standards for population survivorship. One of these gaps is the PEYLL, where the duration of life lost is based on the current period life expectancy of the population. PEYLL for Japan in 1998 is calculated by summing the actual numbers of deaths occurring in 1998 in each age group and multiplying by the Japanese period life expectancy for that age group in 1998. The total PEYLL for Japan in 1998 is 13 million life-years (Table 2). This is 1.84 times larger that the standard expected years of life lost (SEYLL) in 1993, estimated by the National Burden of Disease (NBD) analysis (Table 1). This difference is caused by the increase in deaths at older ages from 1993 to 1998, by not age-weighting these deaths, and by time discounting (at 3%) the years of life lost in the NBD study.

SETTING AN ATTAINABLE SURVIVORSHIP TARGET FOR HEALTH PLANNING

If the Japanese population achieved the survivorship target implied by the current period life expectancy, the Japanese population would have an extremely high average life expectancy. Such a target for life expectancy is not realistically achievable using known interventions. Segami (1999; 2000) has proposed using a SALT mortality index for setting health goals for prefectures in Japan.

Figure 2 uses the box-plotting method to show the distribution of male age-specific mortality rates for cardiovascular diseases (100–159, 170–199) across the 47 Japanese prefectures. The box shows the first quartile rate and the third quartile rate, the whisker lines show the full range of the rates, and the middle lines in the box show the average rates. Circles show outlier rates which varied unexpectedly from the distribution. Figure 2 illus-

Table 2 Japanese mortality gaps based on the 1998 Vital Statistics of Japan

	PEYLL for current mortality[a]	PEYLL for SALT mortality[b]	Mortality benefit (life years) of achieving SALT target		Current mortality gap using SALT standard[c]	Benefit as % of current gap
	A	B	C = B − A	C/A (%)	D	D/A (%)
Males	7 356 019	6 967 226	388 793	5.29	429 590	5.84
Females	5 674 325	5 333 646	340 679	6.00	363 282	6.40
Persons	13 030 344	12 300 872	729 471	5.60	792 873	6.08

a. Calculated using the current period life table to define the loss function for mortality.

b. Calculated using the period life table corresponding to SALT mortality rates to define the loss function for mortality.

c. Calculated using the SALT survivorship curve to define the loss function for mortality (see below).

Figure 2   Distribution of mortality rates for cardiovascular disease in
                      males across 47 prefectures in Japan, by age, 1996–1998

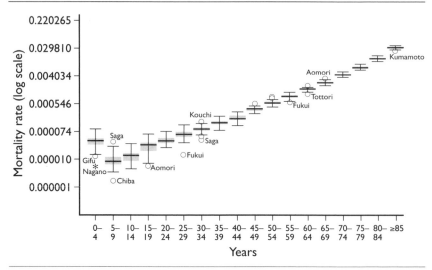

Source: Segami (2000).

Boxes indicate the first quartile and the third quartile of mortality rates.

trates the small range of variances of mortality rates across prefectures of
Japan. The SALT mortality rates are set in terms of the 1st quartile of the
age-sex specific mortality rates for each of the leading causes across the
47 prefectures of Japan. The overall all-cause SALT mortality rate sets a
mortality target that relates to the health goals of the prefectural governments and is realistically achievable within 3–5 years.[1]

If PEYLL is used to calculate the expected gain in life years for Japan,
assuming the SALT mortality rates, the difference between the current
PEYLL (calculated using current mortality and the current period life table
[Column A, Table 2]), and the PEYLL calculated assuming the SALT standard mortality rates, can be calculated. The latter is shown in column B
of Table 2 and is calculated using the mortality implied by the SALT
mortality rates, together with the period life table corresponding to the
SALT mortality rates. The difference between these represents the life years
gained (729 471 years in total for Japan).

SALT SURVIVORSHIP CURVE AS A NORM FOR MORTALITY GAPS

Assuming SALT mortality rates are achieved, the new survivorship curve
can be drawn on the right side of the actual one (Figure 3), and the increase
in life expectancy can be calculated. The SALT survivorship curve can also
be used directly to define a norm for calculating mortality gaps. Such
mortality gaps will directly quantify the benefits in life-years to be gained

from achieving the SALT target through the projected effects of existing and newly introduced health interventions.

Using the SALT survivorship curve as a norm, we can define the loss function in terms of the horizontal gap between the two survival curves. This is defined by finding the age x' on the SALT survival curve which has the same number of survivors (lx') as the actual survival curve at age x (l_x). The years of difference $(x'-x)$ are the years lost by a death at age x (the loss function) that correspond to setting the SALT survival curve as the normative target. When individual loss of life years are multiplied by the actual number of age-specific deaths, the age-specific mortality gap can be obtained.

Column D in Table 2 shows this mortality gap for Japan with a total benefit of 792 873 life years. This is slightly larger than the benefit calculated by taking the difference between the two PEYLL estimates (columns A and B, Table 2).

MORTALITY GAPS FOR 10 LEADING CAUSES OF DISEASE

Table 3 shows the mortality gaps attributable to 10 leading causes of death and to some specific causes. Malignant neoplasms are ranked in first place as a cause of the mortality gap. Specifically, among malignant neoplasms the leading causes of death for women are malignant neoplasms of the stomach, followed by malignant neoplasms of the colon, rectum and anus. For males the leading causes of death are malignant neoplasms of trachea, bronchus and lung, followed by malignant neoplasms of the stomach. Note

Figure 3   The SALT survivorship norm for calculation of mortality gaps

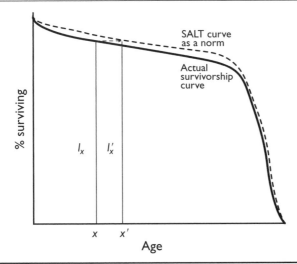

Table 3   Mortality gaps for 10 leading causes of death, Japan 1998

Cause	Males PEYLL	% of total	Rank	Females PEYLL	% of total	Rank	Persons PEYLL	% of total	Rank
Malignant neoplasms C00–C97	145 432	33.9	1	106 781	29.4	1	252 213	31.8	1
Diseases of the circulatory system excluding CVD I00–I59, I70–I99	57 198	13.3	2	54 650	15.0	3	111 849	14.1	2
Cerebrovascular disease I60–I69	51 847	12.1	3	57 867	15.9	2	109 714	13.8	3
Pneumonia J12–J18	27 639	6.4	5	25 540	7.0	4	53 179	6.7	4
Accidents V01–X59	32 628	7.6	4	18 230	5.0	5	50 858	6.4	5
Intentional self-harm X60–X84	21 302	5.0	6	11 808	3.3	6	33 110	4.2	6
Diseases of the liver K70–K76	12 004	2.8	7	5 254	1.4	10	17 258	2.2	7
Senility R54	3 538	0.8	10	9 262	2.5	7	12 800	1.6	8
Renal failure N17–N19	5 623	1.3	9	6 558	1.8	8	12 181	1.5	9
Diabetes mellitus E10–E14	5 805	1.4	8	5 658	1.6	9	11 462	1.4	10
Other causes	28 201	6.6		17 458	4.8		45 658	5.8	
All causes	429 590	100.0		363 282	100.0			100.0	

Table 4   Mortality gaps for 7 specific causes of death, Japan 1998

Cause	Males PEYLL	% of total	Females PEYLL	% of total	Persons PEYLL	% of total
Malignant neoplasm of stomach C16	28 201	6.6	17 458	4.8	45 658	5.8
Malignant neoplasm of trachea, bronchus and lung C33–C34	29 230	6.8	12 114	3.3	41 344	5.2
Malignant neoplasm of colon, rectum and anus C18–C21	15 939	3.7	13 827	3.8	29 766	3.8
Intracerebral haemorrhage I61, I69.1	15 558	3.6	13 065	3.6	28 623	3.6
Subarachnoid haemorrhage I60, I69.0	6 095	1.4	9 155	2.5	15 250	1.9
Acute and subsequent myocardial infarction I21–I22	22 556	5.3	18 242	5.0	40 797	5.1
Transport accidents V01–V98	15 648	3.6	7 247	2.0	22 894	2.9

also the magnitude of acute and subsequent myocardial infarction (Table 4).

DISCUSSION

In the last 20 years, Japan has attained the highest national life expectancies in the world. Reasons for this may include improvements in the standard of living due to economic growth and equity of access to medical resources. But more attention should be given to the competition of prefectural governments to introduce suitable health interventions against many historical health risks. Such efforts have resulted in low mortality rates across prefectures in Japan. Despite the narrowing of mortality differentials among the 47 prefectures, however, there are still differences.

Therefore, prefectural governments need information on the causes of mortality inequalities and on the availability of effective interventions. For effective social involvement in health planning, it is important to get wider participation of residents both in planning and in implementing policy. Especially in planning, participation is a keyword to empower people to follow positive health practices. In this connection, the easier the understanding of health targets, the more effective social involvement can be attained.

Prefectural governments need measures of population health that are generally understandable, and provide guidance for setting priorities for health policy and selecting effective health interventions. Mortality gaps based on the SALT standard provide such information. In this paper, mortality gaps were used to quantify the foreseeable benefits of interventions that reduced the PEYLL for various diseases.

NOTES

1 Editors note: The SALT standard defined in this way is open to criticism, however. The choice of leading causes is arbitrary and the interdependence of death rates is not taken into account. Both of these issues could be avoided by determining SALT rates on the basis of all-cause mortality. This definition, too, has been criticized on the basis that the age-specific selection of minimum death rates is an artificial construct, mixing the experience of several generations.

REFERENCES

Fukuda Y, Hasegawa T, Yatsuya H, et al. (1999) Japanese burden of disease and disability adjusted life years. (In Japanese.) *Kosei-no-sihyo [Journal of Health and Welfare Statistics]*, 46(4):28–33.

Ikeda S (1998) Japanese burden of disease and disability adjusted life years. (In Japanese.) *Medicine and Society*, 8:83–98.

Murray CJL, Lopez AD, eds. (1996) *The global burden of disease: a comprehensive assessment of mortality and disability from diseases, injuries and risk factors in 1990 and projected to 2020.* Global Burden of Disease and Injury, Vol. 1. Harvard School of Public Health on behalf of WHO, Cambridge, MA.

Segami K (1999) Proposal of SALT. (In Japanese.) *Kosei-no-sihyo [Journal of Health and Welfare Statistics]*, **46**(8):3–15.

Segami K (2000) *Tables of health indices towards twenty first century.* (In Japanese.) Kosei Toukei Kyokai [Association of Health and Welfare Statistics], Tokyo.

Chapter 5.4

Shifting the goalpost — normative survivorship goals in health gap measures

Theo Vos

Health gap measures, such as the DALY, are a quantification of the gap between the current health status in a population and a stated goal for population health. This goal can be understood as an ideal situation in which everyone in a population lives into old age free of disease. Health gaps are the addition of time lost due to premature mortality, as measured against the normative survivorship goal and time spent in states of less than full health, weighted for severity. Assuming a stable population, the health gap is shown in Figure 1 as area C, between the survivorship curve and the normative survivorship goal, plus area B indicating the proportion of time lived in less than full health weighted for severity (Murray et al. 2000). This paper examines the mortality component of health gaps and the desirability of the current methods used in burden of disease studies.

Figure I   Survivorship curve

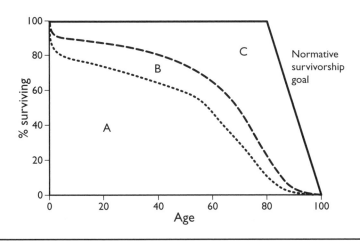

Murray et al. (2000) have suggested five criteria or desirable properties for summary measures of population health that include health gaps.
The first criterion stipulates that if age-specific mortality decreases in any
age group, *ceteris paribus*, a health gap should decrease. The other four
criteria concern incidence, prevalence, remission and severity of states of
ill health and are not relevant to this paper. The first criterion for the
mortality component of health gaps has been restated to the effect that the
loss function for a death at age *a* should be invariant across different
populations. The Global Burden of Disease (GBD) study defined the normative survivorship goal as the gap between age at death and the life
expectancy from a model life table mimicking the high life expectancy of
Japanese women in the early nineties. Thus, for a death at each age, a fixed
number of "lost years" is defined and applied to all regions of the world.
The steering committee for the Australian Burden of Disease study
(Mathers et al. 1999) preferred using the 1996 cohort life expectancy for
Australian men and women, which shows slightly higher life expectancies
than the GBD standard life tables. If future burden of disease studies in
Australia want to retain comparability over time, the same 1996 cohort
life expectancies will need to be applied. For comparisons between the
Australian and GBD studies it is necessary to use an alternative set of
results with Years of Life Lost recalculated using the GBD standard life
tables. If that is taken into account, both studies meet the criterion of
invariant loss function for deaths at each age.

A second criterion has also been suggested, stating that the normative
survivorship should be constant across populations. It was also argued that
the current GBD methods violate this criterion (Figure 2). The Figure
shows the survivorship curves of two populations, one with high mortality and one with low mortality. The horizontal arrows suggest that the gap
between the normative survivorship goal and a death at age sixty years is
greater in the population with high mortality. This is not quite where the
problem lies because we have established that the first criterion holds and
therefore that the gap between a death at age *a* and the normative survivorship goal is equal in both populations.

Figure 3 illustrates that both populations have different normative
survivorship goals. The conclusion is that under the current methods the
normative survivorship goal is greater when mortality in a population is
lower. Thus, if mortality decreases in a population the health gap is calculated against a further removed goal and the second criterion is violated.

To satisfy the second criterion a normative survivorship goal should be
rectangular in shape. In other words, the potential years of life lost (PYLL)
would have to be used with an arbitrary potential limit to life. Murray
(1996) has pointed out that while easy to calculate, PYLL measures have
the drawback that loss of life at ages beyond the arbitrary limit chosen is
ignored. The choice of a very high potential limit to life (e.g. 85, 90 or 100
years) limits the magnitude of this age discrimination problem but does
not take it away. We can formulate a third criterion for health gaps:

Figure 2   Survivorship curves for a high- and low-mortality population

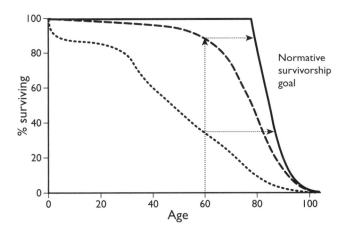

Figure 3   Survivorship curves for a high- and low-mortality population: shifting normative survivorship goals

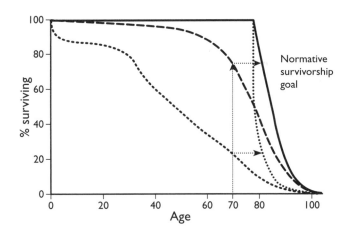

"Health gaps should include all loss of health in a population." Only a PYLL measure with a potential limit to life greater than the oldest age at death observed (121 years?) would meet all three criteria.

However, the choice of the limit to life when calculating PYLLs has a major bearing on how we tend to interpret burden of disease results. To illustrate this, I have recalculated the results of the Victorian Burden of Disease study (Vos and Begg 1999; 2000), using the GBD standard life tables, PYLL 80, PYLL 85, PYLL 90, PYLL 100 and PYLL 120. The first thing to note is that the contribution of Years Lived with Disability (YLD) as a proportion of the total burden of disease varies between 27 and 59% in the non-age weighted scenarios, and between 45 and 64% in the age-weighted scenarios (Figure 4).

A breakdown of the burden by age shows that significant differentials between the scenarios become apparent for age groups 55–64 years and older, with large variations in the 75 years and older age group (Figure 5). In the age-weighted scenarios (Figure 5), the differentials are less extreme than without age weighting (Figure 6), but are still considerable.

The consequences for high mortality countries are small, as the greater part of the burden is experienced at younger ages and therefore hardly affected by the choice of normative survivorship goal. However, in low mortality countries, where a large part of the burden is concentrated at older ages, this choice is important. Because the normative survivorship goal is a social value, there is no right or wrong choice. The GBD standard life tables violate the second criterion that the normative survivorship goal should be constant across populations. If we adopt a third criterion that all loss of health, regardless of the age at which it is experienced, should be included in a health gap measure, a PYLL with a limit to life of 120 or more years is the only measure that satisfies all criteria. However, it is questionable whether epidemiologists and health policymakers feel comfortable with the dramatically greater emphasis on mortality in general, and at older ages in particular, when using a PYLL 120.

Figure 4 Discounted YLL and YLD from the Victorian Burden of Disease study, recalculated using the GBD standard life tables, PYLL 80, 85, 90, 100 and 120 in non-age weighted (3,0) and age weighted (3,1) scenarios

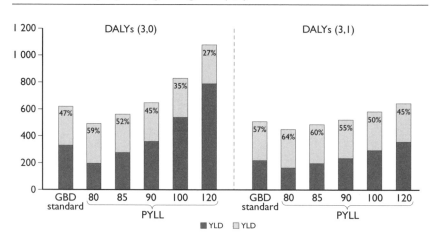

The fact that differentials are smaller, though not trivial, with the controversial age weighting (Anand and Hanson 1997; Barendregt et al. 1996), lends some pragmatic support to their inclusion as a social value in DALYs. From a pragmatic point of view, the compromise for future burden of disease studies may be the use of PYLL 90, because this agrees with the first two criteria and provides results that are closest to those of the Global Burden of Disease study.

Figure 5 Discounted and age-weighted DALYs by age from the Victorian Burden of Disease study, recalculated using the GBD standard life tables, PYLL 80, 85, 90, 100 and 120

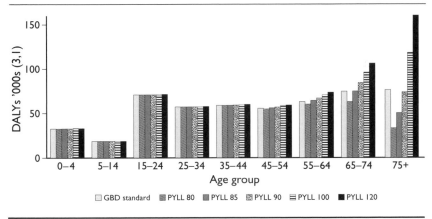

Figure 6 Discounted and non-age weighted DALYs by age from the Victorian Burden of Disease study, recalculated using the GBD standard life tables, PYLL 80, 85, 90, 100 and 120

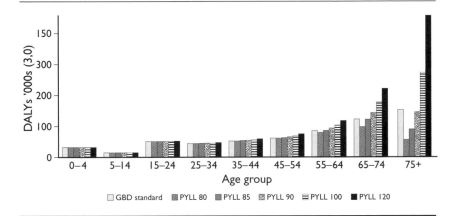

REFERENCES

Anand S, Hanson K (1997) Disability-adjusted life years: a critical review. *Journal of Health Economics,* **16**(6):685–702.

Barendregt JJ, Bonneux L, van der Maas PJ (1996) DALYs: the age-weights on balance. *Bulletin of the World Health Organization,* **74**(4):439–443.

Mathers CD, Vos T, Stevenson C (1999) *The burden of disease and injury in Australia.* Australian Institute of Health and Welfare, Canberra. *http://www.aihw.gov.au/publications/health/bdia.html.*

Murray CJL (1996) Rethinking DALYs. In: *The global burden of disease: a comprehensive assessment of mortality and disability from diseases, injuries, and risk factors in 1990 and projected to 2020.* The Global Burden of Disease and Injury, Vol. 1. Murray CJL, Lopez AD, eds. Harvard School of Public Health on behalf of WHO, Cambridge, MA.

Murray CJL, Salomon JA, Mathers CD (2000) A critical examination of summary measures of population health. *Bulletin of the World Health Organization,* 78(8):981–994.

Vos T, Begg S (1999) *Victorian burden of disease study: mortality.* Public Health Division, Department of Human Services, Melbourne. *http://www.dhs.vic.gov.au/phd/9903009/index.htm.*

Vos T, Begg S (2000) *Victorian burden of disease study: morbidity.* Public Health Division, Department of Human Services, Melbourne. *http://www.dhs.vic.gov.au/phd/9909065/index.htm.*

Chapter 6.1

Causal decomposition of summary measures of population health

Colin D. Mathers, Majid Ezzati, Alan D. Lopez, Christopher J.L. Murray and Anthony Rodgers

Introduction

A fundamental goal of summary measures of population health (SMPH), which may explain the increasing attention given to them, is identifying the relative magnitudes of different public health problems, including diseases, injuries and risk factors. In turn, this will allow the benefits of health interventions to be estimated and used in cost-effectiveness analyses, better planning of public health policy and programmes and in informing public health debates on priorities for research and development (uses 6, 7 and 8 of SMPH identified by Murray, Salomon and Mathers; see chapter 1.2).

Figure 1 provides a simplified conceptual framework for causal analysis of SMPH. This framework identifies four broad categories in the causal chain leading to loss of well-being or death:

- Health determinants (here divided into broad distal determinants and more proximal risk factors at the individual level)

- Diseases and injuries

- Health status (limitations in functioning)

- Death

Figure 1   Relating causes to health outcomes

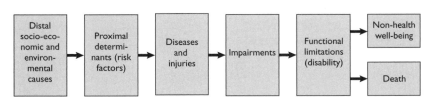

Without intending to pre-empt any conclusions on the components of well-being that are distinct from health, in Figure 1 we have identified impairment and disability (in the sense of functional and activity limitations at the person level) as the components of health status that are causally related to diseases and injury. Other, non-health components of well-being are in turn causally related to health status, as well as being potential causes of health loss themselves (e.g. when social isolation results in depression).[1]

Investigators from a variety of disciplines such as epidemiology, demography, environmental sciences, public health, economics and other social sciences increasingly address similar questions on the relationship between different types of causal factors and human health. The causal factors analyzed by epidemiologists are usually proximate causes of disease and injury; physical, biological, psychological and behavioural risk factors; and more distal health determinants such as social, cultural, economic and environmental factors. Social scientists are predominantly interested in investigating the relationships between the more distal factors and health, as well as other components of well-being. As a result, many epidemiological analyses are restricted to considering health determinants (boxes 1 and 2 in Figure 1) as causes, and disease, injury or death as the consequences (other boxes in Figure 1). In general, however, causal analysis may be carried out between any two (or more) of the domains shown in Figure 1 (e.g. diseases as causes and disability as outcome, or distal determinants as causes and risk factors as outcomes).

Frameworks for better understanding and representing the causal nature of the determinants of health have been proposed in several disciplines. For example, Mosley and Chen (1984) attempted to link the epidemiological and social science approaches by providing a multilayer causal framework for child mortality. The framework for comparative risk analysis (CRA) developed by Murray and Lopez (1999) extends the Mosley and Chen framework to all causes of mortality and disability.

There are two dominant traditions in causal attribution of health determinants, outcomes, or states: categorical attribution and counterfactual analysis. In categorical attribution, an event such as death is attributed to a single cause according to a defined set of rules. In counterfactual analysis, the contribution of a disease, injury or risk factor is estimated by comparing the current or future levels of a summary measure with the levels that would be expected under some alternative hypothetical, or counterfactual, scenario. There has been little discussion of the advantages and disadvantages of the two approaches to causal attribution, or of the issues of comparability or inconsistency that may arise when using both approaches in the same analysis. An example of the latter is provided by the 1990 Global Burden of Disease (GBD) study (Murray and Lopez 1996a), in which the burden attributable to diseases and injuries was estimated using categorical attribution, whereas burden attributable to risk factors or to diseases such as diabetes which act as risk factors, was estimated using counterfactual analysis.

We review these two approaches to causal attribution for SMPH, discuss their relative advantages and disadvantages and the implications for comparability when the two approaches are used in the same analysis.

CATEGORICAL ATTRIBUTION

In categorical attribution, an event such as death or the onset of a disease or health state is attributed categorically to one single cause according to a defined set of rules. Categorical attribution is commonly used in population health statistics that use cause-of-death classification or principal diagnosis for health system encounters. In cause-of-death tabulations, for example, each death is assigned to a unique cause according to the rules of the International Classification of Diseases (ICD), even in cases of multicausal events. For example, in ICD-10, deaths from tuberculosis in HIV-positive individuals are assigned to HIV (WHO 1992). This categorical approach to representing causes is the standard method used in published studies of health gaps, such as the 1990 Global Burden of Disease (Murray and Lopez 1996a).

For data relating to health system encounters, there are a similar set of rules for identifying the principal diagnosis. These rules may apply to the "underlying reason" for the health system encounter in a way similar to the cause of death rules, or may apply to the diagnosis responsible for the largest resource use during the health system encounter. The latter approach would be more relevant if the purpose of analysis is, for example, to attribute health system costs to disease and injury causes.

Categorical attribution requires a classification system with two key components: a set of mutually exclusive and collectively exhaustive categories, and a set of rules for assigning events to them.[2] For diseases and injuries, ICD has been developed and refined over nearly 150 years. No classification system has been developed for other types of causes, such as physiological, proximal or distal risk factors.

Mortality gaps have generally been categorically attributed to the underlying cause of death using ICD rules. Health gaps such as DALYs also have generally used categorical attribution for disease and injury causes. The YLD component is calculated in terms of the loss of health (quantified by a set of disability weights) associated with each of the disease stages, the severity levels and the sequelae caused by the disease (Murray 1996). DALY calculations start from information on diseases and injuries (incidence, prevalence and duration) and use categorical attribution to estimate the associated impairments, disability and mortality (the consequences on the right-hand side of the disease and injury box in Figure 1). Using the counterfactual approach discussed below, it is also possible to estimate the attributable burden of specific risk factors or health determinants (the causes to the left-hand side of the disease and injury box in Figure 1).

COUNTERFACTUAL ANALYSIS

Generally, when examining causality in population health (whether at the disease and injury level, or at the disability level), there is a complex "causal web" connecting the causes and health outcomes. In this causal web of interactions, combinations of component causes may be necessary and/or sufficient for the outcome to take place (Rothman 1976; Rothman and Greenland 1998). Although the terminology of component and sufficient cause is useful in emphasizing that combinations of exposures or factors may be required to cause an outcome, it is less suited to the hierarchical nature of health causation (Figure 2). Because of the large number of pathways and their complexity, it is difficult to apply the terminology of component, sufficient and necessary causes in assessing the burden of risk factors and distal health determinants, which motivates an alternative framework for causal attribution. Two basic approaches can be used to summarize the direction and intensity of the relationship between a given causal variable and an outcome (Figure 2). (As previously noted, the language of risk factors and outcomes can be applied to any part of the causal chain illustrated in Figure 2.) The approaches are:

- To characterize the relationship between change in one variable and change in an outcome variable.

- To compare the magnitude of health outcomes to some counterfactual state where the level of the causal variable has been changed.

If all the links in the causal web shown in Figure 2 were known, we could evaluate the effect of small changes in the causal variable and express the results as the elasticity of the summary measure with respect to changes in the causal variable; or as a numerical approximation of the partial derivative of the summary measure. However, for causal webs of

Figure 2   Simplified causal web linking exposures and outcomes

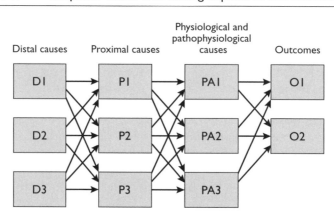

any degree of complexity, this approach is difficult to operationalize. Also, both partial and total derivatives suffer from the problem that they are entirely context specific and any change in any other variables could change the derivative of interest. Furthermore, any change in the expectation of the causal variable itself is likely to be associated with a change in the distribution of the causal variable, so that the task of specifying a "small change" also becomes context specific.

The alternative to complete characterization of the causal web is to estimate the contribution of a disease, injury or risk factor by comparing the current and future levels of a summary measure of population health with the levels that would be expected under some alternative hypothetical scenario, such as a counterfactual distribution of risk factor or the extent of a disease or injury. The models used in such a counterfactual analysis may be extremely simple or quite complex (as in the case of risk factors with complex time and distributional characteristics). The validity of the estimate depends on that of the model used to predict the counterfactual scenarios. Various types of counterfactual distributions may be used for this type of assessment.

The classical approach in epidemiology for causal attribution to a risk factor is to define an attributable fraction, which is the proportion of the outcome in the specific population that would be eliminated in the absence of exposure (e.g. Beaglehole et al. 1993). The concept of attributable risk is therefore implicitly based on a simple dichotomous exposure variable and a particular reference distribution of exposure, namely zero exposure. For many of the health determinants of interest, this approach is either too restrictive or inappropriate, since the comparison is restricted to zero exposure baseline. Murray and Lopez (1999) have suggested generalizing the attributable risk concept by defining attributable burden to be the difference between the burden currently observed and the burden that would be observed under an alternative, or counterfactual, population distribution of exposure. They have also developed a classification of various counterfactual risk distributions that can be used for these purposes, discussed below.

Counterfactual analysis of summary measures has a wide spectrum of uses, from the assessment of specific policies or actions to more general assessments of the contribution of diseases, injuries or risk factors. In intervention analysis the change in a summary measure resulting from the application of a specific intervention may be estimated. Greenland (see chapter 6.2) has argued that counterfactual analysis for policy formulation should measure only the effects of actions that can be operationalized (e.g. anti-smoking campaigns, food-distribution programmes), rather than effects of removing the outcomes targeted by those actions (e.g. smoking cessation, malnutrition). We argue that this is too limiting, and that apart from intervention analysis, counterfactual analysis is useful for the more general assessment of the contribution of disease, injuries or risk factors to population health, even when there is no known intervention for changing the current distribution.

ADDITIVE DECOMPOSITION AND COUNTERFACTUAL ANALYSIS

Murray et al. proposed that, for practical reasons, it would be desirable for summary measures to be linear aggregates of the summary measures calculated for any arbitrary partitioning of subgroups of the population (see chapter 1.2). Many decision-makers, and very often the public, desire information that is characterized by this type of additive decomposition. In other words, they would like to know what fraction of the summary measure is related to health events in the poor, in the uninsured, in the elderly, in children, and so on. Additive decomposition is also often appealing for causal attribution.

Clearly, categorical attribution provides additive decomposition by cause, whereas counterfactual analysis may not. This is because the sum of attributable burden for exposure to various health determinants is theoretically unbounded, since death and disability from many diseases and injuries can result from several exposures acting simultaneously. For example, imagine a disease causation model that requires the coincidence of three factors such as hypertension, alcohol and smoking. If any one of the three is not present, a death will be averted. Using a variety of counterfactual distributions of exposure for each of these three factors, that death is fully attributable to all three risk factors. This implies great caution when interpreting attributable fractions, as the sum of attributable fractions can exceed 100% for any subset of causes.

CAUSAL ATTRIBUTION OF HEALTH EXPECTANCIES

Because health expectancies are positive measures of health, integrated across the life span, they combine the effects of all causes acting at each subsequent age. Therefore, categorical attribution of health expectancies is not possible. Attempts have been made to relate health expectancies back to causes of disease and risk factors, using "disease elimination", a form of counterfactual analysis. Data for the analysis are provided by population surveys of health conditions contributing to the disability (Bone et al. 1995; Mathers 1999; Mathers 1992; Nusselder et al. 1996). The key to all these methods has been estimating the contribution of specific diseases or disease groups to the prevalence of disability. The elimination of a disease then reduces the overall prevalence of disability and also reduces mortality rates, resulting in an increase in disability-free or health-adjusted life expectancy. A related approach is based on a generalization of the concept of entropy or elasticity of life expectancy, defined as the marginal change in life expectancy that results from a small (say 1%) decrease in mortality rates at all ages (Hill et al. 1996).

Attempts have been made to calculate a variety of disease-free life expectancies (together with their complementary expectations of life with disease), but they have not provided a causal decomposition of health expectancy, since each pair of expectancies (with and without disease) form a separate complete decomposition of the total health (or life) expectancy, whose components cannot be compared across diseases.

CALCULATING CAUSE-DELETED HEALTH EXPECTANCIES

Cause-deleted health expectancies estimate the contribution of specific diseases or disease groups to risk of death and the prevalence of disability. The "elimination" of a disease then reduces the overall prevalence of disability and also reduces mortality rates, resulting in an increase in disability-free or health-adjusted life expectancy.

The effect of eliminating a disease or injury on health expectancies is usually calculated assuming the following independence among causes of death and disability:

- Cause-deleted probabilities of dying are estimated with cause-elimination life Tables, assuming independent causes of death (Tsai et al. 1978). Cause elimination is carried out for all age groups, including the final open-ended age group.

- Cause-deleted disability and handicap prevalences are calculated directly from the survey estimates by subtracting the cause-specific disability and handicap prevalences from the total prevalences.

- Cause-deleted health expectancies are calculated by Sullivan's method using the cause-deleted prevalences in the cause-elimination life tables.

Assuming independent causes, Tsai et al. (1978) derive the following formula for the effect of eliminating a fraction of deaths from cause k on the life table probability q_i of dying in the age interval (x_i, x_{i+1}):

$$q_i' = 1 - (1-q_i)^{(D_i - \pi_{ik} D_{ik})/D_i}$$

where D_i is the total number of deaths in the age interval (x_i, x_{i+1}), π_{ik} is the proportion of deaths from cause k that are eliminated $(0 \le \pi_{ik} \le 1)$, and D_{ik} is the total number of deaths from cause k in the age interval (x_i, x_{i+1}).

If the observed prevalence of disability in the age interval (x_i, x_{i+1}) is d_i, and d_{ik} is the prevalence of disability attributable to cause k, then the average expectation of life free of disability at age x_i, after eliminating proportion π_{ik} of cause k, may be calculated using Sullivan's method as:

$$DFLE_x = \frac{\sum_{i=x}^{w}(1 - d_i + \pi_{ik} d_{ik}) L_i}{l_x}$$

where l_i and L_i are the life table functions for the number of persons surviving to exact age x_i and the total number of years lived in the age interval (x_i, x_{i+1}). These functions are calculated using the cause eliminated probabilities of dying q_i' defined above.

Note that this method involves the hypothetical elimination of the disease or injury at all ages. Estimation of the change in a health expectancy due to elimination of a disease in a specific age range would require information on the duration or age of onset of the disability, since the disability may be the result of a disease or injury which occurred many years before (or prior to birth).

Manton et al. (1976) illustrate that even in the presence of dependent multiple causes, mortality (and by extension other health states) can be represented by independent processes which are activated during aging. The contribution of a cause can then be estimated by eliminating all processes that contain that cause.

MAPPING DISABILITY TO DISEASE

To estimate gains in disability-free or handicap-free life expectancy resulting from the elimination of a disease or disease group, the prevalence of disability and handicap attributable to the disease group must be estimated. This is not straightforward because multiple health conditions are common, particularly for older people, but also for younger adults with mental disorders. In British disability surveys, for example, up to 10 separate health conditions were recorded for disabled people and 78% of all disabled people cited multiple health problems as contributing to disability. Two main approaches for classifying multiple disability (co-morbidity) have been used:

The first is to identify the principal cause of disability for each individual (as derived from respondents' self-reports) and attribute all disability for that individual to the principal cause (categorical attribution). Thus, elimination of that cause reduces the prevalence of disability by the number of people for whom that disability was a principal cause. This approach was used by Mathers (1992) and Bone et al. (1995). The main limitation of this categorical approach to cause-deleted health expectancy is the difficulties of mapping disability to diseases and injuries. A significant proportion of respondents in most disability surveys state that they do not know the main cause of their disability, and others undoubtedly give incorrect answers. Additionally, this approach does not take into account co-morbidity situations, where disability is the result of the interaction of a number of health problems. For older people particularly, a number of diseases and impairments may act interdependently to limit activity.

The second approach, developed by Nusselder et al. (1996) uses a multivariate modelling approach to estimate the proportion of disability prevalence associated with each of a number of chronic diseases. If this approach were developed for estimating counterfactual prevalences that resulted from eliminating each chronic disease separately, full disease elimination analysis of the health expectancy could be carried out consistently using counterfactual methods. This has not yet been attempted, however. Similarly, the multiple-cause mortality method of Manton et al. (1976) can, in principle, be extended to disability to estimate the effects of disease elimination on health expectancy through all the disability processes that include the eliminated disease.

COMPARATIVE RISK ASSESSMENT

The first global estimates of disease and injury burden due to different risk factors were reported in the initial round of the GBD study (Murray and Lopez 1996b; 1997). These estimates expand on the many others made for selected risk factors in specific populations, such as tobacco (Peto et al. 1992), environmental factors (Smith et al. 1999), blood pressure (Rodgers et al. 2000) and selected risk factors for certain regions (Mathers et al. 1999; MH-NZ 1999; NIPHS 1997). In the GBD study, risk factors could either be exposures in the environment (e.g. unsafe water), human behaviour (e.g. tobacco smoking) or physiological states (e.g. hypertension). Table 1 summarizes initial estimates of the global burden of disease attributable to 10 major risk factors, together with the exposure measures and counterfactual reference distributions used.

Several issues arose from the initial GBD study estimates, which provided the impetus for developing a Comparative Risk Assessment (CRA) framework. CRA can be defined as a systematic counterfactual approach for estimating health gaps (or changes in health expectancy) causally attributable to a risk factor or a group of risk factors.[3] The advantages of a non-zero counterfactual distribution were discussed earlier. The broad rationale for other developments, based largely on the work of Murray and Lopez (1999), is described in this section and some important theoretical and methodological issues are identified.

ATTRIBUTABLE AND AVOIDABLE BURDEN

CRA distinguishes between the current burden of premature death and disability due to past exposure (i.e. attributable burden), and the future burden due to current exposure (i.e. avoidable burden). When the time lag between exposure and disease or death is short, this distinction is not critical. But if the time lag is long, such as for tobacco, hypertension, unsafe sex, physical inactivity, some occupational exposures and alcohol, there may be a major difference between attributable and avoidable burden. The concepts of attributable and avoidable burden are shown graphically in Figure 3.

Calculating the future burden due to current exposure is inherently more complicated and uncertain, given secular trends in diseases, possible changes in the exposure-outcome relationship, expected socioeconomic changes and likely advances in technology. On the other hand, the future burden of disease and injury due to current exposure is more important for public health planning and prevention than are estimates of current burden due to past exposures, since the latter cannot be altered. Nevertheless, attributable burden may be interesting because it is likely to be a good predictor of avoidable burden.

Table I   Global burden attributable to 10 major risk factors[a]

Risk Factor	Type of risk factor			Measure of exposure	Reference distribution of exposure	Time lag from exposure to burden	Attributable burden
	Exposure	Physio-logical state	Controlled for confounding in relative risk				
Malnutrition		■		Population less than 2 SDs weight-for-age based on extensive national surveys	Population weight-for-age higher than minus 2 SDs	Intermediate	15.9%
Poor water, sanitation and hygiene	■			Based on the theoretical fecal-oral route of transmission	Zero	Short	6.8%
Unsafe sex	■			Based on theoretical model of transmission of STDs and on contraceptive demand surveys for maternal conditions	Zero	Short to long	3.5%
Alcohol (disease)	■		■	Indexed on alcohol consumption, non-hepatitis B cirrhosis, and alcohol dependence sydrome	Zero	Long	3.5%
Alcohol (injury)	■			Indexed on estimate of consumption patterns based on small-scale studies	Zero	Short	
Occupation (disease)	■			Registration data for EME, FSE, and LAC and constant rates for all other regions	Zero	Long	2.7%
Occupation (injury)	■			Registration data for EME and constant rates for all other regions	Zero	Short	
Tobacco	■			Indexed on lung cancer	Zero	Long	2.6%
Hypertension		■	■	Population surveys of blood pressure	Systolic blood pressure of 110 mm Hg	Long	1.4%
Physical inactivity	■			Population surveys of activity patterns	Regular physical activity	Long	1.0%
Illicit drugs	■			Small-scale studies	Zero	Short to intermediate	0.6%
Air pollution	■			Monitoring systems in urban areas for most regions	WHO guidelines	Short to long	0.5%

a. Source: 1990 Global Burden of Disease study (Murray and Lopez 1996b).

Figure 3   The concepts of attributable and avoidable burden

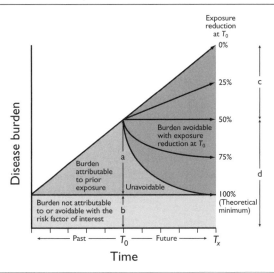

a = disease at T_0 attributable to prior exposure.

b = disease at T_0 not attributable to the risk factor (caused by other factors).

c = avoidable burden at T_x with a 50% exposure reduction at T_0.

d = disease burden at T_x after a 50% reduction in risk factor.

Attributable fraction at T_0 due to prior exposure = $a / (a + b)$.

Avoidable fraction at T_x due to 50% exposure reduction at T_0 = $c / (c + d)$. In general avoidable burden at T_y due to exposure reduction at T_0 is given by the ratio of the darkest shaded area to total burden at T_y.

Note that the burden attributable solely to other risk factors (lightest grey area) may be decreasing, increasing, or constant over time. The last case is shown in the figure.

Because attributable burden is an estimate of the proportion of current burden due to a given risk factor, and is complementary to the main partitioning by disease/injury category, attributable burden might best be principally regarded as *an alternative system for categorizing disease burden*. As such, it should have maximum reliability and the methods should have maximum comparability. In contrast, avoidable burden is an estimate of future burden that might be avoidable with changes in current exposure levels. It can also give an estimate of what the effects of complete primary prevention (also called primordial prevention) might have been. As such, it should primarily be regarded as *an input to prioritization* for health care services and research, together with local costs, preferences, etc. Clearly, the reliability of avoidable burden estimates depends on the reliability of the attributable burden estimates (as well as on the reliability of projections of disease burden and risk reversal estimates).

CHOOSING COUNTERFACTUAL DISTRIBUTIONS

A counterfactual analysis requires that the current distributions of risk factors be compared to some alternative distribution of exposure. Many different counterfactuals are potentially of interest, including four types described by Murray and Lopez (1999):

- *Theoretical minimum risk distribution.* The distribution of exposure which would yield the lowest population risk (for example, zero tobacco use).

- *Plausible minimum risk.* The distribution of exposure among the set of plausible distributions that would minimize overall population risk. Plausible implies that the shape of the distribution can be imaginable in some real population.

- *Feasible minimum risk.* The distribution of exposure that could imply minimum risk under a set of circumstances that are feasible. Feasible implies that there exists or has existed a population with this distribution of exposure. This approach has been used to estimate burden from unsafe water and sanitation. (Note that *plausible* means that the distribution is imaginable or possible, whereas *feasible* means that it has been achieved in some population).

- *Cost-effective minimum risk.* This is the distribution of exposure that would result if all cost-effective interventions (against some reference value) could be implemented. This distribution will depend on what might be considered cost-effective in different populations and is therefore not uniformly applicable to all populations.

The theoretical minimum exposure distribution is more complicated for risk factors for which zero exposure is not defined, such as physiological risk factors (e.g. cholesterol and BMI). In these cases, a distribution or minimum level which results in the lowest overall risk will have to be estimated. For other exposures there may be region/age/sex subgroups for which zero exposure may not always be associated with the lowest risk. An example is alcohol which, at low levels, is found to have protective effects against cardiovascular disease at higher ages. Although the exact level which minimizes population risk may vary from one region to another, the theoretical minimum counterfactual distribution should be the same in all regions to maximize comparability. The question is then: "What is the lowest risk for the whole population if a constant age-sex specific counterfactual is chosen?" Such a global theoretical minimum will avoid problems of "shifting goal posts", yet still allow alternative estimation of minima at non-zero levels. Feasible and cost-effective reductions, however, are likely to vary by age, sex or region.

CHARACTERIZING THE DISTRIBUTIONAL TRANSITION

A shift from current population distribution of exposure to a counterfactual distribution is referred to as the distributional transition. In a distributional transition, exposure may be uniformly shifted or scaled downwards for the whole population, or certain segments of the population may be targeted for exposure reduction, such as those most at risk or those whose exposure may be reduced with the lowest cost. We emphasize that distributional transition (Figure 4) on its own is a methodological tool for representing (incremental) changes in population distribution of exposure and is conceptually independent from the initial (current) and terminal (counterfactual) distributions. In particular, plausible, feasible, and cost-effective risk factor distributions should lie between the current risk factor levels and the theoretical minimum.

In many instances the counterfactual of most relevance will involve small to moderate distributional transitions (e.g. 10%, 20% or 30%), as these are most likely to be feasible, cost-effective, etc. Two other advantages of concentrating on such small-to-moderate transitions are:

• First, these estimates are likely to be most reliable, as the dose-response is often least certain at low exposure levels. Large distributional transitions (e.g. 80% risk factor reduction) would require estimates of dose-response associations at these low levels of exposure.

• Second, small shifts are less susceptible to the influence of arbitrary choices of theoretical minima.

TEMPORAL ISSUES IN COUNTERFACTUAL ANALYSIS

The transition between current and counterfactual exposure distributions often takes place over a time interval. The path between different exposure levels is of little importance if exposure changes over a short time interval, especially relative to the time required for the impact of exposure on disease. Over long time periods, however, the actual path of transition may be as important as the end points in determining the disease burden associated with change in exposure. The complexity of defining the temporal characteristics of the shift to the counterfactual distribution, and the

Figure 4   Example of distributional transitions for blood pressure and for tobacco smoking

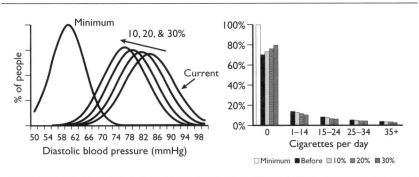

NB: For a categorical exposure variable, distributional transitions can be defined in terms of either shifting to the category below or to the baseline category (e.g. quitting for tobacco).

time during which change is evaluated, can be illustrated using the example of smoking. A counterfactual for smoking, in which the whole population does not smoke for one year, followed by a return to the status quo at the end of this year, could be traced out in terms of changes in future health expectancies or future health gaps. Because of time lags and threshold effects, removing a hazard for such a short duration may lead to little or no change in a summary measure of population health over time. Alternatively, the counterfactual distribution of smoking cessation can last longer, such as a permanent change to a state of no tobacco consumption.

Changes in the counterfactual distribution of exposure in a population may have an impact on summary measures of population health over many years in the future. It may be argued that all changes in future population health should be included in an analysis of avoidable burden. It could also be argued that changes in the distant future should be weighted as less important than more immediate changes, by discounting future changes. Instead of assuming a constant discount rate, an alternative method has been to apply a dichotomous discount rate, such that changes up to time t are counted equally (i.e. zero discount rate) and changes after time t are given zero weight (i.e. infinite discount rate). Although debate continues on the merits of discounting (e.g. chapters 13.1–13.3), choices on the temporal characteristics of counterfactual exposure distribution are intimately linked to whether future changes in population health are discounted. For example, a permanent shift in exposure could lead to an infinite stream of future changes in health expectancies or health gaps in the absence of discounting.

MODELLING THE JOINT EFFECTS OF DIFFERENT RISK FACTORS AND THE FULL EFFECTS OF DISTAL RISK FACTORS

For many diseases or injuries, the underlying exposures do not operate directly to cause disease or injury, but operate through different levels of risk factors. For example, socioeconomic status, including income and education, has been linked to diet, alcohol consumption and smoking, which in turn influence outcomes such as coronary heart disease through physiological processes. The full impact of such proximal risk factors may not be captured in traditional regression analysis methods in which both proximal and distal variables are included. Characterization of the complete causal web of interactions which result in disease, may on the other hand lead to more appropriate estimates in this case.

In addition to estimating the effects of distal risk factors, causal webs can be used to consider the effect of simultaneous changes in two or more risk factor distributions. This has particular significance when a disease is caused by more than one risk factor, such as those in Figure 5, especially if the risk factors are expected to be affected by the same policies, such as smoking and alcohol consumption.

Figure 5 Causal web to estimate full rather than partial effects of a risk factor such as physical activity

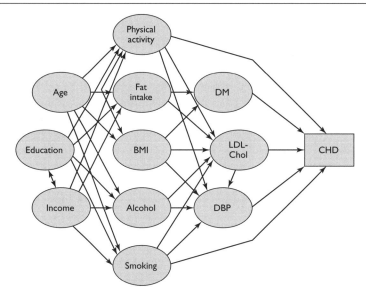

DISCUSSION AND CONCLUSIONS

We have identified a number of possible approaches to analysing the contribution of diseases, injuries or risk factors to summary measures of population health (Table 2). Population health can be summarized using health expectancies and health gaps, and causal attribution for diseases and injuries can be assessed using categorical attribution or counterfactuals. Because there is no established complete classification system for risk factors, they can only be assessed using the counterfactual

Table 2 Approaches to analysing the contributions of diseases, injuries or risk factors to summary measures of population health

	Categorical attribution	Counterfactual analysis
Health expectancies	Health states[a]	Health states Diseases Injuries Risk factors
Health gaps	Health states Diseases Injuries	Health states Diseases Injuries Risk factors

a. May be specific impairments, disabilities, or health states defined on several dimensions (such as EuroQol or HUI).

approach. Even for diseases and injuries, it is not possible to use categorical attribution with a health expectancy, as positive health measures cannot be assigned to specific diseases or injuries.

The advantage of categorical attribution is that it is simple, widely understood and appealing to many users of this information because the total level of the summary measure equals the sum of the contributions of a set of mutually exclusive causes (i.e. categorical attribution produces additive decomposition across causes). The disadvantage is well illustrated by multicausal events, such as a myocardial infarction in a diabetic, or liver cancer resulting from chronic hepatitis B. If additive decomposition is a critical property, the contribution of diseases and injuries can only be assessed using health gaps.

The counterfactual method for calculating the contribution of diseases, injuries and risk factors has different advantages. It is conceptually clearer, solves problems of multicausality and is consistent with the approach for evaluating the benefits of health interventions (Murray et al. 2000).

How can causal attribution be used to inform debates on research and development priorities, the selection of national health priorities for action, and health curriculum development? It can be argued that a method of causal attribution should yield an ordinal ranking of causes which is identical to that of the absolute number of years of healthy life gained by a population through cause elimination (or appropriate counterfactual change for a risk factor). As such, the absolute numbers of deaths or DALYs attributable to a cause are critical where cause decomposition is intended to inform public health prioritization.

Causal attribution is a key aspect of summary measures for several important uses outlined above. For diseases and injuries, ICD allows a choice between categorical attribution and counterfactual analysis. The desirability of additive decomposition strongly favours the use of categorical attribution. However, the results of counterfactual analysis have a more direct and theoretically cogent interpretation. We suggest that in practice the only solution to this dilemma is routine reporting of both categorical attribution and counterfactual analysis for diseases and injuries. All issues of multicausal death, as with diabetes mellitus, would be well captured in counterfactual analysis since categorical attribution tends to underestimate the problem. There is no classification system for risk factors, whether physiological, proximal or distal, and consequently the only option is counterfactual analysis. There are many options for defining counterfactuals, and substantial work is needed to understand more fully the implications of adopting different approaches.

While health expectancy provides a single positive measure of the overall level of health for a population, the use of counterfactual analysis for causal decomposition does not result in additivity. For this reason, we recommend that an initial analysis of the causes of health loss in a population through disease and injury use health gap measures with categorical attribution, followed by counterfactual analysis for proximal and distal risk factors and other structural determinants.

NOTES

1 Figure 1 has been simplified to identify the major causal path; causal arrows of varying importance connect all components of the diagram in both directions.

2 These sets of rules codify a form of counterfactual analysis, where the counterfactual scenario would be approximately: *Would this death have occurred if disease or injury cause x had been absent in this individual, all else (apart from the consequences of x) being the same?*

3 CRA is conceptually distinct from Intervention Analysis. The latter is a time-series based evaluation of the health benefits of a specific intervention. CRA estimates the burden due to different risk factors, each of which may be altered by many different strategies.

REFERENCES

Beaglehole R, Bonita R, Kjellstrom T (1993) *Basic epidemiology.* World Health Organization, Geneva.

Bone MR, Bebbington AC, Jagger C, Morgan K, Nicolaas G (1995) *Health expectancy and its uses.* HMSO, London.

Hill GB, Forbes WF, Wilkins R (1996) *The entropy of health and disease: dementia in Canada.* (Presented at the 9th meeting of the international network on health expectancy and the disability process REVES, December 1996.) Rome.

Manton KG, Tolley HD, Poss SS (1976) Life table techniques for multiple-cause mortality. *Demography,* 13(4):541–564.

Mathers CD (1992) *Estimating gains in health expectancy due to elimination of specified diseases.* (Presented at the 5th meeting of the international network on health expectancy and the disability process REVES, February 1992.) Ottawa.

Mathers CD (1997) *Gains in health expectancy from the elimination of disease: a useful measure of the burden of disease.* (Presented at the 10th meeting of the international network on health expectancy and the disability process REVES, October 1997.) Tokyo.

Mathers CD, Vos T, Stevenson C (1999) *The burden of disease and injury in Australia.* Australian Institute of Health and Welfare, Canberra. *http://www.aihw.gov.au/publications/health/bdia.html.*

Ministry of Health (1999) *Our health, our future. The health of New Zealanders.* Ministry of Health (MH-NZ), Wellington.

Mosley WH, Chen LC (1984b) An analytical framework for the study of child survival in developing countries. In: *Child survival: strategies for research.* Mosley WH, Chen LC, eds. Population Council, New York.

Mosley WH, Chen LC (1984) An analytical framework for the study of child survival in developing countries. *Population and Development Review,* 10(Suppl.):25–45.

Murray CJL (1996) Rethinking DALYs. In: *The global burden of disease: a comprehensive assessment of mortality and disability from diseases, injuries, and risk factors in 1990 and projected to 2020.* The Global Burden of Disease and Injury, Vol. 1. Murray CJL, Lopez AD, eds. Harvard School of Public Health on behalf of WHO, Cambridge, MA.

Murray CJL, Lopez AD, eds. (1996a) *The global burden of disease: a comprehensive assessment of mortality and disability from diseases, injuries and risk factors in 1990 and projected to 2020.* Global Burden of Disease and Injury, Vol. 1. Harvard School of Public Health on behalf of WHO, Cambridge, MA.

Murray CJL, Lopez AD (1996b) Quantifying the burden of disease and injury attributable to ten major risk factors. In: *The global burden of disease: a comprehensive assessment of mortality and disability from diseases, injuries, and risk factors in 1990 and projected to 2020.* Global Burden of Disease and Injury, Vol. 1. Murray CJL, Lopez AD, eds. Harvard School of Public Health on behalf of WHO, Cambridge, MA.

Murray CJL, Lopez AD (1997) Global mortality, disability and the contribution of risk factors: global burden of disease study. *Lancet,* **349**(9063):1436–1442.

Murray CJL, Lopez AD (1999) On the comparable quantification of health risks: lessons from the global burden of disease study. *Epidemiology,* **10**(5):594–605.

National Instititute of Public Health Sweden (NIPHS) (1997) *Determinants of the burden of disease in the European Union.* Folkhälsoinstitutet [National Institute of Public Health], Stockholm.

Nusselder WJ, van der Velden K, van Sonsbeek JL, Lenior ME, et al. (1996) The elimination of selected chronic diseases in a population: the compression and expansion of morbidity. *American Journal of Public Health,* **86**(2):187–194.

Peto R, Lopez AD, Boreham J, Thun M, Heath JC (1992) Mortality from tobacco in developed countries: indirect estimation from National Vital Statistics. *Lancet,* **339**(8804):1268–1278.

Rodgers A, Lawes C, MacMahon S (2000) Reducing the burden of blood pressure related cardiovascular disease. *Journal of Hypertension,* **18** (Suppl.):S3-S5.

Rothman KJ (1976) Causes. *American Journal of Epidemiology,* **104**(6):587–592.

Rothman KJ, Greenland S (1998) Causation and causal inference. In: *Modern epidemiology.* Rothman KJ, Greenland S, eds. Lippincott-Raven, Philadelphia, PA.

Smith KR, Corvalan CF, Kjellstrom T (1999) How much global ill health is attributable to environmental factors? *Epidemiology,* **10**(5):573–584.

Tsai SP, Lee SE, Hardy RJ (1978) The effect of a reduction in leading causes of death: potential gains in life expectancy. *American Journal of Public Health,* **68**(10):966–971.

WHO (1992) *International statistical classification of diseases and related health problems (ICD 10).* 10th edn. World Health Organization, Geneva.

Chapter 6.2

CAUSALITY THEORY FOR POLICY USES
OF EPIDEMIOLOGICAL MEASURES

SANDER GREENLAND

This paper provides an introduction to measures of causal effects and focuses on underlying conceptual models, definitions and drawbacks of special relevance to policy formulation based on epidemiological data. It begins by describing a foundation for critical analysis based on counterfactuals and potential outcomes. It then describes analyses based on hypothetical outcome removal and rejects them as potentially misleading. It is argued that one should analyse measures within a multivariate framework to capture the impact of major sources of morbidity and mortality. This framework can clarify what is captured and missed by any proposed summary measure of population health, and shows that the concept of summary measure can and should be extended to multidimensional indices.

INTRODUCTION

This paper describes a set of fundamental concepts from causality theory that can be used to critically analyse summary measures of population health. It then uses these concepts to argue that health measures based on hypothetical outcome removal are ambiguous and potentially misleading. Thorough analyses require a multivariate framework to capture what is known about sources of morbidity and mortality. Because of the unavoidable shortcomings of single-valued summaries, multidimensional indices should be considered for summary measures of population health.

The first task is to define cause and effect in a manner precise enough for logical manipulation and quantification. Three types of models have achieved widespread usage:

- *Counterfactual or potential-outcomes models.* These models were glimpsed by Hume (1748) and were operationalized by statisticians in the 1920s and 1930s (Rubin 1990). They have also received much attention in philosophy (Lewis 1973; Simon and Rescher 1966), social sciences (Sobel 1994; Winship and Morgan 1999) and epidemiology (see citations below).

- *Structural-equations models.* These models can be traced to early work in path analysis in the 1920s and were given full expression by econometricians in the 1940s.

- *Graphical models* (causal diagrams). These models also originated in path analysis, but were not fully developed until the early 1990s (Greenland et al. 1999; Pearl 1995).

A recent book on causal theory (Pearl 2000) details the above approaches and their histories, and emphasizes that they are logically equivalent (isomorphic) for all practical purposes. This means that an analysis using one approach can be translated into either of the other two approaches, while maintaining logical consistency.

Because of the emphasis on counterfactual models in the literature on measures of cause and effect, the following development is based on them. Further details of counterfactual theory for health science research are described elsewhere (Greenland 1987; Greenland 1990; Greenland 2000; Greenland and Morgenstern 2001; Greenland and Poole 1988; Greenland and Robins 1986; Greenland and Robins 1988; Maldonado and Greenland 2002; Robins and Greenland 1989; 1992; Rothman and Greenland 1998). For details on missing-data models, see Rubin (1991).

BASIC CONCEPTS OF COUNTERFACTUAL CAUSALITY

ACTIONS, OUTCOMES AND COUNTERFACTUALS

To minimize ambiguity, a counterfactual model requires reasonably precise definitions of the following model ingredients:

- At least one *target* subject of interest in whom or which causation is to be studied (e.g. a specific person or population).

- A list of two or more possible alternative actions, x_0, x_1 etc., that could have been applied at or over a span of time, one of which may be the actual action taken.

- An outcome measure, Y, taken at a point in time or over a period of time, following completion of the action.

As an example, the subject could be Kosovo, the action x_1 could be revocation of its autonomy by Yugoslavia in 1988, an alternative x_0 could be that revocation never occurred, and the outcome measure could be the mortality of pre-1999 residents during 1999. Because only one of the possible actions x_0, x_1, etc. can take place, all but one of the actions must become *counterfactual*, or contrary to fact. In the example, the actual (or factual) action was x_1 = "revocation of autonomy"; thus, the action x_0 =

"no revocation" is counterfactual. (This example also illustrates the truism that to do nothing is an action, corresponding to zero on an action scale.)

If x_a is the actual action taken (from the list x_0, x_1, etc.), we may observe the outcome $Y(x_a)$ that follows that action. A *counterfactual outcome model* posits that, for any counterfactual action, x_c (from the same list), there is also a well-defined outcome, $Y(x_c)$, that would have followed *that* action (often called a "potential outcome"; (Rubin 1990; 1991). In the example, the actual action, x_a, was x_1 and was eventually followed by a certain mortality, $Y(x_1)$, in 1999. $Y(x_1)$ is difficult to assess but nonetheless exists as a matter of fact; it is part of what occurred subsequently to the action x_1. A counterfactual model for 1999 mortality posits that, had the counterfactual action x_0 been taken instead (that is, if no revocation had occurred), the mortality would have equaled some number, $Y(x_0)$. Given that x_0 is counterfactual, it is logically impossible for us to observe $Y(x_0)$. Nonetheless, the counterfactual model treats this number as a precise, though unknown, quantity.

The idea of treating the outcome, $Y(x_c)$, under a counterfactual action, x_c, as a precise quantity has been a source of much controversy and misunderstanding (e.g. Dawid 2000; Holland 1986). Some major misunderstandings are addressed below:

- The counterfactual approach does *not* require that the outcome, $Y(x_c)$, be precisely defined for every possible counterfactual action, x_c. In the above example, if we are interested only in contrasting revocation (x_1) with no action (x_0), our model need not mention any other actions. That is, we can limit the action list to just those actions of interest.

- The counterfactual approach is *not* inherently deterministic in either the classical or quantum-mechanical sense. The potential outcomes, $Y(x_0)$, $Y(x_1)$, etc., may represent different values for a statistical parameter in a classical probability model. For example, they may be expected rates in Poisson models. Alternatively, they may represent different mixtures of superposed states (different wave functions) in quantum models. Indeed, some theoreticians regard counterfactuals as essential for formulating coherent explanations of quantum phenomena (Penrose 1994).

- The counterfactual approach extends the partial quantification of outcomes, $Y(x_c)$, under counterfactual actions embedded in ordinary discourse. In the example, some (though not all) observers of the events in Kosovo 1988–1999 speculated that the actual 1999 mortality, $Y(x_1)$, was probably greater than $Y(x_0)$, the mortality that would have occurred had autonomy never been revoked. This speculation arises from the following tentative explanation of actual events in Kosovo: revocation of autonomy, (x_1), caused Albanian resistance to increased Serb authority, which in turn caused Serbian leaders to extend their "ethnic cleansing" policy to Kosovo. Had there been no revocation, (x_0), this tragic causal sequence of events would not have occurred.

CAUSE AND EFFECT

The speculative explanation in the third bulleted item above is an example of an informal causal hypothesis. Consideration of such hypotheses has led to the following definition: An *effect* of taking an action, x_j, rather than another action, x_k, on an outcome measure, Y, is a numerical contrast of that measure (e.g. the difference or ratio) under the two different actions. The contrast is called an *effect measure*. In the example, the contrast $Y(x_1) - Y(x_0)$ is an effect of revocation x_1 versus no revocation x_0; this effect measure is known as the mortality difference due to x_1 versus x_0. Similarly, $Y(x_1) / Y(x_0)$ is the effect measure known as the mortality ratio due to x_1 versus x_0.

Many common ideas and a few surprises follow from the above definitions, among them:

- An effect is a *relation* between the outcomes that would follow *two* different actions, x_j and x_k, in just *one* subject (a population or single person). It is thus meaningless to talk of (say) "the effect of smoking a pack a day"; one must at least imply a reference (baseline) action for "the effect" to have meaning. While smoking a pack a day can cause lung cancer relative to no smoking, it can also prevent lung cancer relative to smoking two packs a day.

- If $Y(x_j) = Y(x_k)$, we say that having x_j happen rather than x_k had no effect on Y for the subject; otherwise, we say having x_j happen rather than x_k caused the outcome to be $Y(x_j)$ and prevented the outcome from being $Y(x_k)$. For example, we may say that smoking prevents survival past age 70 years just as surely as it causes death by age 70. Similarly, we may say that not smoking causes survival past age 70 just as surely as it prevents death by age 70. Thus, the distinction between causation and prevention is merely a matter of whether we are talking of an action, x_j, and *its* consequence, $Y(x_j)$ (causation of $Y(x_j)$), or an action, x_j, and a consequence, $Y(x_k)$, of an alternative action $x_k \neq x_j$ (prevention of $Y(x_k)$).

- At least one of the actions, x_j, x_k, in an effect measure must be counterfactual. Thus, we can never observe an effect measure separate from an outcome measure. In the example, we observed the mortality:

$$Y(x_1) = Y(x_0) + [Y(x_1) - Y(x_0)],$$

so the mortality difference, $Y(x_1) - Y(x_0)$, is mixed with the reference (baseline) mortality rate, $Y(x_0)$, in our observation. The best we can do is make an informed estimate of $Y(x_0)$, which is the outcome that would have happened under the counterfactual action x_0, and from that estimate deduce an estimate of the effect measure (by subtraction, in this example).

CAUSATION, CONFOUNDING AND ASSOCIATION

Problem 6 is considered a fundamental problem of all causal inference. It was recognized by Hume (1739) and is now known as the *identification problem* of cause and effect. All causal inferences (and hence all intervention plans) depend on accuracy in estimating or predicting at least one unobserved potential outcome following one counterfactual action. We ordinarily make this prediction based on observations of other subjects (controls) who experienced actual actions different from the subject of interest. For example, we might estimate that the mortality Kosovo would have experienced in 1999 had been no revocation, $Y(x_0)$, would equal the mortality it experienced in 1988, before violence began growing. In making this estimate, we run the risk of error because, *even under the action* x_0 (no revocation), Kosovo mortality might have changed between 1988–1999. If so, we say our estimate is *confounded* by this unknown change.

Denote by Y_{1988} the mortality experienced by Kosovo in 1988. We can then restate the last problem as follows: we do not observe $Y(x_0)$, so we cannot directly compute a measure of the effect of x_1 versus x_0. If, however, we believed the speculative explanation given in the above third bulleted item, we might also think that Y_{1988} is not too far from $Y(x_0)$, and so substitute Y_{1988} for $Y(x_0)$ in our measures. Thus, if we also observe $Y(x_1)$, the actual 1999 mortality, we would estimate the effect measure $Y(x_1) - Y(x_0)$ with the observed mortality difference $Y(x_1) - Y_{1988}$.

The latter observed difference is called a *measure of association*, because it contrasts two different *subjects* (Kosovo in 1999 versus Kosovo in 1988), rather than one subject under two different *actions* in our list (Kosovo in 1999 under revocation versus Kosovo in 1999 with no revocation). Because of the identification problem (we cannot see $Y(x_0)$), we must substitute a measure of association for the measure of effect. In this usage, the observed difference will misrepresent the effect measure by an amount equal to the difference of the two:

$$[Y(x_1) - Y_{1988}] - [Y(x_1) - Y(x_0)] = Y(x_0) - Y_{1988}$$

This quantity measures the amount of *confounding* in the association measure (the observed difference) when it is used as a substitute for the effect measure. Like the effect measure itself, the confounding measure contains the unobserved $Y(x_0)$ and so can only be estimated, not observed directly. Suppose, however, we know of reasons why $Y(x_0)$ and Y_{1988} would differ, such as changes in age structure over time. We can then attempt to adjust Y_{1988} for these suspected differences, in the hopes of getting closer to $Y(x_0)$. *Standardization* is probably the simplest example of such adjustment (Greenland 2000; Rothman and Greenland 1998).

The presumption underlying use of an adjusted effect measure is that it accounts for all important differences between the unobserved (counterfactual) reference outcome, $Y(x_0)$, and the substitute, Y_{1988}, in the above example. The presumption is debatable in most applications; for example, some would argue that "ethnic cleansing" would have spread to Kosovo even without autonomy revocation and Albanian resistance. This problem of uncontrolled confounding is but one of many methodological problems in estimating effects that are discussed in textbooks (e.g. Rothman and Greenland 1998).

THE EFFECTS OF OUTCOME REMOVAL

Consider a question that asks about the health burden attributable to y_1 versus y_0, where y_1 and y_0 are not actions in the earlier sense, but are themselves alternative *outcomes* such as AIDS death and CHD death. For example, y_1 could be "subject dies of lung cancer" and y_0 could be "subject does not die of lung cancer". As in the earlier framework, these outcomes are mutually exclusive possibilities for just one subject at a time; hence, at least one must become counterfactual. Because they are not interventions, however, there is severe ambiguity in any definition of another outcome, T, as a function of the potential outcomes, y_1 and y_0, because T depends in a critical fashion on *how* y_1 and y_0 are caused.

To see this, suppose T is years of life lived beyond age 50 (which is age at death minus 50). How would one have brought about y_0 (prevented the lung-cancer death) if the subject were a male lifelong heavy smoker who developed lung cancer at age 51 and died from it at age 54 (and so had $T(y_1) = 4$ years of life after age 50)? If y_0 had been achieved by convincing the subject to never start smoking, $T(y_0)$ could be much larger than $T(y_1)$, because the risks of many other causes of death (e.g. CHD) would have been much lower as a consequence of never smoking. But if y_0 had been achieved via an unusually successful new chemotherapy for lung tumors, $T(y_0)$ might be little changed from $T(y_1)$. This would occur if, shortly after remission, the subject had a fatal myocardial infarction whose occurrence was traceable to smoking-induced coronary stenosis.

The problem just described has long been recognized in discussions of estimating the impact of "cause removal" or "removal of competing risks" when the "causes" or "risks" at issue are outcomes rather than actions or treatments (Kalbfleisch and Prentice 1980). These outcomes are not subject to direct manipulation independent of the earlier history of the subject. Therefore, any realistic evaluation of the impact of their removal must account for other effects of the *means* of removal.

A similar problem arises in the evaluation of ordinary treatments whenever noncompliance can occur. In general, only advice or prescriptions are under control of the health practitioner; what a patient actually receives is affected not only by advice or prescription, but also by the many complex social and personality factors that influence compliance. This leads to manifold problems in evaluating the effects of received treatment (Goetghebeur and van Houwelingen 1998), for then the treatment a subject receives is only an outcome, $Y(x_j)$, of an earlier prescriptive action, x_j. In most cases, however, this initial action is unambiguous.

Suppose we could avoid the ambiguity problem by introducing a pair of well-defined alternative actions, x_1 and x_0, such that x_1 causes y_1 and prevents y_0 relative to x_0. That is, suppose y_1 will follow x_1, whereas y_0 will follow x_0, so that we have $y_1 = Y(x_1)$ and $y_0 = Y(x_0)$ with $y_1 \neq y_0$. We may still face a serious confounding problem in the form of "dependent competing risks". Consider again the heavy smoker who develops lung cancer at age 54, with treatment, x_0, being successful chemotherapy. It could be a mistake to calculate this subject's life expectancy, $T(x_0)$, from that of other heavy smokers of the same age and sex who had not developed lung cancer, because such smokers may differ in ways that render them not only less susceptible to smoking-induced lung cancer, but also less susceptible to other smoking-induced cancers (perhaps because they have better DNA-repair mechanisms).

More generally, even if the means of removal is precisely defined, feasible and has no side-effects, there is rarely a basis to believe, and often good reason to doubt, that removal of a particular outcome (such as a particular cause of death) would be followed by risks similar to risks among persons who, in the absence of intervention, do not experience the removed outcome (Kalbfleisch and Prentice 1980; Prentice and Kalbfleisch 1988). Unfortunately, standard statistical procedures for projecting outcomes under cause removal (such as Kaplan-Meier/product limit methods and traditional "cause-deleted" life tables) are based on this similarity assumption.

In view of the problems just described, it is reasonable to conclude the following:

- Projections of the impact of outcome removal (e.g. removal of a particular ICD9 cause of death; Lai and Hardy 1999), rather than an action that brings about outcome reduction, may not be useful for programme planning. Except perhaps in some unusually simple cases (e.g. smallpox eradication), the effects of actions and policies do not correspond to simple cause removal.

- Even when we have a treatment that specifically and completely prevents an outcome, biased effect estimates are likely if one simply projects the experience of those who naturally lack the outcome onto those who avoid the outcome because of the treatment. Only ongoing follow-up of successfully treated subjects can reliably identify the impact of outcome removal.

Problem 7 implies that summary measures for policy formulation should refer to effects of operationalizable actions (e.g. anti-smoking campaigns, food-distribution programmes), rather than effects of removing the outcomes targeted by those actions (e.g. smoking, cancer, malnutrition). Only rarely will the two effects coincide. Furthermore, because any action will have multiple consequences, a thorough analysis must consider outcomes in a *multivariate* framework that accounts for the multiple effects

of actions and the competition among various outcomes. This multivariate perspective raises serious questions about the value of univariate summaries.

ARE SOCIOECONOMIC INDICATORS CAUSES?

The theory outlined above is strictly a theory of effects of *actions* or *interventions*. It does not formalize all ordinary-language or intuitive uses
of the words "cause" and "effect". Two naive extreme reactions to this
limitation have been common: one that denies it is meaningful to talk of
causes that are not actions, and one that rejects counterfactual theory
outright. But two types of constructive reactions have also appeared. The
first type generalizes the theory to encompass nonactions as causes, a prime
example being the many-worlds theory (Lewis 1973). This approach is
very controversial and not suitably operationalized for everyday use.

The second constructive response accepts the limitations of the restricted theory and instead seeks to identify potential actions within ordinary events. This approach recognizes that certain "causes" are best
treated as intermediate outcomes; one then traces the etiology of such
"causes" back to events with intervention potential, or else treats such
"causes" as conditioning events and searches for actions that modify or
prevent the ultimate outcomes. Earthquakes, which cause extensive destruction, provide neutral examples of unmodifiable causes. An earthquake, y_1, is the outcome of a long and complex chain of events with little
intervention potential under today's technology. Perhaps someday we will
be capable of interventions that lead to dissipation of crustal stresses with
less ensuing damage. But for now, mere prediction would be a major
achievement and would facilitate actions to prevent damage when an
earthquake occurs. An example of such an action is the enforcement of
strict building codes in earthquake-prone regions.

More charged examples are provided by common measures of education, such as the classification "No high-school diploma", "High-school
diploma", "Some college, no degree", "Two-year degree", "Four-year
degree" and "Graduate degree". People believe that education leads to
more income and health. But how well do differences in the observed
education measure predict the effects of real interventions such as affir-
mative action, public-school improvements, or scholarship programmes?
For policy purposes, it is the implementation and evaluation of such
programmes that matter; the ensuing changes in education measures are
only intermediates between the programmes and the ultimate goals of
improved social, economic and health outcomes.

Counterfactual models provide a basis for thought experiments that
treat observed associations of socioeconomic indicators and health as
outcomes of potentially intervenable events. Consider a highly charged
example, such as "race", that is commonly measured as "white" or
"black". People talk of race as a "cause". But to do something about racial

disparities in health outcomes (which is to say, to eliminate the observed association of race and health), we must explain their origin in terms of intervenable causes, such as disparities in school funding, availability of individual college funding, prevalence of racist attitudes, etc. Finding feasible interventions and estimating their costs and benefits is required to address observed disparities; asserting or denying that "race" is a cause is helpful in this endeavor.

SHOULD DIFFERENT OUTCOMES BE SUMMARIZED IN A SINGLE NUMBER?

Two distinct connotations of summary measure appear extant: the first and most common presumes that the measure summarizes a single outcome variable with a single number. Classic examples include the mortality rate and the life expectancy. The second connotation, largely confined to statistics and physical sciences, allows a summary to be a vector, that is, an ordered list of numbers that summarize different dimensions of a system. An example of such a *multidimensional* or *multivariate* population summary would be the list containing life expectancy, health expectancy, health gap and the proportions of deaths due to various causes (e.g. starvation, violence, infectious disease, heart disease, stroke, cancer).

It should first be noted that all the earlier concepts and discussion apply equally to any action or outcome, whether unidimensional or multidimensional. In particular, the potential outcomes, $Y(x_j)$, may represent outcome vectors and the alternative actions, x_0, x_1, etc., may also be vectors; for example, x_0 could specify that 30%, 40% and 30% of a fixed budget be allocated to family planning, sanitation and medical supplies, respectively, and x_1 specifies a different allocation scheme. The chief problem in expanding to the multidimensional perspective is the limited number of dimensions that the human mind can contemplate at once. Because that limitation is a key motive for summarization, it is essential to keep track of what is lost in the dimensionality reduction that defines summarization. It also is essential to keep track of the *values* that influence (or should influence) what is kept and what is lost.

Summary measures of population health serve no good purpose when they strongly confound valuations, which vary by individual preference, culture, etc., with measures of occurrence and effect (which are presumably matters of scientific fact, albeit subject to uncertainty). For example, many individuals, in continuing to smoke, explain their behaviour as stemming from a conscious preference to die sooner from cardiovascular disease or cancer than survive until mental or neurological deficit is nearly inevitable. For such individuals, measures such as healthy years of life lost due to smoking represent a conflation of someone else's values with the factual risks of smoking, because that summary ignores preferences among various morbidity and mortality outcomes affected by smoking. To give the individual the information necessary for personal choice, we must supply a multidimensional summary that includes lifetime risks of different diseases.

Moving to the societal level, healthy years of life lost due to smoking not only neglects the differences in resource allocation that must exist between present (actual) society and a counterfactual tobacco-free society, it also neglects differences in absolute and proportional morbidity and mortality with and without tobacco use. This neglect is addressed by measures of the economic cost of tobacco use, and by absolute and proportional morbidity and mortality comparisons. By providing all these measures, we shift to a multidimensional summary of tobacco impact.

The intention in raising these issues is not to offer a solution to a specific summarization problem. Rather, it is to remind those facing a choice among measures that candidates need not (and, for policy purposes, should not) be limited to unidimensional summaries. While our ability to think in several dimensions is limited, it can be improved with practice. That practice has proven crucial in attacking problems in physics and engineering, and there is no reason to suppose it is less important in tackling more complex social policy issues. In instances in which many different people must make informed choices based on the same scientific data, but with different values, multidimensional measures are essential if we are to provide each person and each executive body with sufficient information for rational choice.

REFERENCES

Dawid AP (2000) Causal inference without counterfactuals (with discussion). *Journal of the American Statistical Association*, **95**(450):407–448.

Goetghebeur E, van Houwelingen H (1998) Analyzing non-compliance in clinical trials. *Statistics in Medicine*, **17**(3).

Greenland S (1987) Interpretation and choice of effect measures in epidemiologic analyses. *American Journal of Epidemiology*, **125**(5):761–768.

Greenland S (1990) Randomization, statistics, and causal inference. *Epidemiology*, **1**(6):421–429.

Greenland S (1997) Concepts of validity in epidemiologic research. In: *The Oxford textbook of public health*, Vol. 2. 3rd edn. Detels R, Tanaka H, McEwen J, Beaglehole R, eds. Oxford University Press, New York.

Greenland S (2000) Causal analysis in the health sciences. *Journal of the American Statistical Association*, **95**:286–289.

Greenland S, Morgenstern H (2001) Confounding in health research. *Annual Review of Public Health*, **22**:189–212.

Greenland S, Pearl J, Robins JM (1999) Causal diagrams for epidemiologic research. *Epidemiology*, **10**(1):37–48.

Greenland S, Poole C (1988) Invariants and noninvariants in the concept of interdependent effects. *Scandinavian Journal of Work Environment and Health*, **14**:125–129.

Greenland S, Robins JM (1986) Identifiability, exchangeability, and epidemiological confounding. *International Journal of Epidemiology,* **15**(3):413–419.

Greenland S, Robins JM (1988) Conceptual problems in the definition and interpretation of attributable fractions. *American Journal of Epidemiology,* **128**(6):1185–1197.

Holland PW (1986) Statistics and causal inference. *Journal of the American Statistical Association,* **81**(396):945–970.

Hume D (1739) *A treatise of human nature.* (Reprint 1988, Clarendon Press, Oxford)

Hume D (1748) *An enquiry concerning human understanding.* (Reprint 1988, Open Court Press, LaSalle, IL)

Kalbfleisch JD, Prentice RL (1980) *The statistical analysis of failure-time data.* Wiley, New York.

Lai D, Hardy RJ (1999) Potential gains in life expectancy or years of potential life lost: impact of competing risks of death. *International Journal of Epidemiology,* **28**(5):894–898.

Lewis D (1973) Causation. *Journal of Philosophy,* **70**:556–567.

Maldonado GM, Greenland S (2002) Estimating causal effects. (In press). *International Journal of Epidemiology,* **31**

Pearl J (1995) Causal diagrams for empirical research. *Biometrika,* **82**(4):669–710.

Pearl J (2000) *Causality: models, reasoning and inference.* Cambridge University Press, Cambridge.

Penrose R (1994) *Shadows of the mind.* Oxford University Press, New York.

Prentice RL, Kalbfleisch JD (1988) Author's reply. *Biometrics,* **44**(4):1205.

Robins JM, Greenland S (1989) The probability of causation under a stochastic model for individual risks. *Biometrics,* **45**(4):1125–1138.

Robins JM, Greenland S (1992) Identifiability and exchangeability for direct and indirect effects. *Epidemiology,* **3**(2):143–155.

Rothman KJ, Greenland S (1998) *Modern epidemiology.* 2nd edn. Lippincott-Raven, Philadelphia, PA.

Rubin DB (1990) Comment: Neyman (1923) and causal inference in experiments and observational studies. *Statistical Science,* **5**:472–480.

Rubin DB (1991) Practical implications of modes of statistical inerence for causal effects and the critical role of the assignment mechanism. *Biometrics,* **47**(4):1213–1234.

Simon HA, Rescher N (1966) Cause and counterfactual. *Philosophy and Science,* **33**:323–340.

Sobel M (1994) Causal inference in latent variable models. In: *Latent variables analysis: applications for developmental research.* von Eye A, Clogg CC, eds. Sage, Thousand Oaks, CA.

Winship C, Morgan SL (1999) The estimation of causal effects from observational data. *Annual Review of Sociology,* **25**:659–706.

Chapter 6.3

ON CAUSAL DECOMPOSITION
OF SUMMARY MEASURES
OF POPULATION HEALTH

MICHAEL C. WOLFSON

Summary Measures of Population Health (SMPH) are useful simply to follow trends and reveal patterns in the health of members of a population. For example, an SMPH like health- or disability-adjusted life expectancy (HALE or DALE), will hopefully increase over time for a given population. If this measure increases more rapidly than life expectancy (LE), then we may conclude that not only are we "adding years to life", but also "adding life to years" (Rochon Commission 1987), or in Fries' (1980) sense, we are witnessing a "compression of morbidity".

Moreover, given the ways this kind of SMPH is typically constructed for a country, such as the Sullivan method, increment-decrement life tables, and the Global Burden of Disease (GBD) approach; and given sufficient sample size in the underlying data systems, we should also be able to produce estimates of the measure by sex, geographic area, socio-demographic group and age. These "straightforward" disaggregations rely on the fact that HALE or DALE measures can be produced for constituent subpopulations, and are additive over age groups that together cover the full life cycle (Wolfson 1996). Comparing these disaggregated SMPH and examining their trends over time can help indicate groups or areas for priority health policy attention.

However, expectations for SMPH are much higher than this. It is better if historical changes in SMPH can be ascribed to one or another cause, and the impacts of prospective changes from interventions or other causes can be estimated. SMPH will be most relevant for public policy if their movements or variations can be attributed to causes, and their likely responses to health policy interventions can be explicitly quantified.

For these reasons, there is a desire that SMPH also be disaggregated along another dimension, "causes". The (naive) assumption that this kind of disaggregation is reasonable stems from widely used breakdowns of mortality rates by "cause of death" (i.e. the ICD-defined disease recorded on death certificates). In this case, the sum of all "causes" of mortality equals the overall mortality rate, and the causal attribution of deaths to diseases is additively decomposable. Similarly, the entire burden of health problems measured in DALYs can be exhaustively partitioned among a set of explicit causes (e.g. Table 4 in WHO 2000). This is a convenience, especially when communicating to non-expert journalists and politicians. But it also over-simplifies the meaning of "cause" and gives a false sense of comfort in the precision of the methodology. The ICD is a *classification*, while any particular death is the endpoint of a complex, multifactorial and uncertain causal process.

The LE is a relatively simple SMPH, but it is a good illustration of the basic problem of additive causal decomposition. Period LE answers the question: "What if a cohort was born in year t, and every year of its life was exposed to the age-specific mortality risks observed at this same time, t, for age group a?" Since the mortality rates that enter this calculation are generally also available by "cause", it is possible *mechanically* to ask a family of related "what if" questions. One is: "What would this LE be if no one ever died of lung cancer (and everything else remained unchanged)?" Another is: "What if no one ever died of heart disease?" etc. The result would be a series of incremental "cause-deleted" life expectancies, one for each disease.

However, these increments clearly do not add up to anything sensible. Indeed if we did not die of anything (i.e. if we eliminated all causes of death simultaneously), we would in fact be immortal. Yet the sum of these incremental cause-deleted life expectancies is clearly finite. Thus, even when mortality rates are additively decomposable, cause-deleted life expectancy is not additively decomposable by cause of death, even though this widely used indicator is based on the mortality rates. From this simple example, it should be clear that additive decomposability across "causes" is an unreasonable expectation for SMPH like HALE and DALE, which are generalizations of LE.

A better approach for causal attribution is to think in terms of explicit "what if" simulations—our definition of "counterfactuals"—such as cause-deleted life expectancies. The answers to these "what if" questions are constructed by sets of calculations that constitute a simple simulation model. It is reasonable to demand that SMPH offer a connection to health policy by allowing changes in health outcomes to be linked back to causes or interventions. The way to achieve this is for SMPH to be explicitly embedded in, and estimated by, a simulation model. While this may sound strange or ambitious, it is nothing more than a generalization of current practices, such as the calculation of cause-deleted LE.

At best, cause-deleted LEs are limited "what if" simulations. They give an overall sense of the relative importance of diseases, for example that lung cancer elimination would have roughly half the impact on LE of eliminating coronary heart disease (CHD). However, the lung cancer-deleted

LE measure makes an unrealistic assumption, namely that lung cancer can be eliminated without anything else changing. A more realistic causal assumption would be that smoking in the population was substantially reduced, and that lung cancer incidence and fatality fell as a result. But in this case, CHD would also fall substantially. In other words, the causes of lung cancer and CHD are not independent in practice. (They may be conditionally independent, conditional on smoking history, sex and age, but this should be an explicit part of the posited causal story.) Moreover, co-morbidity is also highly prevalent, as with CHD and diabetes. Yet assumptions of disease independence and no co-morbidity are pervasive in categorical attribution. The fact that these necessary assumptions are manifestly wrong is yet another reason that categorical attribution, though superficially attractive, is a bad idea.

As the smoking example indicates, causality is multilayered. (It is also not deterministic in these cases.) It is true that deaths are assigned causes that are classified by disease. However, the general public certainly understands that various risk factors like smoking and hypertension play a role "upstream" in causing (predisposing toward) specific ICD-defined diseases. And it is also clear that socioeconomic status (e.g. education) is correlated with and likely plays a role in smoking behaviour, as well as other behaviours predisposing to hypertension. Thus, it is much more realistic to think in terms of a "web of causality" (Krieger 1994), such as those shown in Figures 2 and 5 in chapter 6.1 (Mathers et al.), and in Figure 1 below.

Figure 1   An illustrative "Web of Causality" (e.g. excluding breast cancer, osteoporosis, hip fracture)

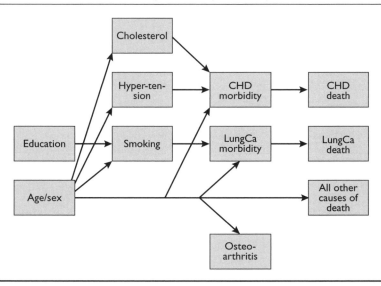

In my comments so far, I would not expect any disagreement from the authors of the two lead chapters in this part. So where do I differ? In the case of chapter 6.1, I am not convinced of the importance of retaining additive decomposition for its ease of communication.

There are three arguments against using additive decomposition in SMPH such as health gaps and health expectancy measures. First, it is not necessary to use additive decomposition for ease of communication with the public, even though this is often cited as a reason. This can be illustrated by the Tax Expenditure Accounts produced by the United States and Canadian governments. These are listings of tax provisions that depart from an ideal straightforward tax base and tax rates, in order to confer programme-like benefits or incentives, such as special treatment of charitable giving or home ownership. Each provision is valued independently in the Accounts by answering the question, "what if the *status quo* tax system were changed to eliminate only that one provision?" Since tax systems are highly non-linear, and provisions frequently interact, the sum of the results of this collection of questions is nowhere near the value of increased tax revenues if all, or even a few, of these provisions were eliminated simultaneously. In other words, the Tax Expenditure Accounts do not satisfy any adding up criterion. Yet, just like cause-deleted life expectancy, the Accounts do give useful estimates.

Second, gap-based SMPH necessarily rely on an arbitrary figure: the target lifespan against which expected health-adjusted life lengths are judged. The other health expectancy group of SMPH needs no such assumption. Given the choice, it seems better not to introduce an arbitrary component into the SMPH. The health expectancy class of SMPH can be readily explained to a broader audience as generalizations of the already familiar life expectancy concept.

Third, the only kind of additive decomposition afforded by these gap measures is causal attribution in terms of ICD-defined diseases. However, it is clear that ICD-defined disease is only one of several legitimate ways to describe causes of health problems. Others include "proximal risk factors" like smoking and hypertension, and "distal" risk factors like socioeconomic status. Too much emphasis is placed on a biomedical model of health if the only kind of "cause" that can be discussed quantitatively within the framework is ICD-defined disease.

In chapter 6.2, Greenland concludes that causal attribution should not be limited to a single summary measure of population health. He rightly observes that a counterfactual analysis should be able to generate multivalued scenarios. This view is taken for granted in finance ministries, for example, whenever they consider tax policy changes. They routinely use large microsimulation models to estimate not only the aggregate revenue impact of a given tax change (e.g. changing tax rate brackets in the personal income tax), but also the disaggregated changes in disposable income that can be expected by family type and income group. Similarly, the global climate models used to assess prospects for global warming have highly multivariate outputs, such as temperature levels in each of a large three-dimensional grid of locations.

However, Greenland's objection to single-valued outcomes in causal decomposition is not entirely reasonable. He is concerned that "they strongly confound valuations [...e.g. preferences] with measures of occurrence and effect (which are presumably matters of scientific fact...)." This concern is misplaced, however, *if* the construction of a counterfactual, or better yet a simulated "what if" value of SMPH, explicitly involves a sequence of intermediate calculations. If the underlying model used to construct the counterfactual simulated SMPH is rich enough, it will be possible to separate the amounts of time various groups of individuals in a representative population cohort spend in each of the range of health states (the sojourn times of the birth cohort by type of health state), from the valuations placed on each of those states. With the underlying sojourn time estimates as an explicit part of the SMPH estimation process, there need be no confounding and it should always be possible to use sensitivity analysis to assess the importance of the microlevel valuation assumptions (see chapter 3.6).

However, in agreement with Greenland (chapter 6.2), it should be possible to disaggregate the impact of a "cause" of health problems by age, sex and population characteristics, whether health problems are defined as an ICD disease, a proximal or distal risk factor, or an explicit health policy intervention. If the counterfactual analysis "engine" is realized as a richly detailed microsimulation model, rather than the kinds of spreadsheets underlying typical GBD analyses, then this multivariate outcome analysis is feasible. An example is the POpulation HEalth Model (POHEM), constructed at Statistics Canada (Wolfson 1994; Will et al. 2001).

Of course, the web of causality and the statistical estimates of its quantitative structure (i.e. the causal story implicit in such a model), will always be imperfect. This is certainly the case with global climate models, for example. But at any moment, the model can and should represent the best of our current state of knowledge. It can be thought of as the result of an exercise in meta-synthesis (i.e. beyond "meta-analysis" as the phrase is used in clinical epidemiology); in other words where the best understanding across a range of diseases, health interventions and risk factors is carefully summarized in terms of formal, empirically-based, quantitative (stochastic) relationships, as a functioning whole. If these quantitative understandings and their realization as a "whole cloth" is published in full, this will provide both replicability and a focus for researchers around the world to test and extend the work. Even though the underlying causal web remains incomplete and tentative in many areas (just as in global climate models), it will be open so that results based upon it can be given appropriate credibility in public and scientific discourse.

REFERENCES

Fries J (1980) Aging, natural death, and the compression of morbidity. *New England Journal of Medicine,* **303**(3):130–135.

Krieger N (1994) Epidemiology and the web of causation: has anyone seen the spider? *Social Science and Medicine,* **39**(7):887–903.

Rochon Commission (1987) *Report of the commission of inquiry on health and social services.* Government of Quebec, Canada.

WHO (2000) *The World Health Report 2000. Health systems: improving performance.* World Health Organization, Geneva.

Will BP, Nobrega KM, Berthelot JM, et al. (2001) First do no harm: extending the debate on the provision of preventive tamoxifen. *British Journal of Cancer,* **85**(9):1280–1288.

Wolfson MC (1994) POHEM – a framework for understanding and modeling the health of human populations. *World Health Statistics Quarterly,* **47**(3-4):157–176.

Wolfson MC (1996) Health-adjusted life expectancy. *Statistics Canada: Health Reports,* **8**(1):41–46.

Chapter 6.4

CAUSALITY AND COUNTERFACTUAL ANALYSIS

DANIEL M. HAUSMAN

In chapter 6.2 of this book, Sander Greenland provides an introduction to contemporary views of causal inference (see also Pearl 2000) and makes two points relevant to summary measures of population health: i) that health gaps are not well-defined; and ii) that a multidimensional index of population health would be superior to a scalar measure. In theory, a multidimensional index of population health is attractive, because health itself is multidimensional. But the theoretical attractions of a multidimensional index have to be balanced against the practical dangers that those who make health policy would ignore most of the dimensions. Greenland and I are not particularly competent to judge these dangers, and I shall focus the remainder of my remarks on matters of causal inference.

Greenland considers how investigators answer counterfactual questions concerning what the consequences would have been had some other action been taken. Such questions are closely related to questions about the consequences of proposed interventions. These are in part questions concerning the *use* of incomplete prior causal knowledge. I do not know how commonly accepted Greenland's views are among epidemiologists, but they are controversial among philosophers.

Given the page constraints, contemporary philosophical controversies concerning the nature of counterfactuals and the relations between causation and counterfactuals will not be discussed in depth. I can only sketch the most influential view, which is due to David Lewis (Lewis 1973a; 1973b; 1979), and explain how it is related to Greenland's position. I shall argue that even a qualified acceptance of Lewis' view undermines Greenland's critique of health gaps. I shall also show that Greenland's own philosophical premises do not support so strong a conclusion as the one he draws.

The general problem is as follows. One begins with a suspicion that there is some relation between a variable, X, and some outcome variable, Y, though one also believes that Y depends on other variables, both known and unknown. The functional relation between X, Y and other variables may be probabilistic or deterministic, but it is never fully known.

One can observe the actual value of X at some particular time, x_1, and the actual value of Y that results, y_1, but not the other values X could have had at that time, or other values that Y would have taken in response. Rather than observing how the outcome would have differed if X had had a different value, x_0 (and everything else at that time and place were the same), one can only observe how the outcome in fact differs when $X = x_0$ at a different time, and when there is no assurance that everything else is just the same. In this way, in Greenland's terminology, "a measure of association" is obtained, from which the "measure of effect" is inferred. As more is known about the functional relation between X, Y, and other variables, for which measures of association constitute evidence, a better answer will be possible to the counterfactual question about what the value of Y would have been if the value of X had been x_0. Although Greenland uses causal language, he is concerned with counterfactuals rather than causation.

Greenland insists that the counterfactual question is well defined only when values of X are *actions*. When the values of X are not actions, the question: "What would the value of Y have been if the value of X had been x_0?" cannot be answered, because it is not known how the value of X became x_0 instead of x_1. If a heavy smoker, P, had not died of lung cancer at age 50 years because (counterfactually) P had never smoked, then P's life expectancy would be much longer than if P had not died of lung cancer because of a successful chemotherapy treatment. There is no answer to the question: "How long would P have lived if P had not died of lung cancer" until one specifies the action or intervention that would have brought it about that P had not died of lung cancer. Calculations of health gaps or years of life lost, such as the number of years of life lost to AIDS, pose exactly such allegedly ill-formed questions. It is unknown how long individuals with AIDS would live if they were not infected with AIDS, because there are different ways in which they might not have had AIDS, and their life expectancies would depend on how they were not infected. Health gaps are thus not well defined and the whole attempt to measure DALYs may be an irretrievable muddle.

Why doesn't this difficulty apply equally to all counterfactuals? How does insisting that the values of X be *actions* circumvent the problems? Consider Greenland's own example: x_1 is the revocation of Kosovo's autonomy in 1988 and Y is mortality in Kosovo in 1999. The actual value of Y can, in principle, be observed. One then asks the counterfactual question: "What would mortality in 1999 have been if Kosovo's autonomy had not been revoked in 1988 (if the value of X were x_0)?" The answer cannot be determined by observation, because no one can observe a counterfactual mortality rate. However, it could be assumed that the counterfactual mortality in 1999 would be the same as the actual mortality in 1988, subject to corrections for factors that are independent of whether autonomy was revoked. In this way, estimates of what mortality would have been in 1999 if Kosovo's autonomy had not been revoked can be obtained and one can offer a fallible answer to the counterfactual question.

Notice that the increased mortality in 1999 was due to the fact that Kosovo's autonomy was revoked *in just the way it was*. If its autonomy were revoked by a Yugoslav government dominated by ethnic Albanians, as part of an effort to impose Kosovo's culture and interests on the whole of Yugoslavia, its effects would presumably have been very different. Consequently, it matters a great deal how x_0, the "non-revocation", is specified. A non-revocation is not of course any specific kind of action, although a specific non-revocation could be identical to some particular action (or actions). The hypothetical non-revocation Greenland refers to, x_0, is presumably a specific complicated set of actions that differs from the actions the Yugoslav government took in 1988 as little as possible, apart from not revoking Kosovo's autonomy.

According to Lewis' theory (Lewis 1973b), a counterfactual such as: "If Yugoslavia had not revoked Kosovo's autonomy in 1988, ethnic cleansing would not have occurred in Kosovo in 1999," is true if and only if some possible world without the revocation and without ethnic cleansing is "more similar" to the actual world than any possible world without revocation and with the ethnic cleansing. Notice that Lewis does not rely on causal knowledge to evaluate the truth of the counterfactual. This is important, because Lewis hopes to define causation in terms of chains of counterfactual dependence (Lewis 1973a). Lewis' account of counterfactuals depends on a theory of "similarity" among possible worlds (Lewis 1979). In its simplest outline, the possible worlds in which Kosovo's autonomy is not revoked that are most similar to the actual world will be identical to the actual world until shortly before the moment in 1988 when Yugoslavia revoked Kosovo's autonomy. Then, despite the occurrence of the causal antecedents for the revocation, the revocation "miraculously" fails to occur. Apart from lacking the revocation, the closest possible worlds will differ very little from the actual world at the moment when Kosovo's autonomy was in fact revoked. History then runs on, according to the same laws as those that govern the actual world. One relies on those laws to predict what the result would be if Yugoslavia had not revoked Kosovo's autonomy when it did. Several quite different possible worlds may be equally similar to the actual world, and the counterfactual will not be true, unless ethnic cleansing does not occur in *any* of those worlds. Although Greenland does not explicitly talk about similarity between possible worlds, he relies implicitly on some such notion in specifying what action x_0, the non-revocation, is.

What then of counterfactuals like those Greenland criticizes, such as: "If P had not died of lung cancer at age 50 years, then P would have lived for at least 20 years more". According to Lewis, this counterfactual is no more difficult to evaluate than the counterfactual concerning what would have been the case if the Yugoslavs had not revoked Kosovo's autonomy. Are possible worlds in which P lives for at least 20 years after not dying of lung cancer at age 50 more similar to the actual world than possible worlds in which P does not die of lung cancer and dies before age 70? Possible worlds in which P never smoked are less similar to the actual world than possible worlds in which P lives just the same life until age 50, contracts lung cancer, but fails to die of it because of a spontaneous remission. We have data on the general life expectancy of people who have lung cancers resembling P's, yet who do not die of them in circumstances like those in which P does in fact die of lung cancer. Thus we have some basis to judge whether it is true that if P had not died of lung cancer at age 50, then P would have lived at least 20 years more.

Since a possible world in which P never smoked would be very unlike the actual world, one does not examine such a world to determine what would be the case if P had not died of lung cancer. In addition, Lewis' framework permits one to consider counterfactuals with more complicated antecedents. For example, consider a counterfactual such as: "If P had not died of lung cancer at age 50 years because P never smoked and never got lung cancer, then P would have lived to age 90." In evaluating this counterfactual, possible worlds that diverged from the actual world long ago when P in fact began smoking are considered. Whatever counterfactual is considered, the indeterminacy that concerns Greenland evaporates.

Lewis' views on similarity among possible worlds and his views of the evaluation of counterfactuals have been questioned elsewhere (Hausman 1998). When the consequence of some counterfactual antecedent depends on how it comes about, it is not always justifiable to suppose that it comes about in just one special way, as if by a miracle or intervention. When it is asked, for example, what is the average number of years of life lost owing to lung cancer, it is necessary to specify the possible state of affairs in which individuals no longer died of lung cancer. For example, do people not die of lung cancer because of interventions designed to stop causes of lung cancer, such as smoking or air pollution; or because of an intervention that interferes with the mechanisms by which these cause lung cancer; or because of improvements in treating lung cancer? Without some such specification, the question: "How much longer (on average) would people live if they did not die of lung cancer?" has no correct answer.

There are, however, two reasons to doubt whether this is a serious problem in practice. First, in some cases the consequence of the non-occurrence of some health state (or some cause of death) will not be so sensitive to the way the health state or cause of death might be prevented. Although the calculation of the health gap caused by malaria will depend on whether one supposes malaria is eliminated by vaccination, by mosquito eradication, or by an effective treatment, the differences are not so large as to make the calculation meaningless. Second, I would conjecture that in assessing health gaps, health analysts typically assume that the counterfactual alternative to the death or disability resulting from a particular disease involves a last-minute intervention of the sort Lewis discusses. For example, one would naturally take the health gap caused by malaria to be the difference between the current state of health where malaria is prevalent and the state of health that would obtain in much the same conditions if there were a vaccine without side-effects or if there were a successful mosquito eradication programme. It is obvious that the benefits of an actual anti-malarial medication might be much less. Greenland's indeterminacy still exists, but at least in cases such as this one the indeterminacy is mild, and ignoring it would not be the greatest of the simplifications and idealizations required in order to define a summary measure of population health.

REFERENCES

Hausman D (1998) *Causal asymmetries*. Cambridge University Press, New York.

Lewis D (1973a) Causation. *Journal of Philosophy*, **70**:556–567.

Lewis D (1973b) *Counterfactuals*. Harvard University Press, Cambridge, MA.

Lewis D (1979) Counterfactual dependence and time's arrow. *Noûs*, **13**:455–476.

Pearl J (2000) *Causality: models, reasoning and inference*. Cambridge University Press, Cambridge.

Chapter 7.1

DEVELOPMENT OF STANDARDIZED HEALTH STATE DESCRIPTIONS

RITU SADANA

INTRODUCTION

Over the past fifty years, a growing number of countries in industrialized and less industrialized countries have been regularly conducting national surveys dedicated to assessing the health of the population, or including health topics in nationally representative household surveys. Examples include the United States' annual National Health Interview Survey (NHIS), carried out since 1957; and the National Sample Survey (NSS), which has been regularly implemented in India since 1950, and has incorporated specialized modules addressing health topics, such as those within Round 28 (1973–1974), Round 35 (1980–1981), Round 42 (1986–1987) and Round 52 (1995–1996).

One of the main advantages of data collected through household surveys is that they provide person- or household-based health statistics. This is in contrast to data collected through health services or disease registries, which are episode- or event-based (UN 1995). Episode- or event-based data are not representative of the population, nor of conditions that are less well defined, or that do not have effective treatments. This is primarily due to population heterogeneity in accessing health services and in health-seeking behavior, as well as the uneven quality of data collected by the health services. Person- and household-based data, on the other hand, provide a different perspective on the health status of a population, one that is independent from data given by health services, professionals or surveillance sites (Kroeger 1988).

Often, the main health topics included in household surveys are an assessment of morbidity; aspects of health status; risk factors and lifestyle practices; utilization of and satisfaction with health services and drugs; and health care expenditures (reviewed in Ferrer 2000; Gudex, Lafortune 2000; Hupkens 1998; Rasmussen et al. 1999). These reviews show that questions specifically addressing health status typically assess the severity and duration of functional or cognitive disability and the impact of the disability on usual activities.

Despite awareness that data collection and analysis need to be standardized, few standardized modules for national health surveys exist or are utilized across countries. Problems of comparability also exist within countries, such as between different geographic areas or time periods. Existing standardized modules developed by international agencies also tend to focus on morbidity or disease classification, rather than on describing health status. The result is that data focusing on morbidity serve as inputs to "policies on curative care" (Ferrer 2000). Other surveys with standardized modules, such as the Demographic and Health Surveys conducted in some 65 countries over the past 15 years, have primarily interviewed women. This paper reviews the domains used to describe health states in health status assessment instruments.

OPERATIONAL APPROACHES TO DESCRIBE HEALTH

Ever since the 1947 World Health Organization (WHO) definition of health, researchers have grappled with operational definitions and methodological approaches to measure health at the population level, particularly health status (Breslow 1972; Chen and Bryant 1975; Moriyama 1968; WHO 1957). In a comprehensive review covering 30 years, Hansluwka (1985) assessed that the challenge remained to develop appropriate measures that are comparable, yet reflect the multi-dimensional nature of health. Most subsequent efforts to assess health combined a range of questions drawn from four categories: i) Items broadly reflecting the WHO definition (i.e. describing physical, mental and social aspects of health); ii) Those that are symptom-oriented or considered indicative of illness or morbidity; iii) Those that focus on fulfilling or performing functions, activities or roles as proximate descriptions of health status; and iv) Those concerned with adaptation to, and coping with, non-fatal health conditions.

Standardized instruments have been developed that combine standard questions with estimates of reliability or validity, and interpret scores based on different subgroups of the population. The first standardized instruments assessed the most severe states of health, particularly among older age groups and individuals living in long-term care institutions. Measures such as the activities of daily living (ADLs) focused on performance in different areas, for example eating; getting in and out of bed; getting around in the home; and dressing, bathing or using the toilet (Katz et al. 1963). The levels of performance in these areas are considered to be proximate descriptions of the severity of health status and the level of assistance required.

These early instruments were enlarged to apply to a broader group of individuals and included questions covering instrumental activities of daily living (IADLs), such as heavy housework; light housework; laundry; shopping for groceries; getting around outside the home; travelling; managing money; taking medicine; and telephoning (Lawton and Brody 1969). Typically, ADL questions measure more severe levels of health and focus on basic physical and cognitive functions, whereas IADL questions are sensitive to less severe levels of health. However, as IADL questions are based on normative roles and activities, the responses are more prone to cultural and gender biases, both within and across populations. As a result, all IADL questions may not be applicable to everyone within populations. For example, in a survey of elderly in four Western Pacific countries, the IADL question "can you prepare your own meals," was only asked to women (Andrews et al. 1986).

The second wave of instruments was developed with clinical and general populations in mind, and combined self-assessment of descriptions on different dimensions of health and of performance in different activities and roles. Data collected by these instruments are often presented as multiple dimensional profiles of health status, further discussed in this section. Several publications catalogue and review the growing number of standardized instruments (Bowling 1991; 1995; McDowell and Newell 1996; Patrick and Erickson 1993). Standardized generic instruments (i.e. those developed to measure health status, regardless of a particular disease or condition) have been used in several studies in different countries and include the Quality of Well-Being Scale (Fanshel and Bush 1970); the McMaster Health Index (Chambers et al. 1976); the Sickness Impact Profile (Bergner et al. 1976); the Nottingham Health Profile (Hunt et al. 1981); the Health Utilities Index Mark 3 (Feeny et al. 1995); EuroQol Quality of Life Scale (Krabbe et al. 1999); Short-Form 36 Health Survey (Ware et al. 1993); the WHO Quality of Life (WHOQOL-BREF) Assessment Instrument (WHOQOL Group 1998); and the WHO Disability Assessment Schedule-II or WHODAS-II (WHO 1999).

Additional instruments that have been used within primary health settings include the Quality of Life Index (Spitzer et al. 1981); the Functional Status Questionnaire (Jette et al. 1986); COOP Charts for Primary Care Practice (Nelson et al. 1987); and the Duke Health Profile (Parkerson et al. 1990). Disease-specific measures are more often used in clinical trials or with individuals receiving specialized treatments. A few of these instruments, such as the Quality of Well-Being Scale or Health Utilities Index, have also been used to classify individuals into different health states indirectly, or combine data from self-reported interviews and other data sources (Grootendorst et al. 2000). Furthermore, the domains included within a few of these instruments have served as the descriptive system for the valuation of health states, including the EuroQol, Health Utilities Index, and a variant of the Short-Form 36 (Brazier et al. 1998).

Each of the 13 instruments noted above provide separate scale scores for each of the domains noted in Table 1. Although each instrument covers multiple domains of health status, few use the same labels for domains or scales, or cover the same content in terms of the questions that make up each domain, reflecting the different empirical approaches to defining and assessing health status. Some instruments use the same domain label, but include different questions (not shown). Some include items focusing on a specific function, such as vision, while others assess a range of complex functions and activities, such as understanding and interacting. Others may create a domain to focus on one aspect, such as performance of activities related to the home, while others may incorporate performance of activities or roles at work, home or recreation in a single domain. The same applies to other domains, such as eating or self-care, with the latter usually incorporating questions addressing eating, bathing, dressing and similar items. Given these differences, Table 1 approximately represents the domains of the 13 instruments included. Note that no one set of domains and questions describing health status is used to compare multi-dimensional profiles of health status across populations.

Furthermore, different instruments claim to assess different aspects of health status or even well-being, such as functional status, health status, well-being, quality of life, or health-related quality of life. Yet operational differences among these measures are not always based on a clear conceptual framework. For this reason, the actual content of an instrument should not be judged solely by its title. It is important to note that the two WHO instruments listed in Table 1 have only some domains in common and use different sets of questions and recall periods for those domains that are similar.

Nevertheless, most instruments include questions addressing general health, physical functioning and mental health state descriptions, as well as the performance of daily activities (ADL and IADL), and the fulfilment of social or other normative roles (Ware et al. 1996). Nearly all instruments are intended to provide data useful for monitoring health status within clinical, research, or evaluation settings, although not all are tested for all purposes. A few of the longer instruments are also available in shorter versions and are promoted for use in large-scale population surveys.

COMPARABILITY OF QUESTIONS

Most efforts to improve the comparability of data have focused on the comparability of surveys, in terms of the health topics covered, the specific wording of questions and the types of response scales. For example, Ferrer (2000) reviews the health topics included in household surveys conducted in Latin American and Caribbean countries on behalf of the Pan American Health Organization. Without publishing details, he reports that questions are not asked in a standardized fashion, are primarily designed to measure morbidity and exclude other aspects of health status. In addition, both the WHO Regional Office for Europe and the European Commission have made progress on reviewing existing European national surveys and standardized instruments for health topics, such as health

Table 1   Domains of 13 generic health status instruments

Health domains (multidimensional profile)	QWB '70	McM '76	SIP '76	QLI '81	NHP '81	FSQ '86	CP '87	Duke '90	SF-36 '92	HUI-III '95	WHOQOL '96	EQ-6D '99	WHODAS II '99
Overall well-being							■						
General health				■			■	■	■				
Change in health							■						
Physical health		■						■			■		
Activities/roles	■			■			■		■			■	■
Work			■			■							
Home			■										
Recreation			■										
Ambulation			■							■			
Eating			■										
Energy/vitality					■				■				
Dexterity										■			
Hearing										■			
Mobility/fitness	■		■		■	■	■	■	■			■	■
Pain/discomfort						■	■	■	■	■		■	
Self-care			■	■		■						■	■
Sleep/rest			■		■								
Speech										■			
Vision										■			
Social health		■						■			■		
Activities/roles	■					■	■		■				
Communication			■										
Interaction			■		■	■							■
Support				■				■					
Mental health						■		■	■		■		
Activities/roles									■				
Alertness			■										
Anxiety/depression								■				■	
Cognition										■		■	
Emotional status		■	■		■		■			■			
Outlook				■									
Self-esteem								■					
Understand/interact													■
Handicap/participation					■								■
Environmental context											■		

QWB: Quality of Well-Being Scale; McM: McMaster Health Index; SIP: Sickness Impact Profile; QLI: Quality of Life Index; NHP: Nottingham Health Profile; FSQ: Functional Status Questionnaire; CP: COOP Charts for Primary Care Practice; Duke: Duke Health Profile; SF-36: Short-Form 36 Health Survey; HUI-III: Health Utilities Index Mark III; EQ6D: EuroQol 6 Domain Quality of Life Scale (5D excludes cognition); WHOQOL: WHO Quality of Life Brief Field Trial Version; WHODAS II: WHO Disability Assessment Schedule.

status (de Bruin et al. 1996; 2000). For example, Hupkens (1998) reviewed the coverage of health topics in 78 national health interview surveys and specific questions in a subset of 52 surveys conducted in the European Union. As is the case for all of these reviews, comparability was assessed in terms of the wording of questions across surveys, not in terms of whether the data across different populations or subpopulations may be interpreted in a comparable fashion. For the ten most commonly included questions in the 52 surveys, only questions on height and weight were considered comparable (Table 2).

A review of 16 national health surveys conducted within 11 European Union countries documented variations among questions, such as recall periods, definition of terms, response categories or qualifications. The surveys specifically included questions addressing aspects of health status, such as limitations in daily activities and functioning (Rasmussen et al. 1999). These authors found that questions addressing chronic and acute sickness, illness and impairment were not comparable across most surveys, primarily due to differences in recall periods. Questions addressing ADLs also were not comparable across most surveys for a variety of reasons, in addition to different recall periods. They include skip patterns, where only subsets of individuals were asked questions (e.g. those with chronic illnesses or not), the types of limitations included, and the response scales. The authors also found that selected questions addressing physical functioning, sensory functions and communication abilities were more comparable across many, but not all surveys. Differences included the level of functioning probed (e.g. different distances for walking) or qualifiers (e.g. with or without resting, with or without glasses).

Gudex and Lafortune (2000) recently extended this review to include another 30 surveys in 23 OECD countries, including non-EU countries as Australia, Canada, the Czech Republic, Japan, the Republic of Korea, New Zealand, Switzerland and the United States. The main finding is that current differences in questions limit comparability only to those countries that have also incorporated standardized health status instruments in national health surveys, such as the SF-36 or EuroQol-5D. Echoing findings from earlier reviews, only a limited number of questions addressing

Table 2   Comparability of the 10 most common health topic questions in 52 European national health surveys[a]

Questions	Comparability
Chronic conditions: disease specific	−
Chronic conditions: open ended	+
General health status	+
Height and weight	++
Missing teeth	−
Toothless persons	−
Dental prosthesis	−
Present and former smoking	− −
In patient care: hospitalization	−
Out patient care: general practitioner consultations	−

Not comparable (− −); comparability limited (−); partially comparable (+); comparable (++).

a. Source: Hupkens 1998.

the prevalence of chronic conditions, or limitations in general activities or roles were considered somewhat comparable.

In a review of national household surveys from both developing and developed countries, Sadana et al. (2000) found a limited number of questions specifically describing health status, including physical or mental health, physical or cognitive functioning, other disability, or the degree and duration of activity or role limitations. Table 3 shows there is considerable variation in the number and types of questions describing health states across typical surveys.

Differences across standardized health status instruments are as great as differences across questions included within nationally representative household surveys. Not shown in Table 1 is that all instruments use different combinations of questions for each domain included, and these vary in range and depth, recall periods, type of response scales and scoring methods. Each of these differences may affect the distribution of responses, comparison among measures and ease of interpretation. For example, within the SF-36 Health Survey, the physical functioning dimension includes ten items assessing whether the person has limitations engaging in vigorous activities such as running, lifting heavy objects, or participating in strenuous sports on the high end of the scale, to limitations in bathing or dressing, on the low end of the scale. Within the EuroQol Quality of Life Scale, each dimension is made up of a single question. Given these differences, it is not surprising that the comparability of questions and domains across standardized health status instruments has also come under scrutiny.

GENERIC DOMAINS FOR THE DESCRIPTION OF HEALTH STATES

A conceptual basis for the description and measurement of health is presented in Figure 1. Broadly, if the objective is to measure health, as opposed to education or other aspects of well-being, health must be distinguished from non-health aspects of well-being. For example, health,

Figure 1   Conceptual model for assessing health

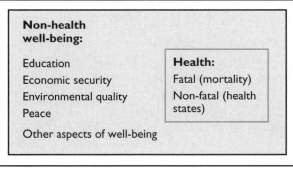

Table 3   Questions describing health status in selected national surveys

Survey	Questions
Integrated Household Survey— LSMS Survey: Paraguay, 1996	• Have you been sick during the past 4 weeks? • Have you been injured in the past 4 weeks? • For how many days during the past 4 weeks were you unable to carry out your usual activities because of this illness or injury?
Longitudinal Integrated Household Survey— LSMS survey: Jamaica 1996, Round 10	• Have you suffered from an injury during the past 4 weeks? • Have you suffered from an illness other than an injury in the past 4 weeks? • Did this injury/illness begin in the past 4 weeks or exist before? • For how many days during the past 4 weeks did you suffer from this illness or injury in the past 4 weeks? • For how many days during the past 4 weeks were you unable to carry out your usual activities because of this illness or injury? • Is a mental or physical disability preventing you from securing and maintaining employment?
Longitudinal Integrated Household Survey: Indonesian Family Life Survey 1993–1994, Wave 1	• In general, how is your health at this time? • If you have to carry a heavy load for 20 meters, could you? • If you have to sweep the house floor or yard, could you? • If you have to walk for 5 kilometers, could you? • If you have to draw a pail of water from a well, could you? • If you have to bow, squat, kneel, could you? • If you have to dress without help, could you? • If you have to stand up from sitting position in a chair without help, could you? • If you have to go to the bathroom without help, could you? • If you have to stand up from sitting on the floor without help, could you? • Have you ever experienced insomnia during the past 4 weeks? • Have you ever experienced fatigue or exhaustion during the past 4 weeks? • Have you ever felt short-tempered or hyper-sensitive during the past 4 weeks? • Have you ever experienced bodily pains in the past 4 weeks? • Have you ever experienced sadness during the past 4 weeks? • Have you ever experienced anxiety or fear during the past 4 weeks?
Longitudinal Integrated Household Survey: European Commission Household Panel 1995, Wave 2	• How is your health in general? • Do you have any chronic physical or mental health problem, illness or disability? • Are you hampered in your daily activities by this physical or mental health problem, illness or disability? • In the past 2 weeks: Have you had to cut down on any of the things you usually do about the house, at work or in your free time because of illness or injury? • In the past 2 weeks: Have you had to cut down on any of the things you usually do about the house, at work or in your free time because of an emotional or mental health problem?
National Health Survey: Pakistan 1990–1994, Adult Module	• Would you say your health in general is excellent, very good, good, fair or poor? • Have you passed/vomited worms during the last 3 months? • Have you had a cough with phlegm in the past 14 days? • In the past 14 days have you had loose stools? • Do you experience sudden shortness of breath at night? • Do you have pain in chest on exertion? • Coming into a house at night would you have trouble seeing anything in the house? • Do you have difficult hearing? • If you had an accident (poisoning, fall, injury, burn etc.) in past 12 months, are you fully recovered, under recovery or recovered with some handicap?

education, economic security, environmental quality and peace are usually considered as some of the important components of well-being (Dasgupta 1993). Across all populations and cultures, some distinction is made between health and other aspects of well-being (Deutsch 1997; Scharfstein 1998). Another way to state this is that health is not the only component of quality of life, and that different components of quality of life are to some degree separable. Others argue that health has some intrinsic value and on pragmatic considerations may be focused on and differentiated from other aspects of well-being (Brock, chapter 3.2, in this volume).

In Figure 1, the distinction between *non-health well-being* and *health* is represented by the outer and inner boxes. This is so even if the boundary between health and non-health well-being is fuzzy or varies across different subpopulations, cultures, geography and by time periods. Some may conceptualize health to include more aspects of well-being, while others may conceptualize it more narrowly. The box delineating the boundary between health and non-health well-being is therefore represented by a gray line (Figure 1). Furthermore, the size of the box is not meant to indicate the relative importance of health in relation to other non-health aspects of well-being.

Although international classifications of disease and disability exist (WHO 1992; 2001), as do local taxonomies of health and illness (Foucault 1973; Kleinman et al. 1978), the only distinction made within the box labeled *health*, is the distinction between *fatal* and *non-fatal* health. As noted, non-fatal health includes all health states for an individual alive; of interest is the description of each state, not a label such as those given by disease or mortality classifications. These can be described either directly or indirectly by a range of domains, such as those included within standardized health status assessment instruments (see Table 1). "Fatal" includes mortality risks. This representation of health excludes determinants or risk factors of health, since the determinants of health must be conceptually separated if we are to be able to empirically assess the relationship between "health" and its determinants.

Given that current measurements used in household interview surveys and standardized health status assessment instruments utilize different operational descriptions of health (see Table 1), WHO has undertaken a survey development programme to establish a core set of generic domains to describe health (Üstün et al. 2001). The term generic conveys that these domains are not associated with any one instrument or survey. The generic domains selected, after appropriate testing, should provide a comprehensive profile of non-fatal health that may describe a broad range of health states. Furthermore, generic domains should lend themselves to cross-population comparison.

Rather than ignoring or suppressing conceptual differences concerning the boundary between health and other aspects of well-being, the cross-population comparison of health states should be based on a core set of generic domains that most agree address non-fatal health. For other purposes, additional domains may be added as deemed necessary. A candidate list of domains that describe non-fatal health, for further testing, is noted in Table 4. Of the 24 candidate domains listed, 18 describe different aspects of non-fatal health directly, such as affect, pain, dexterity or fertility (e.g. domains in the gray shaded box). The remaining six are proximate domains that indirectly assess non-fatal health.

For example, the ability to engage in usual activities does not describe non-fatal health *per se*, but limitations or performance in this area may be associated with a health state. It would be preferable to assess health status directly. However, the self-reporting of limitations in usual activities *may* be reported in a more reliable or consistent manner than the self-reporting of health in some other domain, such as mobility or affect. Although this assumption requires further empirical testing, it is no surprise that proximate domains and questions are often included in standardized health status assessment instruments (see Table 1) and nationally representative survey modules (see Table 3). Even if these proximate domains are reported in a more reliable manner, this does not ensure that they provide a valid representation of non-fatal health across countries.

Specific questions that would actually make up each domain may be culled from existing standardized assessment instruments, national surveys or item banks that document item parameters in different populations. Although a comprehensive multi-dimensional profile of health is highly desirable, a subset of domains or a more parsimonious profile may be preferable for some purposes, such as within surveys that allocate a limited number of items to measuring non-fatal health.

Table 4   Candidate core generic domains for testing that describe health states across countries

Non-health well-being	Health status	
Discrimination/stigma[a]	General health	Sexual activity
Participation barriers[a]	Affect	Fertility
Self-care[a]	Cognition	Hearing
Shame/embarrassment[a]	Communication	Speech
Social functioning[a]	Dexterity	Vision
Usual activities[a]	Mobility	Breathing
	Pain	Eating
	Skin & bodily disfigurement	Digestion
	Energy/vitality	Bodily excretion

a. Proximate domains that may indirectly assess health status. This is not a complete list of domains that would assess other aspects of non-health well-being.

CONCLUSIONS

To promote a standard approach in describing non-fatal health, WHO and its collaborators have drafted a set of comprehensive generic domains, and items measuring these domains, for further testing. A series of surveys in selected countries in each of the six WHO regions are being initiated. The first phase of the studies will be directly supported by WHO. Representative household-based surveys on health of the non-institutionalized population from urban and rural areas have been completed in 10 countries[1] and smaller scale household, postal and telephone surveys have been completed in over 50 additional countries. Based on methods tested and refined, a second round of surveys will be conducted in over 70 countries using standardized methods developed. WHO will provide technical support to future surveys based on these standardized methods.

The main goal of these studies is to develop a module on health that utilizes a standardized descriptive profile of the health state. This module will also incorporate strategies to estimate and adjust for cross-population comparability, in addition to meeting other criteria for validity and reliability. Furthermore, these studies will provide empirical evidence to develop a short list(s) of domains for other purposes. Even if WHO and its collaborating institutions utilize and recommend a standardized module for assessing non-fatal health, it will be up to Member States to integrate this module within national household interview surveys.

NOTES

1   These include: China, Colombia, Egypt, Georgia, Mexico, Nigeria, India, Indonesia, Slovakia and Turkey.

REFERENCES

Andrews GR, Esterman AJ, Braunack-Mayer AJ, Rungie CM (1986) *Aging in the Western Pacific*. World Health Organization Regional Office for the Western Pacific, Manila.

Bergner M, Bobbit RA, Kressel S, et al. (1976) The sickness impact profile: conceptual formulation and methodology for the development of a health status measure. *International Journal of Health Services,* 6(3):393–415.

Bowling A (1991) *Measuring health: a review of quality of life measurement scales*. Open University Press, Buckingham.

Bowling A (1995) *Measuring disease: a review of disease specific quality of life measurement scales*. Open University Press, Buckingham.

Brazier J, Usherwood T, Harper R, Thomas K (1998) Deriving a preference based single index measure from the UK SF-36 health survey. *Journal of Clinical Epidemiology,* 51(11):1115–1128.

Breslow L (1972) A quantitative approach to the World Health Organization definition of health: physical, mental and social well-being. *International Journal of Epidemiology*, 1(4):347–355.

Chambers LW, Sackett DL, Goldsmith C, Macpehrson AS, McAuley RG (1976) Development and application of an index of social function. *Health Services Research*, 11(4):430–441.

Chen MK, Bryant BE (1975) The measurement of health – a critical and selective overview. *International Journal of Epidemiology*, 4(4):257–264.

Dasgupta P (1993) *An inquiry into well-being and destitution*. Clarendon Press, Oxford.

de Bruin A, Picavet HSJ, Nossikov A (1996) *Health interview surveys: towards international harmonization of methods and instruments. European series no 58*. WHO Regional Publications, European Series No. 58. World Health Organization, Regional Office for Europe, Copenhagen.

de Bruin A, Picavet HSJ, Nossikov A (2000) *Common instruments in health interview surveys*. World Health Organization, Regional Office for Europe, Copenhagen.

Deutsch E (1997) *Introduction to world philosophies*. Prentice-Hall, Inc., Upper Saddle River, NJ.

Fanshel S, Bush JW (1970) A health-status index and its application to health services outcomes. *Operations Research*, 18(6):1021–1065.

Feeny D, Furlong W, Boyle M, Torrance GW (1995) Multi-attribute health status classification systems: Health Utilities Index. *PharmacoEconomics*, 7(6):490–502.

Ferrer M (2000) *Health modules in household surveys in Latin America and the Caribbean: an analysis of recent questionnaires*. (Technical report series no 72.) Pan American Health Organization, Public Policy and Health Program, Health and Human Development Division, Washington, DC.

Foucault M (1973) *The birth of the clinic: an archaeology of medical perception. (French original 1963)*. English reprint. Vintage Books Inc., New York.

Grootendorst P, Feeny D, Furlong W (2000) Health utilities index mark III: evidence of construct validity for stroke and arthritis in a population health survey. *Medical Care*, 38(3):290–299.

Gudex C, Lafortune G (2000) *An inventory of health and disability-related surveys in OECD countries (DRAFT)*. (Labour market and social policy, occasional papers no 44.) Organisation for Economic Cooperation and Development, Directorate for Education, Employment, Labour and Social Affairs, Paris.

Hansluwka HE (1985) Measuring the health of populations, indicators and interpretations. *Social Science and Medicine*, 20(12):1207–1224.

Hunt SM, McKenna SP, McEwen J, Williams J, Papp E (1981) The Nottingham Health Profile: subjective health status and medical consultations. *Social Science and Medicine*, 15(3 pt 1):221–229.

Hupkens C (1998) *Coverage of health topics by surveys in the European Union. Population and social conditions.* (Eurostat working papers 3/1998/E/n 10.) European Commission, Luxembourg.

Jette AM, Davies AR, Cleary PD, et al. (1986) The functional status questionnaire: reliability and validity when used in primary care. *Journal of General Internal Medicine,* 1(3):143–149.

Katz S, Ford AB, Moskowitz RW, et al. (1963) Studies of illness in the aged. The index of ADL: a standardized measure of biological and psychosocial function. *Journal of the American Medical Association,* 185:914–919.

Kleinman A, Eisenberg L, Good B (1978) Culture, illness and care: clinical lessons from anthropologic and cross-cultural research. *Annals of Internal Medicine,* 88(2):251–258.

Krabbe PF, Stouthard MEA, Essink-Bot ML, Bonsel GJ (1999) The effect of adding a cognitive dimension to the EuroQol multiattribute health-status classification system. *Journal of Clinical Epidemiology,* 52(4):293–301.

Kroeger A (1988) Modules 10–12, morbidity and specific diseases, conditions and symptoms. In: *Training modules for household surveys on health and nutrition.* WHO/ESM, ed. World Health Organization/Epidemiology and Statistical Methodology Unit, Geneva.

Lawton MP, Brody EM (1969) Assessment of older people: self-maintaining and instrumental activities of daily living. *Gerontologist,* 9(3):179–186.

McDowell I, Newell C (1996) *Measuring health: a guide to rating scales and questionnaires.* 2nd edn. Oxford University Press, New York.

Moriyama IM (1968) Problems in the measurement of health status. In: *Indicators of social change: concepts and measurements.* Sheldon EB, Moore WE, eds. Russell Sage Foundation, New York.

Nelson EC, Wasson J, Kirk J, et al. (1987) Assessment of function in routine clinical practice: description of the COOP chart method and preliminary findings. *Journal of Chronic Diseases,* 40 (1 suppl.):S55–S63.

Parkerson JGR, Broadhead WE, Tse CK (1990) The Duke health profile: a 17 item measure of health and dysfunction. *Medical Care,* 28(11):1056–1072.

Patrick DL, Erickson P (1993) *Health status and health policy: quality of life in health care evaluation and resource allocation.* Oxford University Press, New York.

Rasmussen N, Gudex C, Christensen S (1999) *Survey data on disability.* (Eurostat working papers, Population and social conditions 3/1999/E/n 20.) European Commission, Luxembourg.

Sadana R, Mathers CD, Lopez AD, Murray CJL, Iburg K (2000) *Comparative analysis of more than 50 household surveys on health status* . (GPE discussion paper no 15.) World Health Organization/Global Programme on Evidence for Health Policy, Geneva.

Scharfstein BA (1998) *A comparative history of world philosophy from the Upanishads to Kant.* State University of New York Press, Albany, NY.

Spitzer WO, Dobson AJ, Hall J, et al. (1981) Measuring the quality of life of cancer patients: a concise QL-Index for use by physicians. *Journal of Chronic Diseases,* **34**(12):585–597.

United Nations (1995) *Guidelines for household surveys on health.* UN, Department for Economic and Social Information and Policy Analysis. Statistical Division, New York.

Üstün TB, Chatterji S, Villaneuva M, et al. (2001) *WHO multi-country household survey study on health and responsiveness, 2000–2001.* (GPE discussion paper no 37.) World Health Organization/Global Programme on Evidence for Health Policy, Geneva.

Ware J (2000) SF-36 Health survey update. *Spine,* **25**(24):3130–3139.

Ware JE, Gandeck BL, Keller SD, The IQOLA Project Group (1996) Evaluating instruments used cross-nationally: methods from the IQOLA project. In: *Quality of life and pharmaoeconomics in clinical trials.* 2nd edn. Spilker B, ed. Lippincott-Raven, Philadelphia, PA.

WHO (1957) *Measurement of levels of health: report of a study group.* (Technical report series no 137.) WHO Technical Report Series. World Health Organization, Geneva.

WHO (1992) *International statistical classification of diseases and related health problems (ICD 10).* 10th edn. World Health Organization, Geneva.

WHO (1999) *Disability assessment schedule, version 3.1a (WHODAS-II).* World Health Organization, Geneva.

WHO (2001) *International classification of functioning, disability and health (ICF).* World Health Organization, Geneva.

WHOQOL Group (1998) The World Health Organization quality of life assessment: development and general psychometric properties. *Social Science and Medicine,* **46**(12):1569–1585.

Chapter 7.2

HEALTH-STATUS CLASSIFICATION SYSTEMS FOR SUMMARY MEASURES OF POPULATION HEALTH

DAVID FEENY

Health-status classification systems that use preference-based approaches, including multi-attribute utility functions, are critically examined in this chapter. Five major issues are considered: an underlying conceptual framework; the definition of health status; choice of domains; relationships among the domains; and obtaining data on the quality of population health. (Related issues are discussed in chapter 10.2).

AN UNDERLYING CONCEPTUAL FRAMEWORK

All measurement of health status is based, implicitly or explicitly, on some form of conceptual framework and some set of fundamental normative assumptions (assumptions about fundamental values or objectives – statements about what should be). It is thus important to be explicit about the underlying framework employed. The framework I employ is explicitly based on microeconomic theory, and it is compatible with approaches in the social sciences, epidemiology, health-services research and the health sciences (Becker 1965; Feeny 2000; Grossman 1972; Rosenzweig and Schultz 1982; Rosenzweig and Schultz 1983). Frameworks used in related chapters in this volume are similar to the one presented here. Basic references on utility theory in health economics include: (Torrance 1986; Torrance and Feeny 1989) and (Feeny and Torrance 1989). A simplified version of the framework appears below.

To illustrate the framework, consider a simple world in which there are two final consumption goods, a composite good and health status. Individuals have preferences over each of these final goods, and the utility function summarizes preferences over combinations of the composite final consumption good and health status [equation (1)].

$$U = f(C, HS) \tag{1}$$

where U is utility; C is the composite final consumption good; and HS is health status.

In this framework health status enters the utility function and, together with the composite good, is a fundamental determinant of the level of satisfaction or well-being. Utility functions are defined with respect to consumption of the composite good, or enjoyment of health status over a specified period of time (Henderson and Quandt 1958).

Both of the final consumption goods (C and HS) are produced by the final consumer (within the household) using the time and market goods. The health status production function is given in equation (2). Health status is affected by a number of factors, including medical care.

$$HS = f(C, T_{hs}, MC, GE, PE, SE) \qquad (2)$$

where T_{hs} is time devoted to the production of health status; MC is medical care; GE is genetic endowment; PE is physical environment; and SE is social environment.

Health status depends on the nature and amount of consumption of goods and leisure activities (eating fresh fruits and vegetables, using tobacco); on time spent producing health status (regular exercise, sleep); medical care; genetic predisposition; the physical environment (air and water quality, occupational exposure); and the social environment (degree of inequality, social support).

Similarly, the composite final consumption good uses time and market goods as inputs:

$$C = f(T_c, MG) \qquad (3)$$

where MG represents market goods, and T_c is time devoted to production of composite good.

According to this simple framework, health status is measured because it is of fundamental importance to people. This is both a behavioural proposition (testable hypothesis) and a normative position.

DEFINITION OF HEALTH STATUS

Health status and health-related quality of life (HRQL) are measured for various purposes including description, discrimination, evaluation, and prediction (Guyatt et al. 1993). Discrimination refers to the ability to distinguish among groups at a point in time (cross-sectional study). Evaluation refers to the ability to capture within-person change over time. Prediction refers to the ability of a measure to predict another measure. Prediction may refer to the ability of a short form to predict the score on the corresponding long form of an instrument. Alternatively, prediction may refer to the ability of an assessment with a single measure at one time point to predict health status in subsequent periods. Given the variety of these purposes, measures designed for one purpose may not be ideal for others, and compromise is often involved in deriving summary measures of population health. Thus, it is important to include a variety of measures in population health surveys.

Clinical studies and population health surveys generally rely on self reporting to measure health status, both for practical reasons and on normative grounds. While this may be desirable for some purposes, it will be important to adopt an explicit definition of health status to facilitate comparisons within and between populations, and over time. Also, for the very young and for subjects with particular impairments, such as cognitive or sensory impairments, it is often not possible to rely on self reporting, and proxy assessments must be used instead. In general, self-report and proxy responses are not interchangeable (e.g. Grootendorst et al. 1997).

Ware et al. (1981) have argued for a "within the skin" definition of health status in population health surveys. However, this definition omits social interaction, which clearly affects health status and vice versa. If the "within the skin" definition is adopted, therefore, social interaction should be measured in the same survey. With longitudinal surveys, causation can then be quantified in both directions. (If one includes social interaction in the definition of health status, the examination of these relationships may become tautological. Similar arguments have been made by Colin Mathers). The Health Utilities Index Mark 2 (HUI2) and Mark 3 (HUI3) systems have adopted the "within the skin" approach (Feeny et al. 1992; 1995; 1996; Furlong et al. 1998; Torrance et al. 1992; 1995; 1996).

Another key issue is how to define health status on the impairment, disability and handicap continuum. For health-status classification systems with separate preference-based scoring systems, health status can be defined in terms of impairment or disability. To obtain estimates for preference-based scoring systems, for example, respondents can assess the extent to which disability will involve handicap and the implications of that handicap.

Also important is how capacity and performance contribute to the definition of health status. Performance depends on capacity (ability to run), opportunity (time and place to run) and preference (whether one enjoys running). Again, for health-status classification systems with separate preference-based scoring systems, capacity may be the most appropriate concept (Similar arguments have been made by Dan Hausman and Colin Mathers). This would allow assessors to value capacity according to their own preferences. For example, health status could define whether a subject had a limitation and the extent of that limitation; in a preference survey, the assessor can then decide if the limitation is important.

The task of constructing summary measures of population health has been divided into two parts: developing a multi-attribute health-status classification system (part 7 of this volume); and developing health state valuation methods (part 10). Some important criteria for developing health-status classification systems for population health surveys and clinical studies are described below. This two-part approach is consistent with a definition of the health-related quality of life as the duration of life modified by impairments, functional states, perceptions and social opportunities, all of which are influenced by disease, injury, treatment and policy (Patrick and Erickson 1993).

Finally, an advantage of the multi-attribute approach is that it provides both the disaggregated description of health-profile measures, as well as summary scores. This is illustrated by the 1990 Ontario Health Survey results for arthritis and stroke subjects (Table 1). As expected, stroke subjects often had problems with hearing, speech, ambulation, dexterity, and cognition; while those with arthritis often experienced problems with ambulation, dexterity and pain. Cognitive impairment and problems with speech were more frequently observed in the stroke group. In the arthritis group, by contrast, these problems were no more frequent than in neither the arthritis nor stroke reference group.

Categorical information on health status is presented in Table 1. The same data are represented using single-attribute and overall utility scores in Table 2. The multi-attribute utility functions permit morbidity burdens to be quantified (valued according to community preferences) and facilitate comparisons among groups. A utility function converts the categorical information on health status into interval-scale data that can be used to summarize the relative burden of morbidity in the stroke and arthritis groups.

CHOICE OF HEALTH STATUS DOMAINS

In the conceptual framework discussed above one important criterion in selecting domains (or dimensions or attributes) of health status is the value

Table 1   Health problems for stroke and arthritis subjects[a]

| | Group | | |
| | Stroke only (%) | Arthritis only (%) | Neither stroke nor arthritis (%) |
HUI3 attribute[b]			
Vision	79	76	40
Hearing	14	9	2
Speech	17	1	1
Ambulation	34	11	1
Dexterity	27	4	1
Emotion	35	20	12
Cognition	53	35	20
Pain	33	46	8

a. Source: Grootendorst et al. (1999; 2000). Data are from the 1990 Ontario Health Survey, a population health survey of community dwelling residents in Ontario, Canada. N = 193 for stroke; N = 8584 for arthritis; N = 59 113 for neither stroke nor arthritis. Data for subjects with both stroke and arthritis are not shown (N = 114). Percentages are for HUI3 attributes other than Level 1 (normal, no impairment).

b. The HUI3 health-status classification system is in chapter 10.2, Table 1.

that members of the general population place on that domain. For example, Cadman and Goldsmith (1986), Cadman et al. (1984) and Cadman et al. (1986) assembled a list of 15 domains based on then-prominent measures of health status and on clinical experience.

The 15 domains were physical activity, mobility, school performance (the study was concerned with child health), play, learning ability, happiness, pain or discomfort, sight, hearing, speech, use of limbs, cause of health problem and name of the disorder. A random sample of the general population rated the importance of each of these domains. The top six were sensation (vision, hearing, speech) and communication, happiness, self-care, pain or discomfort, learning and school ability and physical activity ability. These six formed the core of HUI2 and its descendant, HUI3.

If the measure is to be used not only to describe health status but also to value it, such as in health-adjusted life expectancy (Berthelot et al. 1993; Wolfson 1996), quality-adjusted life years, or as an outcome measure in a clinical study, then the health-status measure must be compatible with the valuation process used. Again, following the conceptual framework presented above, it is natural to base the valuations of health status on the

Table 2 Mean HUI3 single-attribute and overall utility scores, by health problem[a]

HUI3 attribute[b]	Group		
	Stroke only (%)	Arthritis only (%)	Neither stroke nor arthritis (%)
Vision	0.941	0.950	0.977
Hearing	0.956	0.968	0.993
Speech	0.934	0.998	0.998
Ambulation	0.785	0.954	0.994
Dexterity	0.851	0.986	0.998
Emotion	0.902	0.968	0.984
Cognition	0.797	0.932	0.964
Pain	0.811	0.818	0.971
Overall utility score	0.538	0.765	0.925

a. Source: Grootendorst et al. (2000). Data are from the 1990 Ontario Health Survey, a population health survey of community dwelling residents in Ontario, Canada. Results are based on linear regression analysis controlling for proxy versus self-report and potential confounding variables that affect health status including age, sex, educational attainment and number of chronic health problems (other than stroke or arthritis). Additional control variables were assessed in sensitivity analyses, including marital status, household income, smoking status, physical activity and body mass index; the results reported above are robust. It is standard practice to report utility scores to two decimal places; scores are reported here to three decimal places to facilitate comparisons.

b. Single-attribute utility scores are on a scale from 0.00 (lowest level, highest degree of impairment, for that attribute) to 1.00 (level 1, no impairment or normal for that attribute). Overall utility scores are on a scale from 0.00 (dead) to 1.00 (perfect health). The single-attribute and overall scoring functions for the HUI3 system are described in Furlong et al. (1998). $N = 173$ for stroke; $N = 7\ 751$ for arthritis; $N = 53\ 838$ for neither stroke nor arthritis. Data for subjects with both stroke and arthritis not shown ($N = 94$).

preferences of the general population. Health status is measured because it is important to people; the system used to value health states should also be based on the preferences of the general population (and/or the recipients of care).

The assessment of preferences for health status is cognitively demanding and a parsimonious number of domains (attributes) should be included in a health-status classification system. In general, people are able to process seven (plus or minus two) concepts at a time (Miller 1956) and the number of attributes for estimating multi-attribute utility functions should therefore be limited. These considerations informed the selection of attributes for the HUI2 and HUI3 systems, which were limited to seven and eight attributes, respectively. Although additional attributes would have provided a more comprehensive description of health status, this was not done because it would have attenuated the ability to develop valid and reliable preference-based scoring systems.

RELATIONSHIPS AMONG HEALTH STATUS DOMAINS

To facilitate preference measurement it is not only important to limit the number of domains, it is also important to select a set of domains that are structurally independent. (Mathers makes a similar argument). Structural independence implies a lack of overlap among attributes, and any combination of levels among domains is logically possible (even if infrequent). For instance, the HUI2 system only had partial structural independence. The combination of Level 5 Mobility (no use of arms and legs) and Level 1 (normal) Self-Care is not logically possible. A lack of structural independence means that certain health states are implausible and complicates preference elicitation when using a decomposed approach for estimating multi-attribute utility functions (see chapter 10.2).

The problem is, however, more fundamental. If the domains overlap are not structurally independent, then preferences among domains will not be independent and it will be more difficult to identify the independent effect of each domain on the overall utility score for each health state (multi-collinearity). Thus, structural independence, while not necessary for descriptive purposes, is crucial for obtaining valid preference-based scoring functions.

There is an additional advantage to designing a health-status classification system with structural independence. Because the domains do not overlap, items in questionnaires based on the system also do not overlap. In a sense, each items generates new information. Results from a recent study at Statistics Canada comparing HUI3 and EuroQol EQ-5D measures illustrate this point. In a pre-test for the third cycle of the National Population Health Survey, both EQ-5D and HUI3 were administered (order randomized) to 1 477 subjects. Kendall correlations between HUI3 attribute levels were generally low (Houle and Berthelot 2000). Correlation coefficients varied from 0.02 (speech and ambulation; speech and vision;

speech and emotion), to 0.35 (cognition and emotion). Juniper et al. (1996) have proposed standards for interpreting the degree of association. Correlations of 0.00–0.19 are regarded as negligible; correlations of 0.20–0.34 are classified as weak; correlations of 0.35–0.50 as moderate; and correlations greater than 0.50 as strong. Using these criteria, 23 (82.1%) of the off-diagonal correlations for HUI3 reported by Houle and Berthelot (2000) indicate a negligible relationship; 4 (14.3%) indicate a weak relationship; and 1 (3.6%) indicates a moderate relationship. Similar results have been found using HUI3 measures in a Japanese general population survey (Uemura et al. 2000).

In contrast, correlations among levels in EQ-5D varied from 0.24 (self-care and anxiety/depression) to 0.64 (mobility and usual activities). Five (50%) of the off-diagonal correlations were weak, 4 (40%) were moderate, and 1 (10%) indicated a strong relationship. Clearly, there is little overlap among levels in HUI3 and considerable overlap among levels in EQ-5D. By designing the system to be structurally independent, each attribute in HUI3 identifies a different dimension of health status and each question provides new information (value added).

Relationships among HUI2 and HUI3

HUI2 and HUI3 are distinct stand alone multi-attribute systems. Each includes a health-status classification system and a multiplicative multi-attribute utility function, and each has advantages and disadvantages. Although there is overlap between the two systems, and although HUI3 was derived from HUI2, there are important differences between the two systems.

HUI2 directly assesses self-care. In many applications this is a clear advantage (e.g. Alzheimer Disease—see Neumann et al. 1999a; 1999b; 2000). The concept of emotion in HUI2 focuses on worry and anxiety; in contrast HUI3 emotion focuses on happiness versus depression. The concept of pain in HUI2 includes the type of analgesia required for relief of pain, which can be an advantage in clinical studies. Pain in HUI3, by contrast, includes the extent of activity disruption due to pain; this approach is well-suited for use in population health surveys. By breaking HUI2 measures of sensation into its constituent parts (vision, hearing, speech), HUI3 measures provide greater descriptive power. The HUI3 index also has 5–6 levels per attribute, whereas HUI2 has only 3–5 levels per attribute. Fertility was included in HUI2 because it was originally developed to assess health-related quality of life in survivors of childhood cancer, and because subfertility and infertility are observed in survivors of some forms of childhood cancers. As a result, HUI2 is used in a number of cancer studies, such as long-term follow-up studies of childhood cancer and prophylaxis studies for some forms of breast cancer. Fertility was omitted from HUI3.

As mentioned above, HUI2 possesses only partial structural independence. In particular, self-care potentially overlapped with a number of

other attributes, including vision, cognition and mobility. When designing HUI3 a concerted effort was made to ensure full structural independence. Thus, self-care was dropped and dexterity was added to capture
an underlying cause of difficulties with self-care not already covered:
impairment in small motor function.

Preliminary assessment of the structural independence for HUI3 included polling experienced clinicians on whether combinations of levels
of attributes were logically possible and whether such combinations had
been observed, particularly "extreme" combinations. The results indicated
that extreme combinations were logically possible and that they had been
observed, although they were rare. These assessment increased confidence
in the structural independence of the HUI3 system (see also Houle and
Berthelot 2000).

OBTAINING DATA ON POPULATION HEALTH QUALITY

Ideally, a compact but comprehensive multi-attribute system, for which
there is a well-validated multi-attribute preference function, should be
included in major population health surveys. For example, the HUI3 sys-
tem was included in the 1990 Ontario Health Survey and the Statistics
Canada 1991 General Social Survey (Statistics Canada 1992; 1994). In
Canada, HUI3 has also been included in the ongoing National Population
Health Survey and National Longitudinal Survey of Children and Youth.
Further, HUI3 will also be included in the Canadian Community Health
Survey. (For examples of analyses based on HUI3 data see Berthelot et al.
1993; Boyle et al. 1995; Grootendorst et al. 1999; 2000; Hood et al. 1996;
Mittmann et al. 1999; Nault et al. 1996; Roberge et al. 1995b; 1996; 1997;
Trakas et al. 1999; Wolfson 1996. Additional references are available at
http://www.fhs.mcmaster.ca/hug/index.htm). Preliminary work on using
HUI3 in population health surveys in Singapore is described in Wang and
Chen (1999). A group at INSERM is developing a French version of the
HUI3 system and a multiplicative scoring function (Costet et al. 1998; Le
Gales et al. 1997). Similarly, questions based on the Years of Healthy Life
measure are included in United States population health surveys, and
EuroQol EQ-5D has been included in British health surveys.

A further advantage of measures like HUI3 is that they are also widely
used in clinical studies. Indeed, in the Institute of Medicine report on
summary measures of population health, Field and Gold (1998) note that:
"It is the consensus of the committee that linking public health and medical care measurement strategies would be of fundamental importance in
assessing the performance of each system individually and in relation to
one another." For HUI3 such linkages are already possible. Speechley et
al. (1999), for example, used HUI2, HUI3, and the Child Health Questionnaire in a survey of survivors of cancer in childhood. The use of the
same measures in clinical and population health surveys provides an im-

portant link and facilitates a number of analyses, including cost-effectiveness and cost-utility studies.

If a multi-attribute system has not been included in a population health survey, it may be possible to map data from the population health survey into an existing multi-attribute system. Although this typically involves some loss of information, the results have often been satisfactory. For example, Erickson et al. (1989) were able to map from United States population health surveys into the Quality of Well Being system and Gold et al. (1996) were able to map into the HUI1 system; and Curtis (1998) was able to map from the Ontario Child Health Survey into the HUI2 system. It was also possible to map from the Minimum Data Set system (widely used in geriatrics) into the HUI2 and HUI3 systems (Wodchis et al. 1999). Other examples include Rizzo et al. (1998) and Rizzo and Sindelar (1999).

Finally, it is important to note that in the approach outlined in this paper the fundamental unit of observation is the person, such as a subject in a population health survey or clinical study. The unit of observation is not the disease or health problem. Further, it is also important to obtain information about the context and community in which the subject lives, as well as information on both the capacity and performance of individuals.

CONCLUSIONS

For the purposes of constructing summary measures of population health it is important to adopt an explicit conceptual framework; define health status; choose a short list of domains of health status that people regard as important; minimize overlap among the domains; and use a system that includes a preference-based scoring system. It is also important that the stimulus used to describe health status and obtain health status information in population health surveys be the same as the one upon which the preference-based scoring system is based. In this manner there is congruence between how subjects are asked to describe their health status and the health status descriptions presented to the general population for valuation. Thus, to assess population health, a brief health-status classification system for which there is a corresponding validated preference-based scoring system should be included.

ACKNOWLEDGMENTS

The author acknowledges the helpful comments of William Furlong and George W. Torrance on an earlier draft.

REFERENCES

Becker GS (1965) A theory of the allocation of time. *Economic Journal*, 75(299):493–517.

Berthelot JM, Roberge R, Wolfson M (1993) The calculation of health-adjusted life expectancy for a Canadian province using a multi-attribute utility function: a first attempt. In: *Calculation of health expectancies: harmonization, consensus achieved and future perspectives.* (Proceedings of the 6th meeting of the international network on health expectancy and the disability process REVES, October 1992, Montpellier.) Robine JM, Mathers CD, Bone MR, Romieu I, eds. John Libbey Eurotext, Paris.

Boyle MH, Furlong W, Feeny D, Torrance G, Hatcher J (1995) Reliability of the health utilities index – mark 3, used in the 1991 cycle 6 Canadian general social survey health questionnaire. *Quality of Life Research,* 4(3):249–257.

Cadman D, Goldsmith C (1986) Construction of social value or utility-based health indices: the usefulness of factorial experimental design plans. *Journal of Chronic Diseases,* 39(8):643–651.

Cadman D, Goldsmith C, Torrance GW, et al. (1986) *Development of a health status index for Ontario children.* McMaster University, Hamilton, Ontario.

Cadman D, Goldsmith CC, Bashim P (1984) Values, preferences, and decisions in the care of children with developmental disabilities. *Journal of Developmental and Behavioural Pediatrics,* 5(2):60–64.

Costet N, Le Gales C, Buron C, et al. (1998) French cross-cultural adaptation of the health utilities index mark 2 (HUI2) and 3 (HUI3) classification systems. Clinical and economic working groups. *Quality of Life Research,* 7(3):245–256.

Curtis L (1998) *The health status of mothers and children.* Doctoral dissertation. McMaster University, Department of Economics, Hamilton, Ontario.

Erickson P, Kendall E, Anderson J, Kaplan R (1989) Using composite health status measures to assess the nation's health. *Medical Care,* 27(3):S66–S76.

Feeny D (2000) A utility approach to the assessment of health-related quality of life. *Medical Care,* 38(9 Suppl.):II-151-II-154.

Feeny D, Furlong W, Barr RD, Torrance GW, Rosenbaum P, Weitzman S (1992) A comprehensive multiattribute system for classifying the health status of survivors of childhood cancer. *Journal of Clinical Oncology,* 10(6):490–502.

Feeny D, Furlong W, Boyle M, Torrance GW (1995) Multi-attribute health status classification systems: Health Utilities Index. *PharmacoEconomics,* 7(6):490–502.

Feeny D, Torrance GW (1989) Incorporating utility-based quality-of-life assessments in clinical trials: two examples. *Medical Care,* 27(3 Suppl.):S190–S204.

Feeny D, Torrance GW, Furlong W (1996) Health Utilities Index. In: *Quality of life and pharmacoeconomics in clinical trials.* 2nd edn. Spilker B., ed. Lippincott-Raven, Philadelphia, PA.

Field MJ, Gold MR, eds. (1998) *Summarizing population health: directions for the development and application of population metrics.* National Academy Press, Washington, DC.

Furlong W, Feeny D, Torrance GW, et al. (1998) *Multiplicative multi-attribute utility function for the health utilities index mark 3 (HUI3) system: a technical report.* (CHEPA working paper no 98/11.) McMaster University, Centre for Health Economics and Policy Analysis, Hamilton, Ontario.

Gold M, Franks P, Erickson P (1996) Assessing the health of the nation: the predictive validity of a preference-based measure and self-rated health. *Medical Care,* 34(2):163–177.

Grootendorst P, Feeny D, Furlong W (1997) Does it matter whom and how you ask? Inter- and intra-rater agreement in the 1990 Ontario health survey. *Journal of Clinical Epidemiology,* 50(2):127–135.

Grootendorst P, Feeny D, Furlong W (1999) *Health utilities index mark III: evidence of construct validity for stroke and arthritis in a population health survey.* (CHEPA working paper no 99/06.) McMaster University, Centre for Health Economics and Policy Analysis, Hamilton, Ontario.

Grootendorst P, Feeny D, Furlong W (2000) Health utilities index mark III: evidence of construct validity for stroke and arthritis in a population health survey. *Medical Care,* 38(3):290–299.

Grossman M (1972) On the concept of health capital and the demand for health. *Journal of Political Economy,* 80 (2):223–255.

Guyatt GH, Feeny DH, Patrick DL (1993) Measuring health-related quality of life. *Annals of Internal Medicine,* 118(8):622–629.

Henderson JM, Quandt RE (1958) *Microeconomic theory: a mathematical approach.* McGraw Hill, New York.

Hood SC, Beaudet MP, Catlin G (1996) A healthy outlook. *Health Reports,* 7(4):25–32.

Houle C, Berthelot JM (2000) A head-to-head comparison of the health utilities mark 3 and the EQ-5D for the population living in private households in Canada. *Quality of Life Newsletter,* (24):5–6.

Juniper EF, Guyatt GH, Jaeschke R (1996) How to develop and validate a new health-related quality of life instrument. In: *Quality of life and pharmacoeconomics in clinical trials.* 2nd edn. Spilker B., ed. Lippincott-Raven, Philadelphia, PA.

Le Gales C, Buron C, Coster N, et al. (1997) Assessment of the multi-attribute preference function for health utilities index mark 3 in France: preliminary results. *Quality of Life Research,* 6(7/8):678

Miller GA (1956) The magical number seven plus or minus two: some limits on our capacity for processing information. *Psychological Review,* 63:81–97.

Mittmann N, Trakas K, Risebrough N, Liu BA (1999) Utility scores for chronic conditions in a community-dwelling population. *PharmacoEconomics,* 15(4):369–376.

Nault F, Roberge R, Berthelot JM (1996) Espérance de vie et espérance en santé selon le sexe, l'état matrimonial et le statut socio-économique au Canada. *Cahiers Québécois de Démographie,* 25(2):241–259.

Neumann PJ, Hermann RC, Kuntz KM, et al. (1999) Cost-effectiveness of donepezil in treatment of mild or moderate Alzheimer's disease. *Neurology,* 52(6):1138–1145.

Neumann PJ, Kuntz KM, Leon J, et al. (1999) Health utilities and health status in Alzheimer's disease: a cross-sectional study of subjects and caregivers. *Medical Care,* 37(1):27–32.

Neumann PJ, Sandberg EA, Araki SS, Kuntz KM, Feeny D, Weinstein MC (2000) A comparison of HUI2 and HUI3 utility scores in Alzheimer's disease. *Medical Decision Making,* 20(4):413–422.

Patrick DL, Erickson P (1993) *Health status and health policy: quality of life in health care evaluation and resource allocation.* Oxford University Press, New York.

Rizzo JA, Pashko S, Friedkin R, Mullahy J, Sindelar JL (1998) Linking the health utilities index to national medical expenditure survey data. *PharmacoEconomics,* 13(5 Part 1):531–541.

Rizzo JA, Sindelar JL (1999) Linking health-related quality-of-life indicators to large national data sets. *PharmacoEconomics,* 16(5 Part 1):473–482.

Roberge R, Berthelot JM, Cranswick K (1996) *Linking disability-adjusted life expectancy with health adjusted life expectancy: calculations for Canada.* (Presented at the 9th meeting of the international network on health expectancy and the disability process REVES, December 1996.) Rome.

Roberge R, Berthelot JM, Wolfson M (1995) Health and socio-economic inequalities. *Canadian Social Trends,* 37:15–19.

Roberge R, Berthelot JM, Wolfson M (1995) The Health Utility Index: measuring health differences in Ontario by socioeconomic status. *Health Reports,* 7(2):25–32.

Roberge R, Berthelot JM, Wolfson MC (1997) Adjusting life expectancy to account for morbidity in a national population. *Quality of Life Newsletter,* (17):12–13.

Rosenzweig MR, Schultz TP (1982) The behavior of mothers as inputs to child health: the determinants of birth weight, gestation, and rate of fetal growth. In: *Economic aspects of health.* Fuchs VR, ed. University of Chicago, Chicago, IL.

Rosenzweig MR, Schultz TP (1983) Estimating a household production function: heterogeneity, the demand for health inputs, and their effects on birth weight. *Journal of Political Economy,* 91(5):723–746.

Speechley KN, Maunsell E, Desmeules M, et al. (1999) Mutual concurrent validity of the child health questionnaire and the Health Utilities Index: an exploratory analysis using survivors of childhood cancer. *International Journal of Cancer,* 12(Suppl.):95–105.

Statistics Canada (1992) *The 1991 general social survey – cycle 6: health – public use microdata file documentation and user's guide.* Statistics Canada, Ottawa.

Statistics Canada (1994) *Health status of Canadians: report of the 1991 general social survey.* Statistics Canada, Ottawa.

Torrance GW (1986) Measurement of health state utilities for economic appraisal: a review. *Journal of Health Economics,* 5(1):1–30.

Torrance GW, Feeny D (1989) Utilities and quality-adjusted life years. *International Journal of Technology Assessment in Health Care*, 5(4):559–575.

Torrance GW, Feeny D, Furlong W, Barr R, Zhang Y, Wang Q (1996) Multi-attribute preference functions for a comprehensive health status classification system: health utilities index mark II. *Medical Care*, 34(7):702–722.

Torrance GW, Furlong W, Feeny D, Boyle M (1995) Multi-attribute preference functions: Health Utilities Index. *PharmacoEconomics*, 7(6):503–520.

Torrance GW, Zhang Y, Feeny D, Furlong W, Barr R (1992) *Multi-attribute preference functions for a comprehensive health status classification system.* (CHEPA working paper no 92/18.) McMaster University, Centre for Health Economics and Policy Analysis, Hamilton, Ontario.

Trakas K, Lawrence K, Shear NH (1999) Utilization of health care resources by obese Canadians. *Canadian Medical Association Journal*, 160(10):1457–1462.

Uemura T, Moriguchi H, Feeny D, et al. (2000) Japanese health utilities index mark 3 (HUI3): measurement properties in a community sample. *Quality of Life Research*, 9(9):1068

Wang Q, Chen G (1999) The health status of the Singaporean population as measured by a multiattribute health status system. *Singapore Medical Journal*, 40(6):389–396.

Ware JE, Brook RH, Davies AR, Lohr KN (1981) Choosing measures of health status for individuals in general populations. *American Journal of Public Health*, 71(6):620–625.

Wodchis WP, Hirdes JP, Feeny D (1999) *A health-related quality of life measure based on the minimum data set.* (Unpublished work).

Wolfson MC (1996) Health-adjusted life expectancy. *Statistics Canada: Health Reports*, 8(1):41–46.

Chapter 7.3

THE INTERNATIONAL CLASSIFICATION OF FUNCTIONING, DISABILITY AND HEALTH — A COMMON FRAMEWORK FOR DESCRIBING HEALTH STATES

BEDIRHAN ÜSTÜN

The *International Classification of Functioning, Disability and Health* (ICF)[1] aims to provide a unified and standard language and framework for the description of health and health-related states. ICF covers all possible components of health, and some health-related components of well-being (such as education, labour, etc) for description and assessment. The ICF domains can, therefore, be seen as *health domains* and *health-related domains*. These domains are described by two basic lists: (1) body functions and structure; (2) activities and participation.[2] As a classification, ICF systematically groups different domains[3] for a person in a given health condition (e.g. what a person with a disease or disorder does do or can do) and renders a useful profile of the individual's functioning in various health and health-related domains.

ICF belongs to the "family" of classifications developed by the World Health Organization (WHO) for application to various aspects of health. In WHO's family of international classifications, health conditions are classified mainly in ICD-10 (International Statistical Classification of Diseases and Related Health Problems, Tenth Revision),[4] which basically provides an etiological framework. The health states associated with diseases, disorders or other health conditions are classified in ICF. The ICD-10 and ICF are therefore complementary. ICD-10 provides a "diagnosis" and this information is enriched by the additional information given by ICF. Together, information on diagnosis plus functioning provides a broader and more meaningful picture that describes the health of persons or populations.

ICF has moved away from a "consequence of disease" classification (in its 1980 version, the International Classification of Impairments, Disabilities and Handicaps [ICIDH]) to a "components of health" classification. "Components of health" defines what constitutes health, whereas "consequences" focus on the impacts of diseases or other health conditions that follow as a result. In this way, ICF takes a neutral stand with regard to etiology and allows researchers to arrive at causal inferences with scientific methods.

Aims of ICF

ICF is a multi-purpose classification designed to serve various disciplines and different sectors. Its specific aim is to provide a scientific basis for understanding and studying health states and health-related outcomes, and their determinants; and to establish a common language for describing health states that will permit comparison of data across countries, health care disciplines, services and time. Since its first publication in 1980, ICIDH has been used for various purposes, such as in health statistics, research, clinical work, and social policy.

Organization of information in the ICF

ICF is a classification of health and health-related domains which are grouped according to their common characteristics (such as their origin, type or similarity) and ordered in a meaningful way.

ICF gives standard operational definitions of the health domains as opposed to "vernacular" definitions of health. These definitions describe the essential attributes of each domain (e.g. qualities, properties and relationships) and contain information as to what is included and excluded in each domain. These definitions contain commonly used anchor points for assessment so that the definitions can be translated into questionnaires, or conversely results of assessment instruments can be coded in ICF terms. For example, "vision" is defined as whether a person can see clearly objects at varying distances, the visual field and the quality of vision; and the severity of vision difficulty can be coded at mild, moderate, severe or total levels.

The ICF codes are only complete by the presence of at least one *qualifier*, which denotes the magnitude of the level of health (e.g. severity of the problem) either in terms of the construct *Performance* or the construct *Capacity* (see below). Qualifiers are coded as one or two numbers after a decimal point. Use of any code should be accompanied by at least one qualifier. Without qualifiers codes have no meaning when used for individuals or cases. A generic qualifier has been developed to describe the extent or magnitude of the problem in that construct.

ICF organizes information in three components:

- The *Body* construct comprises two classifications, one for functions of body systems, and one for the body structure. The chapters of both classifications are organized according to the body systems.

- The *Activities and Participation* constructs cover the complete range of domains denoting aspects of functioning from both an individual and societal perspective.

- A list of *environmental factors* forms part of the classification. Environmental factors have an impact on all three constructs and are organized from the individual's most immediate environment to the general environment.

BODY FUNCTIONS AND STRUCTURE AND IMPAIRMENTS

Body Functions are the physiological or psychological functions of body systems. *Body Structures* are anatomic parts of the body such as organs, limbs and their components. *Impairments* are problems in body function or structure such as a significant deviation or loss. Body functions and body structures refer to the human organism as a whole; hence it includes the brain and its functions, i.e. the mind. Therefore mental (or psychological) functions are subsumed under body functions. Body functions and structure are classified along body systems; accordingly body structures are not considered as organs. Impairments of structure can involve an anomaly, defect, loss or other significant deviation in body structures. Impairments represent a deviation from certain generally accepted population standards in the biomedical status of the body and its functions, and definition of their constituents is undertaken primarily by those qualified to judge physical and mental functioning according to these standards. Impairments can be temporary or permanent; progressive, regressive or static; intermittent or continuous. The deviation from the norm may be slight or severe and may fluctuate over time. These characteristics are captured in further descriptions, mainly in the codes, by means of qualifiers.

ACTIVITIES AND PARTICIPATION

The activity and participation domains are listed in a *single common list* which covers full range of life areas (e.g. basic learning and watching to more composite ones such as social tasks) as a neutral list. These domains are qualified by two basic qualifiers of *Performance and Capacity*. Hence the information gathered from the list provides a solid data matrix which has no overlap or redundancy (see Table 1).

The performance qualifier describes what an individual does in their current environment. Because the current environment brings in a societal context, performance can also be understood as "involvement in a life situation" or "the lived experience" of people in the actual context in which they live.[5] This context includes the environmental factors—all aspects of the physical, social and attitudinal world which can be coded using the Environmental Factors.

The capacity qualifier describes an individual's capability to execute a task or an action described in the classification in a uniform environment. This construct renders an understanding of the highest probable level that a person may reach in a given domain at a given moment. A "uniform environment" as a specific term covers the relevant environmental factors to the specified domain and has to bear no hindrances or barriers so as to allow one to assess the full capability of the individual. Uniform environment is assumed to be the same for all persons in all countries to allow international comparisons.

Difficulties or problems in these domains can arise when there is a qualitative or quantitative alteration in the way in which functions in these domains are carried out. Limitations or restrictions are assessed against a generally accepted population standard. The standard or norm against which an individual's capacity and performance is compared is that of an individual without a similar health condition (disease, disorder or injury etc.). The limitation or restriction records the discordance between the observed and the expected performance. The expected performance is the population norm, which represents the experience of the people without the specific health condition. This is the same norm in the capacity qualifier so that one can make inferences to what can be done to the environment of the person to enhance their performance.

Contextual factors

Contextual factors represent the complete background of an individual's life and living. They include environmental factors and personal factors that may have an impact on the individual with a health condition and that individual's health state.

- *Environmental factors* make up the physical, social and attitudinal environment in which people live and conduct their lives. The factors are external to individuals and can have a positive or negative influence on the individual's participation as a member of society, on performance of activities of the individual or on the individual's body function or structure.

Table 1   Activities and participation information matrix

	Performance	Capacity
1 Learning and applying knowledge		
2 General tasks and demands		
3 Communication		
4 Mobility		
5 Self-care		
6 Domestic life		
7 Interpersonal interactions		
8 Major life		
9 Community, social and civic life		

- *Personal factors* are the individual background of an individual's life and living, composed of features of the individual that are not part of a health condition or health state. These may include age, race, gender, educational background, experiences, personality and character style, aptitudes, other health conditions, fitness, lifestyle, habits, upbringing, coping styles, social background, profession and past and current experience. Personal factors are not classified in ICF.

USE OF THE ICF

In ICF, a person is given an array of codes that encompass the three parts of the classification. In this way the maximum number of codes per person can be 20 at one digit level (e.g. 10 Body Functions, 10 Activities and Participation codes—either as capacity or performance qualifiers). Similarly, at further detail these codes can theoretically be up to 300 or 3 000 depending on the level of detail, however, only some 1 300 are actually filled in the long version of the classification. In real life application of ICF, a set of 3 to 18 codes seem to be used to describe a case with three digit level precision. Generally the more detailed 3-level version is used for specialist services (e.g. rehabilitation outcomes, geriatrics, etc.) whereas the 2-level classification can be used for surveys and clinical outcome evaluation.

In the framework of summary measures of population health (SMPH), ICF provides a useful framework to capture multiple dimensions of *non-fatal health outcomes*. ICF encompasses all aspects of human health and some health-relevant aspects of well-being and describes them as *"health domains"* and *"health-related domains"*. The health states associated with all diseases, disorders, injuries and other health conditions can be described using ICF. The unit of classification is therefore the "domain" of health and health-related states. Descriptions of health states include the information on the disease and the functional abilities affected in various domains. ICF gives a profile of such functional abilities, which are defined in a standard way for observation and measurement (e.g. various body functions, mobility, self-care, cognition, interpersonal relations, etc.). These descriptions can be used as a valuable input for health state valuations for summary health measures. As valuation is expressed as a single numerical value it is obtained through a process where description of health states is given to elicit the values given in terms of importance, time, person, money, probability or risk. The descriptions from ICF provide a useful tool to make the input for the valuation exercises conceptually understandable and culturally meaningful. ICF descriptions provide a common framework with standard definitions and anchor points, which are feasible and scientific.

Using the ICF framework, one can also study the change after a key event such as adaptation, coping, adjustment and accommodation, since ICF allows for the coding and measurement of capacity, environmental factors and personal factors.

Defining the rubrics of health and health-related (non-health) domains, ICF may be useful to draw the line between health and non-health for description of the non-fatal health outcomes. It thus provides a "Rosetta Stone" (e.g. a translation matrix) for various health state description instruments because almost all such instruments could be mapped onto ICF as a common framework.

NOTES

1   The International Classification of Functioning, Disability and Health (ICF) is the second revision of the International Classification of Impairments, Disabilities, and Handicaps (ICIDH), which was first published in 1980 by the World Health Organization for trial purposes. The second revision was developed after systematic field trials and international consultation over the last five years and has been approved by the WHO's World Health Assembly in May 2001 for international use (WHO 2001).

2   These constructs of health-related experience replace terms formerly used- "impairment," "disability" and "handicap" and extend their meanings to include positive experiences. The new terms are further defined in the introduction and detailed within the classification. It is important to note that these terms are used with specific meanings that may differ from their everyday usage. Functioning refers to all body functions, and performance of tasks or actions as an umbrella term; similarly Disability serves as an umbrella term for impairments, capacity limitations or performance limitations. ICF also lists environmental factors that interact with all these constructs.

3   A domain is a practical and meaningful set of related actions, tasks or areas of life.

4   International Statistical Classification of Diseases and Related Health Problems, Tenth Revision, Vols. 1–3. Geneva, World Health Organization, 1992–1994.

5   Some may argue that involvement includes "taking part, being included or engaged in an area of life, being accepted, or having access to needed resources"; these are all covered if one *does* tasks in a domain.

REFERENCES

WHO (2001) *International classification of functioning, disability and health (ICF).* World Health Organization, Geneva.

Chapter 7.4

The 6D5L description system for health state valuation

Prasanta Mahapatra, Lipika Nanda
and K.T. Rajshree

Introduction

When we ask a person to value time spent in a health state without any
information about the key domains of health, (s)he must guess a description of the health state. The description visualized by the valuer would
usually be implicit in the valuation task. This will inevitably introduce
measurement error and a potential for bias in the results. Another consideration is how to convey relevant information about a hypothetical
health state to the individual undertaking the valuation, who might not
have personally encountered the state. Disease labels are short and parsimonious, but do not convey adequate information about functional status. Moreover, disease labels are vulnerable to different interpretations
based on cultural and personal settings. Here we report the 6D5L description system developed and used by the Andhra Pradesh Health State Valuation Study 1999 (APHSV99). Results from this study are presented in
chapter 9.4. More details of design, methods, data collection and analysis have been reported (Mahapatra et al. 2000). We first review current
literature on the theoretical question of how to describe health states for
valuation. We then describe components of the 6D5L system developed
to describe health states for valuation. In the third and final section of this
chapter we present some results about the usage of the 6D5L system by
valuers in the APHSV99 Study.

How to describe health states for valuation

It is now widely recognized that health states should be described in terms
of functional status. Functional status information can be presented either
in a narrative or structured format. For example, Sackett and Torrance
(1978) used brief scenarios written up with help of clinicians, to describe
various health states. EuroQol uses a structured approach where each
health state is described in terms of five dimensions and three severity levels

within each dimension (Brooks 1996). The Health Utilities Index uses a structured approach consisting of an eight dimensions and 5–6 severity levels within each dimension (Boyle et al. 1994). Torrance et al. (1992) have also used structured formats consisting of seven dimensions and 4–5 severity levels within each. Issues relevant to development of a health state description systems have been described by Boyle and Torrance (1984), and Froberg and Kane, I–IV (1989). Briefly, four important considerations guide us in defining the description space (number of dimensions) and the inclusion of specific attributes[1] of human health.

1. Conceptual definitions of health and deduced description systems.

2. Empirically gathered health-related attributes, and description systems induced by them.

3. Attention span and cognitive capacity of the human mind to process multi-dimensional information.

4. Statistical analysis of multi-attribute measurements.

CONCEPTUAL DEFINITIONS OF HEALTH AND DEDUCED DESCRIPTION SYSTEMS

An ideal definition of health provides us the goal towards which a formal health state description system should work. Deductive lineage from an ideal definition gives the description system its content validity. Hence a description system should incorporate as much of our ideal notion of health as is practically feasible. Concepts of health as well as support to and criticism of various definitions of health has been reviewed by Boyle and Torrance (1984); Fanshel (1972); Goldberg and Dab (1987); Noack (1987); Patrick et al. (1973); Stewart (1992) and Patrick and Erickson (1993). Based on an overview of concepts of health Noack (1987), highlighted two common elements in various definitions, namely (a) that health is a holistic concept, and (b) that health is a multidimensional concept. Intuitively appealing this view is invariably shared by researchers dealing with the subject of health and its measurement.

The holistic and multidimensional character of health is emphasized by the World Health Organization (WHO) definition of health. WHO's constitution defines health as a state of complete physical, mental and social well-being and not merely absence of disease or infirmity. This is a very inclusive definition. The definition certainly motivates health workers to integrate their role into a social well-being world-view. From the analytic perspective, there could be some doubt as to whether including social well-being within the health construct helps or hinders analysis. For example, restricting the concept of health status to physical and mental health would allow for testing of research questions as to how actions in the health care sector affect social well-being. On the other hand, an inclusive definition would make it difficult to identify the effect of actions in the health sector on an overall social well-being. Many generic health status measurement tools have drawn inspiration from WHO's definition of health, using the physical, mental and social well-being triad as a starting point for the inclusion of dimensions and items within them. Some examples are: the EuroQol (Brooks 1996), the health status index (Fanshel and Bush 1970), which has since evolved into the more commonly known Quality of Well Being Scale (Kaplan and Bush 1982) and the McMaster Health Index Questionnaire (Chambers et al. 1976). In the EuroQol instrument, for example, mobility and self-care would map to physical functioning; usual activities are linked to social functioning; and anxiety and depression would represent mental health.

EMPIRICALLY GATHERED HEALTH-RELATED ATTRIBUTES AND DESCRIPTION SYSTEMS INDUCED BY THEM

Authors of the Quality of Well Being scale first abstracted "several hundred" case descriptions from medical texts. Then they consulted various survey instruments including the Health Interview Survey of the US National Center for Health Statistics, Alameda County Population Laboratory's community social surveys. Items from the survey instruments were selected to cover the range of disturbances in functional status (Patrick et al. 1973).

Development of the Sickness Impact Profile (SIP) began with accumulation of statements describing behavioural changes attributable to sickness. These statements were collected from a sample of enrolees in a prepaid group practice and persons attending a few other outpatient facilities. Sampling of enrolees in the group practice continued until the yield of new and usable statements diminished markedly (Bergner et al. 1976). A basic catalogue of 1 100 statements was reduced to 312 unique items in 14 categories. The Nottingham Health Profile (NHP) generated its pool of items through a survey of 768 patients with acute and chronic ailments (Hunt et al. 1981). Items from the SIP were used in addition. The NHP contains 38 items grouped into six sections, namely physical abilities, pain, sleep, social isolation, emotional reactions and energy level.

The EuroQol Group (1990) reviewed the health state description systems developed by the above studies to arrive at a parsimonious set of dimensions. The group sought to develop an instrument of generic health status measurement across multiple cultures. Table 1 shows the dimensions arrived at by studies leading to the three scales described above and the five dimensions adopted by EuroQol (EQ-5D). Except alertness and energy level, all other dimensions from SIP, QWB and NHP scales are represented in the EQ-5D system. Note that cognition did not appear as a distinct dimension in any of these scales.

The Rand Health Insurance Experiment, followed by the Medical Outcomes Study (MOS), systematically collected items to describe various aspects of health and studied their properties for construction of a generic health status measurement tool (Brook et al. 1979; Stewart 1992). The Short Form-36 (SF-36) instrument is an outcome of these extensive

Table 1   Mapping of selected health status description systems
                     to EQ-5D

SIP	QWB	NHP	EQ-5D[a]
Ambulation	Mobility	Physical abilities	Mobility
Mobility	Physical activity		
Body care and movements			Self-care
Eating	Social activity—self-care		
Work	Social activity—major		Usual activities
Home management			
Recreation and pastimes	Social activity—other		
		Pain	Pain, discomfort
Emotional behaviour		Emotional reactions	Anxiety—depression
Sleeping and rest		Sleep	
Social interaction		Social isolation	
Communication			
Alertness behaviour		Energy level	

a. Includes main activity and leisure which were separate in early versions of EuroQol.

studies. SF-36 includes multiple items organized under eight dimensions (Table 2). Cognition appeared in these studies as a distinct dimension. Most of these map to the EQ-5D system, except cognition, health perceptions, energy-fatigue, and physical-psychological symptoms.

The EQ-5D description system appears to be strongly rooted in its conceptual lineage to an ideal definition of health and its linkage to empirically rooted health status descriptions. Its emphasis on cross-cultural validity and feasibility of measurement are very attractive. However, the lack of cognitive dimension and the restriction of severity levels within each dimension to three, leaves us with some handicaps. Cognition, hitherto taken for granted, is clearly an important attribute of human health. Diseases affecting cognitive functioning are now being recognized. Recent research in a EuroQol member centre suggests that the addition of cognition as the sixth dimension, would make the EQ-5D system more comprehensive (Krabbe et al. 1998). These authors (Krabbe et al. 1998) found that the inclusion of cognition changed ratings for conditions with lower levels of disability in other dimensions. Valuations for conditions with severe levels of disability in other dimensions did not change much. Restric-

Table 2   Mapping of MOS[a] SF-36 dimensions to EQ-5D

SF-36 domain	Description	EQ-5D
Mobility	Getting around in the community	Mobility
Physical functioning	Walking, climbing stairs	
		Self-care
Self-care		
Role functioning	Performance of usual role activities such as working at a job, housework, child care, community activities and volunteer work	Usual activities
Pain	Subjective feeling of bodily distress of discomfort such as headaches, backaches	Pain— discomfort
Social functioning	Functioning in normal social activities with family, friends, neighbours, marital functioning, sexual problems	Anxiety— depression
Psychological distress/well-being	Positive and negative psychological states including anxiety, depression, behavioural emotional control, loneliness, positive affect, feelings of belonging	
Sleep	Quantity, disturbance, adequacy of sleep	
Health distress	Psychological distress due to health	
Cognitive functioning	Cognitive problems, such as forgetfulness, difficulty in concentrating	
Health perceptions	Personal evaluations of health in general, including current and prior health, health outlook, resistance to illness	
Energy/fatigue	Feelings of energy, pep, fatigue, tiredness	
Physical/psychological symptoms	Subjective perceptions about the internal state of the body, such as stiffness and coughing	

a. Source: Stewart AL (1992) The medical outcomes study framework of health indicators. In: *Measuring Functioning and Well-Being*, Stewart AL and Ware JE eds. Duke University Press, Durham, 1992 (See pp. 23–24).

tion of severity levels to three may be a reason for the insensitivity of EuroQol to minor and trivial illnesses.

ATTENTION SPAN AND COGNITIVE CAPACITY OF HUMAN MIND
TO PROCESS MULTIDIMENSIONAL INFORMATION

Research in the field of psychology suggests that there is a limit to our capacity to process information (Saariluoma 1998). Miller (1956) suggested that human beings process about 5–9 attributes (chunks of information) at a time. More recent evidence from research in working memory suggests that human capacity to simultaneously process multi-attribute information may range from 3 to 5 rather than 5 to 9 as was thought earlier (Halford 1998). These findings imply that the number of dimensions used to describe the states should be kept as minimum as feasible, to allow adequate processing of health state descriptions by valuers. Recognizing the need to keep the information load on valuers within manageable limits, researchers have tried to simplify health state description systems. For example, Brazier et al. (1998) simplified the SF-36 profiles to a six-dimension (SF-6D) description system, which was used to obtain a holistic valuation of health states to be used for estimation of QALYs. Froberg and Kane (1989) propose that the number of dimensions in a description system should not exceed nine, and should preferably be less. Reviewing empirical evidences on the mode of presentation of health states, Froberg and Kane (1989) conjecture that "moderately detailed health state descriptions yield more accurate judgements of preference than either very scant descriptions or very lengthy descriptions that run the risk of overloading the rater's information processing capacity." We believe that the number of dimensions should not exceed six and should preferably be less. We have used six dimensions to describe health states in this study. We hope that future research will help identify more compact description systems with lesser number of dimensions without any loss of descriptive ability.

STATISTICAL ANALYSIS OF MULTI-ATTRIBUTE MEASUREMENTS

The number of dimensions have implications about the type of statistical analyses that can be done on directly measured health state values. Froberg and Kane (1989) have referred to Fischer's overview (1979) which found that with six or fewer dimensions, functional measurement and explicit decomposition procedures assigned similar values to a health state. The reliability of multi-attribute judgements deteriorate with larger number of dimensions. Froberg and Kane have referred to other investigators (Llewellyn-Thomas et al. 1984; Lyness and Cornelius 1982) who found that when only a few dimensions are involved, multi-attribute judgements are more reliable than decomposed judgements. Thus, parsimony of dimensions is important to retain the holistic property of a description used for operational purposes.

HOW TO CONVEY HEALTH STATE DESCRIPTIONS EFFECTIVELY
TO AN INDIVIDUAL UNDERTAKING THE VALUATIONS

Effective communication of the description to individuals acting as valuers has many difficulties. The descriptive system must be comprehensible to the young, middle-aged and older adults with widely varying levels of educational attainment, socio-economic and cultural backgrounds. For example, differences have been found between using paragraphs written in the first person in describing a health state, and using straight lists of levels in each domain of health (Llewellyn-Thomas et al. 1984). The descriptive system should be meaningful across cultures. Translation of instruments should produce equivalence in terms of word meanings and idioms, i.e. semantic and idiomatic equivalence; equivalence in terms of situations and concepts evoked in the descriptions, i.e. experiential and conceptual equivalence, respectively (Guillemin et al. 1993). The description system should enable communication with semi-literate as well as illiterate persons. The description systems used so far have been developed for literate societies like North America and Europe. Even here, studies have experienced communication difficulties due to language barriers. For example, in the Canadian study by Sackett and Torrance (1978), about 12% of the randomly selected sample had to be excluded, because the interviewees could not communicate in English. One way to deal with this problem is to supplement written descriptions with appropriate graphical representations. Some researchers have used multimedia methods for valuation exercises (Lenert and Hornberger 1996; Lenert and Soetikno 1997). One problem with multimedia solutions is that the computer may be a source of distraction, particularly where the general community has limited experience with multimedia. In any case, multimedia solutions need a graphical description system to start with. So description systems for partially literate and multi-lingual communities should ideally include a graphical description sub system.

THE 6D5L HEALTH STATE DESCRIPTION SYSTEM

The 6D5L description system is developed by expanding upon the EuroQol (EQ-5D) description system. Cognition has been added as the sixth dimension. Severity levels in each dimension are described using five levels instead of three. The EQ-5D system allowed for a maximum of 244 distinct health states.[2] This restricted the systems ability to discriminate moderate to small differences in functional status. The 6D5L system will give rise to $5^3 = 15\ 625$ distinct health states. Some of these states may not exist in practice, for example 555555 (a person with total loss of cognitive function would not be anxious). Even then, the system provides for description of a fairly large number of distinct health states. We hope that this will improve 6D5L's sensitivity to minor illnesses.

The 6D5L health state description system, developed for the AP health state valuation study consists of the following distinct parts, each of which is described below.

1. A written description of dimensions and severity levels.

2. A Telugu language version of the dimensions and severity levels.

3. Locally valid graphical representation of dimensions and severity levels.

4. Identification protocols. Procedure to identify health state descriptions of diseases, clinical and epidemiologically encountered conditions.

5. Coding schema to represent different health states.

WRITTEN DESCRIPTION OF DIMENSIONS AND SEVERITY LEVELS

Since most valuers would come in contact with the description system for the first time, we anticipated that they may have difficulty in interpreting the six dimensions and discriminating between them. Hence a set of explanatory notes on "what this dimension represents" were developed to reliably communicate aspects of health represented by respective dimension (Box 1). These notes first explain what are included in the dimension. Then an example of a condition, which does not affect the dimension at all, is given, followed by an example of conditions that may affect the concerned dimension. Published literature on functional status measurement including activities of daily living (ADL), instrumental activities of daily living (IADL), pain measurement questionnaires (McDowell and Newell 1987; 1996), health-related quality of life measurement scales like the EuroQol (Brooks 1996), SF-36 (Ware and Sherbourne 1992), etc. were reviewed to cull out expressions that may explain, elucidate, clarify, or discriminate the concerned dimension. Such expressions have been used in the "what this dimensions represents" part of the descriptive system. These expressions have been taken from many articles and functional status measurement scales. Often more than one article or scale, provided similar expressions. Hence it has not been feasible for us to acknowledge all sources of these expressions. During the study, we found that the expression "usual activities" is easily confused with self-care in the Indian context. Hence the third dimension, namely usual activities, was assigned an alternative label of work and leisure.[3]

TELUGU VERSION OF THE WRITTEN DESCRIPTION SYSTEM

A panel of doctors and nurses practicing in the area were invited for a health state description workshop. Tasks assigned to the workshop included (a) Telugu translation of the 6D5L description system, and (b) Telugu translation of disease labels. The starting document comprised the

Box I   Written description of mobility dimension

Mobility (Position = 1)

A. What this dimension represents

  1. Transfers: Includes the management of all aspects of transfers to and from bed, mat, toilet, etc. More simply, getting in and out of bed.

  2. Ambulation: Includes coming to a standing position and walking about.

  3. Stairs and environmental surfaces: Ability to handle environmental barriers, and includes climbing stairs, curbs, ramps or environmental terrain.

  4. Community mobility: Ability to manage transportation.

  5. Example of a condition that does not affect mobility: Vitiligo

  6. Example of conditions that may affect mobility to various degrees: Backache, paralysis of lower limbs.

B. Severity levels and codes (SLC)

  1. Independent, i.e. no assistance required and no problem with mobility. Ability to run/flight in times of need. SLC = 1

  2. Occasional or very few problems in moving about. SLC = 2

  3. Some problems in moving about. SLC = 3

  4. Many problems in moving about. SLC = 4

  5. Unable to move about, i.e. totally dependent for mobility. SLC = 5

Teluga translations obtained from the health state description panel. The draft translated document was further worked upon with the help of other faculty knowledgeable in Telugu, to arrive at a provisional draft. The provisional draft was then discussed with experts in Telugu literature. They were requested to provide alternate translations. In the next step, persons who were not aware of our list of health states were given the provisional Telugu drafts and were asked to translate them back to English. The back translations that resulted in the original English version were chosen for the Telugu version. The resultant 6D5L written description system in Telugu has been reported in the study report (Mahapatra et al. 2000, appendices 3.4 and 3.5).

LOCALLY APPROPRIATE GRAPHICAL REPRESENTATION OF DIMENSIONS AND SEVERITY LEVELS

To facilitate communication of the 6D5L description system to semi-literate and illiterate valuers in the general population, we planned to develop a graphical description system for the 6D5L profiles. First an Artist brief (reproduced in Mahapatra et al. 2000, appendix 3.5) was prepared explaining the 6D5L description system, and describing the nature of task at hand. The brief gave examples of somewhat similar graphical representations, namely the Dartmouth Coop Function Charts (Nelson et al. 1987) and Faces scale (Andrews and Withey 1976). The art teams task was to arrive at the most appropriate pictorial representation of the severity levels under each of the six health dimensions. A team of fine art students from the University of Hyderabad School of Performing and Fine Arts were identified with the help of the school's faculty. This team of artists worked to draw pictures of the five severity levels in each of the six dimensions. Multiple sets of graphics were drawn by the artist team. We found the scaling and reproducibility of graphics using more of lines and less of shades was better. To facilitate preparation of health state description cards, etc. we preferred art works with more of line drawings and less of shading. Artists were given the following guidelines while preparing the graphics:

1. To minimize gender bias, separate sets of graphics are developed using female and male characters respectively;

2. Features similar to the local population;

3. Dress is consistent with dress pattern prevalent in rural areas of Andhra Pradesh for the respective gender;

4. Background, foreground, and other artefacts in the pictures are consistent with the rural scenario in Andhra Pradesh; and

5. Activities shown in the picture are consistent with usual roles for respective gender, currently prevalent in the state.

The pictures were reviewed many times. Persons not directly involved in the study were shown different sets of the pictures and asked to interpret them. The pictorial systems that were perceived by these judges to represent the severity levels of the corresponding dimension were selected and used. The graphical description system consists of a collection of two sets of pictures, with six sub sets in each. Each sub set in turn represents one of the six health dimensions and consists of five pictures to represent the five severity levels. Thus the basic element of the 6D5L graphical description system is a picture meant to convey a given level of severity in a particular health dimension. Altogether 30 such pictures consisting of five for each of the six health dimensions, and with a female person as the primary character constitutes the graphical description system for females. A similar set is prepared for the males. Figure 1 shows a set of five pictures for a single dimension (self-care) using male characters. A health state can be pictorially described by choosing the appropriate picture from each of the six subsets. So a graphical 6D5L profile would consist of a set of six pictures. For example, Figure 2 shows the 6D5L graphical profiles for continuous moderate back pain in a female character. Figures with Telugu labels were used for the general population survey and those with English labels were used in MDHSV workshops.

IDENTIFICATION OF 6D5L PROFILES

Identification of 6D5L profiles may be required in the following two situations. Firstly, description of typical functional status of disease states.

Figure 1   Self-care

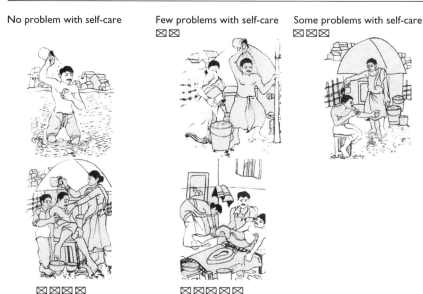

No problem with self-care   Few problems with self-care   Some problems with self-care

Many problems with self-care   Totally dependent for self-care

Figure 2   Continuous moderate back pain

Few problems in walking   No problems in washing or   Few problems in performing
      about   ⊠ ⊠   dressing self   usual activities   ⊠ ⊠

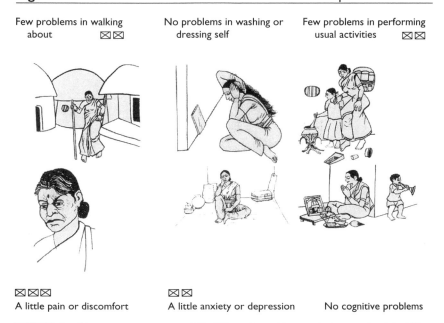

⊠ ⊠ ⊠   ⊠ ⊠
A little pain or discomfort   A little anxiety or depression   No cognitive problems

Here, we use the term disease state to include clinically and epidemiologically encountered conditions, which may not necessarily be considered
disease states. Secondly, identification of labels for specific 6D5L profiles
to facilitate holistic processing of 6D5L information by valuers. The need
for association of labels to 6D5L profiles for purposes of valuation and
how we arrived at the labels used in this study has already been described
earlier. We will discuss here the need for mapping of specific disease states
to 6D5L profiles, and then proceed to describe our efforts to operationalize
the same.

Health state valuations are usually obtained for incorporation into
summary measures of population health status which may be computed
to allow for disaggregated analysis. If disaggregated analysis is required
then identification of 6D5L profiles for disease states becomes necessary.
Summary measures of population health combine cause of death, descriptive epidemiological data on incidence, prevalence, duration, etc. and
health state values. Cause of death data is invariably tabulated according
to disease labels. Descriptive epidemiological information is largely available for health states identified by specific disease labels. The system of
labelling causes of death is usually similar to the system of nomenclature
of morbidities. Where there is some variation, a mapping of disease state
labels to cause of death labels is usually feasible. Hence it becomes imperative for most researchers to use the disease categories as a convenient classification mechanism for disaggregated analysis of summary measures.
Disaggregation by risk factor is usually achieved by tracing incidence of

mortality and morbidity to the risk factor through different disease categories. Thus to incorporate health state values into a summary measure of population health status that allows disaggregate analysis, we need to arrive at health state or disability weights for disease categories included in the computation. If health states were valued separately for each of the disease categories, similar to incidence prevalence measurements, then the computations will be straight forward.

Although valuation of health status of persons suffering specific disease conditions is feasible, such measurements are not used for summary measures of population health status, for various reasons. Valuation of health states is known to be conditioned by the locus of the valuer. Valuation of the same health state by a person in that state is usually different from the valuations given to that state by doctors and nurse. These two valuations differ from the ones given by the general population. Since summary measures are used for health policy analysis and allocation decisions, valuations by the general populations are preferred. To cope with various methodological difficulties, direct measurement of health state values is done for a limited set of indicator conditions followed by statistical modelling to infer health state values for other 6D5L profiles. We need to relate the health state values thus arrived at to disease states used for disaggregated analysis of summary measures. Hence the need for a protocol to identify the 6D5L profile corresponding to disease states. We decided to use expert judgement arrived by a consensus development method for identification of 6D5L profiles for identified disease states. A workshop was organized to bring together a panel of physicians and nurses from various fields working in public and private hospitals. Altogether a group of 19 physicians and 4 clinical nurses participated. All panel members had clinical positions in local hospitals. The panel recommended and assigned 6D5L profiles to each of the 22 diseases.

While planning the study, we had provisionally selected a list of indicator conditions along with their 6D5L profiles. We set aside the 6D5L profile of indicator conditions, until recommendations of the description panel were available. We then compared the provisionally identified 6D5L profiles with the description panel recommendations. In 4 out of 22 cases the two matched. These were: watery diarrhoea 111211, infertility 111131, mild hearing disorder 112121, and paraplegia 444431. There was discrepancy for other conditions. We discussed these discrepancies among ourselves and sought additional expert opinion where necessary. Finally, we accepted panel recommendations for 5 states, adopted a modified profile partially accepting panel recommendations for six cases and maintained our provisional profile for 7 conditions.

LABELS

Ceteris paribus, disease labels have been found to affect the value attached to a health state, by the valuer. For example, Sackett and Torrance (1978) found that labels had statistically significant effects upon health state utilities in both the positive (tuberculosis preferred over an unnamed contagious disease) and strongly negative directions (mastectomy for injury preferred over mastectomy for breast cancer. Pilot testing of the valuation exercises using the descriptions arrived so far, showed that valuers were clearly responding from their stereotyped understanding of the disease labels, without paying much attention to the 6D5L description. For example, people appeared to value tuberculosis much worse that what its 6D5L profile would justify. We could not be sure that the worse valuation was real or an effect, purely, of the label. In any case to minimize effect of label to the extent feasible, we decided to have longer descriptive labels emphasizing the 6D5L profile. Table 3 shows the evolution of labels for selected health states. The leftmost column shows the disease labels that we began with. The next two columns show the label used for the MDHSV workshops and the 6D5L profile, respectively. The last column shows the longer labels used for the household survey.

Table 3   Short and long disease labels used in health state valuation exercises

Disease labels	Labels used in the MDHSV workshops	6D5L Profile	Long labels used in the household survey
Diabetes	Mild diabetes, no symptoms	111121	Mild diabetes with no symptoms controlled with pills
Tuberculosis	Mild tuberculosis with treatment	111221	Tuberculosis under treatment with very mild symptoms limited to occasional cough
Unipolar major depression	Unipolar major depression	124142	Depression, with loss of pleasure from most activities, low energy, and slight difficulties in thinking and concentrating
Congestive heart failure	Severe heart failure (congestive)	434531	Extreme chest pains and failure breathlessness caused by severe heart failure

CODING SCHEMA

A health state is described by a string of six ordered digits, such that position of the digit represents a particular dimension and value of the digit ranging from 1–5 represents the severity level. For example health state 111111 would mean perfect health. Positions in the ordered sequence of six digits first to sixth are respectively, mobility, self-care, usual activities (work and leisure), pain / discomfort, anxiety / depression, and cognition.

RESULTS

USAGE OF SEVERITY LEVELS BY PEOPLE TO DESCRIBE THEIR OWN HEALTH STATE

We used a five levels of functional status within each dimension to improve the description system's ability to discriminate between more number of health states. Table 4 shows usage of severity levels and cognitive functional status by valuers of the Andhra Pradesh Health State Valuation Study, to describe their "Own Health" state. Own health state descriptions by 1 190 persons falls into 295 distinct entities, which is more than the 244 limit in the EQ-5D system. As would be expected lower level severity codes are used more frequently. Given this asymmetry in usage of severity levels only three levels of functional status would lump many milder disabilities with perfect health.

USAGE OF COGNITIVE FUNCTIONAL STATUS BY PEOPLE TO DESCRIBE THEIR OWN HEALTH STATE

The sixth dimension of cognitive function was also used by people to describe their own health. A few persons described their cognitive functioning at levels 4 and 5! (Table 4). This is surprising. One would expect persons with such severe levels of cognitive dysfunction unable to carry out the Own Health description task. To understand this, we first checked if these valuations tasks were done with the help of an assistant. It turns out that only 2 out of the 24 persons who reported a perceived cognitive dysfunction at levels 4 or 5 were assisted (8.3%) compared to 104 out of 1 010 total valuers who communicated through an assistant (10.3%). Each interviewer for the household survey had been instructed to record his/her observation on a few observable health state attributes like hearing impairment, vision defect, usage of walking aid, defective walking, etc. Table 5 shows prevalence of such observed disabilities among the total survey

Table 4   Usage of severity levels and cognitive functional status by valuers to describe "Own Health" states

SLC = Severity Level Code	Distinct health states	Persons
"Own Health" states	295	1 190
with SLC = 2 in at least one dimension	246	678
with SLC = 3 in at least one dimension	202	282
with SLC = 4 in at least one dimension	103	116
with SLC ≥ 2 in D6 (Cognition)	170	325
with SLC = 2 in D6 (Cognition)	98	234
with SLC = 3 in D6 (Cognition)	49	67
with SLC = 4 in D6 (Cognition)	17	18
with SLC = 5 in D6 (Cognition)	6	6

population and the subpopulation who described their own health state to have severe levels of cognitive dysfunction. The subpopulation is clearly worse off than the total survey population in all areas of observed functional status. The pro forma for description of Own Health state included a question asking the valuer to describe his/her current health state in comparison to his/her health over the past year. Answers were coded as 1 for extremely well to 5 for worse. Table 6 (right most four columns) shows that the subpopulation of valuer perceived there current health state to be worse compared to their experience over the past 12 months. Thus this subpopulation does appear to be clearly in a comparatively worse health state than the total survey population.

Table 5   Comparison of observed disabilities for all valuers and those describing their health state to have cognition at severity levels 4 or 5

	Survey all		Own health has 4 or 5 in D6	
	No.	%	No.	%
Observed hearing impairment	38	3.76	10	41.67
Observed vision defect	68	6.73	10	41.67
Observed walking aid	27	2.67	4	16.67
Observed walking defect	34	3.37	7	29.17
Observed paralysis	6	0.59	1	4.17
Observed amputation	6	0.59	1	4.17
Observed cough	8	0.79	1	4.17
Observed shortness of breath	17	1.68	4	16.67
Total valuers	1 010		24	

Table 6   Comparison of total survey population (all) and the sub population describing "Own Health" state with levels 4 or 5 in the cognition dimension (D6 level 4, 5)

| | Perceived accuracy | | | | Respondent cooperation | | | | Current health state | | | |
| | All | | D6 level 4, 5 | | All | | D6 level 4, 5 | | All | | D6 level 4, 5 | |
Code	No.	%	No.	%	No.	%	No.	%	No.	%	No.	%
1	176	17.46	2	8.33	244	24.28	3	12.50	48	4.75	0	0.00
2	397	39.38	7	29.17	375	37.31	8	33.33	379	37.52	3	12.50
3	378	37.50	7	29.17	312	31.04	4	16.67	202	20.00	4	16.67
4	40	3.97	2	8.33	56	5.57	3	12.50	349	34.55	11	45.83
5	17	1.69	6	25.00	18	1.79	6	25.00	32	3.17	6	25.00
Total	1 008		24		1 005		24		1 010		24	

Table 6 also shows the accuracy of Own Health state descriptions by total survey population and the subpopulation with D6 level 4 or 5 in their Own health state descriptions. This is based on the interviewers perception. The accuracy assessment has been coded as 1 for very accurate to 5 for least accurate. Valuations by the subpopulation were assessed as less accurate compared to the total survey population. Similarly the interviewers assessment of respondent cooperation is also slightly worse than that for the total survey population.

These findings suggest that persons describing their own health state to have severe levels of cognitive dysfunction clearly have a poorer health state. The fact that they are able to describe their own health state accurately enough in other dimensions would suggest that their actual levels of cognitive functioning are not as severe as they perceive them to be. It is possible that the depression associated with their poor health status is contributing to such assessments in the cognitive dimension. These issues need to be investigated further.

Valuers feedback on difficulty in describing own health state

One way to assess the usefulness of a description system is the ease with which information about health states was communicated to individual valuers. Valuer's feedback about the difficulty encountered to characterize his/her own health state using the given description system gives us some idea about communicability of a description system. A feedback questionnaire was introduced for the MDHSV workshops, midcourse. Only 34 persons returned responses to this questionnaire. One question was: "Did you encounter any difficulty in description of your own health state?" Thirty-two of the 34 persons who gave feedback said they had no difficulties. The other two had some difficulties and none experienced a lot of difficulty. In the household survey, interviewers were asked to record their observations to determine if the valuer experienced any difficulty in describing his/her own health state. Nine hundred and sixty-two out of 965 returns said the valuers did not have any difficulty. The other three had some difficulty.

Notes

1   "Attributes" and "dimensions" are used in health status measurement literature, and here, interchangeably.

2   Five dimensions with three levels in each give rise to $3^5 = 243$ permutations. To this, death is added.

3   Since this fact was found midway through the study, all instruments and printed material continued to have the label, usual activities, but interviewers and workshop coordinators were instructed to clarify the meaning of this dimension for valuers.

REFERENCES

Andrews FM, Withey SB (1976) *Social indicators of well-being: Americans perceptions of life quality.* Plenum Press, New York.

Bergner M, Bobbit RA, Kressel S, et al. (1976) The sickness impact profile: conceptual formulation and methodology for the development of a health status measure. *International Journal of Health Services,* 6(3):393–415.

Boyle M, Furlong W, Torrance G, Feeny D (1994) *Reliability of the health utilities index – mark 3, used in the 1991 cycle 6 general social survey health questionnaire.* Center for Health Economics and Policy Analysis, Ontario.

Boyle MH, Torrance GW (1984) Developing multiattribute health indexes. *Medical Care,* 22:1045–1057.

Brazier J, Usherwood T, Harper R, Thomas K (1998) Deriving a preference based single index measure from the UK SF-36 health survey. *Journal of Clinical Epidemiology,* 51(11):1115–1128.

Brook RH, Ware JE, Davis-Avery A, et al. (1979) Overview of adult health status measures fielded in Rand's health insurance study. *Medical Care,* 17(7 Suppl.):1–131.

Brooks R (1996) EuroQol: the current state of play. *Health Policy,* 37(1):53–72.

Chambers LW, Sackett DL, Goldsmith C, Macpehrson AS, McAuley RG (1976) Development and application of an index of social function. *Health Services Research,* 11(4):430–441.

EuroQol Group (1990) EuroQol: a new facility for the measurement of health-related quality of life. *Health Policy,* 16(3):199–208.

Fanshel S (1972) A meaningful measure of health for epidemiology. *International Journal of Epidemiology,* 1(4):319–337.

Fanshel S, Bush JW (1970) A health-status index and its application to health services outcomes. *Operations Research,* 18(6):1021–1065.

Fischer GW (1979) Utility models for multiple objective decisions: do they accurately represent human preferences? *Decision Sciences,* 10:451–479.

Froberg DG, Kane RL (1989) Methodology for measuring health-state preferences, part – I: measurement strategies. *Journal of Clinical Epidemiology,* 42(4):345–354.

Froberg DG, Kane RL (1989) Methodology for measuring health-state preferences, part – II: scaling methods. *Journal of Clinical Epidemiology,* 42(5):459–471.

Froberg DG, Kane RL (1989) Methodology for measuring health-state preferences, part – III: population and context effects. *Journal of Clinical Epidemiology,* 42(6):585–592.

Froberg DG, Kane RL (1989) Methodology for measuring health-state preferences, part – IV: progress and a research agenda. *Journal of Clinical Epidemiology,* 42(7):675–685.

Goldberg M, Dab W (1987) *Complex indexes for measuring a complex phenomenon. In: Measurement in health promotion and protection.* European Series no 22. Abelin T, Brzezinski ZJ, Carstairs VDL, eds. World Health Organization, Regional Office for Europe, Copenhagen.

Guillemin F, Bombardier C, Beaton D (1993) Cross-cultural adaptation of health-related quality of life measures: literature review and proposed guidelines. *Journal of Clinical Epidemiology*, **46**(12):1417–1432.

Halford GS (1998) Development of processing capacity entails representing more complex relations: Implications for cognitive development. In: *Working memory and thinking.* Logie RL, Gilhooly KJ, eds. Psychology Press Ltd., Hove, East Sussex.

Hunt SM, McKenna SP, McEwen J, Williams J, Papp E (1981) The Nottingham Health Profile: subjective health status and medical consultations. *Social Science and Medicine*, **15**(3 pt 1):221–229.

Kaplan RM, Bush JW (1982) Health-related quality of life measurement for evaluation of research and policy analysis. *Health Psychology*, **1**:61–80.

Krabbe PFM, Stouthard MEA, Essink-Bot ML, Bonsel G (1998) The effect of adding a cognitive dimension to the EuroQol multiattribute health-status classification system. In: *The valuation of health outcomes.* A contribution to the QALY approach. Erasmus University, Rotterdam.

Lenert LA, Hornberger JC (1996) *Quality of life assessment in clinical trials.* (Proceedings of the Annual Symposium on Computer Applications in Medical Care, 982–996.)

Lenert LA, Soetikno RM (1997) Automated computer interviews to elicit utilities: potential applications in the treatment of deep venous thrombosis. *Journal of the American Medical Informatics Association*, **4**(1):49–56.

Llewellyn-Thomas H, Sutherland HJ, Tibshirani R, Ciampi A, Till JE, Boyd NF (1984) Describing health states: methodologic issues in obtaining values for health states. *Medical Care*, **22**(6):543–552.

Lyness KS, Cornelius ET (1982) A comparison of holistic and decomposed judgement strategies in a performance rating simulation. *Organizational Behavior and Human Performance*, **29**:21–38.

Mahapatra P, Salomon JA, Nanda L, Rajshree KT (2000) *Measuring health state values in developing countries: report of a study in Andhra Pradesh, India.* Institute of Health Systems, HACA Bhavan, Hyderabad, AP 500004, India.

McDowell I, Newell C (1987) *Measuring health: a guide to rating scales and questionnaires.* Oxford University Press, New York.

McDowell I, Newell C (1996) *Measuring health: a guide to rating scales and questionnaires.* 2nd edn. Oxford University Press, New York.

Miller GA (1956) The magical number seven plus or minus two: some limits on our capacity for processing information. *Psychological Review*, **63**:81–97.

Nelson EC, Wasson J, Kirk J, et al. (1987) Assessment of function in routine clinical practice: description of the COOP chart method and preliminary findings. *Journal of Chronic Diseases*, **40** (1 Suppl.):S55–S63.

Noack H (1987) Concepts of health and health promotion. In: *Measurement in health promotion and protection*. European Series no 2. Abelin T, Brzezinski ZJ, Carstairs VDL, eds. World Health Organization Regional Office for Europe, Copenhagen.

Patrick DL, Bush JW, Chen MM (1973) Toward an operational definition of health. *Journal of Health and Social Behavior*, 14(1):6–23.

Patrick DL, Erickson P (1993) Concepts of health-related quality of life. In: *Health status and health policy quality of life in health care evaluation and resource allocation*. Patrick DL, Erickson P, eds. Oxford University Press, New York.

Saariluoma P (1998) Adversary problem-solving and working memory. In: *Working memory and thinking*. Logie RL, Gilhooly KJ, eds. Psychology Press Ltd., Hove, East Sussex.

Sackett DL, Torrance GW (1978) The utility of different health states as perceived by the general public. *Journal of Chronic Diseases*, 31(11):697–704.

Stewart AL (1992) The medical outcomes study for work of health indicators. In: *Measuring functioning and well-being*. Stewart AL, Ware JE, Jr., eds. Duke University Press, Durham/London.

Torrance GW, Zhang Y, Feeny D, Furlong W, Barr R (1992) *Multi-attribute preference functions for a comprehensive health status classification system*. (CHEPA working paper no 92/18.) McMaster University, Centre for Health Economics and Policy Analysis, Hamilton, Ontario.

Ware JE, Sherbourne CD (1992) The MOS 36-item short form health survey (SF-36): I. Conceptual framework and item selection. *Medical Care*, 30(6):473–483.

Chapter 8.1

COMPARATIVE ANALYSES OF MORE THAN 50 HOUSEHOLD SURVEYS ON HEALTH STATUS

RITU SADANA, COLIN D. MATHERS, ALAN D. LOPEZ,
CHRISTOPHER J.L. MURRAY AND KIM MOESGAARD IBURG

INTRODUCTION

Two main challenges exist that prevent the meaningful comparison of household interview data across populations. The first concerns limitations in the cross-population comparability of data since surveys with only self-reported data lack external criteria to calibrate responses across countries. The second is that existing nationally representative surveys use different questions and response scales to assess health. In this chapter, we report recent World Health Organization (WHO) work to assess whether existing data from nationally representative household interview surveys conducted in a large number of countries may be used towards estimating the distribution and levels of severity of health at the population level. Throughout this chapter, we use the term *health* or *health status* in the broadest sense to include illness, impairments, disability and other states of health spanning from the worst health state to full health for an individual alive.

Current empirical approaches to assess health within household surveys are based on the model depicted in Figure 1. A population's underlying *true level of health* may vary on a variety of domains, such as physical or cognitive functioning, or mental health, among others. The true level of health may be reflected by *tested health* (measured through laboratory or functional tests), *observed health* (based on professionals' clinical assessments or other ratings) and *perceived health* (based on individual's knowledge and beliefs) in related domains. No gold standard measurement technique exists to assess all aspects of health or to assess what people perceive. *Self-reported health* is what individuals report within a survey to a lay interviewer. This may differ from what an individual perceives, particularly when specific incentives or sanctions influence reporting behavior. Perceptions may differ from true health due to different definitions of health and well-being, different expectations for health and different cognitive processes. Such differences reflect variations in cultural and

Figure 1   Empirical model for the assessment of health status

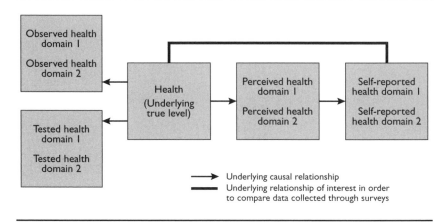

gender norms, knowledge and information, and other factors that shape people's perceptions (Annas 1993; Johansson 1991; Kahneman et al. 1982; Kleinman et al. 1978; Sen 1994). What is observed, tested or reported is not always consistent given these variations in perceptions and differences in the sensitivity and specificity of tests, beyond measurement error (Kempen et al. 1996; Kivinen et al. 1998; Zurayk et al. 1995; Iburg et al. chapter 8.4 and Thomas and Frankenberg chapter 8.2).

Differences in perceptions and subsequent reporting biases may specifically compromise the cross-population comparability of data collected within household surveys. To achieve high cross-population comparability based on self-reported data (1) respondents should interpret identically questions and response scales—such as ordinal scales with response categories of *excellent, very good, good, fair* and *poor*, and (2) for the same true level of health, responses should be identical irrespective of socioeconomic or demographic characteristics (Krosnick 1991; Streiner and Norman 1995; Tourangeau 1984). Not surprisingly, these criteria can not be met in practice (Groot 2000; Idler et al. 1999; Kleinman 1994; Weir and Seacrest 2000).

More surprising is that users of household interview surveys often ignore these limitations and interpret self-reported data at face value. Results reported from the European Community Household Panel survey, relying on self-reported data conducted in 12 countries using identical methodologies, are illustrative. Figure 2 shows the proportion of the population in each country reporting *good* and *very good* health, in response to the question *how is your health in general?* The accompanying article notes that although questions on self-reported health status "may be sensitive to differences in language and 'culture' between Member States, it seems worth noting that for instance 'very good' health is reported by as much as 53% of the Danish and as little as 8% of the Portuguese popu-

Figure 2   Proportion of population ≥ 16 years of age reporting very good and good general health, 12 European countries, age-standardized (EUROSTAT 1997)

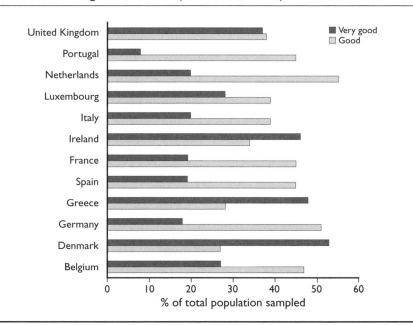

lation" (Eurostat 1997). We believe it is unlikely that differences in the true level of health status, translations or measurement error, account for such large variations between Denmark and Portugal, or other countries within the European Union. Understanding "cultural" and other factors contributing to these differences are crucial before drawing conclusions about comparative health status across populations. Other studies have documented that sub-populations with lower expectations for health (such as the elderly) or less exposure to what constitutes full health (such as those with lower socioeconomic levels) actually report themselves in better health in comparison to tested or observed health status, or other external criteria (Kroeger et al. 1988; Mackenbach et al. 1996; Murray 1996). Such biases reduce the cross-population comparability of data. We recognize that self-reports may be most appropriate for certain domains of health status, such as pain, in comparison to other measurement approaches (Murray and Chen 1992), but may still contain biases.

Most current efforts to enhance comparability of survey data concentrate on improving translation protocols before data collection (Ware et al. 1995) or judging the equivalence of question wording across different national surveys (Robine et al. 2000; Rasmussen et al. 1999). Many have estimated the psychometric properties of the same instrument in different languages and countries (Anderson et al. 1993; Keller et al. 1998;

WHOQOL Group 1998). As no gold standard test exists to measure health status, several weaker forms of validity are estimated for groups of questions hypothesized to assess the same underlying construct (Nunnally and Bernstein 1994). If these weaker tests of validity are met within each population, then an instrument is judged comparable across those populations. More recently, item response theory (IRT) has been used to estimate internal relationships between an individual's response on any one item in a survey and the underlying construct of the domain or scale (Cooke and Michie 1999; Raczek et al. 1998). Proponents of IRT analysis argue that if these relationships are similar in each population tested, then an item acts homogeneously across these populations and provides comparable data on the same scale (Hambleton and Swaminathan 1985). However, one assumption of these IRT models is often violated: that is for individuals with the same level of health status, the probability of answering any item in the same direction should be unrelated to the probability of answering any other item in the same direction (Hambleton et al. 1991; Streiner and Norman 1995). Similar to classical psychometric approaches, IRT analysis does not use external criteria to establish the equivalence of scales across populations. Even though some of the assumptions required to use IRT models are often violated when applied to the measurement of health status, efforts to build on this approach to evaluate the comparability of responses appear worthwhile (see Murray et al. chapter 8.3).

VALIDITY AND CROSS-POPULATION COMPARABILITY

Researchers developing instruments have drawn upon a variety of methods used in behavioral sciences, in particular psychometric tests (see American Psychological Association 1985), in order to provide evidence that instruments consistently measure the true continuum of health status found within a population or sub-population and that scores (e.g. on ordinal or potentially interval scales) may be meaningfully interpreted (see Streiner and Norman 1995). At every stage of the development process, different methods to test reliability and validity are evoked depending upon the intended use of the instrument and the availability of external criteria to estimate the validity of measures. As no gold standard measurement technique exists to distinguish individuals along this true continuum of health status (unlike for the assessment of a specific morbidity, such as anaemia and gonorrhoea), numerous alternative criteria are applied.

Validity is the extent to which an instrument measures what it is intended to measure or more broadly, the range of interpretations that can be reasonably attributed to a measure. Overall, validity estimates for health status measures are reported less frequently than reliability coefficients. Although often stated in this literature, an instrument is never "valid". Instead, evidence supporting and estimating the validity of a particular health status measure is gained when hypotheses about the relationship between scores on specific domains and particular criteria are confirmed.

Several approaches to estimate validity are usually cited as no single aspect of validity provides a definitive evaluation of an instrument within a particular population (Bergner and Rothman 1987; Ware et al. 1996). This partially reflects that the criteria for individual psychometric tests of validity are relatively weak. For example, validity may be assessed in several ways including: content validity (the extent to which an instrument covers all aspects of the topic it purports to measure); construct validity (the extent that abstract constructs—without any external criteria—exist based in turn on comparing the results of several contrasting tests of validity that are based on normative judgements); and criterion validity (the extent that scores are systematically related to one or more other criteria, such as domain scores compared to demographic variables, disease status or clinical measures). Two forms of construct validity are commonly cited: convergent validity is supported when different methods of measuring the same construct provide similar results, whereas discriminant validity estimates whether a measure of one construct can be differentiated from another construct. That these individual criteria may be weak is not to dismiss these approaches to test validity, but to note that more stringent criteria for a validity test would require additional external information most often not collected in health interview surveys or the use of a gold standard test of health status, which does not exist.

Approaches to estimate validity are also used to gauge the interpretation of data collected. For example, criterion-based interpretation provides information on the differences between *known groups* within a particular context, such as individuals with mental illness and those with acute physical impairments. It is expected that these two groups will differ concerning their average score on a scale assessing mental health. These differences may provide guidelines on the meaning of scores measured on ordinal or interval scales. For example, the difference between the average scores observed in these two groups establishes a basis to interpret the size of large differences in scores. Ware and Keller (1996) suggest that comparisons among individuals within a particular category by differing levels of severity or other external criteria may provide guidelines to interpret smaller differences in scale scores. This may be fruitful for within population comparisons, but the ability to interpret scores across populations may not necessarily be facilitated through such comparisons.

Our conceptualization of an underlying true level of health status differs from the concept of a *true score* discussed in psychometric literature.[1] We note that there is no gold standard test to measure the true level of health status in a population (e.g. a test that would measure all aspects of health status), or to know what people perceive. Empirical investigations and the production of knowledge on health status is thus restricted to what is observed or measured and what is reported. Ample evidence exists documenting the differences between these different perspectives on health status (Sadana et al. 2000). Summarizing these differences, Murray and Chen (1992) distinguish three categories of morbidity that are equally relevant to the assessment of health status: 1) those domains of health status that may be both self-reported and professionally observed or tested (i.e. symptomatic conditions, such as impaired physical functioning), 2) those domains which are only self-reported (i.e. pain), and 3) those domains which may only be observed or tested, for example through professional, clinical or laboratory assessments (i.e. asymptomatic conditions, or those requiring external assessment such as severe cognitive impairment). We stress that professional observations and tests, such as laboratory assessment or functioning tests, also differ (see Figure 1). Estimating the relations between self-reported health status and the true level of health status—more practically to observed or tested health status—is important. This information may aid in interpreting data on health status collected through household interview surveys (see chapter 8.4, Iburg et al.). If these relations differ across populations or sub-populations, then these differences may hamper the valid comparison of self-reported health status across these populations or sub-populations.

CROSS-POPULATION COMPARABILITY

An optimal strategy for cross-population comparability of data (see Tourangeau 1984, Krosnick 1991, cited in Streiner and Norman 1995) would require that all individuals with the same true level of health status, irrespective of their age, sex, cultural or geographic context, or other socio-demographic characteristics, or time period, respond to an identical question addressing health status as follows:

- interpret the meaning of the question and response scale identically;

- retrieve all relevant information with no loss of memory;

- process all information, often contradictory, to form a single, integrated judgement or perception, in the same fashion, using cognitive processes that are unbiased; and

- convey this judgement as a final response in each survey context identically.

If so, individuals with exactly the same true level of health status should then respond identically across and within populations. Obviously, this optimal strategy does not exist in practice and is no surprise to those critically assessing methods used within international health and development (Kleinman 1994; Sen 1994; Weir and Seacrest 2000; Wolff and Langley 1968; Zborowski 1952). But what are the likely consequences of the various differences that can and do seep in?

The fact that different strategies are used to respond to questions—and in particular that people interpret the meaning (or health state referents) of questions and response scales differently—suggests that even if questions are equivalent, data collected on identical questions assessing health status may not be equivalent and thus not comparable. These differences are not simply measurement errors. This view is in sharp contrast to those who interpret data collected on self-reported health status, across or within populations, at face value. It is also in contrast to those who focus on improving the comparability of instruments and survey methods, and not on data equivalence, i.e. the comparability of the responses.

A variety of factors may contribute to differences in expectations and norms for health, which will result in systematic differences across populations in the way that response scales are interpreted. Some groups may have different standards for *excellent* health than other groups. Imagine that people around 20 to 25 years of age think that *excellent* mobility is being able to run a marathon while people around 75 to 80 years of age think that excellent mobility is being able to walk a kilometer without pain. If asked about the ability to engage in vigorous activities, the 22 year old who can walk only a half a kilometer before experiencing pain may report his or her health as *poor*, while the 78 year old who had the same experience might report his or her health as *good* or even *very good*.

Several studies from different regions identify that different patterns exist among sub-populations. For example, in Argentina higher socioeconomic groups reported more illness than lower socioeconomic groups in household interview surveys when the reverse was true based on information external to the survey (Kroeger et al. 1988). The same pattern appears to hold true across regions. Based on data collected within the National Sample Survey of India, Round 28, residents of Kerala—the state in India with the lowest levels of infant and child mortality and highest levels of literacy—report the highest incidence of acute morbidity in the country. Conversely, residents of Bihar—the state often with the worst indicators concerning mortality and literacy in India—reported the lowest incidence of acute morbidity in the country (see Murray 1996). Several studies in Europe also document that less educated individuals under-report morbidity conditions to a greater extent than individuals with more education (Heliovaara et al. 1993; Mackenbach et al. 1996). These findings are consistent with the hypothesis that greater awareness of symptoms and higher expectations for good health increases the likelihood of reporting morbidity and health status problems.

Although many studies compare the self-report of morbidity with observed clinical or laboratory findings, few studies provide evidence on the relationship between self-reported health status and observed health status measures, i.e. describing different health states beyond simply reporting morbidity or disease status. Representative of early studies in the United States, Friedsam and Martin (1961) found a positive but weak relationship between self-reported health and physician's ratings. More recently, two studies from the Netherlands and Finland found self-reported health and observed measures to be only weakly correlated (Kempen et al. 1996; Kivinen et al. 1998). These and other studies (Axelsson and Helgadottir 1995; Matthias et al. 1993) indicate that this relationship may be inconsistent and differs across sub-populations. Iburg et al. in chapter 8.4 report a more recent analysis using data from the United States National Health and Nutrition Examination Survey III (1988–94), that compares self-reported physical functioning, physician assessments of physical functioning, and physical functioning tests within the sub-sample of individuals 60 years of age and older. A slightly more complex pattern of reporting emerges from another recent analysis conducted by Thomas and Frankenberg (chapter 8.2), using data from the Indonesian Family Life Survey, 1993.

The biases associated with the self-report of health status and the inconsistent patterns of reporting are a complex function of expectations, norms, exposure to health services, information and judgmental strategies. We do not suggest that these biases render individual assessments of health status less important, but that these biases reduce the cross-population comparability of data. We illustrate the problems of cross-population comparability of self-report health status data through a secondary analysis of household interview surveys that include different questions addressing health. No standard methodologies exist that facilitate the comparability of data from different surveys using different questions. This study represents an initial effort to address the two main challenges that limit the meaningful comparison of household interview data across populations by developing and testing a simple method to compare responses to different questions across surveys, using only self-reported data.

DATA SOURCES AND METHODOLOGY

Unit level data obtained from 64 recent household interview surveys with nationally representative non-institutionalized civilian population samples were collected from 46 countries. Countries from each of the WHO Regions were included (*African*: Côte d'Ivoire, Ghana, South Africa, United Republic of Tanzania; *Pan-American*: Brazil, Guyana, Jamaica, Panama, Paraguay, Peru, United States of America; *Eastern Mediterranean*: Bahrain, Egypt, Jordan, Morocco, Pakistan, Tunisia; *European*: Austria, Belgium, Bulgaria, Denmark, France, Germany, Greece, Ireland, Italy, Kyrgyzstan, Luxembourg, Netherlands, Portugal, Russian Federation, Spain, United Kingdom of Great Britain and Northern Ireland; *South East-Asian*: Bangladesh, Democratic People's Republic of Korea, India, Indonesia, Myanmar, Nepal, Sri Lanka, Thailand; *Western Pacific*: China, Fiji, Malaysia, Philippines, Republic of Korea). Details concerning the surveys, samples and questions are given in Sadana et al. (2000). Questions assessing the level of physical or mental health, physical or cognitive functioning, other disability, as well as the degree and duration of activity or role limitations as a proximate measure of severity, were included. The number of questions meeting the inclusion criteria varied considerably across surveys.

We utilized common factor analysis as an initial attempt to extract information on health status at the individual level from each survey (Sadana et al. 2000). An exploratory factor analysis on several surveys provided evidence that most items meeting the inclusion criteria loaded on one factor. We hypothesized that all questions describing health tap a general health construct, H, and that H is equivalent across populations. Although we believe that health is a multi-dimensional construct, that an underlying factor ties together these domains is concordant with other findings (Keller et al. 1998). We estimated model parameters for each survey and sex using the Mplus statistical analysis program (Muthén and Muthén 1998) which uses specialized estimation techniques for categorical and non-normally distributed data. We calculated a variant of the intraclass correlation coefficient (Werts et al. 1974) to estimate the internal consistency of all variables as a measure of H by survey and sex. Seventy-eight per cent of the models reached 0.7 or higher, the arbitrary cut-off on a zero to one scale suggesting that the variables are tapping a similar construct (Nunnally and Bernstein 1994). This is not, however, an evaluation of the cross-population comparability of data.

We estimated scores for each individual's level of health utilizing survey and sex specific multiple regression models. In general, the factor score for individual i for health, H, can be represented as:

$$\hat{H}_i = \hat{\beta}_1 x_{i1} + \hat{\beta}_2 x_{i2} + \hat{\beta}_3 x_{i3} + \dots \hat{\beta}_p x_{ip}$$

where $\hat{H}_i$ is the estimated factor score (severity level) of health for individual i, $\hat{\beta}_p$ is the sex-specific estimated factor score coefficient (factor loading) for variable p, and x_{ip} is the pth variable included within the survey for individual i. The Mplus statistical analysis program calculates biserial and tetrachoric correlation estimates to produce correlation matrices within factor analyses and requires that all ordered categorical variables are dichotomized.

We attempted to equalize the scale of $\hat{H}$ across populations, while maintaining the relative differences in the level of health and distribution of severity within each population. We first transformed the lowest and highest estimated scores of $\hat{H}$ to zero (e.g. worst living state) and 100 (e.g. full health) respectively. Scores between these values represent the percentage of the highest estimated score. We then adjusted for differences in the end-points of the scale for $\hat{H}$, given no possibility to calibrate end-points or intermediary scores through an external process. We fixed all scores to zero that represent the bottom 0.1% of the cumulative distribution of $\hat{H}$. Although arbitrary, 0.1% maintains a small absolute number of individuals in the worst state across surveys. Fixing the top end-point was more problematic given the highly skewed distribution of $\hat{H}$ towards better levels of health. In one extreme case, 75–80% of males and females within the Pakistan Living Standards Measurement Study Survey of 1991 (5 questions addressing health status) have a transformed score of 99 or 100. We believe that the distribution at the top end is truncated to some degree in all surveys. Several factors contribute to high ceiling effects, including the insensitivity of questions to mild deviations from full health, the relatively small number of questions and non-random reporting differences, among other factors. Given the large variations in ceiling effects (not shown) and no basis to judge what is the true proportion of individuals in each population in full health, we simply fixed 100 to be the highest estimated score of $\hat{H}$.

Given the lack of external criteria, we conducted a series of internal validity and reliability checks (Sadana et al. 2000). The comparison of two different national surveys from Denmark conducted in 1994 serve as one test of convergent validity. Figure 3 shows that the Danish Health and Morbidity Survey (DHMS) (36 questions) provides a relatively smoother distribution of the cumulative frequency of different levels of health than the shorter European Community Household Panel (ECHP) survey (4 questions), as expected. Both surveys have high ceiling effects. Yet the similarity of these distributions provides some evidence that our methods provide a reasonable approach to compare different questions and surveys conducted in the same population.

RESULTS

Figure 4 shows estimates for the level of health, by 10 year age intervals and sex, for selected countries in Africa, South East Asia and Mediterranean Europe, with additional results provided elsewhere (Sadana et al. 2000). A score of 100 is the best level of health, or full health, whereas a score of zero is the worst level of health, excluding death. The level within

Figure 3   Distribution of levels of health status, comparison of two surveys from Denmark, males and females

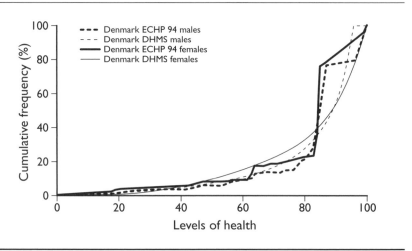

age groups and trends across age groups are generally more similar within regions than across regions, except for the Mediterranean European countries. Greater variation exists at the older age groups than in younger age groups, partially reflecting that at younger age groups little deviation from full health is reported. Furthermore, females generally report worse levels of health in comparison to males, but this is not always the case across all age groups.

Figure 4   Self-reported health status, by age and sex groups, selected countries and regions

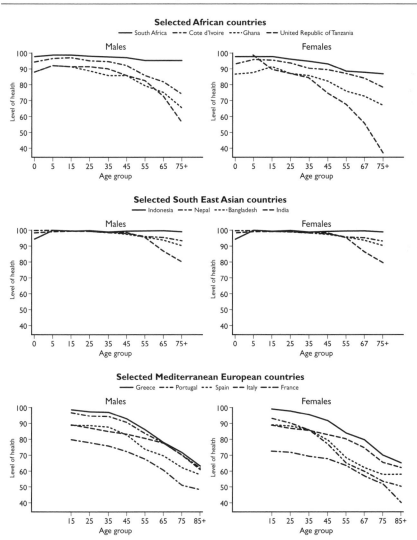

In the African region (Figure 4), very little variation is noted across age groups, except for United Republic of Tanzania, where self-reported health levels drop in the oldest population groups, especially for females. The survey conducted in United Republic of Tanzania (at the sub-national level) included a broader range and depth of items addressing health status than those conducted in the other three African countries. In the European region, for both sexes, the average levels of health vary considerably across age groups, with Greece and Ireland (not shown) at the highest levels

Table I   Rank order of average level of self-reported health in 46 countries, age standardized, by sex[a]

Rank Order	Country	Males	Females	Rank Order	Country	Males	Females
1	Indonesia	99.4	98.5	24	Myanmar	80.0	75.7
2	China	97.9	98.7	25	Tunisia	83.0	72.3
3	Paraguay	93.3	96.8	26	Ireland	78.1	75.1
4	Nepal	94.5	94.9	27	Greece	75.0	75.7
5	Peru	94.0	93.7	28	Denmark	77.5	71.6
6	Bangladesh	92.5	92.4	29	United Kingdom	73.5	74.0
7	South Africa	95.5	87.6	30	United States	76.5	68.7
8	Brazil	90.7	88.9	31	Italy	74.1	71.0
9	Panama	88.4	90.1	32	Netherlands	69.1	75.7
10	Jamaica	88.5	89.0	33	Belgium	73.9	68.6
11	Philippines	91.1	85.4	34	Ghana	71.1	70.8
12	Malaysia	86.2	90.2	35	Egypt	78.0	62.4
13	Bahrain	89.5	86.0	36	Austria	71.3	69.1
14	Bulgaria	87.7	84.2	37	Portugal	74.5	57.3
15	Fiji	86.4	85.1	38	DPR Korea[c]	70.4	61.0
16	Guyana	86.7	82.0	39	Luxembourg	68.5	60.8
17	Morocco	78.3	90.4	40	Pakistan	69.1	58.7
18	Thailand	87.5	80.4	41	Russian Fed.[d]	66.3	61.0
19	India	84.2	83.3	42	Spain	66.7	60.5
20	Rep. Korea[b]	83.5	81.0	43	Sri Lanka	66.5	53.2
21	Germany	78.9	85.0	44	Rep. Tanzania[e]	65.3	47.4
22	Côte d'Ivoire	78.5	82.4	45	France	57.0	54.3
23	Jordan	75.7	82.5	46	Kyrgyzstan	45.1	33.1

a. Among those 65 years and older; 100 = full health.

b. Republic of Korea.

c. Democratic People's Republic of Korea.

d. Russian Federation.

e. United Republic of Tanzania.

across most age groups, and France at the lowest levels across all age groups (Figure 4).

Table 1 summarizes age-standardized[2] estimates for health status across all 46 countries included, for people aged 65 years and older (e.g. the age group common across all surveys) by sex. Considerable variation exists across countries on the aggregate level of health based on self-reported health status. For both males and females, China and Indonesia report the best levels of health (almost at full health), Côte d'Ivoire and Germany report mid range levels of health, while France and Kyrgyzstan report the lowest levels of health (less than half in full health).

Almost no differences are found across age groups in surveys from Bangladesh, Bulgaria, China, Indonesia, Morocco, Nepal, Paraguay, Peru, and South Africa. Self-reported health status is almost at full health in these countries, except for Bulgaria. Not surprisingly, these are the same countries with the highest aggregated health level for the 65 and older population (Table 1).

Figure 5 is a scatter plot of the per capita health expenditures (Poullier and Hernández 2000) and the average level of self-reported health for the over 65 population (males and females combined), for all 46 countries. *Higher* levels of per capita health expenditures are correlated with *lower* average levels of health, an unlikely result.

DISCUSSION AND CONCLUSIONS

Information content. The evidence is rather mixed concerning the information content of surveys within countries. Some surveys clearly appear

Figure 5   Per capita health expenditures vs. average level of self-reported health, 46 countries, age standardized

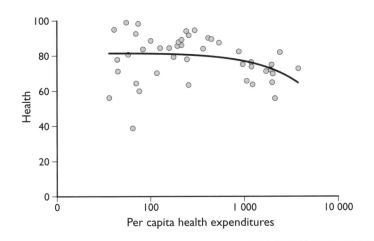

to meet basic criteria, (1) that a range of health states exist at the population level, and (2) that health status declines with age. Even if differences between age groups provide only a weak test of criterion validity, many surveys do not pass this necessary test. Given that different types of surveys have been utilized, some with extensive questions, such as in Indonesia and Bangladesh, and some with more limited questions, such as in Peru or South Africa, we do not conclude that these results only reflect differences in methods. In countries where we would expect worse levels of health for the 0–4 age interval in comparison to the 5–9 age interval, interview reported data do not always conform to expectations, such as in Morocco or Nepal (Sadana et al. 2000). In other countries, such as Belgium, Guyana and Panama, the level of self-reported health status is better in the oldest age group in comparison to the second oldest. Such patterns reduce our confidence in the information content of surveys. Overall, we hypothesize that different norms and expectations by age and potentially other factors contribute to an under-reporting of decrements to full health, particularly at older age groups. We do not assume that non-random reporting differences only exist in surveys that fail the weak test of expected differences across age groups.

Females report more severe levels of health than males, conforming to expected patterns of self-reporting of health status. Whether this is a reflection of non-random reporting differences including different norms and expectations, or differences in the true level of health due to biological or gender-based factors, cannot be addressed given that we only have self-reported data.

Cross-population comparison. We now consider whether the results may be compared across countries within the same region. Differences in survey methodologies may account for some of the differences in the level of health estimated, for example, within the African region. However, given that almost no difference in the level of health was reported across age groups in South Africa, we suggest that some of the differences across these countries are due to non-random reporting differences. We do not conclude that South African females over the age of 55 are significantly healthier than Tanzanian women of the same age group. Similar limitations exist concerning the comparability of data within other regions.

Within Europe, we have the possibility to eliminate differences due to different methodologies, given that the same survey was conducted in 13 European countries. We find it improbable that France has significantly lower levels of health, starting with the 15–24 age interval, in comparison with the other European countries included in the same survey. Instead, we believe that non-random reporting differences are a major factor contributing to these results, beyond variations in the true level of health or measurement error.

Interpretation. The rank order of countries listed in Table 1 raises several issues concerning the meaningful interpretation and use of self-reported data. Can one conclude that the level of health status is much better in Bangladesh or Nepal, than it is in France or Spain, based on self-reported data? We do not. We recommend that non-random reporting differences should be estimated and self-reported data potentially adjusted. This is not to imply that one set of norms or expectations is superior. Rather, we argue that comparisons of health status across populations should compare health, not differences in norms and expectations.

Although not conclusive, Figure 5 suggests that with more information, resources, and exposure to health services, population norms and expectations differ and that these differences are associated with the self-reported level of health across countries. This correlation, even if weak, is consistent with other findings discussed above in the section on cross-population comparability in that sub-populations or countries that are wealthier and spend more resources on health, also self-report worse levels of health in comparison to those with fewer resources. We conclude that the cross-population comparability of existing data from household interview surveys is limited, even where the data collection approaches are standardized. This conclusion is disappointing given WHO's goal to include health, not only mortality levels, in its estimates and comparisons of the level of health status across populations. Given that a growing number of countries implement nationally representative household interview surveys addressing health topics, we believe further investment to improve survey methods is urgently warranted. An innovative and promising new approach to improve the comparability of population health survey data is presented in chapter 8.3 by Murray et al. WHO is currently developing survey instruments to support and test this new approach and surveys have now been carried out in over 70 countries.

NOTES

1   The true score is defined as the average score that would be obtained over repeated self-reports, tests or observations, and measurement error is assumed responsible for differences or fluctuations (Nunnally and Bernstein 1994, p. 211). This differs from the concept we assume, namely that no set of questions, tests or observations provides a complete assessment of non-fatal health status.

2   Age-standardized to the WHO World Standard Population (Ahmad et al. 2000).

ACKNOWLEDGEMENTS

Among several individuals, the authors particularly thank David Cutler and Brodie Ferguson for their contributions.

References

Ahmad O, Boschi-Pinto C, Lopez AD, Murray CJL, Lozano R, Inoue M (2000) *Age standardization of rates: a new WHO standard.* (GPE discussion paper no 31.) World Health Organization/Global Programme on Evidence for Health Policy, Geneva.

American Psychological Association (1985) *Standards for educational and psychological tests.* American Psychological Association, Washington, DC.

Anderson RT, Aaronson NK, Wilkin D (1993) Critical review of the international assessments of health-related quality of life. *Quality of Life Research,* 2:369–395.

Annas J (1993) Women and quality of life: two norms or one? In: *The quality of life.* Nussbaum M, Sen A, eds. Clarendon Press, Oxford.

Axelsson G, Helgadottir S (1995) Comparison of oral health data from self-administered questionnaire and clinical examination. *Community Dentistry and Oral Epidemiology,* 23(6):365–368.

Bergner M, Rothman ML (1987) Health status measures: an overview and guide for selection. *Annual Review of Public Health,* 8:191–210.

Cooke DJ, Michie C (1999) Psychopathy across cultures: North America and Scotland compared. *Journal of Abnormal Psychology,* 108(1):58–68.

Eurostat (1997) *Self-reported health in the European Community. Statistics in focus,* (Population and social conditions, 12.), Eurostat, Luxembourg

Friedsam HJ, Martin HW (1961) A comparison of self and physician's health ratings in an older population. *Journal of Health and Human Behavior,* 179–183.

Groot W (2000) Adaptation and scale of reference bias in self-assesments of quality of life. *Journal of Health Economics,* 19(3):403–420.

Hambleton RK, Swaminathan H (1985) *Item response theory: principles and applications.* Kluwer Nijhoff, Boston, MA.

Hambleton RK, Swaminathan H, Rogers HJ (1991) *Fundamentals of item response theory.* Sage, Newbury Park, CA.

Heliovaara M, Aromaa A, Klaukka T, et al. (1993) Reliability and validity of interview data on chronic diseases. The Mini-Finland health survey. *Journal of Clinical Epidemiology,* 46(2):181–191.

Idler EL, Hudson SV, Leventhal H (1999) The meanings of self-ratings of health: a qualitative and quantitative approach. *Research on Ageing,* 21(3):458–476.

Johansson SR (1991) The health transition: the cultural inflation of morbidity during the decline of mortality. *Health Transition Review,* 1(1):39–68.

Kahneman D, Sovic P, Tversky A, eds. (1982) *Judgement under uncertainty: heuristics and biases.* Cambridge University Press, Cambridge.

Keller SD, Ware JE, Bentler PM, et al. (1998) Use of structural equation modeling to test the construct validity of the SF36 health survey in ten countries: results from the IQOLA Project. *Journal of Clinical Epidemiology,* 51(11):1179–1188.

Kempen GI, van Heuvelen MJ, van den Brink RH, et al. (1996) Factors affecting contrasting results between self-reported and performance-based levels of physical limitation. *Age and Ageing,* **25**(6):458–464.

Kivinen P, Halonen P, Eronen M, Nissinen A (1998) Self-rated health, physician-rated health and associated factors among elderly men: the Finnish cohorts of the seven countries study. *Age and Ageing,* **27**(1):41–47.

Kleinman A (1994) An anthropological perspective on objectivity: observation, categorization, and the assessment of suffering. In: *Health and social change in international perspective.* Chen LC, Kleinman A, Ware NC, eds. Harvard University Press, Boston, MA.

Kleinman A, Eisenberg L, Good B (1978) Culture, illness and care: clinical lessons from anthropologic and cross-cultural research. *Annals of Internal Medicine,* **88**(2):251–258.

Kroeger A, Zurita A, Perez-Samaniego C, Berg H (1988) Illness perception and use of health services in North-East Argentina. *Health Policy and Planning,* **3**:141–151.

Krosnick JA (1991) Response strategies for coping with the cognitive demands of attitude measures in surveys. *Applied Cognitive Psychology,* **5**:213–236.

Mackenbach JP, Looman CWN, van der Meer JBW (1996) Differences in the misreporting of chronic conditions, by level of education: the effect on inequalities in prevalence rates. *American Journal of Public Health,* **86**(5):706–711.

Matthias RE, Atchinson KA, Schweizer SO, Lubben JE, Mayer-Oakes A, de Jong F (1993) Comparisons between dentist ratings and self-ratings of dental appearance in an elderly population. *Special Care in Dentistry,* **13**(2):53–60.

Murray CJL (1996) Epidemiology and morbidity transitions in India. In: *Health, poverty and development in India.* DasGupta M, Chen LC, Krishnan TN, eds. Oxford University Press, Delhi.

Murray CJL, Chen LC (1992) Understanding morbidity change. *Population and Development Review,* **18**(3):481–503.

Muthén LK, Muthén BO (1998) *Mplus. The comprehensive modelling program for applied researchers. User's guide.* Muthén & Muthén, Los Angeles, CA.

Nunnally JC, Bernstein IH (1994) *Psychometric theory.* 3rd edn. McGraw Hill, New York.

Poullier JP, Hernández P (2000) *Estimates of national health accounts. Aggregates for 191 countries in 1997.* (GPE discussion paper no 27.) World Health Organization/Global Programme on Evidence for Health Policy, Geneva.

Raczek AE, Ware JE, Bjorner JB, Gandek B, et al. (1998) Comparison of Rasch and summated rating scales constructed from SF-36 physical functioning items in seven countries: results from the IQOLA project. *Journal of Clinical Epidemiology,* **51**(11):1203–1214.

Rasmussen N, Gudex C, Christensen S (1999) *Survey data on disability.* (Eurostat working papers, Population and social conditions 3/1999/E/n 20.) European Commission, Luxembourg.

Robine JM, Jagger C, Egidi V, eds. (2000) *Selection of a coherent set of health indicators: a first step towards a user's guide to health expectancies for the European Union*. Euro-REVES, Montpellier.

Sadana R, Mathers CD, Lopez AD, Murray CJL, Iburg K (2000) *Comparative analysis of more than 50 household surveys on health status* . (GPE discussion paper no 15.) World Health Organization/Global Programme on Evidence for Health Policy, Geneva.

Sen A (1994) Objectivity and position: assessment of health and well-being. In: *Health and social change in international perspective*. Harvard Series on Population and International Health. Chen LC, Kleinman A, Ware NC, eds. Harvard School of Public Health, Boston, MA.

Streiner DL, Norman GR (1995) *Health measurement scales: a practical guide to their development and use*. 2nd edn. Oxford University Press, New York.

Tourangeau R (1984) Cognitive sciences and survey methods. In: *Cognitive aspects of survey methodology: building a bridge between disciplines*. Jabine T, Straf M, Tanur J, Tourangeau R, eds. National Academy Press, Washington, DC.

Ware JE, Gandeck BL, Keller SD, The IQOLA Project Group (1996) Evaluating instruments used cross-nationally: methods from the IQOLA project. In: *Quality of life and pharmaoeconomics in clinical trials*. 2nd edn. Spilker B, ed. Lippincott-Raven, Philadelphia, PA.

Ware JE, Keller SD (1996) Interpreting general health measures. In: *Quality of life and pharmaeconomics in clinical trials*. 2nd edn. Spilker B, ed. Lippincott-Raven, Philadelphia, PA.

Ware JE, Keller SD, Gandek B, Brazier JE, Sullivan M (1995) Evaluating translations of health status questionnaires: methods from the IQOLA project. *International Journal of Technology Assessment in Health Care*, 11(3):525–551.

Weir C, Seacrest M (2000) Developmental differences in understanding of balance scales in the United States and Zimbabwe. *Journal of Genetic Psychology*, 161(1):5–22.

Werts CE, Linn RL, Jöreskog KG (1974) Intraclass reliability estimates: testing structural assumptions. *Educational and Psychological Measurement*, 34:25–33.

WHOQOL Group (1998) The World Health Organization quality of life assessment: development and general psychometric properties. *Social Science and Medicine*, 46(12):1569–1585.

Wolff BB, Langley S (1968) Cultural factors and the response to pain. A review. *American Anthropologist*, 494–501.

Zborowski M (1952) Cultural components in response to pain. *Journal of Social Issues*, 8:16–30.

Zurayk H, Khattab H, Younis N, et al. (1995) Comparing women's reports with medical diagnoses of reproductive morbidity conditions in rural Egypt. *Studies in Family Planning*, 26(1):14–21.

Chapter 8.2

THE MEASUREMENT AND INTERPRETATION OF HEALTH IN SOCIAL SURVEYS

Duncan Thomas and Elizabeth Frankenberg

INTRODUCTION

Health status is hard to measure. It is widely recognized that health is multi-dimensional reflecting the combination of an array of factors that include physical, mental and social well-being, genotype and phenotype influences as well as expectations and information. A multitude of health indicators have been used in scientific studies drawing on data from both the developed and developing world. Understanding what those indicators measure is central if the results reported in the studies are to be interpreted in a meaningful way. Whether one is interested in summarizing the health of a population or understanding the links between health and other measures of well-being at the individual level, poor measurement will likely yield poor inferences.

There is a large literature that discusses the validity and limitations of different health measures. Murray and Chen (1992) and Sadana (2000) provide excellent reviews and discussion. Some of the most insightful empirical studies have compared indicators of specific morbidities reported by respondents in health interview surveys with indicators based on health examinations of the same individuals conducted by trained healthworkers. Other very influential studies have examined the extent to which self-reported health predicts health problems later in life. A third class of studies contrasts prevalence rates based on health interviews with other sources.

This paper attempts to provide insights into the meaning of a set of relatively general health indicators that are commonly collected in health interview surveys. These self-reports are contrasted with a battery of physical assessments conducted on the same respondents in the same survey, usually a day or two after the interview.

The key complexity that arises from these comparisons is that "true" health status is seldom known. To side-step this complexity, we begin with indicators of health (or, more precisely, nutritional) status which can be measured without any ambiguity: height and weight. Contrasting measurements with self-reports for the same person, we find that self-reports are subject to systematic biases. For example, men are inclined to report themselves as being significantly taller than they actually are; women are inclined to report themselves as significantly lighter than they are. If these were the only differences, it would be simple to adjust reports so they map into measurements. They are not. There is evidence that people are inclined to report their health status as being closer to an "ideal" than it is. This example highlights the complexity of deriving adjustment factors to offset the effects of reporting biases.

We proceed to examine a series of self-reported health indicators collected in the second wave of the Indonesia Family Life Survey (IFLS2). In these cases, truth is not known and so we turn to a comparison of the relationships between health status and socioeconomic status (SES) to provide some insights into the meaning of the health measures. Contrasting the link between SES and physical assessments with the link between SES and self-reported health, we suggest that the more general the health indicator, the more difficult it is to disentangle "true" health status from "reporting effects".[1] However, an examination of the relationships between self-reports and physical assessments suggests that self-reports, particularly more general questions, do contain a good deal of information about the respondent's health.

We conclude that, given the state of knowledge at this time, it would be prudent to invest in the collection of both self-reported health indicators and physical assessments of health status in individual and household surveys. Recent technological advances in health measurement render it feasible to conduct a broad array of assessments in face-to-face surveys at relatively low costs. The benefits are likely to far outweigh the costs.

SELF-REPORTS AND MEASURED HEALTH

Methods that have been used to measure health in social surveys span a wide spectrum, from one or two direct questions asked of individuals about their perception of their overall health to a comprehensive and thorough battery of clinical assessments conducted by physicians or other trained personnel who examine each respondent. For a general review of issues associated with health interview survey implementation, see Kroeger (1985) and Ross and Vaughan (1986). Fischer et al. (1996) provide a discussion in the context of health examination surveys.

The vast majority of surveys in both developed and developing countries have relied on individual responses to a series of questions about their health posed in an interview setting.[2] As a starting point, let self-reported health, θ^S, indicate underlying health, θ^*, with adjustments that are, for simplicity of exposition, assumed to be additive and comprise three parts: an individual idiosyncratic component, ε_i, a factor associated with the specific observable indicator, e_j, and a factor that varies with both the individual and the indicator, e_{ij}:

$$\theta_{ij}^S = \theta_i^* + \varepsilon_i + \varepsilon_j + \varepsilon_{ij} \tag{1}$$

where θ^* is multi-dimensional and hence vector-valued. As a convention, we will treat higher levels of θ as denoting better health status. It is useful to provide concrete examples for the three types of adjustments. First, consider two individuals with the same level of intrinsic health, θ^*; if one is more inclined to report a health problem than the other, then this difference will be reflected in ε_i. Second, say a health state is difficult to detect because it is asymptomatic; self-reports will tend to be noisy indicators of the prevalence of the state as reflected in a relatively large variance component, ε_j. Third, if a health state is better known among some people, relative to others, then these differences will be reflected in the component ε_{ij}. This might arise, for example, if we were to focus on diagnosed health problems; if two people have the same level of intrinsic health, a respondent who has had more contact with health services is more likely to report a diagnosis relative to a respondent who has never seen a trained physician.[3]

Two self-reported indicators, θ_{i1} and θ_{i2}, reported by the same individual will share the common component, ε_i, which, intuitively, may be thought of as the propensity to report oneself as ill. As a result, the two will be positively correlated even if neither is related to θ^*. Clearly, "internal validity" of self-reported measures, based on their being correlated with one another, does not imply they are valid indicators of θ^*. In practice, ε_i does provide information about the respondent's perception of his or her own health which may be an important dimension of health status. Recognizing this, we refer to ε_i as a "(self)-reporting effect" for want of a better shorthand.

There are relatively few examples of examination surveys that have been conducted on a large scale. This presumably reflects the costs and complexity of fielding these sorts of surveys. They are, however, a very rich source of information. One of the best examples, perhaps, is the United States National Health and Nutrition Examination Survey (NHANES) which was started in the late 1950s and is now run on a continuing basis. There are a small number of similar surveys that have been successfully conducted in low income settings which suggest that examination surveys are not only feasible but may also be desirable under certain circumstances (see, for example, Fischer et al. 1996)

In contrast with self-reports, health measurements conducted by a trained nurse or physician will not be affected by reporting error,[4] and for those measures that require no respondent interaction (such as height) there may be no individual-specific measure-specific errors ($\zeta_{ij} = 0$).[5] Some measures do involve respondent interaction (such as blowing into a tube to measure lung capacity) and, like self-reports, they are not perfect indicators of θ^* ($\zeta_j \neq 0$). Thus, in general, measured health, θ^M is:

$$\theta_{ij}^M = \theta_i^* + \zeta_j + \zeta_{ij} \qquad (2)$$

Since interviews are a good deal cheaper to administer and self-reports have been included in a large number of household surveys, it would be very convenient if the relationships between θ^S, θ^M and intrinsic health, θ^*, were mapped out.

Several very important studies have sought to validate self-reports against clinical measurements; typically these studies have contrasted θ_{ij}^M with θ_{ij}^S and assessed the specificity and sensitivity of the self-report. These comparisons tend to be made with specific health indicators such as morbidities associated with particular diseases. It is usually assumed that ζ_j and ζ_{ij} are both zero so that the difference between self-reported and measured health is attributed to the reporting effects, ε. Typically, self-reports tend to understate the incidence of a health problem ($E\varepsilon_i < 0$) and this difference is greater in the case of diseases that are asymptomatic ($E\varepsilon_i < 0$).

Using data from the United States, for example, Krueger (1957) and NCHS (1965) indicate there is a wide gap between respondent perceptions of health and evaluations by a physician and conclude that self-reports are unlikely to serve as a tool for the measurement of diagnosable disease. (See also Pappas et al. 1990). Belcher et al. (1976) provide an early example in a developing country setting. Respondent evaluations of morbidities were compared with physician reports of the same people one to four days later in a study conducted in Ghana. They treat the physician assessment as truth and conclude there is a tendency for self-reports to understate the incidence of health problems and that the extent of understatement is greater the less readily observed the ailment.

There are, however, several problems that are difficult to detect in a clinical setting (such as problems that emerge intermittently) in which case ζ_j will not be zero. Moreover, even in a clinic, many health problems involve eliciting information from the respondent (such as pain) in which case ζ_{ij} may not be zero. More generally, it is reasonable to argue that clinical measures are not perfect and that in some instances, one's perception of one's health is of legitimate concern to health professionals and policy-makers. (See, for example, Younis et al. 1993 and Zurayk et al. 1993; 1995, for an illuminating discussion in the context of reproductive morbidity.) In general, it is going to be very difficult to separately distinguish the components ε and ζ in equations (1) and (2).

To illustrate some of the complexities, we begin with a very simple case in which θ^* and θ^M are identical and so ζ is zero; we consider height and weight of adults which are considered to be indicators of nutritional status. (Since our attention is focused on measurement, we put aside the question of whether anthropometrics are indicative of health status.) The difference, equation (1) – equation (2),

$$\theta_{ij}^S - \theta_{ij}^M = \varepsilon_i + \varepsilon_j + \varepsilon_{ij} \tag{3}$$

is reported in Figure 1 using measures and self-reports for the same individuals age 20 through 90 in the third round of NHANES (conducted between 1988 and 1994).[6] For prime age adults, height is fixed and so any difference between reported and measured height must be due to reporting effects. As seen in the upper panel of the figure, men tend to overstate their height—by around 1 cm until age 50 when the overstatement increases with age. Apparently, as men shrink with age, they do not update their height. Women also overstate their height but the extent of overstatement is small (and not significant) until they reach age 50.

The difference between reported and measured weight is presented in the lower panel. Weight does vary through the day and between days

Figure 1   Height and weight of adults—differences between self-reports and measurements by age (NHANES 3)

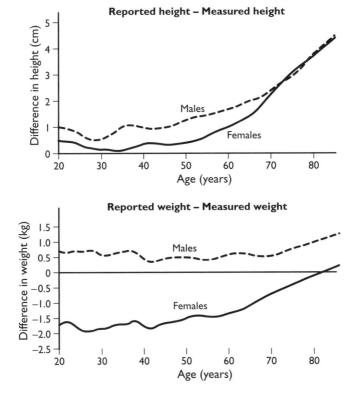

which will affect the variance of the deviation; it should not, however, affect the first moment of the difference which we would expect to be zero. It is not. Whereas, on average, men tend to overstate their weight by nearly two-thirds of a kilogram, women tend to understate weight by nearly 1.5 kg. (The standard errors are 0.07 kg in each case and so the differences are significant.) Weight under-reporting is greatest among younger women, declines with age and, among women in their 80s, reported weight exceeds measured weight.

In principle, if it is known that men tend to report themselves as taller and heavier than they are and that women report themselves as lighter than they are, it would be possible to adjust reported height and weight (taking account of differences by age group) and not incur the costs of conducting anthropometric measures. That conclusion would be premature.

Table 1 reports the correlates associated with the difference between reported anthropometry and measured anthropometry ($\theta_{ij}^S - \theta_{ij}^M$). The age splines essentially replicate the shapes in Figure 1. In household surveys, it is often argued that better educated respondents provide more accurate answers; in the health measurement literature this might be attributed to the better educated having a more complete set of information. However,

Table 1   Difference between reported anthropometry and measured anthropometry, United States NHANES 3

	Reported height minus measured height		Reported weight minus measured weight		Reported BMI minus measured BMI	
	Male	Female	Male	Female	Male	Female
Age 20–40 years (spline)	0.002	−0.009	0.024	0.027	0.009	0.011
	[0.17]	[0.91]	[2.10]	[1.96]	[1.97]	[1.71]
Age 40–60 (spline)	0.035	0.025	−0.011	0.010	−0.016	−0.005
	[3.56]	[2.39]	[1.24]	[0.75]	[3.69]	[0.80]
Age 60–80 (spline)	0.113	0.152	0.003	0.032	−0.030	−0.033
	[9.85]	[12.08]	[1.86]	[3.20]	[6.24]	[5.56]
Years of education	0.050	−0.104	−0.053	−0.072	−0.035	0.013
	[2.75]	[4.12]	[2.95]	[3.32]	[4.18]	[0.94]
ln (per capita income)	−0.085	−0.109	−0.057	−0.020	0.002	0.031
	[1.28]	[1.56]	[0.73]	[0.23]	[0.06]	[0.70]
(1) If self-report as overweight	0.120	0.047	−1.541	−1.430	−0.627	−0.645
	[1.14]	[0.39]	[12.07]	[10.43]	[11.74]	[9.35]
underweight	0.048	0.017	1.253	1.069	0.471	0.447
	[0.24]	[0.05]	[6.19]	[5.47]	[5.77]	[4.25]
Intercept	0.920	2.630	1.413	−0.737	0.246	−1.102
	[1.38]	[4.21]	[1.95]	[0.93]	[0.82]	[2.84]
F (all covariates)	44.51	59.13	40.58	41.13	50.21	27.43
R^2	0.10	0.15	0.06	0.06	0.09	0.04

Notes: Sample is 3 870 males and 3 682 females age 20 through 90 interviewed and measured in NHANES 3 (1988–1994). Height measured in cm, weight in kg and BMI in kg/m². t-statistics in brackets based on Huber-type variance-covariance estimates. F test for all covariates significant at <1% size of test in all regressions.

we see that better educated men tend to over-report height more than those who are less educated. Better educated women, on the other hand, tend to report heights that are closer to the truth. For weight, the reverse is true. Better educated men tend to report weights that are closer to the truth whereas better educated women tend to understate their weight more than those with less schooling. Apparently the link between education and accuracy of reporting is not simple.

To probe more deeply, the regressions also include controls for whether the respondent feels he or she is underweight or overweight. They are powerful predictors of the difference between reported and measured weight: those who feel they are overweight tend to understate their weight whereas those who feel they need to put on weight tend to overstate their weight. The same result emerges if we replace these controls with indicators for respondents who are trying to gain or lose weight (hope springs eternal?).

Apparently, even in the case of indicators that are easily verified, such as height and weight, the gap between perceptions and reality is large, significant and depends on a host of factors. Putting aside the fact that older respondents, whose height declines with age, do not appear to update their perception of their height, one is tempted in this example to conclude that self reports reflect not only θ^* but also the respondent's own perception of some ideal health status. Men want to be taller and as education increases their ideal height increases; women want to be thinner and as their education increases their ideal weight decreases. And those whose weight deviates from their ideal want to move towards that ideal.

Body mass index (BMI), which is weight (in kg) divided by height^2 (in metres^2) is often used as a summary indicator of current nutritional status and reflects, in part, net energy intake. The gap between reported and measured BMI is presented in the third panel of Table 1. Since women tend to under-report weight, BMI tends to be understated with the magnitude of the gap being approximately constant until around age 50 when the gap rises (because under-reporting of weight diminishes while over-reporting of height emerges). Women around age 60 tend to under-report BMI by 1 kg/m^2. Reported and measured BMI of males are very similar for men under age 40. Among older men, the effect of over-stating height results in BMI being under-stated and, for those around age 70, the average understatement is 0.5 kg/m^2. Better educated men tend to understate BMI more (reflecting the combined effect of understating weight and overstating height more as education rises). Among women, education is not related to mis-reporting BMI (as the understatement of both height and weight cancel each other out). Perceptions of ideal weight also significantly affect errors in reported BMI. Respondents who consider themselves to be overweight tend to report their BMI is 0.6 kg/m^2 less than is measured and those who consider themselves underweight underestimate BMI by almost 0.5 kg/m^2. BMI based on self-reported height and weight clearly contains measurement error that is not trivial and varies systematically with the characteristics of the respondent in a complex way.

Using the same source of data but examining child height, Strauss and Thomas (1996) observe that the gap between maternal reports and measurements tend to be smaller among higher income and better educated mothers and the gaps are smaller among older children. They suggest this likely reflects differences in the frequency that children are measured and would arise if mothers of higher socioeconomic status (SES) measure their children (or visit health centers that measure their children) more frequently than women of lower SES. The declining gap across the age distribution is consistent with this interpretation since the rate of growth in height declines with age.

Taken together, these results suggest mapping the association between self reports of health and "true" health will be difficult—even in cases in which there is no argument about the meaning of "truth". Things become even more complicated in the more general case in which the terms ζ in equation (2) are not reasonably assumed to be zero.

REPORTED HEALTH, MEASURED HEALTH AND RESPONDENT CHARACTERISTICS

The majority of studies that cross-validate reported health with measures of health have contrasted specific symptoms or diagnoses reported by a respondent in an interview with clinical assessments. Many of the health indicators recorded in health interviews are, however, very difficult to cross-validate because there is no obvious clinical counterpart. This is, perhaps, least controversial in the case of general health indicators which are often collected in interview surveys; indeed, many multi-purpose surveys focus primarily on "global" or "summary" health status indicators precisely because the number of items required to "fully" characterize health status is large.

The most commonly collected item is self-reported general health status (GHS). One of the most extensively documented relationships to emerge in the literature on health status is that self-reported GHS is a significant predictor of subsequent mortality. McCallum et al. (1994) and Idler and Benyamini (1997) provide a recent review.

It is not obvious what accounts for the strong relationship between self-rated health and subsequent mortality. It is likely that self-reported health is very inclusive with respect to both the range and severity of conditions that it reflects.[7] Respondents may incorporate knowledge of family history (and thus genetic health endowment) into their answer.[8] Possibly self-rated health is associated with practices and resources that affect subsequent health. In-depth interviews suggest that the presence or absence of particular health problems or of positive and negative health behaviour shapes the responses of the majority of answers to questions on general health status. Moreover, this work suggests that factors which lead to a rating of good health differ from those associated with a rating of poor health (Krause and Jay 1994). Respondents in "good" health reported choosing this rating on the basis of comparisons with other people far more frequently than did respondents who rated themselves in fair or poor health. All of the respondents in poor health cited health problems or difficulty with physical functioning (not health comparisons or health behaviours) as the reason for their choice of rating (Krause and Jay 1994). Several studies confirm these findings and the results indicate that it would be incorrect to treat "good" and "poor" health symmetrically (Smith et al. 1994).

While one can certainly ask a physician to provide an assessment of an individual's overall health, θ^M, unless the physician has a complete individual and family history, a good working relationship with the respondent, and knows a considerable amount about the respondent's life style, θ^M will measure "true" health, θ^*, with error. Given the model outlined above, it is not clear what to make of comparisons between θ^S and θ^M since we know nothing about ε and ζ.

To provide an illustration, we draw on data from the second wave of the Indonesian Family Life Survey (IFLS2).[9] In the survey, respondents were asked a long battery of health questions that included their current general health status, difficulties with a series of Activities of Daily Living (ADLs), questions on specific morbidities (including probes to obtain details) and extensive questions about use of health care. In addition, a trained healthworker (a nurse or recently qualified doctor) visited the household separately and conducted a series of physical assessments. These measures were selected to represent different dimensions of health that are of epidemiological relevance to Indonesia (and most developing countries) while also being feasible to field in a household survey setting. For each adult respondent, the healthworker measured height, weight, haemoglobin status, lung capacity, blood pressure and the speed with which the respondent was able to stand up five times from a sitting position.[10] Additionally, at the end of the assessment and after a brief discussion with the respondent, the healthworker rated the person's health relative to someone of average health of the same age and sex using a scale of 1 (for very poor) through 9 (for excellent).

Figure 2 presents the joint distribution of self-reported GHS and healthworker rating. It is comforting that the mean healthworker score declines as self-reports move from good to average and then to poor. As noted above, it has often been observed that the distinction between "good" and "average" is less clear-cut than the difference between "average" and "poor". This is reflected in the scores assigned by the healthworkers. The marginal distributions of the healthworker scores within each GHS category demonstrate that there is a good deal of heterogeneity within each category. There has to be: it is hard to imagine that a construct as complex as health status will be adequately summarized by one trichotomous indicator. The extent of overlap in the marginal distributions across the

Figure 2   General health status—joint distribution of self-reported
               GHS and healthworker evaluation

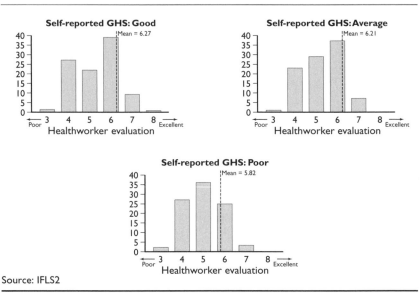

Source: IFLS2

GHS categories is, however, very substantial and is, perhaps, cause for
pause. While it is likely that a complete physical examination, the results
of a battery of tests and a family history would reduce the variance in the
healthworker scores, the central issue will likely remain: it is not possible
to separately identify ε and ζ when comparisons are made between self-
reports and measures of health when neither can legitimately be construed
as revealing some intrinsic level of health.

We turn, therefore, to an alternative strategy in order to better understand the nature of information contained in self-reported and measured
health indicators. Contrasting the correlations between respondent characteristics and self-reported health with the correlations between the same
characteristics and measured assessments affords an opportunity to provide a characterization of how the meaning of health varies with those
characteristics. For concreteness, consider education as an example. The
correlation between it and self-reported health will reflect at least two
components: the influence of education on underlying intrinsic health and
also the relationship between education and the respondent's perception
of his or her own health. In the context of the additive model above, both
the underlying dimensions of health and the components associated with
reporting effects may depend on socioeconomic characteristics, x:

$$\theta_{ij}^S = \theta_{ij}^*(x) + \varepsilon_i(x) + \varepsilon_j + \varepsilon_{ij}(x) \qquad (4)$$

Education will be associated with an individual's reporting propensity, ε_i, if better educated people are better informed about their health and are, therefore, more likely to identify a health problem (conditional on a particular level of θ^*). If what is construed as "normal" (or "difficult") varies with education, then that too will be captured in $\varepsilon_i(x)$.

The relationship between "reporting effects" and education is likely to differ depending on the particular self-reported indicators and so ε_{ij} is allowed to be a function of x. For example, a person with little or no education may not know about health ailments that afflict him or her and so may report GHS as very good; a better educated person, however, with the same level of θ^* but more information about it may perceive himself or herself to not be in very good health. In contrast, whether a person has difficulty breathing—a relatively obvious problem—may be less prone to "reporting effects" of this form. In general, the more "objective" the indicator—or the more objectively defined the reference category—and the more obvious the health problem, the less likely that "reporting effects" will vary with education or any other element of the vector of socioeconomic characteristics, x.[11]

In contrast to self-reports, correlations between socioeconomic characteristics and physical assessments will not be affected by individual characteristics unless the assessment involves participation of the respondent (such as performing the puff test) and that participation is related to the characteristic. Thus

$$\theta_{ij}^M = \theta_{ij}^*(x) + \varepsilon_j + \varepsilon_{ij} \tag{5}$$

and so differences in the effects of x on elements of θ^S and θ^M that are closely related to the same underlying health may be interpreted as being informative about $(\partial \varepsilon_j/\partial x + \partial \varepsilon_{ij}/\partial x)$, that is the "reporting effects" in self-reports. These comparisons will be contaminated if the health indicators differ in their utility as measures of θ^* which argues for basing inferences on multiple health status indicators.

Table 2 presents results of the correlations between a series of health indicators and respondent characteristics for adults aged 20 through 80 years in IFLS2. In addition to gender, we focus on four respondent characteristics: per capita expenditure (PCE) levels in the household which is a measure of longer-run household resources and can be thought of as an indicator of SES; the education and height of the respondent, both of which reflect human capital investments earlier in life and, finally, age. The models include splines in the covariates to permit non-linearities in their effects and controls location of residence of the respondent.

Table 2a focuses on physical assessments conducted by the health-worker. The first two reflect nutritional status of the respondent. BMI is thought to be correlated with physical capacity and VO_2max, and extremes of BMI have been shown to be related to elevated morbidity and mortality. For both males and females, BMI tends to increase as household resources

Table 2a   Physical health assessments and respondent characteristics—IFLS2

	BMI kg/m²		Haemoglobin g/dL		Lung capacity		Sit→stand secs		Blood pressure mm Hg		HW evaln	
	Male (1)	Female (2)	Male (3)	Female (4)	Male (5)	Female (6)	Male (7)	Female (8)	Male (9)	Female (10)	Male (11)	Female (12)
ln (PCE)												
Below median (spline)	0.170 [6.62]	0.216 [7.47]	0.042 [1.48]	0.057 [2.10]	0.021 [0.76]	-0.004 [0.19]	-0.002 [0.05]	-0.006 [0.18]	0.013 [0.56]	0.002 [0.07]	0.200 [4.97]	0.184 [5.00]
Above median (spline)	0.107 [3.41]	0.117 [3.64]	0.055 [1.74]	-0.014 [0.65]	0.041 [1.58]	0.014 [0.85]	0.025 [1.02]	0.018 [0.62]	0.020 [0.61]	0.074 [1.96]	0.066 [1.73]	0.084 [2.30]
Education 0–5 yrs (spline)	0.023 [3.31]	0.072 [8.30]	0.037 [4.17]	0.020 [2.65]	0.032 [4.19]	0.011 [2.07]	-0.019 [1.96]	-0.010 [0.97]	0.021 [2.70]	0.017 [1.95]	0.019 [1.70]	0.028 [2.97]
Education ≥ 6 yrs (spline)	0.034 [7.74]	-0.029 [5.40]	0.020 [4.62]	-0.001 [0.15]	0.030 [7.10]	0.014 [4.16]	-0.018 [4.49]	-0.020 [4.17]	0.002 [0.47]	-0.012 [2.54]	0.028 [4.96]	0.029 [4.87]
Height (cms)	-0.002 [0.95]	-0.003 [1.06]	0.006 [2.83]	0.003 [1.82]	0.025 [11.60]	0.016 [11.27]	0.001 [0.46]	-0.001 [0.35]	0.001 [0.48]	-0.004 [1.48]	0.014 [5.53]	0.010 [4.03]
Age 20–30 (spline)	0.040	0.047	0.000	-0.007	-0.004	0.011	0.016	0.014	0.002	0.008	-0.006	0.002
Age 30–40 (spline)	0.022	0.032	-0.016	-0.004	-0.011	-0.006	0.016	0.015	0.011	0.010	-0.006	-0.001
Age 40–50 (spline)	-0.010	-0.018	-0.019	-0.001	-0.029	-0.022	0.020	0.022	0.012	0.022	-0.016	-0.011
Age 50–60 (spline)	-0.023	-0.031	-0.020	0.005	-0.049	-0.026	0.037	0.061	0.018	0.031	-0.002	-0.006
Age 60–70 (spline)	-0.009	-0.001	-0.012	-0.014	-0.034	-0.018	0.040	0.041	0.006	-0.007	-0.012	-0.007
Age 70–80 (spline)	-0.050	-0.05	-0.021	0.002	-0.037	0.000	0.051	0.051	0.029	0.057	-0.023	0.013
(1) urban	0.116 [4.24]	0.269 [6.75]	0.045 [1.03]	-0.006 [0.16]	0.067 [1.63]	0.035 [1.09]	-0.015 [0.27]	-0.026 [0.43]	0.072 [3.05]	0.068 [2.28]	-0.063 [0.88]	-0.028 [0.43]
F (all covariates)	30.34	37.03	31.95	8.59	107.43	75.17	50.27	54.38	6.86	11.02	57.13	79.14
R²	0.13	0.12	0.12	0.03	0.34	0.26	0.29	0.30	0.04	0.05	0.31	0.28

Notes: Sample is 6 435 males and 7 658 females age 20 through 80 interviewed and measured in IFLS2 (1997). t-statistics in parentheses based on Huber-type variance-covariance estimates allowing within-cluster correlation. Regressions include province controls which are jointly significant at < 5% in all models except female blood pressure. Age effects jointly significant at < 5% size in every regression except the healthworker evaluation (HW evaln). F test for all covariates significant at < 1% size of test in all regressions.

increase, particularly among the poorest, and as education increases, at least for those with less than 6 years of schooling. (Among better educated women, BMI declines with education after controlling PCE.)

Low levels of haemoglobin indicate iron-deficiency which has been shown to be linked to susceptibility to disease, fatigue and lower levels of productivity. Haemoglobin levels likely reflect the combination of a diet that is higher in animal proteins (a primary source of iron) and greater absorption capacity (which is reduced by disease insults, loss of blood and also by diets that are high in rice). As with BMI, better educated men have higher levels of haemoglobin; the same is true of women in the lower half of the SES spectrum. Greater attained height is associated with elevated haemoglobin counts suggesting that the effects of early childhood nutrition experiences may reach into adulthood; an alternative interpretation that height is capturing the influence of SES is not very appealing given the latter's relatively modest effect in the regression. Haemoglobin levels of men tend to decline with age; this may reflect the impact of better nutrition among more recent cohorts or the cumulative effect of disease insults among older cohorts. This pattern among women is complicated by the fact that reproductive age women are prone to elevated levels of anaemia.

Stature and lung size are positively correlated and so height is a very good predictor of lung capacity. Lung capacity is also higher among better educated and younger males and females. Although urban dwellers tend to be taller, and have higher BMI, there is no difference in lung capacity between urban and rural residents which presumably reflects lower air quality in many urban areas in Indonesia.

The time it takes for a respondent to stand from a sitting position is intended to capture muscular-skeletal problems and primarily reflects lower body motor functioning. Each respondent was asked to repeat the test five times and the total time taken was recorded in seconds. As with lung capacity, better educated and younger respondents perform better on this test.

The fifth physical measure is blood pressure; in the regressions, we estimate the probability that a respondent's measured blood pressure is high (≥ 150 mm Hg, ≥ 90 mm Hg). For both men and women, blood pressure is elevated among urban residents and tends to rise with age until around 60. Blood pressure also increases with education until completion of primary school; among better educated males, the probability of high blood pressure is constant and declines with education among women. Since elevated blood pressure tends to be correlated with weight (and thus rise with SES) and with stress (and thus possibly rise with wages), it is plausible that the relatively modest relationships between SES and blood pressure reflect the effect of treatment among the better off and the better educated.

Finally, the healthworker's evaluation of each respondent's general health status is positively associated with PCE, especially among the poorest, with education and with height. There is little association with age—which is as it should be since the healthworker was instructed to compare the respondent's health with the average for a person of the same age.

Of these measures, only BMI and haemoglobin satisfy the condition that measurement error, ζ, is unlikely to be related to respondent characteristics. For the others, things are a bit more complicated. Lung capacity and sit-to-stand times require interaction between the healthworker and respondent. In the field, not all respondents approached these tests the same way: older, higher SES women were sometimes more tentative than other respondents. In our judgement, the impact of these differences is relatively modest. Health interventions that moderate blood pressure are more likely among higher SES respondents, and so we are cautious in our interpretation of those results. While the healthworkers were instructed to only evaluate the health of the respondent, we cannot rule out the possibility that the healthworker was influenced by the respondent's demeanor and attitude which is likely to be linked to SES.

With this in mind, there are several general observations that might be drawn from table 2a. First, measured health tends to be positively associated with SES—PCE or education—particularly in the case of those indicators that do not involve respondent interaction. Second, except in those cases where there are reasons to expect otherwise, the measured indicators suggest that health status declines with age.

Table 2b presents comparable regressions drawing on some of the self-reports of health status collected in IFLS2. Many health interview surveys include questions about activities of daily living (ADLs), the respondent's perception of his or her ability to perform physical activities such as walking or lifting heavy items, or activities that are necessary in daily life such as bathing or dressing, instrumental activities of daily living (IADLs). We examine two of the questions included in IFLS2 and report in the first columns of the table, the characteristics associated with a higher probability that a respondent reports having difficulty walking 5 km (columns 1 and 2) and difficulty carrying a heavy load (columns 3 and 4).

It has been argued that questions about ADLs are easy for respondents to understand as they ask about activities that are well-defined and capture (or are good proxies for) important dimensions of functional health status. Theoretical work has related ADLs to the underlying health dimensions they are intended to tap (Johnson and Wolinsky 1993; Kopec 1995; Nagi 1965). While there is controversy in the literature regarding the success with which ADLs do (and should) match objective measures of functioning (Daltroy et al. 1995; Hoeymans et al. 1996), if predictive power of future health problems is a metric against which to evaluate health indicators, ADLs appear to perform fairly well. Studies have found that scales of physical functioning based on ADLs are significant predictors of subsequent mortality, net of covariates such as age and even self-reported GHS (Reuben et al. 1992; Scott et al. 1997). Nevertheless, they are not without problems. The notions "difficulty" and "heavy" are not

Table 2b Self-reported health and respondent characteristics—IFLS2

	Walk 5 kms with difficulty		Carry heavy load with difficulty		GHS good		GHS poor		Number of days limited activity		Number of days in bed	
	Male (1)	Female (2)	Male (3)	Female (4)	Male (5)	Female (6)	Male (7)	Female (8)	Male (9)	Female (10)	Male (11)	Female (12)
ln (PCE)												
below median (spline)	−0.008 [0.35]	0.042 [1.39]	−0.012 [0.53]	−0.030 [1.05]	0.028 [0.84]	0.000 [0.00]	−0.050 [1.58]	0.034 [1.30]	−0.012 [0.37]	0.079 [3.20]	−0.004 [0.12]	0.018 [0.72]
above median (spline)	−0.017 [0.96]	0.017 [0.56]	0.007 [0.37]	0.078 [2.30]	0.007 [0.22]	0.013 [0.49]	0.002 [0.07]	−0.031 [1.25]	−0.047 [1.54]	−0.040 [1.62]	−0.031 [0.82]	−0.047 [2.54]
Education 0–5 yrs (spline)	−0.008 [1.03]	0.001 [0.07]	−0.019 [2.32]	−0.008 [0.95]	0.001 [0.07]	0.005 [0.77]	−0.015 [1.55]	0.010 [1.25]	0.004 [0.42]	−0.019 [2.59]	0.000 [0.02]	−0.018 [2.54]
Education ≥ 6 yrs (spline)	−0.004 [1.20]	−0.005 [1.03]	0.004 [1.33]	−0.002 [0.41]	−0.002 [0.44]	0.003 [0.52]	−0.010 [2.36]	−0.019 [4.01]	−0.006 [1.30]	−0.003 [0.73]	−0.001 [0.17]	−0.001 [0.26]
Height (cms)	−0.002 [1.14]	−0.005 [2.26]	−0.003 [1.73]	−0.008 [3.60]	0.002 [0.89]	0.001 [0.30]	−0.001 [0.18]	−0.002 [0.71]	0.001 [0.19]	−0.003 [1.16]	−0.001 [0.31]	−0.001 [0.20]
Age 20–30 (spline)	−0.005	0.000	−0.001	−0.013	−0.016	0.009	0.003	0.000	0.003	−0.007	−0.001	−0.010
Age 30–40 (spline)	0.009	0.003	0.004	0.011	−0.005	−0.006	0.001	0.012	−0.007	0.007	−0.004	0.009
Age 40–50 (spline)	0.006	0.036	0.003	0.024	−0.002	−0.010	0.010	0.015	0.012	0.001	0.011	−0.005
Age 50–60 (spline)	0.051	0.048	0.042	0.061	−0.019	−0.011	0.029	0.012	0.021	0.005	−0.009	0.015
Age 60–70 (spline)	0.040	0.029	0.052	0.044	−0.002	−0.005	0.026	0.013	0.000	0.013	0.025	−0.005
Age 70–80 (spline)	0.065	0.038	0.073	0.070	0.000	0.005	−0.013	0.060	0.004	0.043	−0.008	0.052
(1) urban	0.019 [0.92]	0.068 [2.02]	0.022 [1.04]	0.103 [2.94]	0.024 [0.61]	0.056 [1.81]	−0.036 [1.22]	0.046 [1.41]	0.002 [0.05]	0.027 [0.90]	−0.008 [0.23]	−0.002 [0.07]
F (all covariates)	35.74	66.77	0.35	57.54	14.46	19.06	12.99	12.92	4.06	8.23	3.11	2.75
R^2	0.22	0.16	0.20	0.19	0.09	0.06	0.07	0.05	0.02	0.02	0.01	0.01

Notes: Sample is 6 435 males and 7 658 females age 20 through 80 interviewed and measured in IFLS2 (1997). t-statistics in brackets based on Huber-type variance-covariance estimates allowing within-cluster correlation. Regressions include province controls which are jointly significant at < 1% in all models. Age effects jointly significant at < 1% size of test in all regressions. F test for all covariates significant at < 1% size of test in all regressions.

explained in the survey and depend on the respondent's own perception. For some respondents, the ADLs are outside of the range of their own experience. And, for many of the ADLs that are commonly included in surveys, few prime age respondents report difficulties completing the activity.[12] This is reflected in the regressions in Table 2b which indicate that the incidence of difficulties increases substantially with age although the age at which difficulties emerge is lower than that typically observed in higher income countries (see Strauss et al. 1993, for a detailed discussion).

The striking result in the regressions in Table 2b is the absence of a negative correlation between SES and difficulty with either ADL (except in the case of men with little education and carrying a heavy load). In fact, among women in the top half of the distribution of PCE, a higher level of PCE is associated with more difficulty carrying a heavy load. The same is not true of walking 5 km nor is it true of men; one is tempted to conclude that the act of carrying a heavy load is not something higher income women view as part of their daily activities, and reporting difficulties is more a reflection of perception of the appropriateness of the activity than physical constraints.

Columns 5 through 8 report the relationship between GHS and respondent characteristics. The characteristics associated with respondents who report themselves as being in good health are in the first two columns; the characteristics associated with being in poor health are in the second pair. Two issues cloud interpretation of these responses. First, it is unclear what reference the respondent uses as the benchmark: is it the average person in the survey (country), in the community or someone in the respondent's peer group? While this can, in principle, be addressed by explicitly specifying the reference group in the interview,[13] it is likely that a respondent's notion of "good" health will be influenced by his or her own experience and will thus vary with socioeconomic status, interaction with the health system and so on.

Results for physical assessments and ADLs indicate that health status tends to decline with age; the age profile for GHS is substantially more muted, especially in the case of respondents who report themselves as being in good health. If all respondents use the average in the country as the reference, we would expect a decline in health status with age that is comparable with the declines observed for physical assessments and ADLs; if the respondents use someone of the same age as the reference, there would be no systematic relationship with age. The estimated age profile suggests that no single reference is used by all respondents and that the reference health amounts to some combination of the national average and the respondent's peer group. This complicates drawing inferences about θ^* with these sorts of data.

Moreover, even among those who report themselves in poor health, there are marked differences between males and females. A significant incidence of poor health emerges much earlier among females (during their thirties) than males (during their fifties)—a pattern also observed for carrying a heavy load. Waldron (1983) and others have written extensively on this topic and suggest that perceptions of health (ε_i) differ systematically between men and women. Contrasting the age profiles in Table 2b, it appears that these differences vary with the specific health measure (i.e. in context of the model above, ε_{ij} differs between men and women).

The issue of the reference health emerges again when we consider the relationship between GHS and SES. If the reference is the national average, we would expect GHS to improve with SES; if the reference is one's peer group (which is typically comprised of people with similar levels of SES), there is no reason to expect an association. We find no association between SES and the probability that a respondent reports himself or herself as being in good health. There is, however, a negative association between the probability of reporting poor health and education, but only among those who have completed primary school. If these patterns reflect differences in the reference health, they suggest a complex interaction among different measures of SES, levels of SES, age and gender.

The lack of a clearly defined reference health status is not the only problem with interpreting GHS. Rather, the observed patterns probably also reflect differences in perceptions of what is "good" or "poor" health as well as differences in the information respondents have about their health.

Dow et al. (1997) present some evidence supporting the second contention. Drawing on data from two social experiments, one conducted in the United States and one conducted in Indonesia, they show that as the price of health care is increased, there is a decline in use of care. However, GHS tends to improve where prices are raised and, conversely, GHS worsens where prices are lowered. If one were to interpret that evidence at face value, one would conclude that raising the price of health care improves health. In fact, when physical assessments of health are examined, the evidence suggests that θ^* improved when prices were reduced and respondents saw health professionals more often. Dow et al. conclude that it is not seeing the doctor that makes one sick, but seeing the doctor does increase one's information set and thereby influences one's perception of one's health. Since both experiments involved randomization of the treatment, the analyses are not contaminated by the potential for reverse causality—that those who see the doctor more often are more likely to report themselves as ill. See Newhouse et al. (1993) for a fuller description of the US experiment.

The last two health indicators in Table 2b are the number of days the respondent reports having had to limit his or her normal activity in the previous four weeks and the number of days spent in bed during that time. Many studies have argued that because these indicators are conceptually very clear and do not demand judgements of the respondent about the meaning of "poor" or "difficulty", they are likely to be rather good measures of health. We are more sanguine.

It is well known in developed countries that the incidence of reporting limited activity rises substantially when people are applying for or are receiving public assistance that is linked to disability. This is less likely to be a problem in most developing countries where such assistance is not common. It has also been suggested that people who are unemployed (or who have retired) are more likely to report limited activity as a rationalization for their not working.

In low income settings, however, it is not obvious that "limited activity" is well-defined. Moreover, it is quite likely that health problems that limit the activity of a labourer are quite different—and possibly more serious—than those that limit the activity of a sedentary worker. The meaning of "limited activity" is likely to vary across SES. It is also likely to vary with employment status: a self-employed person whose income is directly tied to his or her being actively at work is less likely to have limited normal daily activities (failed to go to work) than someone whose income includes such benefits as sick pay (and so may miss a day of work without incurring an income penalty). The meaning of "limited activity" is likely, once again, to vary systematically with SES.

The regression results support this view. In contrast with the physical assessments, for males, there is no association between SES and either the number of days of limited activity or the number of bed days. Among females, the number of days of limited activity declines with education but increases with PCE (among women in the lower half of the PCE distribution) suggesting that among these women, as income increases, they are more likely to be sick. We suspect that is not the case and that, rather, they are more likely to report their activities are limited by health problems.

As Sadana (2000) shows, it is possible to construct questions about specific activities which are informative about health. As she notes, these kinds of questions need to be tailored to the particular context and sub-population of interest which limits their value in national and cross-national studies.

To summarize, the evidence in Table 2b suggests that it is difficult to interpret self-reports about the kinds of general indicators of health status that are commonly collected in health interviews. The more specific the question, there may be less ambiguity in the interpretation of the question by the respondent, but, unfortunately, that does not necessarily translate into a more readily interpreted answer by the analyst.

Table 2c turns to specific questions about morbidities. As discussed above, it is these sorts of questions that have been the basis for the majority of the cross-validations of self-reports and clinical assessments and several studies have described their strengths and weaknesses. We will not, therefore, dwell on them.

In IFLS2, questions were asked about whether the respondent had experienced a particular morbidity, reading down a list of 30 items. If so, additional questions were asked about the nature of the morbidity in some cases—such as the type of coughing—to elicit more information. Six mor-

Table 2c Self-reported morbidities and respondent characteristics—IFLS2

	Cough		Breathing difficulty		Joint pain		Fever		Diarrhoea		Nausea	
	Male (1)	Female (2)	Male (3)	Female (4)	Male (5)	Female (6)	Male (7)	Female (8)	Male (9)	Female (10)	Male (11)	Female (12)
ln (PCE)												
Below median (spline)	-0.006 [0.19]	0.080 [3.03]	-0.035 [1.09]	0.030 [1.20]	-0.022 [0.74]	0.037 [1.32]	-0.020 [0.63]	0.046 [1.78]	-0.008 [0.24]	0.034 [1.36]	0.051 [2.03]	0.114 [4.29]
Above median (spline)	-0.001 [0.03]	0.036 [1.21]	0.010 [0.27]	-0.013 [0.46]	-0.017 [0.58]	0.026 [1.00]	-0.034 [1.30]	-0.001 [0.02]	0.017 [0.55]	0.053 [1.48]	0.007 [0.24]	-0.029 [0.95]
Education 0–5 yrs (spline)	-0.020 [2.06]	-0.020 [2.60]	-0.040 [3.42]	-0.019 [2.65]	0.006 [0.60]	-0.003 [0.33]	-0.011 [1.06]	-0.025 [2.97]	-0.006 [0.77]	-0.001 [0.16]	-0.005 [0.63]	0.010 [1.30]
Education ≥ 6 yrs (spline)	-0.013 [2.85]	-0.006 [1.20]	-0.012 [3.00]	-0.015 [3.65]	-0.012 [2.73]	-0.006 [1.19]	-0.016 [3.56]	-0.014 [2.72]	0.002 [0.45]	-0.009 [1.83]	-0.006 [1.48]	-0.012 [2.26]
Height (cms)	-0.003 [1.21]	-0.004 [1.62]	-0.004 [1.83]	0.003 [1.42]	-0.001 [0.36]	-3.720 [0.00]	0.001 [0.26]	-0.004 [1.74]	-0.001 [0.38]	0.001 [0.38]	-0.001 [0.39]	-0.002 [0.60]
Age 20–30 (spline)	0.002	-0.002	0.002	-0.004	0.014	0.009	-0.006	-0.002	0.006	0.010	-0.007	0.004
Age 30–40 (spline)	-0.009	0.005	0.002	0.007	0.006	0.027	-0.005	-0.003	-0.008	-0.005	0.000	-0.007
Age 40–50 (spline)	0.013	0.009	0.000	0.008	0.020	0.032	-0.004	0.005	0.008	0.001	-0.008	-0.002
Age 50–60 (spline)	0.012	0.000	0.024	0.013	0.018	0.023	0.008	0.003	-0.011	0.005	0.000	-0.003
Age 60–70 (spline)	0.017	0.013	0.034	-0.008	0.032	0.010	-0.008	-0.014	-0.003	-0.009	-0.006	-0.012
Age 70–80 (spline)	0.018	0.011	-0.027	0.028	-0.028	0.035	0.019	0.007	0.010	-0.011	0.002	0.011
(1) urban	0.005 [0.14]	0.028 [0.89]	-0.007 [0.23]	0.037 [1.34]	-0.052 [1.74]	0.011 [0.35]	0.001 [0.02]	0.057 [1.69]	0.029 [0.92]	0.010 [0.32]	-0.017 [0.69]	-0.002 [0.08]
F (all covariates)	10.78	7.67	12.21	10.56	25.48	41.91	6.97	8.81	4.75	3.04	6.84	11.93
R^2	0.04	0.03	0.05	0.04	0.09	0.14	0.03	0.03	0.01	0.01	0.03	0.04

Notes: Sample is 6 435 males and 7 658 females age 20 through 80 interviewed and measured in IFLS2 (1997). t-statistics in brackets based on Huber-type variance-covariance estimates allowing within-cluster correlation. Regressions include province controls which are jointly significant at < 1% in all models. Age effects significant at < 1% size of text except fever and diarrhoea. F test for all covariates significant at < 1% size of test in all regressions.

bidities are included in Table 2c. In general, the better educated are less likely to report the presence of a morbidity; there is little association with PCE.

The contrast between coughing and breathing difficulties is informative. The regressions suggest higher PCE women are more likely to report they suffer from coughing problems. They are not, however, more likely to report having breathing difficulties and, recall, they do not tend to have lower levels of lung capacity. One suspects that the positive link between SES and reported coughing reflects, in part, differences in what is considered to be a "cough" across the SES distribution, a difference that does not carry through to the more general term, "breathing difficulty". A similar argument might be made for the incidence of reported "nausea" which rises with PCE for both men and women (among those below median PCE). Why does the incidence of coughing differ across the SES distribution? It is possible that poorer women are not aware of coughing whereas higher income women are; while we cannot rule that out, it seems more likely to us that poorer women consider a particular amount of coughing to be normal whereas higher income women report that same amount of coughing as an illness (See Bhatia and Cleland 1995). It is clear that the precise nature of questions about morbidities makes a difference. Sindelar and Thomas (1991) argue that evidence from Peru suggests relative to diagnoses (which often involve interaction with the health system) questions about symptoms are less prone to differences in interpretation across the SES distribution. See also Zurayk et al. (1995) and Murray and Chen (1992).

SELF-REPORTS AND PHYSICAL ASSESSMENTS

If self-reports are contaminated by ε, can they be used to say anything about θ^*? To address this question, tables 3 and 4 present the relationships between self-reports and physical assessments. Substituting equation (5) in equation (4) we estimate:

$$\theta_{ij}^S = \beta'\theta_{ij}^M + \varepsilon_i(x) + \varepsilon_j + \varepsilon_{ij}(x) + \varepsilon_j + \varepsilon_{ij} + u_{ij} \tag{6}$$

to provide an empirical assessment of the links between self-reports of health, θ^S and physical measures, θ^M. If they are unrelated, then β will be zero indicating that the self-report conveys no information about any of the physical assessments.

We begin with GHS in Table 3.[14] The physical assessments do not do a good job of discriminating between respondents who report themselves to be in average health and those in good health. Even the healthworker evaluation is unable to discriminate between these states. (In fact, those who take longer to stand from a sitting position are more likely to report themselves in better health!) In contrast, the assessments, θ^M, do much better in isolating those who report themselves as being in poor health; this is true for lung capacity, blood pressure, haemoglobin levels and BMI. It is also the case that the healthworker evaluation has predictive power

Table 3   General health status, physical health and SES

	GHS Good				GHS Poor			
	Male (1)	Male (2)	Female (1)	Female (2)	Male (1)	Male (2)	Female (1)	Female (2)
In (PCE) (spline)								
Below median	—	0.588 [0.63]	—	−0.268 [0.34]	—	−0.960 [0.93]	—	1.702 [2.02]
Above median	—	−0.061 [0.07]	—	0.265 [0.36]	—	0.435 [0.50]	—	−0.740 [0.95]
Education (spline)								
0–5 yrs	—	−0.008 [0.03]	—	0.094 [0.47]	—	−0.176 [0.55]	—	0.478 [1.91]
≥ 6 yrs	—	−0.095 [0.70]	—	0.083 [0.57]	—	−0.197 [1.45]	—	−0.571 [3.72]
Lung capacity (spline)								
≤ median	−0.006 [0.68]	−0.008 [0.83]	0.003 [0.40]	0.002 [0.20]	−0.098 [4.99]	−0.096 [4.75]	−0.021 [2.05]	−0.017 [1.71]
> median	0.011 [2.12]	0.012 [2.19]	0.009 [0.58]	0.010 [0.62]	0.000 [0.03]	0.000 [0.03]	−0.018 [1.40]	−0.015 [1.16]
Sit→stand time (spline in seconds)								
≤ median	0.903 [1.69]	0.938 [1.72]	1.268 [2.47]	1.294 [2.48]	0.559 [1.29]	0.554 [1.25]	0.763 [1.44]	0.818 [1.54]
> median	0.102 [0.55]	0.119 [0.61]	−0.165 [0.99]	−0.136 [0.80]	0.454 [1.40]	0.494 [1.46]	0.376 [1.47]	0.305 [1.19]
BP diastolic (spline)								
≤ 150 mm Hg	0.078 [2.09]	0.079 [2.09]	−0.051 [1.49]	−0.051 [1.44]	−0.069 [1.53]	−0.068 [1.47]	−0.062 [1.61]	−0.066 [1.68]
> 150 mm Hg	−0.080 [2.09]	−0.078 [2.01]	−0.024 [0.91]	−0.022 [0.85]	0.163 [2.52]	0.166 [2.54]	0.115 [2.41]	0.112 [2.32]
BP systolic (spline)								
≤ 90 mm Hg	−0.025 [0.46]	−0.035 [0.63]	0.057 [1.17]	0.051 [1.04]	0.140 [2.51]	0.143 [2.51]	−0.077 [1.26]	−0.079 [1.27]
> 90 mm Hg	0.074 [0.74]	0.077 [0.75]	−0.102 [1.48]	−0.108 [1.55]	−0.054 [0.41]	−0.074 [0.55]	0.175 [1.52]	0.183 [1.58]
Haemoglobin (spline)								
≤ 12 g/dL	−0.632 [1.07]	−0.552 [0.92]	0.296 [0.94]	0.312 [0.98]	−1.435 [1.58]	−1.199 [1.31]	−1.618 [2.95]	−1.606 [2.89]
> 12 g/dL	0.634 [2.26]	0.725 [2.52]	0.650 [1.68]	0.701 [1.80]	−0.241 [0.88]	−0.209 [0.76]	0.724 [1.63]	0.762 [1.70]
BMI (spline)								
<18 kg/m²	1.079 [1.63]	1.012 [1.48]	0.484 [1.09]	0.501 [1.11]	−4.233 [3.29]	−4.428 [3.38]	−3.363 [3.63]	−3.670 [3.85]
18–28 kg/m²	0.038 [0.24]	0.055 [0.32]	0.166 [1.27]	0.156 [1.15]	−0.411 [2.48]	−0.359 [2.16]	−0.137 [0.99]	−0.182 [1.30]
>28 kg/m²	−0.391 [0.42]	−0.347 [0.36]	0.668 [1.28]	0.673 [1.28]	0.410 [0.45]	0.584 [0.62]	−0.227 [0.48]	−0.286 [0.61]
Height (cms)	0.022 [0.35]	0.018 [0.28]	0.005 [0.09]	−0.006 [0.11]	0.012 [0.16]	0.024 [0.33]	−0.004 [0.06]	0.001 [0.01]
Healthworker evaluation	0.286 [0.51]	0.286 [0.50]	0.096 [0.23]	0.088 [0.21]	−1.601 [3.58]	−1.429 [3.17]	−1.580 [3.20]	−1.551 [3.07]

continued

Table 3   General health status, physical health and SES *(continued)*

	GHS Good				GHS Poor			
	Male (1)	Male (2)	Female (1)	Female (2)	Male (1)	Male (2)	Female (1)	Female (2)
Age 20–30 (spline)	−0.415	−0.460	0.195	0.214	0.085	0.092	0.140	0.090
Age 30–40 (spline)	−0.127	−0.142	−0.196	−0.187	0.009	−0.029	0.417	0.380
Age 40–50 (spline)	−0.036	−0.021	−0.213	−0.216	0.185	0.165	0.298	0.337
Age 50–60 (spline)	−0.486	−0.496	−0.232	−0.234	0.514	0.563	0.124	0.144
Age 60–70 (spline)	−0.043	−0.058	−0.129	−0.118	0.535	0.431	0.211	0.281
Age 70–80 (spline)	0.054	0.057	0.217	0.210	−1.217	−1.157	1.775	1.694
(1) urban	0.638	0.658	1.544	1.471	−2.008	−1.325	1.414	1.810
	[0.64]	[0.62]	[1.86]	[1.65]	[2.18]	[1.36]	[1.43]	[1.70]
F (all covariates)	12.12	10.95	14.27	13.41	12.87	11.28	10.43	10.83
R^2	0.09	0.09	0.06	0.06	0.09	0.09	0.07	0.07

Notes: Sample is 6 435 males and 7 658 females age 20 through 80 interviewed and measured in IFLS2 (1997). *t*-statistics in brackets based on Huber-type variance-covariance estimates allowing within-cluster correlation. Regressions include province controls which are jointly significant at < 1% in all models. Age effects jointly significant at < 1% size of test in every model. F test for all covariates significant at < 1% size of test in all regressions.

that is independent of these assessments (this does not reflect reverse causality since, recall, the healthworker does not know how the respondent answered the questions about self-assessed health). There can be little argument that poor GHS does contain information about θ^*.

There is, however, cause for caution. In the model (6), SES will predict θ^S if there are unmeasured aspects of health that are correlated with SES. In that case, given the positive correlation between SES and physical assessments, we would expect $\partial\theta^S/\partial x$ to be positive. If, conditional on measured health, there are differences in perceptions of health across the SES distribution, then those will enter through ε in (6). Those effects are likely to be negative as higher SES is likely associated with a greater propensity to report poor health. Thus, if $\partial\theta^S/\partial x$ is negative, then the reporting effects must dominate the role of unobservables. For the case of females who report themselves as being in poor health, this turns out to be the case: among those below median PCE, as PCE increases, women are more likely to report themselves as being in poor health. A similar pattern emerges among women with 5 years or less of schooling, although the reverse is true among the better educated. We conclude that for GHS the links between θ^S, θ^M and ε are complex and complicate interpretation of self-reported GHS.

Table 4a focuses attention on the two ADLs. The first regression in each pair includes the physical assessments. They all tend to predict difficulties with walking and carrying a heavy load suggesting that the ADLs are also doing a good job of capturing some dimensions of these assessments. (There are, however, some instances in which the relationships are not as

Table 4a Self-reported ADLs, physical health and GHS

	Walk 5 km with difficulty				Carry heavy load with difficulty			
	Male (1)	Male (2)	Female (1)	Female (2)	Male (1)	Male (2)	Female (1)	Female (2)
Lung capacity (spline)								
≤ median	−0.080	−0.057	−0.016	−0.013	−0.051	−0.033	−0.016	−0.013
	[4.11]	[2.94]	[1.24]	[0.98]	[2.82]	[1.74]	[1.52]	[1.25]
> median	0.005	0.005	0.003	0.006	0.009	0.008	0.013	0.015
	[1.02]	[1.00]	[0.16]	[0.31]	[2.44]	[2.39]	[0.92]	[1.12]
Sit→stand time (spline in seconds)								
≤ median	0.600	0.466	1.077	0.945	0.560	0.452	0.345	0.209
	[1.58]	[1.29]	[1.49]	[1.31]	[1.78]	[1.54]	[0.51]	[0.32]
> median	1.369	1.263	0.971	0.907	0.839	0.753	1.239	1.189
	[4.05]	[4.07]	[3.46]	[3.28]	[2.44]	[2.35]	[4.52]	[4.45]
BP diastolic (spline)								
≤ 150 mm Hg	−0.065	−0.049	−0.037	−0.026	−0.052	−0.039	−0.017	−0.007
	[1.48]	[1.20]	[0.76]	[0.54]	[1.52]	[1.19]	[0.39]	[0.15]
> 150 mm Hg	0.170	0.132	0.129	0.109	0.176	0.145	0.119	0.103
	[2.60]	[2.12]	[2.35]	[2.01]	[3.03]	[2.66]	[2.35]	[2.08]
BP systolic (spline)								
≤ 90 mm Hg	0.130	0.097	−0.006	0.008	0.067	0.041	−0.029	−0.019
	[2.20]	[1.71]	[0.07]	[0.10]	[1.54]	[0.94]	[0.43]	[0.29]
> 90 mm Hg	−0.042	−0.030	0.100	0.071	−0.075	−0.065	0.065	0.042
	[0.31]	[0.23]	[0.77]	[0.55]	[0.67]	[0.59]	[0.55]	[0.36]
Haemoglobin (spline)								
≤ 12 g/dL	−1.217	−0.879	0.236	0.510	−1.037	−0.763	−0.905	−0.680
	[1.56]	[1.25]	[0.36]	[0.79]	[1.38]	[1.09]	[1.76]	[1.37]
> 12 g/dL	0.077	0.131	−1.175	−1.299	0.375	0.419	−0.795	−0.913
	[0.30]	[0.51]	[1.94]	[2.15]	[1.85]	[2.06]	[1.65]	[1.91]
BMI (spline)								
< 18 kg/m²	−3.896	−2.909	−3.602	−3.033	−4.037	−3.240	−2.546	−2.075
	[3.64]	[2.81]	[3.61]	[3.03]	[3.74]	[3.28]	[2.39]	[1.96]
18–28 kg/m²	−0.063	0.034	0.024	0.047	−0.137	−0.059	−0.320	−0.304
	[0.37]	[0.21]	[0.12]	[0.24]	[1.00]	[0.46]	[2.00]	[1.92]
>28 kg/m²	1.067	0.972	2.020	2.057	0.340	0.263	2.169	2.187
	[0.92]	[0.87]	[2.73]	[2.79]	[0.49]	[0.38]	[3.22]	[3.22]
Height (cms)	−0.094	−0.097	−0.177	−0.176	−0.107	−0.109	−0.232	−0.231
	[1.51]	[1.61]	[1.96]	[1.96]	[1.96]	[2.04]	[3.15]	[3.17]
Healthworker evaluation	−0.166	0.207	0.953	1.220	0.003	0.305	0.512	0.736
	[0.42]	[0.53]	[1.57]	[2.02]	[0.01]	[0.90]	[0.86]	[1.25]
(1) Self-report								
Poor GHS	—	0.234	—	0.170	—	0.190	—	0.143
		[12.45]		[9.77]		[11.86]		[10.01]
Good GHS	—	0.004	—	0.002	—	0.003	—	0.021
		[0.38]		[0.08]		[0.46]		[1.27]
Age 20–30 (spline)	−0.254	−0.272	−0.068	−0.092	−0.032	−0.047	−0.439	−0.463
Age 30–40 (spline)	0.357	0.356	0.127	0.057	0.139	0.138	0.325	0.270
Age 40–50 (spline)	0.086	0.043	1.388	1.338	0.014	−0.021	0.711	0.673
Age 50–60 (spline)	1.818	1.700	1.734	1.714	1.192	1.096	1.783	1.770

continued

Table 4a   Self-reported ADLs, physical health and GHS *(continued)*

	Walk 5 km with difficulty				Carry heavy load with difficulty			
	Male (1)	*Male* (2)	*Female* (1)	*Female* (2)	*Male* (1)	*Male* (2)	*Female* (1)	*Female* (2)
Age 60–70 (spline)	1.398	1.273	1.035	0.999	1.510	1.409	1.188	1.161
Age 70–80 (spline)	2.085	2.369	1.403	1.102	1.984	2.214	2.210	1.951
(1) urban	0.183	0.651	2.862	2.619	0.557	0.935	3.447	3.212
	[0.22]	[0.80]	[2.07]	[1.92]	[0.81]	[1.44]	[2.97]	[2.78]
F (all covariates)	29.33	36.28	54.16	61.73	15.53	19.15	46.47	50.47
R²	0.24	0.28	0.17	0.18	0.22	0.26	0.19	0.21

Notes: Sample is 6 435 males and 7 658 females age 20 through 80 interviewed and measured in IFLS2 (1997). *t*-statistics in brackets based on Huber-type variance-covariance estimates allowing within-cluster correlation. Regressions include province controls which are jointly significant at < 1% in all models. Age effects jointly significant at < 1% size of test in every model. F test for all covariates significant at < 1% size of test in all regressions.

one might expect—higher lung capacity is associated with greater difficulty carrying a heavy load among men.)

The second regression in each pair adds self-reported GHS to the list of covariates. We have two motivations. First, we wish to assess the extent to which GHS is able to soak up the predictive power of the physical assessments. Given that all the assessments are continuous indicators and GHS is simply a trichotomous variable, the fact that significant coefficients decline by between 10 and 30 per cent indicates GHS does contain information about θ^*.

Our second motivation for including GHS in the regression is to examine the extent to which it is correlated with other self-reported health measures after controlling measured health. The correlation is high and, for the case of poor health, significant. There are two possible interpretations. Poor GHS is reflecting unmeasured aspects of health which are also reflected in the ADLs. Or, we are simply picking up the effect of individual idiosyncratic reporting effects, ε_i, which are common to both GHS and the ADLs. It is not possible to distinguish between these hypotheses with these data.

Table 4b presents results for morbidities and activity limitations; we report only those specifications that include all physical assessments and GHS. Height and the healthworker evaluation are included in the model but suppressed in the table. Neither is significant in any model. Respondents with low lung capacity (and women with low BMI) are more prone to coughing and breathing difficulties; fever likely emanates from a number of sources and is associated with most of the physical assessments; neither joint pain nor nausea are well-predicted with the physical assessments included in IFLS2; BMI appears to predict the number of days of limited activity. For all of these self-reports, GHS is significantly correlated with the self-reports. In the case of days of limited activity, the inclusion

Table 4b Self-reported morbidities, physical health and GHS

	Cough		Breathing difficulty		Joint pain		Fever		Nausea		No. days limited activity	
	Male	Female	Male	Female	Male	Female	Male	Female	Male	Female	Male	Female
Lung capacity (spline)												
≤ median	-0.071	-0.035	-0.137	-0.048	0.016	0.002	-0.024	-0.020	-0.013	-0.007	-0.088	-0.012
	[3.07]	[2.36]	[6.89]	[5.40]	[0.80]	[0.15]	[1.26]	[1.54]	[1.01]	[0.75]	[0.40]	[0.12]
> median	-0.021	-0.046	-0.009	-0.008	-0.014	0.001	0.002	0.013	0.001	-0.012	0.005	-0.142
	[2.53]	[2.38]	[1.91]	[0.79]	[1.95]	[0.06]	[0.31]	[0.78]	[0.22]	[0.73]	[0.08]	[1.34]
Sit→stand time (spline in seconds)												
≤ median	1.781	0.201	0.109	0.147	-0.523	-0.750	1.967	2.210	-0.135	0.500	-1.804	4.129
	[2.29]	[0.25]	[0.25]	[0.34]	[0.81]	[1.01]	[3.22]	[3.02]	[0.33]	[0.88]	[0.41]	[0.80]
> median	-0.923	-0.148	-0.053	-0.152	0.573	0.060	-0.241	0.012	-0.026	-0.299	2.008	3.516
	[2.35]	[0.48]	[0.16]	[0.83]	[1.48]	[0.19]	[0.76]	[0.05]	[0.12]	[1.51]	[0.60]	[1.30]
BP diastolic (spline)												
≤ 150 mm Hg	-0.088	-0.051	-0.054	-0.046	0.015	-0.016	-0.115	-0.073	-0.038	-0.080	-0.872	-0.115
	[1.34]	[0.89]	[1.41]	[1.52]	[0.23]	[0.33]	[1.86]	[1.36]	[0.91]	[1.93]	[1.69]	[0.29]
>150 mm Hg	-0.087	0.050	0.052	0.006	0.029	0.025	0.076	-0.034	0.064	-0.038	0.262	-0.131
	[1.02]	[0.79]	[0.98]	[0.14]	[0.41]	[0.39]	[1.20]	[0.71]	[1.59]	[1.03]	[0.35]	[0.26]
BP systolic (spline)												
≤ 90 mm Hg	0.039	0.070	0.073	0.052	-0.066	-0.052	0.091	0.074	-0.001	0.050	0.443	-0.880
	[0.42]	[0.86]	[1.30]	[1.15]	[0.71]	[0.73]	[1.10]	[0.97]	[0.01]	[0.79]	[0.64]	[1.35]
> 90 mm Hg	0.294	-0.161	-0.002	0.116	0.117	0.074	0.026	-0.011	-0.127	0.084	1.051	1.644
	[1.53]	[1.10]	[0.02]	[1.15]	[0.71]	[0.56]	[0.18]	[0.09]	[1.42]	[0.85]	[0.66]	[1.32]
Haemoglobin (spline)												
≤ 12 g/dL	-1.031	0.602	-0.335	-0.398	-1.464	-0.614	-0.559	-0.158	-0.135	0.266	-8.544	6.741
	[0.98]	[0.97]	[0.52]	[1.03]	[1.56]	[1.07]	[0.61]	[0.27]	[0.22]	[0.61]	[0.84]	[1.53]
> 12 g/dL	-0.511	-1.223	-0.189	-0.131	-0.217	0.289	-0.521	-0.972	0.569	-0.651	-2.654	-8.846
	[1.23]	[1.87]	[0.76]	[0.40]	[0.61]	[0.56]	[1.35]	[1.68]	[2.01]	[1.50]	[0.96]	[2.30]

continued

Table 4b   Self-reported morbidities, physical health and GHS (continued)

	Cough		Breathing difficulty		Joint pain		Fever		Nausea		No. days limited activity	
	Male	Female	Male	Female	Male	Female	Male	Female	Male	Female	Male	Female
BMI (spline kg/m²)												
< 18 kg/m²	0.122	-4.451	-0.123	-3.784	2.095	-0.099	-2.089	-2.725	0.676	-0.507	-14.193	-4.309
	[0.08]	[4.31]	[0.12]	[3.77]	[1.59]	[0.10]	[1.68]	[2.59]	[0.80]	[0.56]	[0.95]	[0.39]
18–28 kg/m²	-0.127	0.249	-0.100	-0.122	0.039	0.434	-0.294	-0.461	0.093	0.030	-2.936	-0.752
	[0.48]	[1.14]	[0.69]	[1.02]	[0.16]	[2.35]	[1.25]	[2.43]	[0.60]	[0.20]	[1.55]	[0.44]
>28 kg/m²	1.200	0.523	-0.312	0.626	1.537	0.152	1.034	0.701	1.665	0.328	25.737	4.985
	[0.75]	[0.66]	[0.37]	[1.46]	[1.24]	[0.22]	[0.82]	[1.06]	[1.50]	[0.62]	[1.75]	[0.81]
(1) Self-report												
Poor GHS	0.214	0.157	0.198	0.121	0.220	0.182	0.215	0.197	0.126	0.118	3.679	2.787
	[10.78]	[8.63]	[10.84]	[9.03]	[11.92]	[10.75]	[10.73]	[10.80]	[8.01]	[7.48]	[12.93]	[14.19]
Good GHS	-0.098	-0.096	-0.020	-0.119	-0.016	-0.343	-0.049	-0.061	-0.032	-0.048	-4.271	-0.484
	[4.73]	[4.91]	[2.18]	[1.22]	[0.92]	[2.02]	[2.92]	[3.77]	[3.30]	[4.14]	[4.32]	[5.66]

Notes: Sample is 6 435 males and 7 658 females age 20 through 80 interviewed and measured in IFLS2 (1997). t-statistics based on Huber-type estimates allowing within-cluster correlation. Regressions control height (not significant), healthworker evaluation (not significant), age of respondent as a spline, significant at < 5% on all models except female (cough, breathing difficulty, fever, nausea and days of limited activity), urban and province of residence (significant in all models at < 1%). F test for all covariates significant at < 1%.

of GHS increases the regression R^2 by a factor of four. We suspect that correlated reporting effects, ε_p, is the driving force behind that observation.

The regressions have been re-estimated including PCE and education of the respondent to determine whether reporting differences that are correlated with SES persist after controlling measured health and GHS. The results are reported for a subset of the self-reported health indicators in Table 5; all regressions also include the full set of covariates listed in Table 4.

Controlling measured health and GHS, better educated men are more likely to report having difficulty carrying a heavy load. As PCE increases, women in households with PCE above the median are more likely to report having difficulty carrying a heavy load. It would seem that this ADL is not immune to differences in perceptions of what is meant by the question across the SES distribution for both men and women.

Women in households with PCE below the median are more likely to report having a cough and suffering from nausea as PCE increases; the same is true for the probability a male reports suffering from nausea. Increases in PCE in these households is also associated with a greater probability a woman reports health has limited her activities.

The fact that SES is not correlated (or is negatively correlated) with the other self-reported health indicators does not mean that those indicators are not contaminated by reporting effects. Rather, the evidence in Table 5 indicates that the propensity to report health problems increases with SES and this propensity dominates the positive relationship between SES and improved health evident in Figure 2. This provides a powerful test of the hypothesis that interpretation of self-reported health indicators is far from straightforward.

CONCLUSIONS

Using data from NHANES 3 and IFLS2, we have examined the links between self-reported health status, physical assessments of health and SES. The empirical results highlight the complexity of the interactions among these indicators—without even venturing into the even more complex arena of mental health, pain and health difficulties that are very difficult to diagnose.

There can be little doubt that self-reports of health obtained in health interview surveys contain important information about the health status of respondents. There is, however, evidence that the self-reports also contain information about the respondents' own characteristics—their education, their standard of living, their interaction with the health system and their beliefs about what is "good health". Disentangling these pieces is not straightforward (see also Sadana 2000; Sadana et al. 2001).

There are likely to be very substantial pay-offs to investments in collecting and disseminating more experimental and quasi-experimental evidence on the links between self-reports, physician assessments and

Table 5 Self-reported health, physical health and SES

	Carry heavy load with difficulty		Cough		Breathing difficulty		Nausea		No. days limited activity	
	Male	Female	Male	Female	Male	Female	Male	Female	Male	Female
ln (PCE) (spline)										
Below median	-0.020	-1.054	0.234	3.783	-0.633	0.848	1.711	3.534	4.941	26.606
	[0.03]	[1.09]	[0.15]	[2.93]	[0.71]	[1.19]	[2.22]	[4.08]	[0.45]	[3.09]
Above median	0.270	2.764	0.036	1.981	0.361	-0.175	0.100	-0.761	-14.789	-10.990
	[0.43]	[2.46]	[0.02]	[1.45]	[0.39]	[0.23]	[0.11]	[0.80]	[1.52]	[1.31]
Education (spline)										
0–5 yrs	-0.460	-0.230	-0.674	-0.833	-0.791	-0.452	-0.096	0.340	3.889	-6.906
	[1.79]	[0.81]	[1.48]	[2.35]	[2.47]	[2.32]	[0.43]	[1.35]	[1.40]	[2.70]
≥ 6 yrs	0.188	0.025	-0.498	-0.138	-0.254	-0.368	-0.196	-0.322	-0.808	0.887
	[2.06]	[0.14]	[2.20]	[0.55]	[2.21]	[3.14]	[1.51]	[1.93]	[0.48]	[0.59]
F (all covariates)	17.72	47.33	14.60	11.33	12.33	10.83	7.35	10.62	7.41	11.10
R^2	0.27	0.21	0.07	0.05	0.12	0.07	0.05	0.06	0.12	0.10

Notes: Sample is 6 435 males and 7 658 females age 20 through 80 interviewed and measured in IFLS2 (1997). t-statistics in brackets based on Huber-type variance-covariance estimates allowing within-cluster correlation. Regressions control lung capacity, time to stand from sitting position, blood pressure, haemoglobin, BMI, height, GHS, healthworker evaluation, age, urban and province of residence. F test for all covariates significant at < 1% test in all models.

respondent characteristics. Studies of the introduction of disability income for workers whose health prevented them from working has yielded important insights into the way self-reports have responded to changes in economic incentives (Parsons 1991). There are a large number of other potential quasi-experiments—health interventions, introduction of new or improved services, information campaigns, changes in prices of care or changes in health insurance schemes, economic shocks, and financial crises. By exploiting the variation induced by such (quasi-) exogenous changes in the environment that people live in, and by contrasting the impact of the changes on perceptions of health and health assessments, it should be possible to shed some light on the mechanisms that underlie the evolution of self-reported health status.

Now is a good time to conduct these sorts of studies. The rate of technological advances in the measurement of health status is nothing short of stunning, and it is becoming increasing feasible to conduct tests for many common ailments in a field setting as part of a large-scale household survey that also contains a battery of self-reported health indicators, information about respondent behaviours (such as use of health care, employment, daily activities) and good measures of socioeconomic status. If these data are collected longitudinally, it will be possible to exploit the variation that arises as social, economic and demographic environments change either because of shifts in policy or because of external forces. There also seems to be considerable scope for learning about the meaning of self-reports through increased experimentation in questions included in interview surveys that contain large samples of respondents who span a wide spectrum of SES and behaviour.

The collection of survey data that integrates self-reports of health, clinical or physical assessments and includes substantial heterogeneity in respondent backgrounds is an important first step. As those data are placed in the public domain and extensively analysed, so they will surely serve as powerful tools for scientists to make more headway in understanding the meaning of health status indicators collected in social surveys and, thereby, reveal information about the health of a population that can be interpreted with confidence.

ACKNOWLEDGEMENTS

Comments of Ritu Sadana and the editors of this volume have been very helpful. Financial support from the National Institute on Aging (NIA P01-AG08291), the National Institute of Child Health and Human Development (NICHD P01-HD28372) and the National Science Foundation (SBR-9512670) is gratefully acknowledged.

NOTES

1   Iburg et al. (chapter 8.4) present related evidence from the United States in
    which observed health is contrasted with both self-assessments and physician-
    assessments.

2   The content and quantity of those questions depends on the number of different
    dimensions of health that are of interest and, within each dimension, on the
    desired sensitivity to different levels of well-being. Standard health assessment
    instruments include, for example, the Sickness Impact Profile, the Quality of
    Well-being Scale, and the Nottingham Health Profile. A well-known study (and
    resulting instrument) is the RAND Medical Outcomes Study (MOS). The full
    version of the MOS questionnaire contains 149 items and requires an estimated
    30–40 minutes to administer (Stewart and Ware 1992). A reduced instrument,
    SF-36, has been widely adopted and is advocated as a good basic tool for multi-
    purpose surveys. For a good discussion of issues about wording, recall periods,
    etc., see Murray and Chen (1992).

3   It is straightforward to allow the adjustments to depend on the level of intrinsic
    health, in which case the effects become multiplicative. This would make sense
    if respondents are inclined to report their own health as close to the norm
    (average health) so that the adjustment would be largest for those in poorest (or
    best) health. Below, we will allow θ and ε to depend on a common character-
    istic, x, below which also unties the additivity assumption.

4   There may be healthworker-specific measurement error, although that can be
    minimized by good training, field practice and supervision.

5   This restriction will not apply if the amount of information about health
    contained in any measure varies with individual characteristics.

6   The figures relate the gap between reported and measured anthropometry with
    respondent age. The non-parametric locally weighted smoothed scatterplots
    (Cleveland 1980) use a tricube weighting function and 20% bandwidth.

7   Self-reported health may pick up diseases that have begun to affect respondents'
    health but that have not yet been diagnosed. However, one of the studies that
    found significant impacts of GHS on subsequent mortality found no effects of
    GHS on the onset of chronic diseases (Pijls et al. 1993).

8   This is not the entire explanation. Even after controlling family history, several
    studies demonstrate that GHS continues to be a significant predictor of
    mortality (Borawski et al. 1996; Deeg et al. 1989; Pijls et al. 1993).

9   The IFLS is an ongoing longitudinal survey of individuals, households, families
    and communities in Indonesia. The first wave was conducted in the last half of
    1993 and included a sample of 7 224 households in 321 communities in 13 of
    the archipelago's provinces; the sample is representative of 83% of the popula-
    tion of Indonesia. The second wave sought to re-interview IFLS1 respondents
    four years later in 1997: 94.5% of the IFLS1 households were located and
    interviews were completed with more than 30 000 respondents. Enumerators
    interviewed all household members (apart from young children who were
    interviewed by proxy) to obtain comprehensive information on consumption,
    income and wealth of the family, labour market histories, education histories,
    migration histories, marriage histories and fertility histories of each household

member. While the survey is fundamentally multi-purpose, it does contain a good deal of detail on health status and health behaviours. Each respondent completed a battery of questions about personal health, use of health care, health insurance, smoking and the health of non-coresident family members. In addition, a trained healthworker visited each household and conducted a series of physical assessments in the home. IFLS2 was coming out of the field as Indonesia fell into the biggest economic and financial crisis in three decades and so we returned to the field and conducted a re-survey of 25% of the enumeration areas included in IFLS. That survey, IFLS2+, was completed in late 1998 and the next wave, IFLS3, was completed during the last half of 2000. The surveys provide a unique opportunity to assess the impact of the crisis on the health and well-being of the Indonesian population.

10 Height is measured with Shorr wooden measuring boards, weight with SECA scales specially designed for field anthropometry surveys conducted by UNICEF. Blood haemoglobin levels are measured using the Hemocue portable photometer. Lung capacity is measured with Personal Best peak flow meters; each respondent performs the test three times and the top score is used in the analyses below. Blood pressure is measured using an Omran self-inflating meter with a digital readout.

11 See, for example, Mackenbach et al. (1996) who report greater under-reporting of chronic conditions by those with less education in the Netherlands.

12 This suggests there would be a substantial pay-off to the development of ADL-type questions that discriminate among prime age adults.

13 See, for example, the Matlab Health and Social Survey in Bangladesh and pilot studies conducted by WHO.

14 The regressions include controls for age (spline) and location of residence, which are suppressed from the tables.

REFERENCES

Belcher DW, Neumann AK, Wurapa FK, Lourie IM (1976) Comparison of morbidity interviews with health examination survey in rural Africa. *American Journal of Tropical Medicine and Hygiene*, 25(5):751–758.

Bhatia JC, Cleland J (1995) Self-reported symptoms of gynecological morbidity and their treatment in South India. *Studies in Family Planning*, 26(4):203–216.

Borawski EA, Kinney JM, Kahana E (1996) The meaning of older adults' health appraisals: congruence with health status and determinant of mortality. *Journals of Gerontology. Series B, Psychological Sciences and Social Sciences*, 51(3):S157–S170.

Cleveland WS (1980) Robust locally weighted regression and smoothing scatterplots. *Journal of the American Statistical Association*, 74(368):829–836.

Daltroy LH, Phillips CB, Eaton HM, et al. (1995) Objectively measuring physical ability in elderly persons. The physical capacity evaluation. *American Journal of Public Health*, 85(4):558–560.

Deeg DJH, van Zonneveld RJ, van der Maas PJ, Habbema JD (1989) Medical and social predictors of longevity in the elderly: total predictive value and interdependence. *Social Science and Medicine,* **29**(11):1271–1280.

Dow W, Gertler P, Schoeni R, Strauss J, Thomas D (1997) *Health prices, health outcomes and labor outcomes: experimental evidence.* (RAND working paper, DRU-1588-NIA)

Fischer G, Pappas G, Limb M (1996) Prospects, problems, and prerequisites for national health examination surveys in developing countries. *Social Science and Medicine,* **42**(12):1639–1650.

Hoeymans N, Feskens EJM, van den Bos GAM, Kromhout D (1996) Measuring functional status: cross-sectional and longitudinal associations between performance and self-report (Zutphen Elderly Study 1990–1993). *Journal of Clinical Epidemiology,* **49**(10):1103–1110.

Idler EL, Benyamini Y (1997) Self-rated health and mortality: a review of twenty-seven community studies. *Journal of Health and Social Behavior,* **38**(1):21–37.

Johnson RJ, Wolinsky FD (1993) The structure of health status among older adults: disease, disability, functional limitation, and perceived health. *Journal of Health and Social Behavior,* **34**(2):105–121.

Kopec JA (1995) Concepts of disability: the activity space model. *Social Science and Medicine,* **40**(5):649–656.

Krause NM, Jay GM (1994) What do global self-rated health items measure? *Medical Care,* **32**(9):930–942.

Kroeger A (1985) Response errors and other problems of health interview surveys in developing countries. *World Health Statistics Quarterly,* **38**(1):15–37.

Krueger DE (1957) Measurement of prevalence of chronic disease by household interviews and clinical evaluations. *American Journal of Public Health,* **47**:953–960.

Mackenbach JP, Looman CWN, van der Meer JBW (1996) Differences in the misreporting of chronic conditions, by level of education: the effect on inequalities in prevalence rates. *American Journal of Public Health,* **86**(5):706–711.

McCallum J, Shadbolt B, Wang DL (1994) Self-rated health and survival: a 7-year follow-up study of Australian elderly. *American Journal of Public Health,* **84**(7):1100–1105.

Murray CJL, Chen LC (1992) Understanding morbidity change. *Population and Development Review,* **18**(3):481–503.

Nagi SZ (1965) Congruency in medical and self-assessment of disability. *Industrial Medicine and Surgery,* **38**(3):27–36.

NCHS (1961) *Health interview responses compared with medical records.* Vital Health Statistics. (Series D no 5.) Public Health Service Publication, United States National Center for Health Statistics, Washington, DC.

Newhouse J, et al. (1993) *Free for all? Lessons from the RAND health insurance experiment.* Harvard University Press, Cambridge, MA.

Pappas G, Gergen PJ, Carroll M (1990) Hypertension prevalence and the status of awareness, treatment, and control in the Hispanic health and nutrition examination survey (HHANES), 1982–84. *American Journal of Public Health*, 80(12):1431–1436.

Parsons D (1991) Self-screening in targeted public transfer programs. *Journal of Political Economy*, 99(4):859–876.

Pijls LT, Feskens EJM, Kromhout D (1993) Self-rated health, mortality, and chronic diseases in elderly men. The Zutphen study, 1985–1990. *American Journal of Epidemiology*, 138(10):840–848.

Reuben DB, Siu AL, Kimapu S (1992) The predictive validity of self-report and performance-based measures of function and health. *Journals of Gerontology, Series A, Biological and Medical Sciences*, 47(4):M106–M110.

Ross DA, Vaughan JP (1986) Health interview surveys in developing countries: a methodological review. *Studies in Family Planning*, 17(2):78–94.

Sadana R (2000) Measuring reproductive health: review of community-based approaches to assess morbidity. *Bulletin of the World Health Organization*, 78(5):640–654.

Sadana R, Mathers CD, Lopez AD, Murray CJL, Iburg K (2000) *Comparative analysis of more than 50 household surveys on health status* . (GPE discussion paper no 15.) World Health Organization/Global Programme on Evidence for Health Policy, Geneva.

Scott WK, Macera CA, Cornman CB, Sharpe PA (1997) Functional health status as a predictor of mortality in men and women over 65. *Journal of Clinical Epidemiology*, 50(3):291–296.

Sindelar J, Thomas D (1991) *Measurement of child health: maternal response bias*. Mimeo (Discussion paper.) Yale University, Economic Growth Center, New Haven, CT.

Smith AM, Shelley JM, Dennerstein L (1994) Self-rated health: biological continuum or social discontinuity? *Social Science and Medicine*, 39(1):77–83.

Stewart A, Ware J, eds. (1992) *Measuring functioning and well-being: the medical outcomes study*. Duke University Press, Durham.

Strauss J, Gertler P, Rahman O, Fox K (1993) Gender and life-cycle differentials in the patterns and determinants of adult health. *Journal of Human Resources*, 28(4):791–837.

Strauss J, Thomas D (1996) Measurement and mis-measurement of social indicators. *American Economic Review*, 86(2):30–34.

Waldron I (1983) Sex differences in illness incidence, prognosis and mortality: issues and evidence. *Social Science and Medicine*, 17(16):1107–1123.

Younis N, Khattab H, Zurayk H, et al. (1993) A community study of gynecological and related morbidities in rural Egypt. *Studies in Family Planning*, 24(3):175–186.

Zurayk H, Khattab H, Younis N, et al. (1993) Concepts and measures of reproductive morbidity. *Health Transitions Review*, 3(1):17–40.

Zurayk H, Khattab H, Younis N, et al. (1995) Comparing women's reports with medical diagnoses of reproductive morbidity conditions in rural Egypt. *Studies in Family Planning,* **26**(1):14–21.

Chapter 8.3

NEW APPROACHES TO ENHANCE CROSS-POPULATION COMPARABILITY OF SURVEY RESULTS

CHRISTOPHER J.L. MURRAY, AJAY TANDON, JOSHUA A. SALOMON, COLIN D. MATHERS AND RITU SADANA

INTRODUCTION

In constructing summary measures of population health, there is a fundamental need for cross-population comparable data on the health states of individuals. In the broadest sense, comparability is required not only across countries, but also within countries over time, or across different sub-populations delineated by age, sex, education, income or other characteristics.

The primary challenge in seeking cross-population comparable measures is that the most accessible sources of data relating to health domain levels are categorical self-reported data. When categorical data are used as the basis for understanding quantities that are determined on a continuous, cardinal scale, the problem of cross-population comparability emerges from differences in the way different individuals use categorical response scales. Efforts to ensure linguistic equivalence of questions across different settings may improve the psychometric properties of these questions in terms of traditional criteria such as reliability and within-population validity, but they will not resolve problems stemming from non-comparability in the interpretation and use of response categories. There has been great progress over the past three decades in developing health status measurement instruments that are reliable and demonstrate within-population validity (Bergner et al. 1976; Chambers et al. 1976; Fanshel and Bush 1970; Feeney et al. 1995; Hunt et al. 1981; Krabbe et al. 1999; Ware 1993; reviewed in Sadana, chapter 7.1). Even with these advances, however, results obtained using these instruments are usually not comparable across populations (Sadana et al., chapter 8.1), or across different socio-economic subgroups within populations (Iburg et al., chapter 8.4). Thus, cross-population comparability represents a more stringent criterion for evaluation of measurement instruments, beyond the traditional concepts of reliability and validity.

In this paper, we begin by reviewing the general problem of cross-population comparability using a series of empirical examples. We introduce a conceptual framework for understanding the comparability problem in terms of differences in response category cut-points. We then examine the limitations of existing approaches to the problem. Finally, we outline a series of new strategies for enhancing the cross-population comparability of health measures using both new measurement instruments and new analytical tools.

THE PROBLEM OF CROSS-POPULATION COMPARABILITY

Empirical examples suggesting that self-reported categorical data on health lack cross-population comparability abound. A number of different studies have pointed to likely differences in the use of response categories on self-reported assessments of general health, morbidity or levels on particular domains of health:

- In Australian national health surveys comparing the self-reported health status of Aboriginals with that of the general population, only around 12% of the Aboriginal population characterized their own health status as fair or poor, while more than 20% of the general population rated their health in these low categories. By any other major indicator of mortality and morbidity, the Aboriginal population fares much worse than the general population, which suggests that there may be important differences in the interpretation of categorical responses in the different sub-populations due to shifts in response category cut-points (Mathers and Douglas 1998).

- Residents of the state of Kerala in India—which has the lowest rates of infant and child mortality and the highest rates of literacy in India—consistently report the highest incidences of morbidity in the country (Murray 1996).

- A series of studies from the Living Standards Measurement Surveys has examined the gradient of reported illness as a function of income and found that individuals in higher income quantiles consistently report more illness than those with lower income levels (Murray and Chen 1992).

- A recent study presenting self-reported data from 12 countries in the European Union showed implausibly wide cross-country disparities in the proportion of the population reporting *bad* and *very bad* general health, ranging from a high of 19 percent in Portugal to a low of 5 percent in Ireland (Eurostat 1997). Such wide variation in levels of health within the European Union is unlikely, given other major health indicators, and cannot be explained solely by linguistic differences or measurement error.

- A critical review and re-analysis of 64 data sets covering self-reported health status from population-based surveys in 46 countries provide similar results (Sadana et al., chapter 8.1). Data concerning the level and distribution of health do not appear comparable across or even within populations, leading the authors to conclude that the information content of these surveys is suspect. Many surveys do not meet even the weakest form of criterion validity, i.e. that some decrements from "full health" are noted, and that self-reported health decreases with age, particularly in the oldest age groups.

Response category cut-point shifts

The problem of comparability can be conceptualized in terms of response category cut-point shifts across populations, across subgroups within a population, or within the same population over time. Figure 1 illustrates the primary challenge of using self-reported levels on a health status domain (even when reliability and within-population validity have been well established). For each domain, there is some true or latent scale for that domain that is, by definition, unobserved. So, for instance, imagine that there is a latent mobility scale, depicted in the first column of Figure 1. Now imagine a self-reported survey question that asks respondents how much difficulty they have walking up stairs and offers five response categories: "no difficulty", "mild difficulty", "moderate difficulty", "severe difficulty", and "extreme difficulty/cannot do". The second column in the figure shows the response category cut-points for population A. These are

Figure 1   Mapping from latent mobility scale to categorical responses

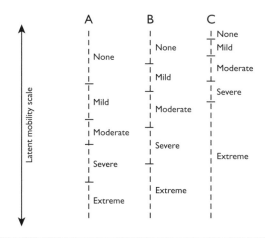

levels of mobility at which an individual will shift from one response category to another. The lowest cut-point in the figure shows the transition from answering "extreme/cannot do" to "severe difficulty". In population B, the response category cut-points are shifted relative to those in population A so that a higher level of mobility is associated with each of the response categories. Population C shows a third example with even more shift in the cut-points. The implication is dramatic. A response of "mild difficulty" walking up stairs, for instance, maps to a different level of mobility in populations A, B and C. In this example, survey results may be reliable and valid within each population, but the results cannot be compared across populations without adjustment.

We can hypothesize that cut-points may vary between populations because of different cultural expectations for domains of health. Cut-points are also likely to vary within a cultural group. The cut-points for older individuals may shift as their expectations for a domain diminish with age. Men may be more likely to deny declines in health so that their cut-points may be systematically shifted as compared to women. Contact with health services may influence expectations for a domain and thus shift cut-points (Caldwell and Caldwell 1991; Johansson 1991; Johansson 1992; Murray and Chen 1992; Riley 1992). Response category cut-point shifts can make crude comparisons of results across populations nearly meaningless, even when exactly the same questions are used, as illustrated by some of the examples already provided.

STRATEGIES TO ENHANCE CROSS-POPULATION COMPARABILITY

Comparable measurement of individual health and population health in different settings requires using the same questions or items in similar surveys. In addition, it requires explicit strategies to measure the response category cut-points of each item in different populations and socio-demographic groups. Methods to establish cut-points fall into two basic categories, each of which is discussed below. The first strategy is to establish a scale that is strictly comparable across individuals and populations. Measurements on the comparable scale can then be used to establish the response category cut-points for each survey item. The second approach is to elicit categorical responses from different groups for a fixed level on the latent scale. If the level is fixed, variation in the responses provides information on the differences in cut-points across individuals and populations.

USING A COMPARABLE SCALE TO ESTABLISH RESPONSE CATEGORY CUT-POINTS

There are at least two main strategies for establishing a comparable scale of measurement: (a) the use of multiple items (i.e. questions) for measuring a particular domain; and (b) the incorporation of exogenous information such as a measured performance test. In the following section, we begin by describing the general approach of using multiple domain items, consider the limitations of this approach and introduce an alternative approach using measured tests to establish a comparable scale.

Item response theory

Psychometricians have over several decades developed powerful statistical models to establish response category cut-points for different items in a survey instrument by comparing each response category to the underlying factor in the data. This body of work is often associated with the term item response theory (IRT). IRT has been used widely, for example, to establish the difficulty of different standardized scholastic test items. There are many different statistical models used in the application of IRT, and the field is rapidly expanding (Thissen and Steinberg 1986; van der Linden and Hambleton 1997). The basic building block for many of these models is the one-parameter Rasch model, which is a variant of the conditional logit with a fixed effect. With more than two response categories, the Rasch model generalizes to the partial credit model (PCM) (Masters 1982).

Estimation of the partial credit model is based on specification of the probability of responding in a particular category rather than in the previous category, which is modelled as an increasing function of a person's "ability" (level on a particular domain) and a decreasing function of the item response "difficulty". The "difficulty" parameters specify the level on the latent variable at which an individual is more likely to respond in a particular category than in the previous category. It is worth noting that these difficulty parameters do not correspond exactly to the notion of response category cut-points described above, but they are conceptually related in that they refer to the probabilities of responding in each category.

The individual "ability" is captured through a fixed effect for each individual, although in practice the use of the conditional logit means that these fixed effects are not directly estimated. The key insight in the model is that the response data can be used to estimate both the difficulties of various questions and the abilities of various individuals because the difficulties *for a particular question* are assumed to be the same for all individuals, and multiple responses per individual allow for estimation of their ability.

The key challenge in developing cross-population comparable measures from survey data is to detect systematic shifts in cut-points across different populations, or what is known as differential item functioning (DIF) in psychometric parlance. A variety of methods have been developed to identify DIF, but these methods all assume that DIF applies only to a subset of items used to measure a domain, so that a comparable scale can be established using the underlying factor in the data from the remaining items. If all items suffer DIF in a systematic and correlated fashion, IRT is unable to identify this problem (Holland and Weiner 1993).

A simple thought experiment can prove that no statistical procedure can deal with this problem in its extreme form without the addition of exogenous information. Imagine a domain such as mobility. In population A the distribution of mobility on the latent scale is normal with mean 5 and standard deviation 2 (in units with interval scale properties on some arbitrary scale). In population B, the distribution of mobility is normal with mean 8 and standard deviation of 2. In population B, all the response category cut-points on all items about mobility are exactly 3 units higher than in population A. The net result is that the distribution of responses on all items in the survey in the two populations will be identical. In other words, population B has much higher mobility than A but the survey gives identical responses. No statistical method can identify this difference because the data are completely identical.

Because we have strong prior beliefs that cut-points on items are likely to shift systematically for a domain, we suspect that the potential to establish cross-population comparability using only the underlying factor in the response data without additional information is limited. For this reason, exogenous information is needed to aid in establishing cross-population comparability.

Measured tests and the HOPIT model

One type of exogenous information that could be used to establish a comparable scale is a measured calibration test for a particular domain. A calibration test can establish a comparable scale if: (a) it adequately captures a domain, and (b) it can be implemented in different settings without systematic bias in the results.[1] Such calibration tests are not feasible for a number of domains of health such as pain or affect. For some domains such as vision, hearing, cognition, mobility and others, calibration tests are feasible. In the WHO Multi-Country Household Survey Study on Health and Responsiveness (Üstün et al. 2001), low-cost calibration tests have been included for three domains of health:

- The Snellen's chart to measure visual acuity (distant vision). Since cross-national surveys include a range of literacy levels, we have selected the "tumbling E's" version of the Snellen's chart (Coren 1987).

- In the domain of cognition, verbal fluency has been tested with a category naming task, vigilance with color-shape cancellation and short term memory with verbal recall (Wilson et al. 1987; Spreen and Strauss 1998).

- A modified version of the posturo-locomotion-manual (PLM) test for mobility has been implemented (Kokko et al. 1997). Though the original version of the test was designed for use in sophisticated laboratory conditions with computerized equipment, it has been adapted for use in survey settings to obtain gross measures of mobility.

Test-retest reliability was found to be acceptable in pilot tests of these performance measurements. With more careful quality control on the calibration tests, we expect that test-retest will rise substantially. Further work on other calibration tests for other domains or alternatives for these domains will be needed. Additional calibration tests could be considered for hearing (audiometry), sleep (polysomnography), or exercise tolerance (treadmill).

Given a reliable and valid measured test for a domain, variation in response category cut-points for the self-reported items on these domains may be estimated using the heirarchical ordered probit (HOPIT) model (Tandon et al. 2001). The HOPIT model is a variant of the standard ordered probit model, which assumes that there is an unobserved latent variable that is normally distributed. Observed categorical responses depend on the categorical cut-points on this latent scale. The key difference between HOPIT and the standard ordered probit model is that these cut-points are allowed to vary as a function of covariates in the HOPIT model. In essence, this means that the mapping from the underlying latent variable to the categorical responses depends on individual characteristics. As illustrated in Tandon et al. (2001), the HOPIT model is able to recover the cut-points in simulated data sets quite well using exogenous information (such as measured test results) to fix the scale of the latent variable, and consistently outperforms models that do not incorporate this exogenous information.

USING FIXED ABILITY COMPARISONS TO ASSESS VARIATION IN CUT-POINTS

For some domains of health such as pain, reliable and valid measured tests may not exist, may not be affordable, or may be unethical, even for a subsample. An alternative strategy for establishing cross-population comparability is to fix the level of health on a domain and assess variation in the response categories across individuals, groups and populations. In other words, if the level of mobility is fixed but one group says that this level maps to a response category of "no difficulty" and another says it maps to the category "some difficulty", this information can be used to assess the response category cut-points. Two strategies are available for fixed ability comparisons: vignettes and comparable homogeneous groups.

Establishing cross-population comparability using vignettes

The primary strategy for using fixed ability comparisons to establish comparable scales is the use of vignettes, as described in detail in Salomon et al. (2001). A vignette is a description of a concrete level of ability on a given domain that individuals are asked to evaluate using the same question and response scale as the self-report question on that domain. For example, one self-report question on health in the WHO survey instrument is: *Overall in the last 30 days how much difficulty did you have with self-*

care? (1 = None, 2 = Mild, 3 = Moderate, 4 = Severe, 5 = Extreme/cannot do).

To assess the response category cut-points, each respondent is also asked to assess levels of self-care for hypothetical cases described with vignettes, for example:

> [John] cannot wash, groom or dress himself without personal help. He has no problems with feeding.

> How would you rate his difficulty with *self-care*?

None	1
Mild	2
Moderate	3
Severe	4
Extreme/cannot do	5

The vignette fixes a given level of self-care so that variation in the response categories is attributable to variation in the response category cut-points. When individuals are asked to evaluate a series of vignettes of varying severity, the cut-points can be evaluated using the HOPIT model (Tandon et al. 2001). The vignette version of the HOPIT model is constructed such that the dependent variable is the categorical response for a given vignette, and the independent variables are simply indicator variables for each vignette. An underlying latent variable representing level of ability on self-care is assumed to exist, with a fixed value associated with each vignette. The probability of responding in a particular category is then modelled in reference to individual cut-points expressed as a function of covariates such as country of residence, age, sex, education and income.[2]

Using comparable homogeneous groups to establish cross-population comparability

Another way to evaluate a fixed ability and thus variation in cut-points is to identify comparable homogeneous groups in different populations and compare their responses to an item. Recent acute changes in health status from injuries such as fractures might be used to identify reasonably comparable groups. Alternatively some lifestyle or occupational characteristic might be used such as elite athletes.

There are two main limitations to this strategy. First, identifying groups needs to be independent of any measurement of health status. Even when groups are identified through some factor such as an injury, doubts can always be raised about the true comparability of groups. It may be difficult to persuade people that apparent differences in the responses are due to cut-point shift as opposed to differences in that domain between groups. Second, to be able to assess variation in response category cut-points for all response categories, a series of homogeneous groups must be used. Analytically, each homogeneous group is like one vignette. This means that the comparable group strategy can only work if several comparable groups are studied. Despite these limitations, it may be worthwhile assessing comparable groups as an adjunct to other methods.

Discussion

One of the key conclusions of this paper is that adjustments are needed to make survey results comparable across populations. In particular, when categorical variables are involved, it is essential to account for differences in response category cut-points. There is considerable evidence that suggests that response category cut-points vary across countries, and even across subgroups within a country. Therefore, until cut-points are assessed, analysts must start from a presumption that results are not comparable across populations.

Four strategies were identified to enhance cross-population comparability; of these, we believe that the most promising are the use of vignettes and the inclusion of measured performance tests on some domains where possible. The use of vignettes is especially attractive because vignettes are low cost and involve no special measurement techniques. This makes them potentially easy to implement across a variety of survey settings and domains.

We emphasize that the problem of cross-population comparability applies not only to cross-country comparisons but also to comparisons within countries across different socioeconomic and demographic groups. This problem has important implications for the measurement of inequality, which may be greater or smaller than measured before accounting for response category cut-point shifts. It also has critical implications for comparisons over time. Cut-points may shift systematically over time (e.g. due to rising income, education, and health norms), so long term trends may be difficult to assess without correction.

There are several avenues to explore for further development of the strategies discussed here. In the area of measured calibration tests, a number of additional analyses are warranted: different tests could be identified for calibration purposes, test-retest reliability needs to be investigated further, and strategies for eliminating systematic biases in implementation of these tests need to be examined. Another area of development is to strengthen the connection between the HOPIT model and IRT. Further research is also required for the strategy of using vignettes. The performance of different vignettes, individually and as sets, should be evaluated systematically in order to identify vignettes that perform best on each domain. Cross-validation of vignette results and measured tests where available may also be useful.

Notes

1   As long as the measurement error in the measured tests is randomly distributed it should not create much bias in the results. However, the estimation will

be more complicated if the measurement error is explicitly accounted for in the likelihood process (e.g. by using an errors-in-variables type approach to estimation).

2   Vignettes can also be used with the PCM model. For details see Tandon et al. (2001).

References

Bergner M, Bobbit RA, Kressel S, et al. (1976) The sickness impact profile: conceptual formulation and methodology for the development of a health status measure. *International Journal of Health Services*, **6**(3):393–415.

Caldwell J, Caldwell P (1991) What have we learnt about the cultural, social and behavioral determinants of health? From selected readings to the first health transition workshop. *Health Transition Review*, **1**(1):3–20.

Chambers LW, Sackett DL, Goldsmith C, Macpehrson AS, McAuley RG (1976) Development and application of an index of social function. *Health Services Research*, **11**(4):430–441.

Coren S (1987) Reporting the visual acuity of groups: the relation among alternate measures. *American Journal of Optometry and Physiological Optics*, **64**(12):897–900.

Eurostat (1997) *Self-reported health in the European Community. Statistics in focus.* (Population and social conditions, 12.) Eurostat, Luxembourg.

Fanshel S, Bush JW (1970) A health-status index and its application to health services outcomes. *Operations Research*, **18**(6):1021–1065.

Feeny D, Furlong W, Boyle M, Torrance GW (1995) Multi-attribute health status classification systems: Health Utilities Index. *PharmacoEconomics*, **7**(6):490–502.

Holland PW, Wainer H (1993) *Differential item functioning.* Lawrence Erlbaum Associates, Hillsdale, NJ.

Hunt SM, McKenna SP, McEwen J, Williams J, Papp E (1981) The Nottingham Health Profile: subjective health status and medical consultations. *Social Science and Medicine*, **15**(3 pt 1):221–229.

Johansson SR (1991) The health transition: the cultural inflation of morbidity during the decline of mortality. *Health Transition Review*, **1**(1):39–68.

Johansson SR (1992) Measuring the cultural inflation of morbidity during the decline of mortality. *Health Transition Review*, **2**(1):78–89.

Kokko SM, Paltamaaa J, Ahola E, Malkia E (1997) The assessment of functional ability in patients with Parkinson's disease: the PLM-test and three clinical tests. *Physiotherapy Research International*, **2**(2):29–45.

Krabbe PF, Stouthard MEA, Essink-Bot ML, Bonsel GJ (1999) The effect of adding a cognitive dimension to the EuroQol multiattribute health-status classification system. *Journal of Clinical Epidemiology*, **52**(4):293–301.

Masters GN (1982) A Rasch model for partial credit scoring. *Psychometrika*, **47**(2):149–174.

Mathers CD, Douglas RM (1998) Measuring progress in population health and wellbeing. In: *Measuring progress: is life getting better?* CSIRO Publishing, Collingwood, Victoria.

Murray CJL (1996) Epidemiology and morbidity transitions in India. In: *Health, poverty and development in India.* DasGupta M, Chen LC, Krishnan TN, eds. Oxford University Press, Delhi.

Murray CJL, Chen LC (1992) Understanding morbidity change. *Population and Development Review,* **18**(3):481–503.

Riley JC (1992) From a high mortality regime to a high morbidity regime: is culture everything in sickness? *Health Transition Review,* **2**(1):71–78.

Salomon JA, Tandon A, Murray CJL (2001) *Using vignettes to improve cross-population comparability of health surveys: concepts, design, and evaluation techniques.* (GPE discussion paper no 41.) World Health Organization/Global Programme on Evidence for Health Policy, Geneva.

Spreen O, Strauss E (1998) *A compendium of neuropsychological tests.* Oxford University Press, New York.

Tandon A, Murray CJL, Salomon JA (2001) *Statistical methods for enhancing cross-population comparability.* (GPE discussion paper no 42.) World Health Organization/Global Programme on Evidence for Health Policy, Geneva.

Thissen D, Steinberg L (1986) A taxonomy of item response models. *Psychometrika,* **51**(4):567–577.

Üstün TB, Chatterji S, Villanueva M, et al. (2001) *WHO multi-country household survey study on health and responsiveness, 2000–2001.* (GPE discussion paper no 37.) World Health Organization/Global Programme on Evidence for Health Policy, Geneva.

van der Linden WJ, Hambleton RK (1997) *Handbook of modern item response theory.* Springer-Verlag, New York.

Ware JE, Snow KK, Kosinski M, Gandek B (1993) *SF-36 Health survey manual and interpretation guide.* The Health Institute, New England Medical Center, Boston, MA.

Wilson B, Cockburn J, Halligan PW (2002) Development of behavioural test of visuospatial neglect. *Archives of Physical Medicine and Rehabilitation,* **68**:98–102.

Chapter 8.4

CROSS-POPULATION COMPARABILITY
OF PHYSICIAN-ASSESSED AND SELF-
REPORTED MEASURES OF HEALTH

KIM MOESGAARD IBURG, JOSHUA A. SALOMON,
AJAY TANDON AND CHRISTOPHER J.L. MURRAY

INTRODUCTION

Assessing levels of health on various domains is a key component of measuring population health, evaluating the impact of health interventions and monitoring individual health levels. Meaningful comparisons across countries are useful in setting goals for the improvement of population health and charting progress towards attaining these goals. Comparisons are also useful within countries in order to understand differences in health levels across subpopulations and to measure health inequalities.

Efforts to compare self-reported health status across population subgroups often have indicated major differences between males and females, high and low income, between different ethnic groups, or across various other demographic and socioeconomic variables. One of the challenges in the measurement of individual health, however, has been in interpreting self-reported health data in a way that allows meaningful comparisons. Empirical evidence pointing to concerns about the comparability of self-reported data on health abounds. Substantial evidence shows that disability rates have been falling rapidly over the last two decades while trends in self-reported health have been more mixed. In some studies, higher income groups report higher morbidity than lower income groups, even though observed disability declines rapidly with income (Murray and Chen 1992). The challenge is to ascertain how much of the difference is determined by real differences in health and how much is due to differences in the way individuals report on their health relative to different norms and expectations. Previous studies describing comparisons of self-reported health have raised concerns about the face validity of some of these measures, highlighting the fundamental challenge of cross-population comparability.

A number of different approaches have been taken to improve comparability of self-reported data both across and within countries. One approach has been to ensure that specific survey items have the same meaning across languages and different cultural settings. Variations among questions used in health surveys, such as recall periods, definitions of terms, and response categories are documented for 16 surveys conducted in 11 European Union countries (Rasmussen et al. 1999) and another 30 surveys from 23 OECD countries (Gudex and Lafortune 2000). The main findings were that variations in question content are prevalent in nearly all health surveys, with the exception of those that use standardized health status instruments such as the SF-36 or EuroQol. The best example of attempts to minimize differences in items in health surveys is probably the adaptation of the standardized SF-36 questionnaire to more than 40 countries (Ware 2000). But while this may help to remove one important barrier to comparisons, it does not account for the fact that individuals may have different expectations for health that are unrelated to linguistic differences in the phrasing of questions.

A key obstacle to cross-population comparability that remains even after reliability and within-population validity of instruments is established relates to the fact that survey questionnaires most commonly elicit categorical responses, which do not provide cardinal values for levels of health; i.e. distances between response categories are not equal, and are unknown. Comparisons are complicated by the fact that different individuals use the categorical response scales in different ways. We may conceptualize these differences in terms of variation in individual response category cut-points, which mark the boundaries between categories in reference to an unobserved, continuous latent scale. Attempts to establish equivalent scale endpoints across different questions may offer some benefits in enhancing comparisons, but they cannot account for cut-point shifts. A recent study by the World Health Organization (Sadana et al., chapter 8.1) described a confirmatory factor analytic approach to fix the endpoints of self-reported data in order to improve the comparability of estimated health levels from household interview surveys in 64 countries. Despite efforts to improve comparability of endpoints, the study concluded that a valid and meaningful comparison of existing data on non-fatal health from household interview surveys across countries was limited.

Even in cases where cut-point differences would seem unlikely, as in binary questions about clearly defined physical phenomena, surprising results have been reported. For example, a study from Ghana (Belcher et al. 1976) showed that missing body parts very rarely were self-reported. Other studies have found large differences between self-reported morbidity and clinical examinations (Krueger 1957), and cross-cultural differences in people's experiences of illness severity and norms for when to seek health services are well-documented (Bletzer 1993; Hunt et al. 1981; Tsuji et al. 1994). When are people feeling sick enough to label themselves as sick persons—or healthy enough to say that they have excellent health? Clearly these differences may depend not only on cultural influences but also on age, sex, race and socioeconomic status. In order to gauge these differences in scale references, exogenous information is required in order to translate categorical responses into comparable cardinal measures.

It is worth noting that problems stemming from the non-comparability of categorical response data apply not only to self-reported information but to any source of data that uses categorical responses. Thus, while it may be useful to distinguish self-reported data from physician assessments, both forms of information are subject to the constraints of the question format that they employ. In both cases, responses to categorical questions will depend critically on the individual cut-points for a particular question.

Murray et al. (chapter 8.3) have outlined a series of different strategies for enhancing cross-population comparability of survey results through the formal analysis of systematic cut-point shifts. One way to address this problem, whether it arises in self-reported or physician-assessed data, is by fixing the levels of the unobserved latent variable of interest in order to isolate cut-point differences as the source of variation in assessments of these levels. There are several ways of fixing the scales, including the use of vignettes (Salomon et al. 2001) or the inclusion of measured tests. In combination with new statistical models described by Tandon et al. (2001), the incorporation of this exogenous information allows estimation of variation in cut-points attributable to socio-demographic or other factors.

In this paper, we describe the application of this new approach to the publically-available Third National Health and Nutrition Examination Survey dataset. Using the results of performance tests on the domain of mobility from this survey, we estimate differences in cut-points for various sub-groups in the United States population on a range of self-reported and physician-assessed items relating to this domain. The objective of this paper is to examine whether sex, race/ethnicity and income affect self-reports and physician-assessments of mobility through predictable differences in the use of categorical responses.

MATERIALS AND METHODS

DATA

Data originate from the Third National Health and Nutrition Examination Survey (NHANES III), conducted in the United States from 1988 to 1994 (NCHS 1999). NHANES is a periodic survey conducted by the National Center for Health Statistics, Centers for Disease Control and Prevention, designed to obtain health information on the non-institutionalized civilian population through interviews, physical examinations and laboratory tests. The full data set includes information on approximately 40 000 respondents aged 2 months and older, based on a complex stratified sampling design.

NHANES III includes items relating to a large number of different health domains. For this study, the objective was to identify one domain to illustrate a new approach to estimating cut-point differences in both self-reported descriptions and physician assessments of health levels. The approach relies on the availability of measured tests that can be used to fix the scale of the unobserved latent variable (level of ability on a particular domain) in order to understand systematic differences in response category cut-points across different sub-populations.

Our choice of domain for this analysis was guided by a review of existing health status instruments in order to develop an extensive list of candidate domains, followed by a systematic inventory of the number of self-reported, physician assessed and measured items available on various domains. This inventory is summarized in Table 1 using a listing of domains from the Health Utilities Index Mark III (Feeny et al. 1995) as a parsimonious catalogue of key health domains, as well as other components

Table 1   Numbers of items in NHANES III by domain and mode of assessment

Domains	Self-reported	Physician-assessed	Measured tests
Key domains			
Vision	9	3	
Hearing	6	1	2
Speech	1	1	
Getting around (physical ability)	15	5	7
Hands and fingers (dexterity)	5	4	1
Feelings (emotional function)	12	5	
Memory and thinking (cognitive function)	9	1	2
Pain and discomfort	22	2	
Other components of health			
General health	5	9	
Social functioning	12		
Body mass index	2	1	1
Height	1		1
Weight	2	1	1
Dental status	3	1	
Blood pressure	1		1
Pulse			1
Lung function	3	1	1
Allergy	2	1	1
Blood	2		1
Urine	1		1
Gall bladder	1		1
Ocular photo	1		1

of health captured by various items in the survey. Across different domains, there are varying numbers of items on self-reports, physician assessments and measured performance tests. The domain in NHANES III with the largest number of available items across the three assessment types is physical ability.

The choice of the domain of physical ability leads to a more narrow focus on those examinees aged 60 years and older, as the physical performance tests in NHANES III are confined to this subsample. In total, the final study population includes 5 724 respondents who completed the battery of physical performance measures. Within the domain of physical ability, we have identified the questions of interest more precisely as those pertaining specifically to mobility or ambulation, which resulted in

Table 2   Mobility items and response codes from NHANES III

Item	Response codes
Self-reported	
Difficulty walking for a quarter of a mile (about 2 or 3 blocks)	(Note *a*)
Difficulty walking up 10 steps without resting	(Note *a*)
Difficulty stooping, crouching or kneeling	(Note *a*)
Difficulty lifting or carrying something as heavy as 10 pounds (like a sack of potatoes or rice)	(Note *a*)
Difficulty doing chores around the house (like vacuuming, sweeping, dusting or straightening up)	(Note *a*)
Difficulty walking from one room to another on the same level	(Note *a*)
Difficulty getting in or out of bed	(Note *a*)
Physician-assessed	
Estimated level of difficulty: walking ¼ mile	(Note *b*)
Estimated level of difficulty: running 100 yards	(Note *b*)
Estimated level of difficulty: stooping, crouching, or kneeling	(Note *b*)
Estimated level of difficulty: doing heavy housework, gardening, exercise or play	(Note *b*)
Measured tests	
Right shoulder external rotation	(1) full, (2) partial, (3) unable
Left shoulder external rotation	(1) full, (2) partial, (3) unable
Right hip and knee flexion	(1) full, (2) partial, (3) unable
Left hip and knee flexion	(1) full, (2) partial, (3) unable
Time to complete 8-foot walk (mean time from 2 trials)	2–60 seconds
Time tandem stand held	(1) 10 or more seconds, (2) 1–9 sec, (3) not able
Time to complete five stands (from an armless chair)	2–93 seconds

a. Response codes for self-reports were (1) unable to do, (2) much difficulty, (3) some difficulty, and (4) no difficulty.

b. Response codes for physician assessments were (1) could not be done, (2) moderate difficulty, (3) some difficulty, and (4) no difficulty.

the selection of seven self-reported items, four physician-assessed items, and seven measured tests (Table 2). Self-reported items concern ability to walk, climb stairs, bend down, carry heavy objects, do household chores, and get in and out of bed. Physician assessments refer to abilities to walk, run, bend down, and perform heavy housework and exercise. Selected physical tests relate to shoulder movements, hip and knee flexibility and timed performance measurements, such as walking eight feet and rising repeatedly from an armless chair.

As independent variables, we include sex, race/ethnicity, and median family income in the last 12 months, all defined as dichotomous variables. Thus, the combinations of these three variables delineate eight different population sub-groups for examination of differences in response category cut-points for each of the 11 self-reports and physician-assessments.

STATISTICAL ANALYSIS

Missing data. Across the variables included in our analysis, only approximately 64% of the observations include complete information on all variables. In order to address the problem of missing data, we adopt a multiple imputation approach as described by King et al. (2001), using the software program Amelia (Honaker et al. 1999). Five different completed data sets are imputed in order to reflect the uncertainty around the missing values, and all analyses are run separately on each dataset. The results of the five sets of analyses are then combined using standard methods (King et al. 2001).

HOPIT model. The goal of the analysis is to estimate differences in cut-points across different population sub-groups for either self-reported or physician-assessed categorical questions. The conceptual basis for the

Figure I   Illustration of cut-point differences for physical ability
                 at different sex, race and income combinations

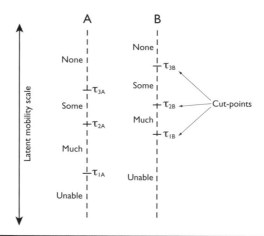

statistical model is illustrated in Figure 1. Consider as an example the following question: "How much difficulty do you have in walking for a quarter of a mile?" with response categories "unable to do", "much difficulty", "some difficulty" and "no difficulty". If we assume that there is an unobserved latent variable that represents an individual's true mobility level, then each individual's response to this question will depend on his or her cut-points, which are the threshold levels on the latent scale at which an individual will transition from one category to the next. In Figure 1, we imagine two hypothetical individuals (A and B) who have different response category cut-points for this question. At the same true mobility level, individual A may respond that she has no difficulty, while individual B reports some difficulty in walking for a quarter of a mile. With some knowledge of true mobility levels, it is possible to understand differences in responses to a particular question in terms of cut-point shifts. In this study, we use results from measured performance tests as a source of information on the unobserved mobility levels of individuals in order to quantify these cut-point shifts.

In order to estimate cut-point differences, we apply the hierarchical ordered probit (HOPIT) model, an extention of the ordered probit model described in more detail elsewhere (Tandon et al. 2001). The HOPIT model, like the standard ordered probit model, assumes that there is an unobserved latent variable Y_i^* (e.g. level of mobility) that is distributed normally with mean μ_i and variance 1, where i is an indicator for the respondent.[1] The mean level of the latent variable is described by a function of some set of covariates, in this case a vector of measured test results X_i,

$$Y_i^* \sim N(\mu_i, 1)$$

$$\mu_i = X_i' \beta$$

If we define y_i as the observed categorical response for individual i on the question of interest (either a self-report or physician assessment), the HOPIT model stipulates an observation mechanism such that, for questions with four response categories:

$$
\begin{aligned}
y_i &= 1 &&\text{if} &&-\infty \le Y_i^* < \tau_{1i} \\
y_i &= 2 &&\text{if} &&\tau_{1i} \le Y_i^* < \tau_{2i} \\
y_i &= 3 &&\text{if} &&\tau_{2i} \le Y_i^* < \tau_{3i} \\
y_i &= 4 &&\text{if} &&\tau_{3i} \le Y_i^* < \infty
\end{aligned}
$$

where τ_{1i}, τ_{2i} and τ_{3i} are the response category cut-points for individual i. The key difference between the HOPIT model and the standard ordered probit model is that these cut-points are allowed to vary as a function of covariates such as sex, race and income:

$$\tau_{ki} = Z_i'\gamma_k$$

Maximum likelihood methods are used to derive estimates of the β and γ coefficients, along with the variance-covariance matrix for these estimators. In this study, the HOPIT model is run on all seven self-reports and all four physician-assessed questions simultaneously, in order to fix the scale of the estimates across questions while allowing cut-points to vary across questions.

Uncertainty analysis. After the model is run, numerical simulation methods are used in order to compute estimated cut-points by question for the different sub-populations delineated by sex, race and income, as well as ranges around these estimates. Simulation allows the combination of the results from the five different imputed data sets in a way that reflects the uncertainty of the estimated coefficients both within and across data sets. For each separate data set, ten different draws of the vector of coefficients are generated by sampling from the joint distribution defined by the maximum likelihood estimates of the parameters and their variance-covariance matrix. For each draw, we calculate the predicted cut-points for the eight different sub-populations defined by the three covariates included in the model (sex, race and income), for each of the self-reported or physician assessed questions. The final distributions for these cut-points are produced by combining the draws from the five different analyses (creating a total of fifty draws), and we report the median value and the confidence intervals defined by values at the the 2.5th percentile and 97.5th percentile of this distribution. These estimated cut-points have been rescaled such that 0 corresponds to the point on the latent scale defined by the worst possible scores on all measured performance tests, and 1 corresponds to the point on the latent scale defined by the best possible scores on all measured tests.

RESULTS

Characteristics of the study population appear in Table 3. The study includes nearly equal numbers of men and women. The median reported income in the sample is between US $16 000 and US $17 000. Non-hispanic whites make up approximately 59% of the study population. For purposes of subgroup analyses of cut-point differences, we have defined both race and income dichotomously: race as either white (non-hispanic) or non-white, and annual family income as either above or below US $17 000 per year.

Table 4 presents a summary of the HOPIT results on cut-point differences by sex, race and income for both self-reported and physician-assessed items. For each question, the direction and magnitude of shifts are reported for the three response category cut-points: τ_3 marks the transition from "no difficulty" to "some difficulty"; τ_2 the transition from "some" to "moderate/much difficulty"; and τ_1 the transition from "moderate/much diffi-

Table 3   Characteristics of the study population ($N = 5\,724$)

	Number	Per cent
Sex		
Males	2 756	48.2
Females	2 968	51.9
Race-ethnicity		
Non-hispanic white	3 364	58.8
Non-hispanic black	1 125	19.7
Mexican-American	1 067	18.6
Other	168	2.9
Family income (last 12 months)		
Less than US $10 000	1 397	24.4
US $10 000 to 16 999	1 191	20.8
US $17 000 to 29 999	1 290	22.5
US $30 000 to 49 999	706	12.3
US $50 000 and over	438	7.7
Unknown	702	12.3

culty" to "unable to do". Of most interest in a general health survey like NHANES III is perhaps τ_3 because the largest proportion of respondents is often found in the mildest category of many questions—a phenomenon characterized as a "ceiling effect" in population surveys.

The HOPIT regression results show that there are significant differences by sex, race and income in individual cut-points separating "no difficulty" from "some difficulty" (τ_3) for all physician-assessed questions. In all cases, the direction of the effects are the same, with lower cut-points for males compared to females, for non-whites compared to whites, and for high income respondents compared to low income respondents. A lower cut-point may be interpreted as a lower standard for defining excellent mobility levels; in other words, given the same level of mobility, an individual with a lower cut-point will be more likely to characterize this level of mobility favourably than an individual with a higher cut-point.

For self-reported items, only income is a statistically significant predictor of differences in τ_3 for all questions. Sex is statistically significant for five out of seven questions and race for four out of seven questions. Where coefficients are significant, the directions of the effects are the same as in the physician assessments for all cases except for race in the items relating to walking 10 steps and walking from room to room.

Similar patterns emerge with respect to systematic differences in τ_2 for both physician assessments and self-reports, although the overall magnitude of the differences tends to be slightly smaller. A notable exception is the effect of race on physician assessments, where the size of the differences is greater for τ_2 than τ_3 on all but one question. There are fewer sig-

Table 4   Results from HOPIT analysis of self-reported and physician-assessed mobility: cutpoint differences by sex, race and income

Item	Sex (male = 1)		Race (non-white = 1)		Income (high = 1)	
	Coef.	p-value	Coef.	p-value	Coef.	p-value
Self-report						
τ_3 Walking ¼ mile	−0.171	< 0.001	−0.016	0.682	−0.287	< 0.001
Walk up 10 steps	−0.290	< 0.001	0.187	< 0.001	−0.275	< 0.001
Stooping, crouching, kneeling	−0.219	< 0.001	−0.203	< 0.001	−0.179	<0.001
Carrying 10 pounds	−0.476	< 0.001	−0.189	< 0.001	−0.253	< 0.001
Chores around the house	−0.287	< 0.001	−0.031	0.438	−0.182	< 0.001
Walking room to room	−0.081	0.123	0.165	0.002	−0.152	0.004
Getting in or out of bed	−0.075	0.084	−0.064	0.147	−0.121	0.005
τ_2 Walking ¼ mile	−0.175	< 0.001	−0.077	0.079	−0.232	< 0.001
Walk up 10 steps	−0.227	< 0.001	0.108	0.017	−0.235	< 0.001
Stooping, crouching, kneeling	−0.253	< 0.001	−0.180	< 0.001	−0.187	< 0.001
Carrying 10 pounds	−0.312	< 0.001	−0.159	< 0.001	−0.192	< 0.001
Chores around the house	−0.127	0.011	−0.068	0.184	−0.154	0.002
Walking room to room	0.050	0.522	0.068	0.388	−0.084	0.282
Getting in or out of bed	−0.079	0.268	0.112	0.111	−0.032	0.649
τ_1 Walking ¼ mile	−0.135	0.006	−0.316	< 0.001	−0.231	< 0.001
Walk up 10 steps	−0.211	< 0.001	−0.019	0.741	−0.246	< 0.001
Stooping, crouching, kneeling	−0.208	< 0.001	−0.063	< 0.001	−0.175	< 0.001
Carrying 10 pounds	−0.231	< 0.001	−0.082	0.242	−0.093	0.079
Chores around the house	0.002	0.976	0.062	0.185	0.009	0.879
Walking room to room	0.141	0.189	0.082	0.567	−0.044	0.683
Getting in or out of bed	0.009	0.947	−0.238	0.526	−0.010	0.940
Physician-assessment						
τ_3 Walking ¼ mile	−0.114	0.002	−0.171	< 0.001	−0.381	< 0.001
Running 100 yards	−0.197	< 0.001	−0.148	0.001	−0.422	< 0.001
Stooping, crouching, kneeling	−0.208	< 0.001	−0.129	< 0.001	−0.386	<0.001
Heavy housework, exercise, etc.	−0.190	< 0.001	−0.153	< 0.001	−0.394	<0.001
τ_2 Walking ¼ mile	−0.092	0.019	−0.185	< 0.001	−0.369	< 0.001
Running 100 yards	−0.170	< 0.001	−0.163	< 0.001	−0.343	< 0.001
Stooping, crouching, kneeling	−0.210	< 0.001	−0.171	< 0.001	−0.354	< 0.001
Heavy housework, exercise, etc.	−0.112	0.002	−0.131	< 0.001	−0.397	< 0.001
τ_1 Walking ¼ mile	0.063	0.206	−0.238	< 0.001	−0.296	<0.001
Running 100 yards	−0.142	< 0.001	−0.136	< 0.001	−0.300	<0.001
Stooping, crouching, kneeling	−0.059	0.258	−0.192	< 0.001	−0.244	< 0.001
Heavy housework, exercise, etc.	0.012	0.774	−0.135	0.002	−0.343	< 0.001

nificant effects on τ_1 in both self-reported and physician-assessed items. Nevertheless, there is remarkable consistency in the direction of the effects on nearly all of the significant results on all cut-points and questions.

Based on the results from the HOPIT regression, we can estimate predicted cut-point values on each question for different subgroups in the sample, as well as ranges around these estimates (Figure 2). The pattern for the estimated cut-points for population groups is quite similar for all

Figure 2 Estimated cut-points and ranges by population subgroup for self-reports and physician assessments of difficulties in walking one-quarter mile

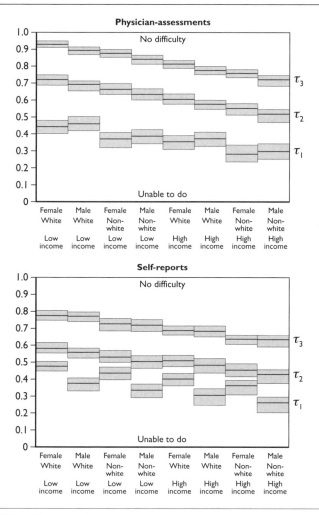

Bars indicate 95% confidence intervals.

seven self-reported and four physician-assessed items. The example in Figure 2 depicts cut-points on two parallel questions relating to difficulties in walking one-quarter mile. The cut-points are located on the latent mobility scale that emerges from HOPIT, after rescaling based on anchors defined by the best and worst results on the range of performance tests, as described above. While the 95% confidence intervals show that there is some overlap between estimated cut-points in different groups, significant differences remain between various subgroups in the study population. Thus, for example, at the same level of health, a white female with low income will report some difficulties in walking one-quarter mile, while a non-white male with high income will report no difficulties.

This example highlights two key findings:

1. that the ordering of cut-points across the eight subgroups is almost identical in physician assessments as compared to self-reports. In other words, the variation in norms and expectations associated with sex, race and income may apply not only to individuals assessing their own health levels, but also to medical professionals making these assessments for their patients. In fact, judging by the range in cut-points across subgroups, differences in norms and expectations may even be larger for physicians than for self-reporting individuals;

2. that physician cut-points tend to be higher overall for the threshold between "no difficulty" and "some difficulty", but slightly lower overall for the threshold between "much/moderate difficulty" and "unable to do"; in other words, given a relatively high level of health, physicians will be more likely to characterize individuals as having difficulties on this domain than the individuals themselves, whereas physician appraisals of low levels are more generous.

Discussion

Self-reported health is a complex function of observed morbidity, health expectations, contact with health services or other sources of health knowledge, and social and cultural context. A number of studies have illustrated the difficulties of comparing responses to self-reported health questions across individuals who differ in terms of various socioeconomic, demographic or cultural factors. A classic example is from Kerala state in India, where rates of self-reported morbidity have been found to be higher than anywhere else in India, despite the fact that Kerala has the lowest mortality rates in India (Murray and Chen 1992). Another noteworthy example comes from a study in Australia (Mathers and Douglas 1998) in which the Aboriginal population describe their health levels much more favourably than the general population, even though the opposite would be expected given incidence rates of major health problems and other key health indicators. Survey results such as these ones suggest that there are major problems of comparability that make meaningful cross-population analyses difficult.

One important strategy to improve cross-population comparability of health surveys has been to improve the standardization of questionnaires across countries. Even if cross-cultural standardization in questions could be achieved, however, a major challenge to comparability remains in the reliance on categorical responses, which will be subject to individual variation in the use of the available response categories, even for instruments with established reliability and validity. An individual's use of categories such as "no difficulties", "some difficulties", etc. will depend on their norms and expectations for health along a particular domain. Johansson (1991) has pointed to a "cultural inflation of morbidity", through which expectations for health rise in countries as they undergo the health transition to lower rates of mortality, but even within populations, it is easy to imagine that expectations will vary according to age, sex, education, income, and a host of other variables. It is therefore essential to adjust categorical questions to a comparable cardinal scale before attempting comparisons between countries or across population groups within countries.

In this paper, we describe the application of a new method for addressing the problem of comparability in categorical responses to health questions, using measured tests to capture fixed levels on a latent health domain in order to quantify individual differences in response category cut-points. We apply the hierarchical ordered probit (HOPIT) model described in Tandon et al. (2001) to information from the Third National Health and Nutrition Examination Survey in the United States to develop empirical estimates of cut-point differences in population subgroups defined by sex, race and income. This study focuses on the domain of mobility, using information from almost six thousand adults aged 60 years and older, but any data set containing both self-reports or physician-assessments and measured performance tests relating to the same domain of health could be analysed using the same approach.

The results of this study point to significant differences in individual response category cut-points as a function of sex, race and income, on several different questions relating to mobility levels. Across different questions, the nature of the differences are largely consistent. There is a strong tendency for males to have lower cut-points on mobility questions than females, which implies that males are less likely to report difficulties given the same levels of mobility. The frequently observed pattern in many health surveys in which women report worse health than men may therefore be understood not simply as an indicator of lower health levels, but of higher expectations for health (i.e. higher cut-points). Our findings also point to lower cut-points for non-white respondents relative to white respondents, which again may suggest important differences in expectations for health that lead to different characterizations of the same fixed levels on a particular domain.

A somewhat surprising finding is that individuals with higher income levels tend to have lower cut-points for mobility than individuals with lower income levels. This result runs counter to the notion that standards for excellent health increase with rising income, but might be understood in terms of a "wishful thinking" scenario in which wealthier individuals have a belief that they *should* be in excellent health and therefore use liberal standards for excellence in reporting on their own health. These findings may have important implications for the measurement of social inequalities in health where these measures rely on categorical self-reported data. If wealthier respondents use more lenient standards in reporting on their own health levels, this could exaggerate disparities in health between the rich and poor.

It is interesting to observe that both self-reported and physician-assessed health measures are subject to the same variations in cut-points relating to socio-demographic factors such as sex, race and income. In this study, the differences were even more marked for physician assessments than for individual self-reports. Thus, the way physicians characterize the mobility levels of different individuals with the same performance levels on measured tests will depend on whether the examinee is a man or woman, white or non-white, and of higher or lower economic status. The results from our study add to previous work that has examined potential biases in physician evaluations according to certain patient characteristics. For example, a study from Norway found that general practitioners' awareness of their patients' psychosocial problems were dependent on the age and sex of both the doctor and the patient, as well as the patient's educational level and living conditions (Guldbrandsen et al. 1997). Our study also finds that physicians and patients, when asked the same question (such as the one relating to difficulties in walking one-quarter mile), will characterize the same fixed mobility levels in different ways. A previous study has noted that patients with multiple sclerosis appear less concerned than their clinicians about physical disabilities caused by their illness (Rothwell et al. 1997), and significant differences have also been found between patients and geriatric experts in Europe and United States when comparing the importance of functional status items (Kane et al. 1998). Understanding how patient characteristics influence physician evaluations, and how these evaluations differ from those of the patients themselves, remain important topics for further study.

Notes

1   Since the latent variable is unobserved, the variance of the latent variable conditional on determinants is arbitrarily set to 1 in the ordered probit model. In addition, in order to identify the model, the constant term is set to 0. These conventions produce a scale that is unique up to any positive affine transformation, i.e. the latent scale has so-called *interval* properties.

References

Belcher DW, Neumann AK, Wurapa FK, Lourie IM (1976) Comparison of morbidity interviews with health examination survey in rural Africa. *American Journal of Tropical Medicine and Hygiene,* 25(5):751–758.

Bletzer KV (1993) Perceived severity: do they experience illness severity as we conceive it? *Human Organization,* 52(1):68–75.

Feeny D, Furlong W, Boyle M, Torrance GW (1995) Multi-attribute health status classification systems: Health Utilities Index. *PharmacoEconomics*, 7(6):490–502.

Gudex C, Lafortune G (2000) *An inventory of health and disability-related surveys in OECD countries (DRAFT)*. (Labour market and social policy, occasional papers no. 44.) OECD, Directorate for Education, Employment, Labour and Social Affairs, Paris. *www.oecd.org/els/health/docs.htm*.

Guldbrandsen P, Hjortdahl P, Fugelli P (1997) General practitioners' knowledge of their patients' psychosocial problems: multipractice questionnaire survey. *British Medical Journal*, 314(7086):1014–1018.

Honaker J, Joseph A, King G, Scheve K, Naunihal SA (1999) *Amelia: a programme for missing data*. (Software).

Hunt SM, McKenna SP, McEwen J, Williams J, Papp E (1981) The Nottingham Health Profile: subjective health status and medical consultations. *Social Science and Medicine*, 15(3 pt 1):221–229.

Johansson SR (1991) The health transition: the cultural inflation of morbidity during the decline of mortality. *Health Transition Review*, 1(1):39–68.

Kane RL, Rockwood T, Philip I, Finch M (1998) Differences in valuation of functional status components among consumers and professionals in Europe and the United States. *Journal of Clinical Epidemiology*, 51(8):657–666.

King G, Honaker J, Joseph A, Scheve K (1999) *Analysing incomplete political social science data: an alternative algorithm for multiple imputation*. Harvard University, Department of Government, Cambridge, MA.

King G, Honaker J, Joseph A, Scheve K (2001) Analysing incomplete political social science data: an alternative algorithm for multiple imputation. *American Political Science Review*, 95(1):49–69.

Krueger DE (1957) Measurement of prevalence of chronic disease by household interviews and clinical evaluations. *American Journal of Public Health*, 47:953–960.

Mathers CD, Douglas RM (1998) Measuring progress in population health and wellbeing. In: *Measuring progress: is life getting better?* CSIRO Publishing, Collingwood, Victoria.

Murray CJL, Chen LC (1992) Understanding morbidity change. *Population and Development Review*, 18(3):481–503.

Murray CJL, Tandon A, Salomon JA, Mathers CD (2000) *Enhancing cross-population comparability of survey results*. (GPE discussion paper no. 35.) World Health Organization, Geneva.

NCHS (1999) *The third US national health and nutrition examination survey (NHANES III) 1988–94*. National Center for Health Statistics, Washington, DC.

Rasmussen N, Gudex C, Christensen S (1999) *Survey data on disability*. (Eurostat working papers, Population and social conditions 3/1999/E/n 20.) European Commission, Luxembourg.

Rothwell PM, McDowell Z, Wong CK, Dorman PJ (1997) Doctors and patients don't agree: cross sectional study of patients' and doctors' perceptions and assessments of disability in multiple sclerosis. *British Medical Journal,* **314**(7094):1580–1583.

Salomon JA, Tandon A, Murray CJL (2001) *Using vignettes to improve cross-population comparability of health surveys: concepts, design, and evaluation techniques.* (GPE discussion paper no 41.) World Health Organization/Global Programme on Evidence for Health Policy, Geneva.

Tandon A, Murray CJL, Salomon JA (2001) *Statistical methods for enhancing cross-population comparability.* (GPE discussion paper no 42.) World Health Organization/Global Programme on Evidence for Health Policy, Geneva.

Tsuji I, Minami Y, Keyl PM, et al. (1994) The predictive power of self-rated health, activities of daily living, and ambulatory activity for cause-specific mortality among the elderly: A three-year follow-up in urban Japan. *Journal of the American Geriatrics Society,* **42**(2):153–156.

Ware J (2000) SF-36 Health survey update. *Spine,* **25**(24):3130–3139.

How to derive disability weights

Marie-Louise Essink-Bot and Gouke J. Bonsel

Introduction

"Summary measures of population health are measures that combine information on mortality and non-fatal health outcomes to represent the health of a particular population" (Murray et al. 2000). Technically, summary measures combine mortality data and data on non-fatal health outcomes. Such data is usually of a cross-sectional nature, i.e. annual mortality data and an array of prevalence/incidence data from various sources.

In the original disability-adjusted life year (DALY) approach in the Global Burden of Disease (GBD) 1990 study, the mortality component was reflected as years of life lost (as recognized by Barendregt, the choice of this metric implies a normative choice for age-at-death, Barendregt and Bonneux [1998]). The morbidity component consisted of years lived with disability (YLD). Years lived with a specified disability were combined with a disability weight ranging from 0 (no disability) to 1. These disability weights again implied value choices. The methodology to arrive at DALYs closely resembled QALY-computations commonly in use in cost-effectiveness analysis, based on the summation of separately weighted one-year periods. This again implied critical assumptions: independence of the disability weight from the total duration in that disability, absence of sequence effects, and absence of uncertainty and prognosis. Additional values in the GBD 1990 were the age-weights and discounting, but these are not essential to the DALY concept.

The present chapter deals with the empirical assessment of disability weights in the context of DALYs. The choices to be made in the empirical design of a strategy for deriving disability weights are to be guided by certain assumptions and by the intended use of the summary measures in which disability weights will be applied. Given different uses, the choices have different outcomes.

We will outline the types of uses of summary measures and the essential link between disability weights and descriptive epidemiological data as the points of departure for empirical assessment of disability weights. Then we will discuss some of the consequences of these two points for the strategy for empirical derivation of disability weights. Although the choice of the most appropriate valuation method often seems to draw much of the attention, we emphasize the importance of looking at complete research designs for empirical valuation studies, i.e. including the stimulus (the states to be presented for valuation; in short, "what?") and the subjects who perform the valuation task (in short, "who?"). These issues are highly interrelated.

The paper ends by summarizing the conclusions and listing a research agenda for the near future.

USES OF SUMMARY MEASURES OF POPULATION HEALTH

As pointed out by Murray et al. (2000), different uses for summary measures can be distinguished. The first is "descriptive use", e.g. comparing the health of populations in different regions or countries at the same point in time; and comparing the health of the same population at different points in time. Descriptive use compares variability over time and place. A second type of use is to decompose the burden of disease into the contributions of various diseases, injuries and risk factors. This could be labelled "causative use", because it analyses burden of diseases by cause. A third category of use is the quantification of potential benefits of health interventions in cost-effectiveness analysis and health care priority-setting. This could be called "evaluative use".

The desirable properties of summary measures vary with their intended use. Descriptive uses may require value sets that differ from those included in cost effectiveness analysis. We will explore this view for descriptive and evaluative use.

DESCRIPTIVE USE

Disability weights in summary measures for comparative use can be regarded as no more than an extension of epidemiological frequency measures. Disability weights in this context should reflect as much as possible "only" the relative severity of the health-related consequences of various diseases and disease stages. In epidemiological descriptions of burden of disease, disability weights are needed if the severity of the consequences varies *between* diseases and, *within* a disease, between various stages of that same disease, *and* if it is considered necessary to take these differences into account.

Descriptive estimates of the burden of disease in this context are used for comparisons over time or between populations (please note that "descriptive" is not intended as a synonym of "objective"). A prerequisite for useful comparisons of burden of disease over time or between countries is that any divergence can be reasonably attributed to differences in incidence, prevalence, duration, or severity of specified diseases and disease-stages over time or between countries, and not to changes over time or cross-national differences *in values* included in the summary measure.

This implies that the disability weights included in summary measures for descriptive purposes should be *in*variant over time and *in*variant between countries to the largest possible extent. The question remains whether it is at all "possible to agree on a universal weighting of disability" (James and Foster 1999; Üstün et al. 1999). If agreement is insufficient, this poses certain limits to comparability across cultures and over time of burden of disease as expressed by summary measures that include disability severity weights.

A further implication is that basic epidemiological data and disability weights underlying the composite burden of disease estimates must be transparent, to enable interpretation of changes or differences.

Evaluative use

In resource allocation debates the relative severity of disability also plays a vital role, but additionally other values are at stake. In other words, the epidemiological description of the health of a nation or a region may be a necessary but insufficient piece of information for priority setting. Assuming that cost-effective interventions exist, the values held by the society involved regarding the distribution of health become important. (Nord et al. 1999) These can be called "social distributional values": values of the distribution of health gains or prevented health losses in a population. Examples are socioeconomic status (e.g. priority to raise the health of the poor, irrespective of their level of health), ethnic group (priority to improve the health of specific ethnic groups), age (e.g. priority to save the productive ages), sex, medical history (e.g. priority to help the worst-off), level of health to be reached (e.g. priority to equalize the state of health of the subjects in the population) or number of persons (e.g. priority to improve the health of relatively few people a lot instead of improving the health of many people a little).

These social distributional values will probably depend on regional circumstances and may change over time (e.g. when the circumstances change). But as far as we are aware, systematic research in this respect is scarce.

For use of summary measures in allocation debates, three choices seem to be open regarding social distributional values:

- They can be included directly in the summary measures, i.e. in the derivation of the components and/or in combining these into summary measures. However, it will be difficult to disentangle the different effects of different components (as shown by the GBD 1990 results), so that results may be difficult to interpret.

- They can be applied *ex post*, similar to applying separate "equity weights" to descriptive burden data (as proposed by Williams (1999), and by others). Preferably, all components of the summary measures (basic epidemiology, disability severity weights, social distributional weights) are reported both as summarizing figures *and*, separately, in a modular fashion. This provides insight into the contribution of different components to the summary results. Potential users can decide which values to use for any particular aim. (Please note that the *sequence* of applying various value functions may also affect the result; Barendregt et al. [1996].)

- They can be excluded, and the debate is then left to the decision-makers.

LINK TO EPIDEMIOLOGY

Perhaps this is an appropriate place to repeat that disability weights are not a goal in themselves. They are meant to be combined with epidemiological data on incidence, duration, age at onset, or prevalence of non-fatal, disease-related outcomes to form summary measures. However, one of the lessons to be learned from GBD 1990 is that descriptive epidemiological data (incidence, prevalence, duration) of disability by cause, age and sex are at best incomplete and often inconsistent (Murray and Lopez 1996), even in developed countries such as The Netherlands. There is no use in deriving disability weights for detailed disease stages if there is nothing to multiply them with, that is, if corresponding epidemiological data on the frequency of occurrence of these stages is not available. The level of detail and reliability of the disability weights should approximately equal that of the epidemiological data.

But if we have epidemiological data, there must be a precise link between the states that were valued and the epidemiological registries. Finding the optimal way of covering the often complex changes in health status over time (even within a year) in a disability description to be presented for valuation is a formidable task. A further prerequisite for useful comparisons of burden of diseases between countries is that comparable epidemiological data is available in these countries or populations.

SUMMARIZING THE POINTS OF DEPARTURE

- Disability weights in summary measures for descriptive purposes must reflect, if possible, only the relative severity of the consequences of different diseases and disease stages. They must be, as much as possible, universal across time and over the globe, i.e. invariant over time and cross-nationally stable.

- Summary measures for use in resource allocation debates should allow for inclusion of additional social distributional values. These can be separately added or be integrated from onset.

- There is no use in deriving detailed disability weights if the corresponding epidemiological data are not available. If epidemiological data are available, there must be a precise link between these and the disability weights.

In the following three sections, some of the consequences for the design of empirical studies to assess disability weights, and associated problems to be solved, will be worked out.

Valuation methods

Current valuation methods include rating scales (e.g. visual analogue scaling or VAS) and trade-off methods (e.g. standard gamble [SG], time trade-off [TTO], willingness-to-pay [WTP] and person trade-off [PTO]). For a review, see Brazier et al. (1999). Many versions of each method are available and many more are imaginable.

VAS

The respondent's task in VAS valuation is to locate health state descriptions on a scale with anchored end-points (commonly "full health" at one end and "dead" or "worst imaginable health state" at the other) in order of preference. VAS does not include a trade-off. This is probably the cause of the repeatedly found result of relatively high VAS disability weights for relatively mild conditions. It is also questionable whether VAS values have interval properties, that is, if state A is valued as x and B as $2x$, that respondents are prepared to state the equivalence between differences in the values and the value of those differences, additional to the statement that B is better than A. Major advantages are that VAS is relatively easy to use, and to understand, particularly by less educated raters.

Trade-off methods

These share the feature that the respondent is asked to trade-off hypothetically "something valuable" in exchange for improvement of the state-to-be-valued to full health or, in the reverse, in exchange for prevention of loss of health. The "something valuable" is called the calibrator of the method.

Below we list general operationalizations of each of the trade-off methods:

- In *SG*, the amount of risk of immediate death (e.g. operative mortality) a respondent is hypothetically willing to take in order to be restored from the state to be valued is the calibrator. The worse the disability, the more (hypothetical) risk of immediate death the respondent is willing to take.

- In *TTO*, the calibrator is the number of life-years (or the proportion of life expectancy) a respondent is hypothetically willing to sacrifice to be restored from the state to be valued. The more years the respondent is prepared to sacrifice hypothetically, the worse the disability of the state to be valued.

- In *WTP,* a subject is asked how much he would be willing to pay from a hypothetical budget to be restored from the state to be valued.

- In *PTO,* a subject is asked hypothetically to trade numbers of persons in good health for numbers of persons in the state to be valued, or for an improvement to full health of persons in the state to be valued.

Some general remarks can be made.

- Trade-off methods share a degree of cognitive complexity that limits large-scale unsupported data collection and even raises doubts about whether the task can be performed by less well-educated subjects. To some extent, trade-off tasks may work as IQ-tests. There appears, as shown in the York MVH study (Dolan et al. 1996), much to be gained from operationalizing the task to be as simple as possible, ("stripping it to its bare bones"), carefully designing instructions, providing interviewer support, using props, computer-assisted interviewing techniques, etc. One of the difficulties is caused by the fact that valuing hypothetical health states is a complex task in any case. We have found repeatedly that in valuation studies where a written questionnaire is provided, *usable* responses are associated with higher educational levels, even if the task consisted of "simple" VAS valuation (Essink-Bot et al. 1993).

- It has proved difficult to design operationalizations of trade-off methods that suit all types of diseases and disease states, especially in cases of attack-wise or short-duration diseases, and in those generally associated with a sequence of different levels of disability within a relatively short time period (see below).

- Each of the trade-off methods can be operationalized for valuation from a third person's perspective, i.e. for "someone like you".

- Originally, PTO differed from the other trade-off methods because subjects were asked to state preferences between persons instead of within a single person. However, TTO can be framed easily for groups of persons ("social TTO"). This is also possible with the other methods.

- All methods introduce a bias because the calibrator itself has a value. For example, risk-aversive people are less willing to accept even hypothetical risks, hence their SG values are higher (implying a lower disability weight). Rich people are generally prepared to spend more money on health improvement, so their WTP values will be worse (implying higher disability weights). Similar reasoning holds for the other trade-off methods. This effect may only partly be avoided by design or it can be adjusted for, but it cannot be avoided completely because trading-off something valuable is the essential characteristic of these methods.

- All methods suffer from ceiling and threshold effects, that is, some states of health are considered not bad enough for trading-off anything, hence mutual relationships cannot be determined.

Games or reality?

One view on valuation methods is to regard them as hypothetical games to be played by the respondent in order to elicit the real value of the state in question. In this approach, which has its roots in psychology and psychophysics, a valuation method is regarded as a guide to the cognitive process in eliciting valuation responses. The intention is to help the respondent concretize the valuations by providing him with a "realistic" situation. Providing "realistic" situations is, hopefully, a way of making the always difficult task of evaluating health states a little less abstract (Anderson 1971, cited by Krabbe 1998).

Another view regards valuation methods as a species of reality. Considerable debate has focused on which method is best for deriving disability weights. "Best" is in this view to be judged from the viewpoint of similarity of the method to real-world decision-making (either individual or population-wide). However, as pointed out by Richardson (1994), the p-value in SG (the method probability) is generally not the same as probability (risk) associated with the outcome of a particular medical intervention under study. Hence, method-uncertainty is not equal to stimulus uncertainty. Similarly, Krabbe (1998) and others (Essink-Bot 1998) showed the same arguments to hold for WTP (the method's money bears no direct relationship to the health care budget); TTO (calibration years are not equal to real life-time perspective) and PTO (method-number of persons bears no relationship to real populations). We have no preference in favour or against any valuation method, but we prefer a deliberative process that includes a combination of multiple valuation methods.

Does having so much choice of methods create difficulties? Mostly not. It has been repeatedly reported in the literature that, although different methods yield different absolute values, ranking remains largely unaffected (Krabbe et al. 1997). Admittedly, as mentioned above, each trade-off method introduces a bias in the shape of the value of the calibrator (risk, time, money, persons and numbers). Absolute differences can be ascribed to different method effects:

- SG-values are confounded by risk posture;

- TTO-values by time-preference;

- WTP-values by the value attached by the respondent to money; and

- PTO-values by distributional preferences (Williams 1999).

Or, conversely: SG is suitable for measuring a subject's risk-posture *and* valuation of health states; TTO for empirically measuring time preference *and* valuation of health states; PTO for measuring social distributional preferences *and* valuation of health states. Keeping the state to be valued but varying the time horizon turns TTO into a tool to measure time preference. In fact, values elicited by each of the trade-off methods can be said to consist of a "real disability severity value component", a method-specific component and an error term. Apart from the method-specific component, each of the trade-off methods provide reasonably similar results.

Which valuation method is the most suitable depends on intended use of the values. As indicated in the points of departure, disability weights for descriptive uses of summary measures should only reflect levels of disability (if that is at all possible), i.e. the disability weights should be largely neutral. Further research should focus on obtaining values for health states by using three or more methods, followed by careful modelling of the components of the resulting values. Suitable statistical techniques are available, such as General Linear Modelling with hierarchical models. In theory, this approach would enable "isolation" of the ultimate disability severity weights. To some extent, this approach approximates what Murray has named "the importance of deliberation". By applying multiple valuation methods, respondents look at the same health state from different angles, and by so doing, they finally are able to attach a value they feel comfortable with.

WHAT IS TO BE VALUED?

DEFINITION OF DISABILITY

One of the issues at stake here is the definition of "disability". It is self-evident that the disability weights must largely be cross-culturally stable for meaningful cross-cultural comparisons of burden of disease. This requires a cross-culturally equivalent definition of disability (if this is at all possible) and investigation of whether the values are cross-culturally invariant. Definition difficulties arise because disability depends on the level of treatment available, and this differs around the globe. This issue is being dealt with elsewhere in this book.

DISEASE-SPECIFIC OR GENERIC?

We can see two arguments in favour of the derivation of disease-specific disability weights. The first is that the disease label may be a vital piece of information for valuation. The second but less important is that the precise link between the state that was valued and the epidemiological frequency data can be ascertained more easily. There is also a reverse side of these advantages.

It is obvious that a disease label adds information. Generic health state descriptions rarely contain a clue towards the underlying disease, hence much of the specific health status consequences of the disease that causes the health state are—by definition—left out of consideration. We have empirical evidence that it matters for the valuation whether a disabled state is associated with, for example, low back pain or prostate cancer (Stouthard et al. 2000). This is because the diagnostic "label" *adds* information to the state to be valued. In the example, the prostate cancer is obviously associated with a different *perceived* prognosis than low back pain. The questions at stake are:

- whether a disease label provides information that is essential for valuation of the state, and if so,

- whether adding a disease label is the most appropriate way to provide this vital information (whatever its exact nature) to the raters.

What is precisely added by a disease label has not been investigated empirically. It may add essential information, or introduce undesired effects, or both. Systematic research comparing valuations of disease-specific and generic health states has not yet been published.

As stated above, descriptive epidemiological data on non-fatal health outcomes must be available for use of disability weights in summary measures (e.g. a prevalence distribution of cases across the disease stages for which disability weights were derived). Assuming that such epidemiological data is available, the link between disability weights and disease-specific data from epidemiological registries and cohort studies must be established. The second advantage of deriving disease-specific disability weights appears to be the straightforward direct link between epidemiological data and disability weights. For a correct appreciation of this advantage it is necessary to understand and balance the two strategies that are available to arrive at such a link. Either strategy is associated with different routes of data collection and processing:

1. *Derivation of disease-specific disability weights using health state descriptions with disease label.* In this case a two-stage procedure is needed. First, a disease is subdivided into stages that can be matched precisely to the registry data, assuming that these stages represent a clinically interpretable state that is associated with a stable level of disability. In the second step these stages are valued. A strategy-specific disadvantage emerges.

   A disease stage described in standardized clinical terms may, for various reasons, produce different mental "images" of the disability across the subjects who conduct the valuation. Take, for example, uncomplicated diabetes mellitus. In the Dutch Disability Weights study, where we applied a valuation strategy with disease labels, we added a standardized health status description in functional terms to the clinical disease stage to be valued (Stouthard et al. 1997; 2000).

   Related to this disadvantage, the suboptimal performance of the disease-specific valuation strategy among medically uneducated respondents remains a factor, even if generic information is added (see below). A second strategy-specific problem occurs if disease labels affect the valuations (e.g. by adding prognostic information) that were theoretically assumed not to play a role in the model of summation of separately valued periods of time.

2. *Derivation of disability weights using generic descriptions of the health states associated with specific diseases* (empirical mapping of generic health states to diseases).

This second strategy is routinely applied in cost-effectiveness analysis using QALYs. It includes a three-step procedure. In the first step, the disability associated with the disease is described using a generic health classification (e.g. the Health Utilities Index or EQ-5D). Preferably a mapping procedure is carried out using empirical survey data regarding patients. Second, this descriptive generic data is reduced to one or more representative one-year descriptions covering the disability of the disease over time. In the third step, one-year generic descriptions (for which the links to particular disease stages are hidden to the rater) are valued directly by raters or by applying some already available formula (such as the algorithms available for the Health Utilities Index and the EQ-5D). An obvious disadvantage is the complexity of a valid projection of disease stages on generic health state descriptions. The advantage is the transparency of the valuation task itself, and, in the presence of a formula, the facility to cover any generic health state without additional valuation studies, which explains its current popularity in economic evaluation work.

STAGES

A third issue is whether it is desirable to elicit one disability weight per disease. Consider a comparison of burden of disease over time within a population, using one disability weight for the disease as a whole. Assume that incidence, prevalence and mortality of disease X have remained constant. However, a successful new treatment was introduced in the period between the two assessments of burden. The duration of the disease remained the same, but on average the disability associated with the disease decreased, perhaps because of slower progression from mild to severe stages. The actual burden of disease decreased, but if the original disability weight had been used, this improvement in population health could not be expressed (similar to concluding that as a result of the new treatment the disability weight for disease X changed over time).

In order to take changes in disease epidemiology over time by, for example taking therapeutic innovations, into account, we need to define disease *stages*. Each disease is subdivided in a number of stages, preferably of the type "mild", "moderate", "severe", if this is compatible with epidemiological data sources. Each stage is valued separately. In a prevalence approach to DALYs, prevalent cases are distributed across all stages. If at all possible, stages must be defined in such a way that a therapeutic innovation causes a shift in the distribution of prevalent cases across the stages instead of changing the stages themselves.

There is a secondary argument for presenting disease stages instead of diseases for valuation. The sequelae of a disease are often not a homogenous category. Dementia, for example, causes a broad array of disabilities. If respondents are asked to assign a single weight to dementia, it must be assumed that the respondent knows the contribution of each disability to the total morbidity burden (which assumes insight into incidence, prevalence and duration), and furthermore that the respondent is capable of arriving at a single weight by means of an averaging routine. By defining stages, respondents can be presented with a more singular stimulus.

Duration, annual states and annual profiles

When evaluating health states, it is essential to define their duration. As shown by Bala et al. (1999), health status values are not "timeless". What is valued by respondents is a combination of a health state and a duration, whether this duration is specified or not.

A fixed duration of one year, during which the health state is considered to remain constant, is realistically imaginable for a majority of chronic disease stages. This format is less appropriate in the following categories:

- attack-wise diseases (e.g. asthma, epilepsy);

- short-duration diseases, followed by complete recovery in the majority of cases (e.g. influenza); and

- conditions of short duration followed by incomplete recovery and hence a permanently impaired health status (e.g. acute myocardial infarction followed by post-infarct angina).

The duration problem also occurs with "whole disease" disabilities, but on a more refined time axis. The standard QALY/DALY approach of summing up periods of separately valued stages here meets its limits. Even if we can find respondents willing to attach a value to one year in a state of epilepsy, asthma or the like, the resulting disability loss in patients will be minimal if we apply the rules of independent adding up of value periods. However, one must be aware that this splitting up into one-year parts is much of a matter of convenience that is supported by the availability of annual epidemiological data. Its validity depends on strong assumptions of the independence of the disability weight and the duration of the disability, which obviously do not hold in the case of durations much shorter than a year. Imagine a disease presenting as one week of excruciating pain, so terrible that one is unable to imagine having to suffer it ever again. Assume the pain to start and end instantaneously. If duration and disability weight were independent, the maximum disability weight for this disease would be $[(1/52 * 1) + (51/52 * 0) = 0.019$, corresponding to almost perfect health. Or imagine an epilepsy attack: following the same arithmetic, halving its duration would halve the associated disability weight. These problems originate in the basic QALY/DALY assumption of independence of the disability weight and the duration of the disability.

In the Dutch Disability Weights study, we tested an innovative approach to cover these problems. Attack-wise diseases were presented as what they really are—attacks occurring at unpredictable moments but with a defined frequency on a baseline of, here, one year. The value for such an annual profile is of course not equal to what would have been arrived at after summation of separate smaller periods (10 minutes epilepsy plus 364.99

days of normal life). This implies that the attacks themselves were not valued, but being in a state of having to take regular preventive medication, having to avoid attack-provoking situations, fear of recurrent attacks, etc.

For the two types of conditions of short duration, we developed a similar annual profile approach. Short duration conditions with full recovery (e.g. influenza) were presented for valuation as "one year in good health with two weeks of influenza". The approach was well accepted by the respondents and is currently under further development. Some have argued that the resulting disability weights for this type of disease were too high (e.g. acute sinusitis [two weeks in an otherwise healthy year] being valued at 0.02, and acute gonorrhoea [one week in an otherwise healthy year] at 0.01). This may be true (although difficult to test), but it is a problem of lack of differentiation at this end of the scale. The problem is one of assigning disability weights to diseases with high prevalence and low severity, and by no means specific for the annual profile approach. If, as an afterthought, we *model* the annual profile data as a simple summation of value periods, either the Q of the disease episode has to be assigned a negative value, or the Q of the normal period must be valued lower, which is conflicting with the standard assumptions of a value range between 0 and 1, and of period independence.

Short duration diseases characterized by a sequence of shorter periods of different disability levels (e.g. acute myocardial infarction) were in the Dutch Disability study also presented as what they are: a defined period in hospital with defined disability, followed by a defined period of rehabilitation associated with defined disability. Although realistic and methodologically superior, it has been shown that at present it is difficult to find the associated epidemiological data (but this problem is not specific for the annual profile approach either).

We conclude that many questions remain about whether the currently available methods for valuation of health states, originally developed in health economics for aggregate categorical decision-making, lend themselves sufficiently for valid valuation of "real" disease stages in burden of disease and economic evaluation studies. The annual profile approach seems a promising alternative approach.

WHOSE VALUES?

The question of whose values should be included in summary measures is determined by the perspective of its intended use. For all uses described in the second section of this chapter, the societal perspective is the appropriate one. The subsequent question is then what panel can be regarded as providing values that reflect this perspective? It has often been argued that a representative sample of the general population, including sufficient numbers of subjects of both sexes, different ages, income groups, and healthy persons as well as patients and ex-patients, is the most appropriate (Gold et al. 1996). There are two obstacles to this. Most of these subjects will not be well-informed about the total array of conditions that contribute to burden of disease at an (inter)national level. Furthermore, many subjects scarcely will have witnessed severe states. The alternative of approaching broadly educated and experienced medical professionals, because they have professional third-party experience with a broad range of health states including severe ones, has also evoked objections because health care professionals may have a non-representative value structure due to their origins and education. There is accumulating evidence that health-state valuations vary by age, education and disease experience (Brazier et al. 1999). The sizes and consequences of this have still to be quantified and documented.

The current political viewpoint seems to be that the general population's views should be included in burden of disease measures. The consequences for the design of the valuation procedure are twofold.

- Most important, the general public may have only the vaguest notion of, for example, the "average" diabetes patient—perhaps at best a relative or friend with the disease, or they do not know anything about it and may only focus on the fact that it is an illness, "something with syringes". If the general public is to value disease-specific health states, this information gap is a major issue. The subjects must somehow be "educated" about the consequences of each disease stage they are supposed to value, by information that is standardized across diseases. Standardized video presentations may be an (expensive) option.

- The complexity of the trade-off valuation methods probably limits their applicability. This issue was dealt with above.

EMPIRICAL DISABILITY WEIGHTS

A comprehensive, coherent series of disability weights, based on relative severity for a large number of diseases, are currently available from the GBD 1990 and from the Dutch Disability Weights study.

For the GBD 1990, a disability scale was derived from valuations by the famous Geneva panel of 22 indicator conditions in a deliberative procedure including two operationalizations of person trade-off. In a separate step, the distribution of prevalent cases across the seven classes of the disability scale was estimated by disease experts (Murray 1996).

In the Dutch Disability Weights study, a disability scale was calibrated by values for 16 indicator disease *stages*; in a similar procedure involving three panels of medical experts, VAS was added. The separate step in the DDW included direct interpolation of 175 remaining disease stages on the disability scale (Stouthard et al. 1997; 2000). The resulting disability weights were applied in the Dutch Public Health Status and Forecast 1997 study (Melse et al. 2000; Ruwaard and Kramers 1998).

In 2000, the cross-cultural stability of disability weights in a set of developed countries was investigated empirically in the European Disability Weights project (BIOMED II BMH4-98-3253). Participating countries included Denmark, England, France, The Netherlands, Spain, and Sweden. Project coordinator is Paul van der Maas from the Department of Public Health, Erasmus University Rotterdam, The Netherlands. In each country, a number of disease-specific states have been valued by panels of experts and of laymen using several valuation methods (including VAS, TTO and PTO). The values were applied in burden of disease estimations of, for example, dementia and breast cancer in the six participating countries. The sensitivity of DALYs to variation and uncertainties in epidemiological data and disability weights has been analysed (Essink-Bot et al. 2002).

CONCLUSIONS AND RESEARCH AGENDA

The main conclusions can be listed as:

1. For descriptive use of summary measures, we need disability severity weights as an extension of descriptive epidemiological data. These weights must be invariant over time and across regions of the world.

2. Social distributional values are important in resource allocation. Such values can be included in summary measures, preferably *ex post* by separate empirically-based value functions.

3. Modular reporting of the constituting elements of summary measures is required. Insight in the basic epidemiologic and value data underlying the composite burden of disease estimates is essential for the interpretation of changes or differences in burden of disease.

4. The most important factor limiting the applicability of disability weights is the lack of comprehensive, consistent and internationally comparable epidemiological data on non-fatal health outcomes.

5. Defining the states to be valued and how to present them for valuation are the crucial issues in the empirical design for the derivation of disability weights.
   a. The exact nature of the information contained in a disease label, whether this information is essential for valuation, and whether there are better alternative ways to convey this information remains to be established.
   b. If the general public is to value disease-specific health states, the presentation is an issue of major concern.
   c. There must be a direct link between the states that were valued and epidemiologic data.
   d. Disability weights must be derived for disease stages that enable the taking of dynamic changes in disease epidemiology over time by, for example, therapeutic innovations, into account.

6.   As for valuation methods, the approach to be tested includes application of multiple methods, first to enhance deliberation, and secondly to enable separation of method effects from disability severity weights by a modelling approach.

We would suggest the following research agenda:

DEFINING THE STATES TO BE VALUED AND HOW TO PRESENT THEM

1.   Empirical investigation of the information contained in a disease label, whether this information is essential for valuation, and whether there are different ways to convey this information. This would start with an empirical comparison of generic and disease-specific valuation of health states.

2.   Systematic development of standardized procedures to present health states including medical aspects for weighting by non-medically educated subjects.

3.   Further development of a systematic approach to disease staging, and founding this empirically.

4.   Further work on the valuation of health profiles versus the standard QALY/DALY approach.

VALUATION METHODS

5.   Empirical testing of the "multiple method + modelling the disability severity weight" approach.

6.   Developing and testing operationalizations of valuation methods that are understandable and acceptable to the general public (the proper understanding by experts will probably improve as well).

7.   Qualitative research on subjects' interpretation of trade-off valuation methods (do the raters perform the tasks as we designed the tasks to be performed?).

SUBJECTS

8.   Systematic empirical comparisons of valuations from different groups of raters (experts, general public, patients).

APPLICATION OF DISABILITY SEVERITY WEIGHTS IN SUMMARY MEASURES

9.   Investigate the stability of disability weights over time.

10. Investigation of cross-cultural stability of disability weights in a wider-than-European context.

11. Systematic, internationally comparable, descriptive epidemiological research regarding non-fatal health outcomes. There is no use at all in the work stated in the other points of this research agenda if we

do not "count the noses", that is, collect systematic data on incidence and prevalence of important diseases and injuries, and on their medium and long-term disabling sequelae.

SOCIAL DISTRIBUTIONAL VALUES

12. Empirical studies of age preferences (Tsuchiya 1999).

13. Empirical studies of other social distributional values.

ACKNOWLEDGEMENTS

We are grateful to Erwin Birnie, Luc Bonneux and Paul van der Maas for constructive comments on earlier versions of this paper.

REFERENCES

Anderson NH (1971) Integration theory and attitude change. *Psychological Review,* 78(3):171–206.

Bala MV, Wood LL, Zarkin GA, Norton EC, Gafni A, O'Brien BJ (1999) Are health states "timeless"? The case of the standard gamble method. *Journal of Clinical Epidemiology,* 52(11):1047–1053.

Barendregt JJ, Bonneux L, van der Maas PJ (1996) DALYs: the age-weights on balance. *Bulletin of the World Health Organization,* 74(4):439–443.

Barendregt JJ, Bonneux LGA (1998) *Degenerative disease in aging populations – models and conjectures.* [Dissertation]. Erasmus University, Rotterdam.

Brazier JE, Deverill M, Green C (1999) A review of the use of health status measures in economic evaluation. *Journal of Health Services Research and Policy,* 4(3):174–184.

Dolan P, Gudex C, Kind P, Williams A (1996) The time-trade-off method: results from a general population study. *Health Economics,* 5(2):141–154.

Essink-Bot ML (1998) *Soci(et)al disability weights?* (Paper presented at the first meeting of the international burden of disease network.) Stowe, VT.

Essink-Bot ML, Pereira J, Packer C, Schwarzinger M, Burström K, and the European Disability Weights Group (2002) Cross-national comparability of burden of disease estimates: the European disability weights project. *Bulletin of the World Health Organization,* 80(8):644–652.

Essink-Bot ML, Stouthard MEA, Bonsel GJ (1993) Generalizability of valuations on health states collected with the EuroQol questionnaire. *Health Economics,* 2:237–246.

Gold MR, Siegel JE, Russel LB, Weinstein MC, eds. (1996) *Cost-effectiveness in health and medicine.* Oxford University Press, New York.

James KC, Foster SD (1999) Weighing up disability. (Editorial). *Lancet,* 354(9173):87–88.

Krabbe PFM (1998) *The valuation of health outcomes.* Erasmus University, Rotterdam. (Citing Anderson, NH., Integration theory and attitude change. Psychological Review 19971;77:153–169.)

Krabbe PFM, Essink-Bot ML, Bonsel GJ (1997) The comparability and reliability of five health-state valuation methods. *Social Science and Medicine,* 45(11):1641–1652.

Melse JM, Essink-Bot ML, Kramers PGN, Hoeymans N (2000) A national burden of disease calculation: Dutch DALYs. (On behalf of the Dutch burden of disease group). *American Journal of Public Health,* 90:1241–1247.

Murray CJL (1996) Rethinking DALYs. In: *The global burden of disease: a comprehensive assessment of mortality and disability from diseases, injuries, and risk factors in 1990 and projected to 2020.* The Global Burden of Disease and Injury, Vol. 1. Murray CJL, Lopez AD, eds. Harvard School of Public Health on behalf of WHO, Cambridge, MA.

Murray CJL, Lopez AD (1996) Global and regional descriptive epidemiology of disability: Incidence, prevalence, health expectancies and years lived with disability. In: *The global burden of disease: a comprehensive assessment of mortality and disability from diseases, injuries, and risk factors in 1990 and projected to 2020.* Global Burden of Disease and Injury, Vol. 1. Murray CJL, Lopez AD, eds. Harvard School of Public Health on behalf of WHO, Cambridge, MA.

Murray CJL, Salomon JA, Mathers CD (2000) A critical examination of summary measures of population health. *Bulletin of the World Health Organization,* 78(8):981–994.

Nord EM, Pinto JL, Richardson J, Menzel P, Ubel P (1999) Incorporating societal concerns for fairness in numerical valuations of health programmes. *Health Economics,* 8(1):25–39.

Richardson J (1994) Cost-utility analysis: what should be measured? *Social Science and Medicine,* 39(1):7–21.

Ruwaard D, Kramers PGN (1998) *Public health status and forecasts. Health prevention and health care in the Netherlands until 2015.* National Institute of Public Health and Environmental Protection, Elsevier.

Stouthard MEA, Essink-Bot ML, Bonsel GJ (2000) Disability weights for diseases: a modified protocol and results for a western European region. (On behalf of the Dutch disability weights group). *European Journal of Public Health,* 10:24–30.

Stouthard MEA, Essink-Bot ML, Bonsel GJ, et al. (1997) *Disability weights for diseases in the Netherlands.* Erasmus University, Department of Public Health, Rotterdam.

Tsuchiya A (1999) Age-related preferences and age weighting health benefits. *Social Science and Medicine,* 48(2):267–276.

Üstün TB, Rehm J, Chatterji S, et al. (1999) Multiple-informant ranking of the disabling effects of different health conditions in 14 countries. WHO/NIH joint project CAR study group. *Lancet,* 354(9173):111–115.

Williams A (1999) Calculating the global burden of disease: time for a strategic reappraisal? *Health Economics,* 8(1):1–8.

Chapter 9.2

THE CASE AGAINST ANNUAL PROFILES FOR THE VALUATION OF DISABILITY WEIGHTS

THEO VOS

The quantification of disability in burden of disease studies relies on coupling severity weights to time spent in less than full health. In the Australian Burden of Disease studies (Mathers et al. 1999; Vos and Begg 2000) a conscious choice was made to spend the available research time in collecting plausible and internally consistent estimates of incidence, prevalence and duration. For the severity weights we relied mostly on the weights generated by the Dutch Disability Weight Study (Stouthard et al. 1997) and supplemented these with weights from the Global Burden of Disease (GBD) Study (Murray and Lopez 1996) or generated new, interpolated weights for conditions not covered by the Dutch study. The Dutch weights were attractive to use as they: i) covered the range of conditions contributing most to the burden of disease in Australia; ii) allowed more detailed disease modelling because weights for the most common disabling conditions were available by several levels of severity; iii) had described each of the disease states valued with a EuroQol—with a sixth dimension for cognitive functioning (EQ5D +)—notation which facilitated matching disability weights to epidemiological data for comparable health states.

A small set of weights from the Dutch study appeared to be outliers. These are the conditions of short duration for which annual profiles were presented to the valuation panels. For example, symptomatic acute gonnorrhoea was described as "one year of which during one week symptomatic acute gonorrhoea is present" with an EQ5D + description of 111211 (indicating moderate pain/discomfort and no problems in the other five dimensions of mobility, self-care, usual activities, anxiety/depression and cognitive functioning). The Dutch weights were subsequently applied in a national burden of disease calculation for the Netherlands, which estimated the burden from non-fatal conditions by multiplying prevalence with a one-year duration and the corresponding disability weights (Melse and Kramers 1998). This is a different approach from that used in most other burden of disease studies, including the GBD, which calculate the disability burden from the multiplication of incidence, duration and a disability weight. The burden from short duration conditions for which disability weights were derived from annual profiles was calculated by multiplying the number of incident cases by a one-year duration and the disability weight. In the example of the one week with gonnorrhoea in an annual profile of a year this means that for each case the duration of disability was taken as 52 weeks and coupled with the disability weight for the annual profile. In personal communication, two of the authors of the Dutch study have stated that it is not valid to "back-calculate" the values of the constituting elements of a profile from the profile value. However, from the way these weights have been applied in the Dutch burden of disease study, I can only conclude that an annual profile weight for one week with gonnorrhoea must be the equivalent of 1/52 of the weight implied for the one week of disability. The only reason not to do so would be to argue that the 51 weeks following an episode of one week of gonnorrhoea are different from 51 weeks of healthy life. With some creativity one could argue that a bout of gonnorrhoea may cause anxiety about marital strife or the risk of having contracted other sexually transmitted diseases leading to loss of health-related quality of life beyond the one week of symptoms. If this is considered an important "health state", I would argue that it ought to be valued separately to be matched with epidemiological data on how frequently it occurs. It is a lot harder to imagine that a bout of nasopharyngitis would cause disability beyond the symptomatic period. Yet, each incident case of common cold in a year was multiplied with the annual profile's weight. If the Dutch annualized weights for common cold, sinusitis and tonsillitis had been used in the Victorian Burden of Disease Study the contribution of upper respiratory tract infections to Years Lived with Disability (YLD) would have increased six-fold and raised the ranking from 54 to 12. Similarly, lower respiratory tract infections (pneumonia and influenza) would increase eight-fold and change in YLD ranking from position 45 to 9. This indicates that the adoption of annualized weights can have more than trivial consequences on burden of disease results.

Let us examine the Dutch weights for annual profiles after "back-calculation" to a value for the implied severity for the duration of the short illness. This involves a simple transformation of the weights to the common GBD notation where 0 indicates full health and 1 complete loss of health and then multiplication by 52 divided by the duration in weeks. Figure 1 shows the implied weights for the short duration of these condition and illustrates how the annual profiles have failed to produce plausible weights. First, the weights for pneumonia and cystitis are greater than one and thus imply that these conditions are worse than being dead. Second, it is hard to imagine that the members of the valuation panels would have valued, for example, the loss of health due to urethritis as worse than that of paraplegia if they had realized this is the consequence of the value of their annual profile. In general, each of the annual profile disability

Figure 1   Duration-specific Dutch disability weights (95% confidence interval) for three selected chronic conditions and annual profiles of conditions of short duration

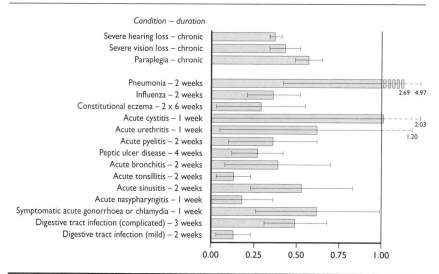

weights appear to be considerably overvalued. Their use in burden of disease assessments would give undue weight to short duration conditions.

Essink-Bot and Bonsel (chapter 9.1) state that the annual profile approach worked reasonably well. This may be the case for the valuation procedure. It is indeed a bit uncomfortable for panel members to imagine living a full year with pneumonia. However my experience as a member of a valuation panel in the past is that it is feasible to imagine living for a year in a state as severe as during a bout of pneumonia and to compare it with a year with a chronic condition.

A reason for the high values given to the annual profiles may be that valuation procedures have problems in determining accurate weights for low-severity conditions. Specifically, in the PTO_1 and PTO_2 methods the Dutch study replicated from the GBD protocol, the numbers of people to trade off against 1 000 healthy persons for a low-severity condition is close to 1 000 for the PTO_1 method and a very high number in the PTO_2 method. For example, the equivalent for a condition with a disability weight of 0.01 in the PTO_1 trade-off is 1 010 and in the PTO_2 trade-off is 100 000 (Table 1). What probably happens is that most people find it hard to make a distinction between one large and another even larger number in the PTO_2 trade-off and similarly consider the difference trivial between trading off 1 010 or 1 005 people with a minor disease against 1 000 healthy people in the PTO_1 version. Unfortunately, at the lower end of the severity spectrum these seemingly trivial differences in PTO values translate into a doubling of the corresponding disability weight. As a conse-

Table I   Trade-off equivalents in PTO₁ and PTO₂ methods for disability weights of a selected number of severity levels

Disability weight	PTO₁ trade-off equivalent	PTO₂ trade-off equivalent
0.005	1 005	200 000
0.01	1 010	100 000
0.02	1 020	50 000
0.45	1 818	2 222
0.50	2 000	2 000

quence when applied in a burden of disease calculation this also means a doubling of the DALY estimate for that condition.

This is a recognized problem of the current valuation methods for which no alternative has yet been developed and tested. It is therefore not a wise practice to put relatively severe conditions of short duration, such as myocardial infarction and pneumonia, artificially into a low-severity category by presenting them as an annual profile.

From comparisons of burden of disease results between different settings and time periods, it is desirable that disability weights relate to health states in their "purest" form and that variations in numbers of cases and durations drive the differentials in the calculations. Stipulating a duration in the description of conditions for which weights are derived reduces their applicability to making these comparisons. To illustrate this point, let us look at peptic ulcer disease. The Dutch study valued this health state as an annual profile with four weeks of peptic ulcer disease in an otherwise healthy year. If an intervention becomes available that reduces the average duration to three weeks, a new weight would have to be generated for a profile of one year with three weeks of peptic ulcer disease unless the true weight for the symptomatic period is back-calculated from the annualized weight. We have seen above that this did not give very credible results. The simple solution to this problem is to keep duration out of the description of disease states for which disability weights are generated. Any changes in the duration of the condition can then be driven by the epidemiological findings.

It becomes even messier when annual profiles are valued for a combination of a short duration condition followed by a chronic complication. Let us take acute myocardial infarction (AMI) and heart failure as an example. An annual profile would be, say, six weeks of AMI followed by heart failure for the rest of the year. You would also need to have a separate weight for AMI not followed by heart failure and another weight for heart failure for those who continue to have heart failure past the first year. If these three are valued separately it is more than likely that the composite weight for AMI + heart failure will differ from six weeks at the weight for AMI alone and 46 weeks with heart failure. That would be an untenable position unless you want to argue that heart failure in the 46 weeks following AMI is different from the heart failure at week 47 post-AMI. Again, from an epidemiological point of view it is desirable to have a separate weight for AMI that can be applied for the estimated duration of six weeks and another weight for heart failure, preferably with distinctions for mild, moderate and severe. These weights for heart failure can then also be applied to heart failure arising from other diseases such as cardiomyopathy or valvular heart disease.

Another issue is related to chronic diseases of an episodic nature, which include a lot of mental disorders (major depression, bipolar disorder, schizophrenia, a lot of the anxiety disorders), asthma and epilepsy. These conditions differ considerably in the length of episodes: minutes in the case of epilepsy, hours to days in asthma, months to years in the mental disorders. Furthermore, the length of an episode may vary between countries and over time. For example, the proportion of time spent in a psychotic episode during five years of follow-up in the International Pilot Study of Schizophrenia of WHO (Leff et al. 1992) varied considerably between countries. Thus, one disability weight for schizophrenia assuming an average split between time spent in psychosis and in between psychotic episodes would be time and context specific and thus unable to reflect differences between countries and over time. This problem is circumvented by having a weight for the symptomatic episode and another weight for the time in between episodes if there is considered to be "rest-disability". Existing differentials between countries and over time can then be reflected in the estimates of incidence and duration. This becomes more problematic the shorter the average duration of an episode. In the case of asthma there is some information on the average time spent with symptoms of wheeze and shortness of breath (e.g. Bauman et al. 1992) that would allow valuation of time spent while asthmatic with symptoms (with an appropriate disability weight) and time without symptoms (at an appropriate much lower weight). This would allow capturing changes over time. For instance, if through a concerted effort the coverage of preventive therapy for asthma with steroid inhalers dramatically increases one would expect the average proportion of time asthmatics are symptomatic to decrease and you would want your burden of disease methodology to be able to capture that change.

An alternative method for the disease with short episodic intervals is to develop weights for different levels of severity. An example is the following staging for epilepsy: i) mild, asymptomatic for most of the time; ii) moderate, moderate symptoms most of the time; iii) severe, uncontrolled. A similar staging for asthma is also possible: i) mild, asymptomatic for most of the time; ii) moderate, moderate symptoms at least half of the time, e.g. coughing at night, wheezing at any time and feeling of breathlessness; iii) severe symptoms most of the time, necessitating repeated hospitalizations or visits to emergency departments. I would prefer the first option with weights for symptomatic asthma and asymptomatic periods as that would give more flexibility to combine with epidemiological estimates (if available, of course!) of average time spent with symptoms, while the second option restricts you to making assumptions on the proportions of asthmatics in each severity category.

In conclusion, the Dutch Disability Weight Study has made a great contribution by developing weights for different levels of severity for important disabling conditions and by adding a generic health state description to the disease labels of the conditions valued. However, their use of annual profiles for short duration conditions has rendered implausible weights. Even if the weights would have been more credible, stipulating a certain duration in the description of health states to be valued severely limits the application of such weights in burden of disease studies.

REFERENCES

Bauman A, Mitchell CA, Henry RL, et al. (1992) Asthma morbidity in Australia: an epidemiological study. *Medical Journal of Australia*, **156**(12):827–831.

Leff J, Sartorius N, Jablensky A, Korten A, Ernberg G (1992) The international pilot study of schizophrenia: five-year follow-up findings. *Psychological Medicine*, **22**(1):131–145.

Mathers CD, Vos T, Stevenson C (1999) *The burden of disease and injury in Australia*. Australian Institute of Health and Welfare, Canberra. *http:// www.aihw.gov.au/publications/health/bdia.html*.

Melse JM, Kramers PGN (1998) *Berekening van de ziektelast in Nederland. Achtergronddokument bij VTV-1997; deel III, hoofdstuk 7, [Calculation of the burden of disease in the Netherlands. Background document to VTV-1997; part III, chapter 7]*. Rijksinstitut voor Volkgezondheit en Milieu [National Institute of Public Health and the Environment], Bilthoven.

Murray CJL, Lopez AD, eds. (1996) *The global burden of disease: a comprehensive assessment of mortality and disability from diseases, injuries and risk factors in 1990 and projected to 2020*. Global Burden of Disease and Injury, Vol. 1. Harvard School of Public Health on behalf of WHO, Cambridge, MA.

Stouthard MEA, Essink-Bot ML, Bonsel GJ, et al. (1997) *Disability weights for diseases in the Netherlands*. Erasmus University, Department of Public Health, Rotterdam.

Vos T, Begg S (2000) Victorian burden of disease study: morbidity. Public Health Division, Department of Human Services, Melbourne. *http:// www.dhs.vic.gov.au/phd/9909065/index.htm*.

Chapter 9.3

MEASURING HEALTH STATE VALUES IN DEVELOPING COUNTRIES — RESULTS FROM A COMMUNITY SURVEY IN ANDHRA PRADESH

PRASANTA MAHAPATRA, JOSHUA A. SALOMON
AND LIPIKA NANDA

INTRODUCTION

There have been few attempts to elicit health state valuations from the general population, and previous studies typically have focused on fully literate populations in economically developed countries such as Canada (Sackett and Torrance 1978) and the United Kingdom (Gudex et al. 1996). Because population-based empirical assessments of health states are extremely limited, new surveys are needed. A study was conducted in Andhra Pradesh (AP) state, India to measure individual preferences regarding various health states. To the best of our knowledge, this is the first community-based health state valuation study in the developing world. Details of the study design, methodology, data collection, analysis and results are reported elsewhere (Mahapatra et al. 2000). In this paper we review the study methodology and the reliability and validity of the measurements very briefly. Results from the community survey are reported in greater detail, including an examination of the distributions of valuations for different health states, and comparison of the disability weights obtained from this study with results from previous valuation studies.

MATERIALS AND METHODS

The study was conducted in the year 1999 and included two components. The first arm of the study consisted of a series of multi-method deliberative health state valuation workshops for educated persons from different backgrounds. The 180 participants for the workshops were urban professionals recruited by convenience, although efforts were made to include a broad spectrum of different professional backgrounds. Participants in these workshops valued health states using four procedures: card sort, visual analogue scale (VAS), time trade-off (TTO), and person trade-off (PTO).

The second arm of the study consisted of a household survey in Kondakkal village of Ranga Reddy district in AP, in which health state valuations were elicited using a card sort exercise followed by the VAS. The sample of 1 010 persons for the community survey was drawn randomly from the list of voters, with balanced representation of males and females and adults in all age groups.

Twenty-two health states were selected to represent a broad range of severity levels. These 22 states were organized into four sets. Each set included six core states common to all four sets, plus four set-specific health states. Each study participant was asked to value a total of 11 states including his or her own health state. A six-dimension, five-level (6D5L) system was used to describe the health states to respondents. The 6D5L descriptive system was adapted from the EuroQol EQ-5D system (Brooks 1996) by adding cognition as a sixth dimension (Krabbe et al. 1999) and expanding the descriptions of severity levels to five (rather than three) categories. In addition, our implementation of the 6D5L system included a graphic description system to assist in conveying the health state descriptions to partially-literate and illiterate respondents (see chapter 7.4). Results from the multi-method workshops and test-retest data from a subset of the community survey respondents were used in assessing the reliability and validity of the measurements.

RELIABILITY AND VALIDITY

Analysis of test and retest data on ordinal rankings of health states, individual valuations of their own health states, and differences in distributions of valuations at the community level, led us to hypothesize that an individual's true health state valuations may be characterized by multi-valued fuzzy sets with different degrees of clarification for different states rather than as single-valued quantities for each state. The rank orderings in test and retest measurements provide one means of examining this hypothesis. In the community survey, none of the 100 test-retest respondents exactly reproduced their original rank orderings in the retest, and 31% of the respondents showed no statistically significant correlation between the test and retest rankings. In comparison, two (13%) of the 15 test-retest respondents in the multi-method workshops had no statistically significant relationship between the test and retest rank orders. If we assumed that ordinal rankings suffer from minimal measurement error, then major changes in rankings from test to retest would support the notion that valuations arise from a fuzzy set of values with different degrees of clarification for different health states. In fact, there is likely to be at least some measurement error associated with ordinal rankings, and the different levels of consistency in the workshops and community surveys suggest that the level of measurement error may be related to the education level of the respondents.

Reliability of the health state valuations in this study was judged as moderate based on generalizability coefficients (0.56 to 0.67) and conventional reliability measures such as the intraclass correlation coefficient (ICC) (0.6), within-valuer correlation (around 0.6 to 0.8) and within-valuer ICC (0.6 to 0.8). It is worth noting, however, that existing reliability measures are typically used in measurement models that seek to discriminate personality characteristics between individuals, while many applications of health state valuations focus on the measurement of values in a community. If a health state is invariably perceived by members of a community to be a severe disability, for example, health state valuations will vary little across individuals in the community. Existing measurement models that have been developed primarily for educational testing do not account for the fact that different health states may have different degrees of crystallization of valuations in a community. A more appropriate measurement model for health state valuations would improve the interpretation of reliability measures.

The health state valuation instruments used in this study have good content validity, as they represent the product of numerous efforts by researchers working from similar conceptual definitions of health and are based on empirical catalogues of health state attributes by some large studies. The criterion validity of health state valuation instruments cannot be tested, since we do not have a gold standard for this purpose. The instruments have shown good convergent validity. Measurements from multiple methods including the VAS, TTO, and PTO agreed reasonably well with each other.

Incorporation of an ordinal rank consistency requirement in valuation tasks appeared to facilitate deliberation. Overall, the incidence of counter-intuitive valuations (better valuations for states whose profiles were unambiguously worse than other states) was lower for VAS than for other methods. Considering its simplicity and feasibility for community surveys, VAS appears to be the instrument of choice for the collection of data on health state valuations in the general community, although responses elicited by VAS may need to be transformed to account for scale distortions and other possible sources of bias.

RESULTS FROM THE COMMUNITY SURVEY OF HEALTH STATE VALUATIONS

DISTRIBUTION OF VALUATIONS FOR DIFFERENT HEALTH STATES

Figures 1 to 3 plot the distribution of VAS scores in the community survey for 22 health states. The VAS scores are plotted on a scale in which higher numbers represent more severe health levels. The total number of valuations ranged from 230 to 280 for health states other than the core conditions (watery diarrhoea, mild diabetes, mild tuberculosis, severe continuous migraine, unipolar major depression and quadriplegia), which were included in all four sets and therefore provided approximately 1 010 valuations. Most health states in this study have unimodal distributions, although a few states, such as continuous moderate back pain and severe heart failure, show bimodal distributions, with two modes that are reasonably close to each other. Unimodal distributions for most health states would suggest that members of the community share some commonality in the valuation of health states. This is important for the application of health state valuations in summary measures of population health. Without any consensus on valuations to be assigned to different health states, it would be impossible to combine non-fatal health outcomes into a summary measure of population health.

The degree of crystallization clearly varies across different health states. Health states in this study have been categorized into three groups based on the level of diffuseness in valuations across respondents (Table 1). The classification was based on a visual examination of the frequency plots for each health state and hence is subjective. As we gather more experience from examination of health state valuation distributions, it will be useful to develop objective criteria for the classification. We have used the height of the tallest frequency bin as one criterion to aid our judgement. The valuations for group A health states in Figure 1 are all quite diffused. The tallest frequency bin is approximately 0.2 or less. For example, the valuation for infertility appears to be distributed more or less uniformly between 0 and 0.7 and tapers off thereafter. This tells us that most people would not consider infertility to be worse than 0.7, but within the broad range between 0 and 0.7 wide variation remains.

The eight health states that comprise group B in Figure 2 show more crystallized valuations. The tallest frequency bin for all these plots is about 0.2 or less, i.e. the same as in the case of group A. However, the distributions are less diffuse and show increasing mass around the peaks. The Group C plots in Figure 3 show more peaked distributions, usually skewed to the right or left. The distribution for quadriplegia is unique in that

Table 1   Classification of health states by degree of crystallization of community valuations

Group A: Diffused	Group B: Intermediate	Group C: More crystallized
Infertility	Watery diarrhoea	White marks on face
Angina	Urinary incontinence	Two broken arms in cast
Unipolar major depression	Mild hearing disorder	Mild diabetes
Bronchitis	Continuous moderate back pain	Quadriplegia
Severe hallucinatory fever	Mild tuberculosis with treatment	Below knee amputation: two legs
Pain and stiffness in joints	Sever continuous migraine	Severe heart failure
	Schizophrenia	Below knee amputation: one leg
	Peptic ulcer	Blindness

approximately 70% of the valuers rated quadriplegia in the narrow range between 0.9 and 1. The fraction of valuations in the tallest bin for all other health states in group C is in the range of 0.25 to 0.4.

The observed variation in the extent to which valuations of different health states are well-crystallized in the community is consistent with the notion that individual-level valuations are drawn from fuzzy sets with different degrees of clarification. The degree of crystallization of valuations in the community for different health states has important implications for disease-burden assessment. The range of disability weight inputs for each of the health states included in sensitivity analyses should reflect the distribution of valuations in the community. Health states with diffused valuations merit a wider range of disability weight inputs, while narrower ranges will suffice for health states with well-crystallized valuations in the community. Parametric description of the distributions should fa-

Figure I   Distribution of disability weights—group A health states

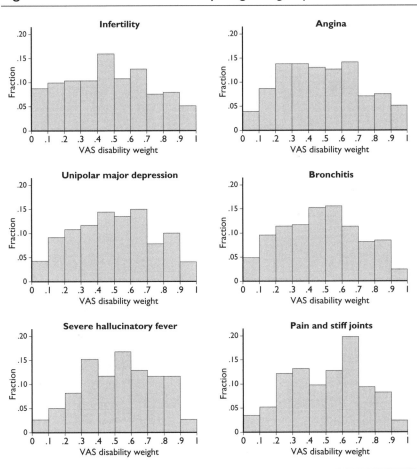

Figure 2   Distribution of disability weights—group B health states

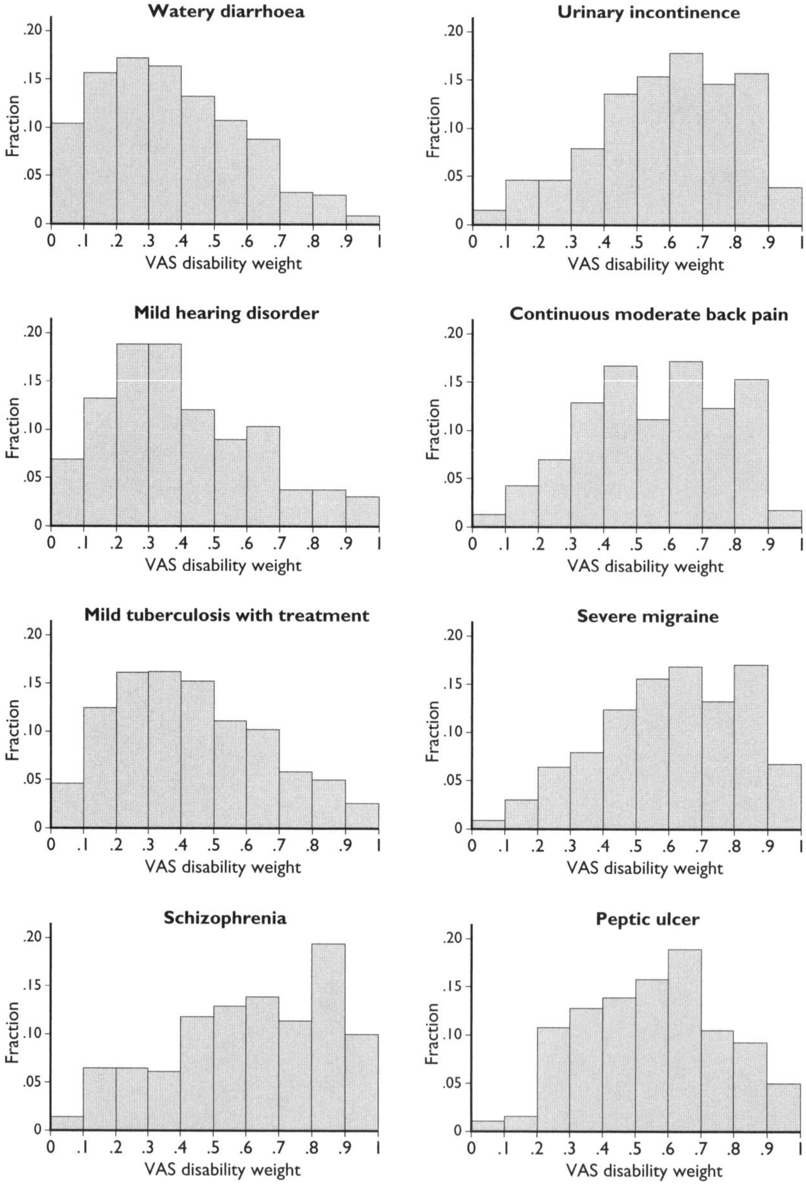

Figure 3   Distribution of disability weights—group C health states

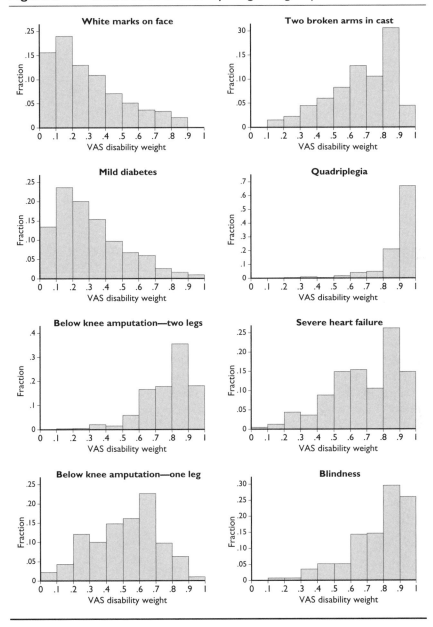

cilitate uncertainty analysis of disease-burden estimates, and will enable further analysis to improve our understanding of what contributes to diffuseness and crystallization of community valuation of health states.[1]

COMPARISON WITH DISABILITY WEIGHTS REPORTED BY OTHER STUDIES

The Global Burden of Disease Study 1990 (Murray and Lopez 1996) developed a set of disability weights using a deliberative group exercise among health professionals based primarily on alternatively-framed PTO questions (the results are referred to hereafter as the GBD96 disability weights). More recently, a set of Dutch disability weights were estimated using VAS and PTO methods (Stouthard et al. 1997). In the Dutch study, the 38 valuers were urban professionals, most from medical and health backgrounds and some from other areas.

Table 2 shows the 6D5L profiles and disability weights obtained in the present study (APHSV99) alongside the GBD96 weights and Dutch disability weights for the closest comparable conditions.[2] For the Dutch disability weights, the health state profile for each state is indicated using the EQ-5D + C system (Stouthard et al. 1997), which consists of the same six domains used in this study but has three rather than five severity levels. We have labelled these profiles as 6D3L rather than EQ-5D + C to provide a shorthand indication of the similarity and differences between the descriptive systems used in the Dutch study and the current study.

The GBD96 and Dutch disability weights are quite similar to each other. They differ from the weights obtained in this study by a fairly wide margin in most cases (Figure 4). For many states, GBD96 weights are higher than APHSV99 weights by approximately 0.3. At the lower end of the disability scale (between 0.1 and 0.4), a few health states are given much higher disability weights by the APHSV99 study, for example, bronchitis, two broken arms in casts, peptic ulcer, and severe heart failure. At the upper end of the scale, the gap between the two studies is relatively smaller. Unfortunately there are not many common estimates in the middle range with disability weights around 0.5, but additional states in the mid-range might suggest a non-linear functional relationship between results from the two studies.

One explanation for the higher disability weights in the current study is that these weights were obtained primarily using the VAS. Although we did not find much difference in the magnitude of the VAS and TTO weights in this study, we cannot rule out the possibility that the VAS provides an overestimate of the severity level for milder conditions. To see how APHSV99 weights compare with VAS measurements elsewhere, results were compared to those in a different study that included VAS measures in a group of public health professionals attending a training workshop on burden of disease analysis in November 1999 (Figure 5) (see chapter 9.4

Table 2 Comparison of mean disability weights from different studies

Health state	This study 6D5L	Wkshp	Survey	GBD96	Dutch study 6D3L	Mean
Angina	111321	0.460	0.480	0.227	111121	0.080
Below knee amputation: one leg	322211	0.510	0.510	0.300		
Below knee amputation: two legs	433221	0.690	0.780			
Blindness	323122	0.640	0.770	0.600	123121	0.430
Bronchitis	112311	0.350	0.470	0.099	112211	0.170
Common cold	112211	0.120		0.000	111211	0.020
Continuous moderate back pain	212321	0.360	0.550		212211	0.060
Infertility	111131	0.370	0.460	0.180		0.110
Mild hearing disorder	112211	0.210	0.390		112111	0.110
Mild tuberculosis with treatment	111221	0.420	0.420	0.264	112211(40%) 222221(60%)	0.290
Moderate anaemia	112121	0.290		0.011		
Mild diabetes	111121	0.290	0.300	0.012	111111(90%) 112221(10%)	0.070
Peptic ulcer	112321	0.360	0.550	0.115	111111(20%) 111211(60%) 112211(10%) 112221(10%)	0.020
Pain and stiffness in joints	222331	0.490	0.510	0.233	122211	0.210
Quadriplegia	554341	0.860	0.900	0.895	332111(70%) 333221(30%)	0.840
Severe hallucinatory fever	444333	0.770	0.530			
Severe heart failure	434531	0.730	0.690	0.323	223321	0.650
Severe migraine	113431	0.500	0.600	0.738		
Schizophrenia	234244	0.790	0.610	0.627–0.667	222223	0.810
Two broken arms in cast	154321	0.590	0.680	0.137–0.180		
Unipolar major depression	124142	0.600	0.490	0.600	223232	0.760
Urinary incontinence	113331	0.500	0.590			
Watery diarrhoea	111211	0.250	0.360	0.086–0.119		
White marks on face	111131	0.240	0.290	0.020		

The following mappings are used for comparisons with GBD96 disability weights:

Bronchitis = Lower respiratory infections – chronic sequelae
Common cold = Upper respiratory infections – episodes
Below knee amputation: one leg = Amputated leg
Mild tuberculosis = Tuberculosis, HIV sero-negative cases, ages 15–44
Mild diabetes = Diabetes cases
Severe heart failure = Congestive heart failure

Figure 4   Scatterplot of GBD96 disability weights versus APHSV weights

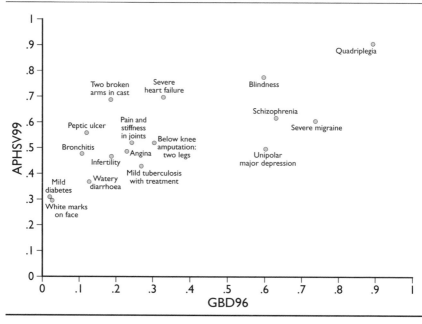

for a description of the study). For most of the nine common states in these two studies, APHSV99 weights are higher by about 0.1.

We can also compare the APHSV99 disability weights to the weights obtained using VAS in the Dutch study. Table 3 shows the mean disability weights for the five states common to these two studies, as well as the 6D3L (in the case of the Dutch study) and 6D5L (for APHSV99) descriptions. For four out of five conditions APHSV99 VAS weights are higher than the corresponding Dutch study weights. The difference is 0.17 for mild diabetes and more than 0.2 for the remaining three conditions. In the case of pain and stiffness of joints (rheumatoid arthritis), the Dutch study weight is higher. This exception can be explained by the fact that the Dutch study valued severe rheumatoid arthritis, while the AP study used a less severe description of pain and stiffness of joints. Overall, APHSV99 VAS disability weights appear to be higher than the Dutch disability weights by approximately 0.2.

It is worthwhile to consider several possible explanations for higher disability weights assigned by the community in the APHSV99 study. Firstly, measurement error attributable to differences in study implementation likely contributed to part of the disparity in results. Further improvements in descriptions of the health states may increase the spread of valuations toward the endpoints of the scale, particularly on the low disability end. Secondly, differences in valuation methods probably explain

Figure 5   Mean VAS disability weights from APHSV study and 1999 burden of disease training workshop

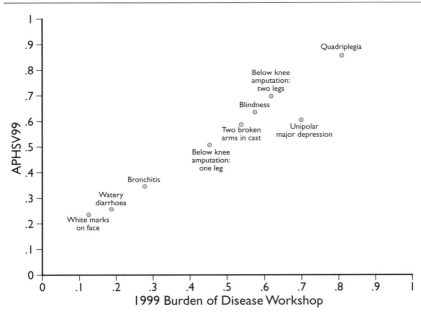

part of the difference between the APHSV99 and GBD96 weights. Thirdly, real differences between valuations by the community and valuations given by public health experts are also possible. Furthermore, it may be the case that the community in AP views any disruption in perfect health as a more serious loss than in the other study settings. This difference in AP might be conceptualized as a fixed effect that assigns a certain decrement to any departure from perfect health in addition to the health loss specific to the state. Based on the comparisons of APHSV99 data with results from other studies, the size of this fixed effect may be somewhere between 0.1 and

Table 3   Mean VAS disability weights from APHSV99 and Dutch health state valuation study 1997

| Health state | Dutch study 1997 | | APHSV99 | |
	6D3L	Disability weight	6D5L	Disability weight
Angina	111211	0.16	111321	0.46
Blindness	123121	0.38	323122	0.64
Back pain	212211	0.13	212321	0.36
Mild diabetes	112221	0.12	111121	0.29
Pain and stiff joints	222331	0.70	222331	0.49

0.3. Each of the above possibilities and other unknown factors need to be investigated further to give a clearer picture of the determinants of differences in valuations of health states by different persons and at different sites.

SUMMARY AND SOME CONCLUSIONS

An important contribution of this study is the advancement of methodological aspects of health state valuation in developing country communities. A health state descriptive system incorporating a graphical description component was developed to facilitate communication in partially literate communities. Some deliberative tools for conducting health state valuation workshops for educated persons were also developed. We hope that the experience gained in this project will aid in future research on the valuation of health states in developing country settings.

Health state valuation studies will have to contend with the problem of measurement error, as is the case in most other areas of psychometric measurement. Unfortunately, we do not yet have a fully specified measurement model for health state valuations. Most studies use reliability measures conceived under classical test theory developed in the context of educational testing and measurement. In the field of educational measurement, it is generally assumed that the object of measurement is distributed normally with some variance. If the variance component attributable to subjects is high, then educational tests are considered reliable. We have seen that community valuations of different health states follow different distributions. Health state valuations are not personal endowments that can be assumed to be distributed normally in a fashion similar to, say, intelligence. If the community valuation for a particular health state is well crystallized, then the true variance of subjective valuations will be less as compared to health states where the valuation is more diffused. Generalizability theory allows for a more realistic modelling of the measurement process.

The incidence of measurement error and our present understanding about the nature of the valuation process would suggest that community level valuation of health states requires a large sample size and also repeated measurements. Large sample sizes would help minimize the measurement error for mean values estimated from community surveys. We would expect that repeated measures would occasion repeated deliberation by the valuers and thereby help in the clarification of their value sets. The tradeoffs between sample size and repeated measurements will have to be studied.

To date, researchers have focused largely on mean valuations within their study populations. This study has demonstrated that community valuations of different health states do not all follow the same distribution. Valuations for some states, such as infertility, are quite diffused, while valuations for others, such as quadriplegia, are well crystallized. To the extent that the variance of different health state valuations may relate systematically to their mean values, it may be possible to characterize these different distributions parametrically. A better understanding of the distributions of valuations remains a priority for research, as differences in these distributions for different health states can have important policy implications.

NOTES

1 We conjecture that the sub-family of unimodal beta distributions may serve well to describe distribution of health state valuations. Further work is needed to examine goodness-of-fit, estimate the distributions and study factors that may contribute to differences in the distribution of health state values.

2 Note that the Dutch study results were reported as health state weights, so the scale was transformed (disability weight = 1 − health state weight) for purposes of this comparison.

REFERENCES

Brooks R (1996) EuroQol: the current state of play. *Health Policy,* 37(1):53–72.

Dolan P (1997) Modelling valuations for EuroQol health states. *Medical Care,* 35(11):1095–1108.

Gudex C, Dolan P, Kind P, Williams A (1996) Health state valuations from the general public, using the visual analogue scale. *Quality of Life Research,* 5(6):521–531.

Krabbe PF, Stouthard MEA, Essink-Bot ML, Bonsel GJ (1999) The effect of adding a cognitive dimension to the EuroQol multiattribute health-status classification system. *Journal of Clinical Epidemiology,* 52(4):293–301.

Mahapatra P, Salomon JA, Nanda L, Rajshree KT (2000) *Measuring health state values in developing countries: report of a study in Andhra Pradesh, India.* Institute of Health Systems, HACA Bhavan, Hyderabad, AP 500004, India.

Murray CJL, Lopez AD, eds. (1996) *The global burden of disease: a comprehensive assessment of mortality and disability from diseases, injuries and risk factors in 1990 and projected to 2020.* Global Burden of Disease and Injury, Vol. 1. Harvard School of Public Health on behalf of WHO, Cambridge, MA.

Sackett DL, Torrance GW (1978) The utility of different health states as perceived by the general public. *Journal of Chronic Diseases,* 31(11):697–704.

Stouthard MEA, Essink-Bot ML, Bonsel GJ, et al. (1997) *Disability weights for diseases in the Netherlands.* Erasmus University, Department of Public Health, Rotterdam.

ESTIMATING HEALTH STATE VALUATIONS
USING A MULTIPLE-METHOD PROTOCOL

JOSHUA A. SALOMON AND CHRISTOPHER J.L. MURRAY

INTRODUCTION

In any summary measure of population health such as healthy life expectancy (WHO 2000), disability-adjusted life years (Murray 1996), quality-adjusted life expectancy (Kaplan and Erickson 2000) or health-adjusted life expectancy (Rosenberg et al. 1999), one essential data input is a set of valuations that assign weights to health states that are worse than ideal health. These health state valuations provide the critical link between information on mortality and information on non-fatal health outcomes. In order to serve as the basis for the combination of these two types of information, health state valuations must provide a cardinal measure of the value placed on time spent in a particular health state, relative to time spent in ideal or full health. It is important that any discussion of health state valuations in summary measures begins with a clear understanding of this requirement. As Essink-Bot and Bonsel point out in chapter 9.1, much of the confusion in the research on health state valuations has resulted from the failure to recognize that strategies for measuring these valuations may differ depending on their intended use.

A range of different methods for eliciting health state valuations have been proposed and used widely, including the standard gamble, time trade-off, visual analogue scale and person trade-off (Froberg and Kane 1989; Nord 1992). Thus far, there has been little agreement as to which method is most appropriate, stemming in part from the lack of clarity regarding the need to tailor the approach to the application. Arguments for and against different methods have been based on ethical grounds (Arnesen and Nord 1999), economic theory (Torrance 1976), and comparisons of psychometric properties (Krabbe et al. 1997). Many of the proponents of different approaches, however, have implicitly acknowledged that perhaps none of the available approaches is ideal.

In a number of empirical studies in which multiple methods have been used, the different methods have yielded different valuations for the same set of states (Dolan et al. 1996; Torrance 1986), although high correlations between the different measures have been observed. In some studies, mathematical relationships between responses on different types of valuation questions have been estimated (Dolan and Sutton 1997). This strategy is motivated by the assumption that one of the available methods must be selected for practical purposes, and it may be useful to develop a convenient function that would allow the transformation of valuations obtained using another method to the equivalent valuations that would be expected from the chosen method. Yet, if in fact none of the available measurement techniques provides the cardinal valuation measure that is required for summary measures of population health, it is worth considering whether transformations from one to another of these techniques is the most appropriate way to proceed.

In this paper, we propose an alternative, which acknowledges that none of the available methods gives us the exact quantity of interest, but that each of them produces responses from which this quantity may be imputed. By formalizing our understanding of how each of the valuation techniques captures other values or sources of bias in addition to the value of the health state itself, we aim to recover the underlying health value function from responses to four different types of valuation questions applied to a range of different health states.

This paper presents our approach to estimating health state values using a multiple-method exercise and describes the design, implementation and analysis of a first study of this approach.

METHODS

HEALTH STATE VALUATION EXERCISE

A multiple-method health state valuation exercise was implemented among a convenience sample of 69 public health professionals from 28 different countries.

Twelve health states were selected to span a range of different severity levels. The states were described by brief labels and standardized descriptions of levels on six dimensions of health (mobility, self-care, usual activities, pain/discomfort, anxiety/depression and cognition) based on the modification of the EuroQol EQ-5D classification system that increases the number of levels in each domain from three to five and includes cognition as an additional domain (Brooks 1996; Krabbe et al. 1999).

The exercise consisted of 5 different tasks:

- ordinal ranking of the 12 states with the aid of index cards;

- valuation of the 12 states using a visual analogue scale (VAS) anchored by the best imaginable health state at 100 and death at 0, and with 100 equally-spaced tick marks, labelled at every even number;

- valuation of the 12 states using a time trade-off (TTO) question and self-completed worksheets, followed by the opportunity to examine and revise all 12 TTO valuations;

- valuation of the 12 states using a standard gamble (SG) question and self-completed worksheets, followed by the opportunity to examine and revise all 12 SG valuations; and

- valuation of the 12 health states using a person trade-off (PTO) question and self-completed worksheets, followed by the opportunity to examine and revise all 12 PTO valuations.

The format of each of the valuation tasks was as follows:

1. *Ordinal ranking*. Respondents were asked to consider each health state, imagining what it would be like for them to live in that health state. They were asked to assume that the life expectancy in each health state would be the same (10 years). They were then asked to rank them from the most desirable to the least desirable state.

2. *Visual analogue scale*. Respondents again were asked to imagine what it would be like for them to live in each of the health states for a duration of 10 years. The instructions reminded them to try to use the actual distances on the scale in a meaningful way, such that states that are similarly attractive would be placed close together while states that are very different would be placed far apart. They were asked to indicate the exact point on the scale where they would place each state, relative to the best imaginable health, death and all of the other states.

3. *Time trade-off*. Respondents were asked to imagine that they were living in the health state with a life expectancy of ten years, and faced a choice between 2 options: (1) to remain in that health state for the 10 remaining years of life; or (2) to be restored to perfect health but live for a shorter period of time. A worksheet for each health state guided the respondents through a series of trade-offs in which the number of years of shortened life expectancy in return for improved health was varied. The worksheet was designed to help respondents determine their indifference point, which consisted of the number of years in perfect health that would make the two options equally attractive.

4. *Standard gamble*. Respondents were again asked to imagine that they were living in the health state with a life expectancy of 10 years, but this time the choice was between: (1) remaining in that health state with 100% certainty for the 10 remaining years of life; or (2) accepting a risky procedure that offers some probability of being raised to perfect health for the remaining 10 years but also carries some risk of immediate death. A similar worksheet was used in which the respondents answered a number of different trade-offs with varying levels of risk,

in order to identify the indifference point where the risky option would be equally attractive as the certain option.

5. _Person trade-off._ Respondents were asked to imagine that they were decision-makers facing a difficult choice between two different programmes, with only enough money to fund one of them. The first programme would prevent the deaths of 100 perfectly healthy individuals, thereby extending their lives for 10 years, while the second programme would prevent the onset of some health problem in a certain number of healthy people, thereby improving their health expectancy from 10 years in a state worse than perfect health to 10 years lived in perfect health. A worksheet was provided to help respondents identify their indifference point, where the number of cases of prevented health problems would balance the prevention of 100 deaths.

Before beginning each task, basic instructions were given, and two volunteers were led through examples. After the instruction, individuals were allowed to complete each task for the 12 states. For the time trade-off, standard gamble and person trade-off, once respondents had completed the exercise for all 12 states, they were presented with their responses for all 12 conditions and allowed to revise any of the values if they wished to do so.

ANALYSIS

The goal of the analysis was to use the entire collection of responses for each individual to impute the health state values required in the construction of summary measures. In order to achieve this goal, the first step was to formalize the relationship between responses on each type of measurement method and the underlying values of interest using flexible parametric forms.

For each of the four measurement methods—visual analogue scale, time trade-off, standard gamble and person trade-off—we assumed that responses were described by an increasing function of the underlying value for the state (i.e. more severe states would be ranked as such by all methods), with specification of the functional form guided by relevant theoretical and empirical findings. We describe these functions briefly in this section and include complete mathematical details in the Technical Appendix.

For each measurement method, at least one auxiliary parameter was needed to describe the transformation from the underlying value function to the response function:

- Based on the common observation that the standard gamble reflects both strength of preference for a health state and an individual's attitude towards risk, we modelled standard gamble responses as a function of the underlying valuation and a risk aversion parameter. We examined several different formulations including exponential, logarithmic and power functions, based on the theoretical framework presented in Bell and Raiffa (1998).

- For the person trade-off, proponents have recognized that responses depend both on the level of health in a particular state and on distributional concerns (Arnesen and Nord 1999). In responding to person trade-off questions, some individuals may be reluctant to choose to prevent large numbers of non-fatal health outcomes when the option of preventing deaths is available. We have therefore modelled the person trade-off responses using similar functions as those used for the standard gamble, but allowing for a distinct parameter to capture this "rule of rescue" (Hadorn 1991).

- For the visual analogue scale, a long-standing result from psychophysics suggests that individual perceptions of sensory stimuli of varying intensities tend to follow a power function transformation of the true intensity levels (Stevens 1957). We have based the model for the VAS responses on this finding, including a coefficient that determines the amount of curvature in the power function.

- For the time trade-off, responses will vary depending on the degree of time preference that individuals exhibit. If individuals have non-zero discount rates, then the two streams of life that are compared in the time trade-off (e.g. 10 years in state X and 5 years in perfect health) must first be translated into their equivalent present values in order to compute the implied health state value. We have assumed an exponential discounting model, with a single parameter to capture the discount rate.

Given the specification described above, the model included a total of 16 parameters of interest: 12 health state values, plus 4 auxiliary parameters.

We used maximum likelihood methods to estimate the parameters in the model. It was assumed that the stochastic component of the model followed a truncated normal distribution constrained between 0 and 1. Inspection of the distributions of responses on the different measures suggested strong heteroskedasticity, which was confirmed in regressions of the standard deviation of responses by the mean values for each method. We therefore specified the variance of the truncated normal distribution as a linear function of the expectation, and allowed the slope and intercept of the function to differ by valuation method.

In order to represent the uncertainty around the model estimates, we undertook numerical simulations of the results by sampling from the joint distribution of the estimated parameters obtained from the maximum likelihood estimation, and recalculating the quantities of interest for each set of sampled parameters. This approach allowed us to develop bounds around the estimated strength of preference values and auxiliary parameters in the model that reflected important estimation uncertainties.

Results

Responses from the four different measurement methods are summarized in Figure 1.

Overall, the visual analogue scale tends to give the lowest values for a given health state, with the smallest variance across respondents. Time trade-off values tend to be slightly higher than VAS values, followed by standard gamble and finally, person trade-off. For severe states, the standard gamble and person trade-off methods both produce considerably higher variance across respondents than either the time trade-off or visual analogue scale.

Figure 2 plots the mean valuations against the standard deviations for each of the different methods. As this figure illustrates, there are systematic differences in the standard deviations for the four different methods. Furthermore, the standard deviations appear to be strongly associated with the mean level, especially for the time trade-off, standard gamble and

Figure 1   Mean response and interquartile range across 69 respondents for 12 states and 4 valuation methods

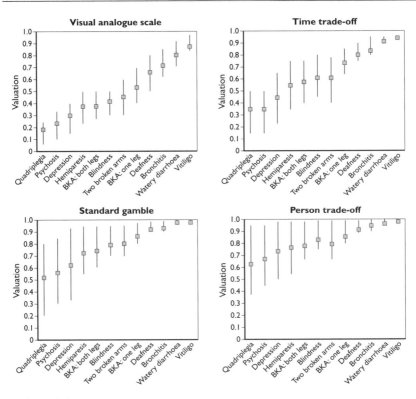

BKA: Below the knee amputation.

person trade-off. This relationship formed the basis for the heteroskedastic formulation of the stochastic model in the estimation procedure.

Table 1 lists the estimated severities for the 12 states in this study, along with the approximate 95% confidence interval for each estimate. The rank order of the estimated severities is consistent with the rankings from the four measurement methods. Because the methods have distinguished the effects of risk aversion and equity concerns from the severity of the health state, mild health states have a lower rating than the valuations in previ-

Figure 2   Mean valuations and standard deviations by method and state

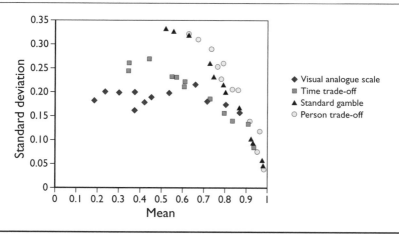

Table 1   Estimated health state valuations and ranges based on multiple-method protocol using visual analogue scale, time trade-off, standard gamble and person trade-off techniques

State	Severity	Range[a]
Quadriplegia	0.29	0.23–0.37
Active psychosis	0.31	0.24–0.39
Major depression	0.36	0.28–0.44
Hemiparesis	0.43	0.35–0.52
Below the knee amputation, both legs	0.45	0.36–0.54
Blindness	0.50	0.40–0.59
Two broken arms	0.49	0.41–0.59
Below the knee amputation, one leg	0.60	0.50–0.68
Deafness	0.71	0.62–0.79
Chronic bronchitis	0.77	0.68–0.84
Watery diarrhoea	0.84	0.76–0.89
Vitiligo on face	0.89	0.83–0.94

a. 95% confidence interval.

ous studies (Murray 1996). This has important implications for the economic analysis of preventive and curative health interventions.

The estimated values for the auxiliary parameters (Table 2) imply that the respondents are strongly risk averse and have preferences consistent with strong distributional concerns. The results point to a moderate degree of scale distortion in VAS responses. For the TTO, the model results indicate negative time preference. The unusual finding of a negative discount rate would imply that individuals consider a unit of health in the future as more valuable than a unit of health today. While this finding has been demonstrated in other empirical studies of individual discount rates (Dolan and Gudex 1995; Ganiats et al. 2000; van der Pol and Cairns 2000), it runs against conventional health economics wisdom. It would be possible to add further constraints to the model, for example that only non-negative time preference would be allowed, but the results presented here are for the unconstrained model. Consideration of alternative functional forms for each of the different measurement methods remains an important area for further research.

Based on the maximum likelihood estimates of the underlying health state valuations for the 12 states and the auxiliary parameters, we have estimated predicted responses for each of the 12 states using the four different methods. The predicted responses fit the observed distributions of responses quite closely (Figure 3).

DISCUSSION

In this paper, we have demonstrated that it is possible to explain responses to the standard gamble, time trade-off, person trade-off and visual analogue scale based on a consistent set of health state valuations for a range of states. None of these methods provides a pure measure of strength of preference, but we may explicitly model the process by which individuals respond to different types of measurement techniques given the underlying valuation of a health state. The multiple-methods approach presented here also allows the measurement of levels of risk aversion, time prefer-

Table 2   Maximum likelihood estimates of auxiliary parameters[a]

State	Estimate	Standard error
Risk attitude (SG)[b]	2.6	0.43
Distributional concerns (PTO)	2.9	0.44
Discount rate (TTO)	−0.089	0.039
Scale distortion (VAS)[c]	0.83	0.10

a. See Appendix for complete description of parameters.

b. A number > 0 indicates risk aversion. The parameter for distributional concerns in the PTO has a similar interpretation.

c. A number < 1 indicates a convex curve.

ence, visual analogue scale distortion and distributional concerns in a group of respondents. One important benefit of this approach is that it will facilitate the mapping between different measurements and the underlying health state valuations that may be needed for comparison of different studies.

With wider use of summary measures of population health and economic appraisal of health interventions, there is considerable interest in the extent of cultural variation in valuations of health states (e.g. Üstün et al. 1999). Variation across individuals in responding to different types of questions may be due to at least three different factors: different interpretation of the health state description; differences in risk aversion, time preference, distributional concerns or visual analogue scale distortion; or differences in the valuation assigned to the same health state.

One important component of the current research agenda on health state valuations is to improve the mode of description of health states as stimuli for valuation. In the study described here, each of the state descriptions included domain levels from a standardized descriptive system. There may be some doubts, however, as to how much of this information was actually reflected in the valuations; the extent to which individuals substitute their own preconceptions about health states for the descriptions that are provided is an important concern. In ongoing studies, we are experimenting with alternative modes of description, including the use of respondents' own ratings of each health state on a range of domains.

Using a multiple-methods approach as outlined here, it should be possible to disentangle cultural or individual variation in factors such as risk aversion or time preference from variation in the value assigned to a health state. This will require larger datasets and the elaboration of the statisti-

Figure 3   Underlying health state valuations and predicted responses for 12 states using 4 different valuation methods

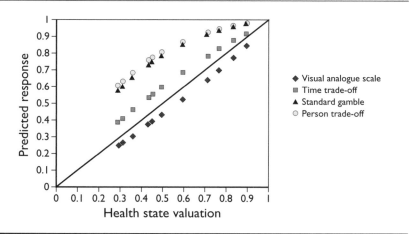

cal model used here to allow for variation in the health state values and auxiliary parameters. One implication is that observed cross-cultural variation in the results from one method such as the VAS or TTO should be interpreted with caution, as it does not necessarily indicate cultural variation in the health state valuation itself.

A number of limitations in this preliminary study are worth noting. First, it is important to recognize that different results might be obtained depending on the functional form of the models that are used. We have selected models based on previous theoretical and empirical work, but other plausible alternatives should be considered. As other model formulations are explored, it will be necessary to examine the sensitivity of the results to the choice of models. The model used for the time trade-off may require particularly careful inspection. Other methodological advances may be fruitful, for example, in using Bayesian statistical methods for incorporating additional prior information into the estimation framework. The nature of measurement error in the application of these methods also merits further examination. While the truncated normal distribution improves on the traditional assumption of normality by accounting for the natural constraints of the data, more work is required before the most appropriate choice of error distributions is clear.

Despite these limitations, the results of this study suggest that new approaches to health state valuations may hold promise. We are hopeful that wider application of these methods can lead to significant improvements in the development of valid, reliable and comparable health state valuations for use in summary measures of population health and evaluations of the benefits of health interventions.

TECHNICAL APPENDIX

Each measurement technique produces a response for each state, x, on a scale particular to that method:

Method	Response	Units and Scale	Interpretation
VAS	s	0 to 100	Rating of health state x
TTO	y	years, 0 to 10	Years of perfect health equivalent to 10 years in state x
SG	p	risk, 0 to 100%	Risk of death at which treatment is equivalent to certainty in state x
PTO	n	persons, 100 to ∞[a]	Number of averted cases of x equivalent to 100 deaths averted

a. In principle, n may be less than 100, which would imply that preventing cases of health state x is preferred to preventing deaths of individuals in ideal health. In practice, all respondents indicated values greater than 100 for all states.

These responses may be rescaled such that each one ranges from 0 to 1, with 1 being the highest valuation:

$$SG_x = 1 - p$$

$$PTO_x = 1 - \frac{100}{n}$$

$$VAS_x = \frac{s}{100}$$

$$TTO_x = \frac{y}{10}$$

We then assume that each one of these rescaled responses is an increasing function of the underlying value for the health state v_x and an auxiliary parameter.

The standard gamble has one parameter θ_1 that represents an individual's risk aversion. The formulation is derived from utility theory, as described by Bell and Raiffa (1998).

$$SG_x = \frac{-e^{-\theta_1 v_x} + 1}{-e^{-\theta_1} + 1}$$

The person trade-off formulation is parallel to the standard gamble formulation, but in this case the parameter θ_2 represents aversion to decisions resulting in loss of life, the so-called "rule of rescue" (Hadorn 1991).

$$PTO_x = \frac{-e^{-\theta_2 v_x} + 1}{-e^{-\theta_2} + 1}$$

The visual analogue scale is a power function with one parameter θ_3. This formulation is based on results from psychophysics experiments (Stevens 1957) and has been suggested by Torrance (1976) in modelling the functional relationship between VAS and SG.

$$VAS_x = 1 - [1 - v_x]^{\theta_3}$$

The function for the time trade-off is derived from the following relation, in which θ_4 characterizes an individual's rate of time preference:

$$v_x = \frac{\dfrac{1}{\theta_4} - \dfrac{1}{\theta_4}\left(e^{-10\theta_4 TTO_x}\right)}{\dfrac{1}{\theta_4} - \dfrac{1}{\theta_4}\left(e^{-10\theta_4}\right)}$$

If people have some rate of time preference, then both alternatives in the TTO should be converted to their present values, so the formula for discounting a continuous stream of life is applied. The function for the time trade-off simply solves the above equation for TTO_x.

$$ TTO_x = - \frac{1}{10\theta_4} \ln \left[1 - (1 - e^{-10\theta_4}) v_x \right] $$

References

Arnesen T, Nord E (1999) The value of DALY life: problems with ethics and validity of disability adjusted life years. *British Medical Journal,* 319(7222):1423–1425.

Bell DE, Raiffa H (1998) Marginal value and intrinsic risk aversion. In: *Decision making: descriptive, normative and prescriptive interactions.* Bell DE, Raiffa H, Tversky A, eds. Cambridge University Press, Cambridge.

Brooks R (1996) EuroQol: the current state of play. *Health Policy,* 37(1):53–72.

Dolan P, Gudex C (1995) Time preference, duration and health state valuations. *Journal of Health Economics,* 4(4):289–299.

Dolan P, Gudex C, Kind P, Williams A (1996) Valuing health states: a comparison of methods. *Journal of Health Economics,* 15(2):209–231.

Dolan P, Sutton M (1997) Mapping visual analogue scale health state valuations onto standard gamble and time trade-off values. *Social Science and Medicine,* 44(10):1519–1530.

Froberg DG, Kane RL (1989) Methodology for measuring health-state preferences, part – II: scaling methods. *Journal of Clinical Epidemiology,* 42(5):459–471.

Ganiats TG, Carson RT, Hamm RM, Cantor SB, et al. (2000) Population-based time preferences for future health outcomes. *Medical Decision Making,* 20(3):263–270.

Hadorn DC (1991) Setting health care priorities in Oregon. Cost-effectiveness meets the rule of rescue. *Journal of the American Medical Association,* 265(17):2218–2225.

Kaplan RM, Erickson P (2000) Gender differences in quality-adjusted survival using a health utilities index. *American Journal of Preventive Medicine,* 18(1):77–82.

Krabbe PF, Stouthard MEA, Essink-Bot ML, Bonsel GJ (1999) The effect of adding a cognitive dimension to the EuroQol multiattribute health-status classification system. *Journal of Clinical Epidemiology,* 52(4):293–301.

Krabbe PFM, Essink-Bot ML, Bonsel GJ (1997) The comparability and reliability of five health-state valuation methods. *Social Science and Medicine,* 45(11):1641–1652.

Murray CJL (1996) Rethinking DALYs. In: *The global burden of disease: a comprehensive assessment of mortality and disability from diseases, injuries, and risk factors in 1990 and projected to 2020*. The Global Burden of Disease and Injury, Vol. 1. Murray CJL, Lopez AD, eds. Harvard School of Public Health on behalf of WHO, Cambridge, MA.

Murray CJL, Salomon JA, Mathers CD (2000) A critical examination of summary measures of population health. *Bulletin of the World Health Organization*, 78(8):981–994.

Nord EM (1992) Methods for quality adjustment of life years. *Social Science and Medicine*, 34(5):559–569.

Read JL, Quinn RJ, Berrick DM, Fineberg HV, Weinstein MC (1984) Preferences for health outcomes: comparison of assessment methods. *Medical Decision Making*, 4(3):315–329.

Rosenberg MA, Fryback DG, Lawrence WF (1999) Computing population-based estimates of health-adjusted life expectancy. *Medical Decision Making*, 19(1):90–97.

Stevens SS (1957) On the psychophysical law. *Psychological Review*, 64(3):153–181.

Torrance GW (1976) Toward a utility theory foundation for health status index models. *Health Services Research*, 11(4):349–369.

Torrance GW (1986) Measurement of health state utilities for economic appraisal: a review. *Journal of Health Economics*, 5(1):1–30.

Üstün TB, Rehm J, Chatterji S, et al. (1999) Multiple-informant ranking of the disabling effects of different health conditions in 14 countries. WHO/NIH joint project CAR study group. *Lancet*, 354(9173):111–115.

van der Pol MM, Cairns JA (2000) Negative and zero time preference for health. *Health Economics*, 9(2):171–175.

Weinstein MC, Siegel JE, Gold MR, Kamlet MS, Russel LB (1996) Recommendations of the panel on cost-effectiveness in health and medicine. *Journal of the American Medical Association*, 276(15):1253–1258.

WHO (2000) *The World Health Report 2000. Health systems: improving performance*. World Health Organization, Geneva.

Chapter 10.1

MODELLING THE RELATIONSHIP BETWEEN THE DESCRIPTION AND VALUATION OF HEALTH STATES

PAUL DOLAN

A number of health state descriptive systems have been specifically designed for calculating a single index value for every state defined within the system. Since most descriptive systems define more health states than it is feasible to elicit direct valuations for in an empirical study, choices have to be made about how best to estimate values for all states from direct observations on a subset of those states. This paper discusses the relative merits of the decomposed and composite approaches to modelling health state valuations. The choice of approach to modelling depends partly on the extent to which there is a pre-commitment to a particular axiomatic model of preferences. The paper also considers various decisions that have to be made when attempting to generate valuation "tariffs" and looks at how such tariffs have been estimated for the HUI3 and EQ-5D descriptive systems. It is argued that a fruitful avenue for future research in this area would be to directly compare the predictive ability of the decomposed and composite approaches.

INTRODUCTION

It is now widely recognized that, to capture the health effects of different policies and programmes, it is necessary to say something about their effects on life expectancy and on health-related quality-of-life (HRQoL). As a result, there are now a number of approaches which try to combine these two attributes into a single composite measure. For example, the disability-adjusted life year (DALY) has been developed in order to calculate the loss associated with premature mortality and morbidity (see Murray 1996) while the quality-adjusted life year (QALY) approach has been used to measure the health outcomes associated with different health care interventions (see Weinstein and Stason 1977).

Whichever approach is adopted, the central question is how to attach values to different levels of HRQoL. For the purposes of this paper, it will be assumed that these values should reflect the preferences of actual or hypothetical patients regarding their own HRQoL. In this context, a decision about the way in which health is to be described is required. One way is as a scenario in which a relatively detailed description of a state of health is presented to respondents, but this suffers from generalizability problems. More often, states of health have been described using a health state descriptive system, and there now exists a number of different types, each designed for a particular purpose (see Streiner and Norman 1995). In order to serve as a summary measure of population health, any measure must allow for the different dimensions (or attributes) of HRQoL to be combined to form an overall single index.

There now exist a number of health state descriptive systems that have been specifically designed for calculating a single index value for each of the generic health states generated by the system (for the most comprehensive review of these descriptive systems to date, see Brazier et al. (1999). Table 1 shows that the different descriptive systems contain different numbers of attributes, as well as different numbers of levels (or items) within each attribute. Consequently, the number of health states each system generates is shown to vary enormously. In general, however, most descriptive systems define more health states than it is feasible to elicit direct valuations for in an empirical study (the possible exception being the Rosser Index). Therefore, a number of important choices have to be made about how best to estimate values for all states from direct observations on a subset of those states.

This paper discusses the relative merits of alternative approaches to modelling health state valuations. It then considers a number of choices that have to be made when attempting to generate a "tariff" of values for

Table 1   Number of health states generated by different descriptive
                systems

Descriptive system	Attributes	Items per attribute	Health states
QWB[a]	4	3, 5 and 27	1 215
Rosser[b]	2	4 and 8	29
15-D[c]	15	5	> 30 billion
HUI3[d]	8	5 or 6	972 000
EQ-5D[e]	5	3	243
AQoL[f]	15	4	> 1 billion
SF-6D[g]	6	2 to 5	9 000

a. The Quality of Well-Being Scale, see Patrick et al. (1973).

b. See Rosser and Kind (1978).

c. See Sintonen (1994).

d. Health Utilities Index Mark 3, see Furlong et al. (1998).

e. See Brooks (1996).

f. The Assessment of Quality of Life, see Hawthorne et al. (1997).

g. See Brazier et al. (1998).

any descriptive system. Finally, it looks at how such tariffs have been estimated for the HUI3 and EQ-5D.

APPROACHES TO MODELLING

There are essentially two approaches that can be adopted when attempting to model health state valuations. The *decomposed* approach involves asking respondents to value each item within a particular attribute by holding the items of all other attributes constant, often at their best level. The resulting single-attribute utility functions are then used to generate valuations for composite health states by specifying a multi-attribute utility function (MAUF). The *composite* approach requires respondents to value a subset of composite health states. The values for each attribute, and possible interaction effects, are then obtained by using appropriate regression or statistical techniques. (There is some ambiguity in the literature regarding precisely which terms should be used to describe each of these approaches; this paper follows Dolan [2000a]).

There is no consensus regarding which of the two approaches ought to be used in the context of modelling health state valuations since each has a number of advantages and disadvantages. The decomposed approach might reduce the complexity of the valuation task since, when valuing single-attribute health states, respondents are required to consider only one dysfunctional attribute at a time rather than attempt to simultaneously weigh up different items on different attributes. On the other hand, respondents might be more likely to doubt the plausibility of health states in which one attribute is at very low levels while all others are at their best level, e.g. the state in which severe pain prevents most activities but there are no problems with ambulation and emotion (see part 5).

By making simplifying assumptions about the relationships between attributes, the decomposed approach has the advantage that it reduces the total number of valuations required. Moreover, these assumptions are consistent with a well-specified and explicit theoretical model; namely, multi-attribute utility theory (MAUT) (see Keeney and Raiffa 1976). However, the functional forms admissible under MAUT place stringent restrictions on the way in which different items on different attributes can be related to one another. Precisely how stringent these restrictions are depends on which of three functional forms is employed (see Torrance 1982).

The most restrictive functional form is the *additive* one that does not allow for any interactions between attributes; that is, the weights given to each item are simply added to one another. The *multiplicative* model allows for interactions between attributes but forces all interactions to be of the same kind. This means that the combined weights for all pairs of items across attributes must always be more than the sum of the weights for each item alone (in which case the attributes are complements for one another), or they must always be less than the sum of the weights for each item (in which case the attributes are substitutes for one another). The least restrictive functional form is the *multilinear* one that allows some pairs of items across attributes to be complements and other pairs to be substitutes. However, the weights for the items on any one attribute are still required to be independent of the items that are fixed on the other attributes. In practice, a full multilinear model would require direct valuations on a large number of states and therefore often only a subset of possible interactions is allowed for.

In comparison, the composite approach has the distinct advantage that fewer *a priori* restrictions need to be placed on the model. In principle, many first-order and higher-order interactions between items and attributes can be taken into account, although in practice the model often produces a highly simplified account of the data and thus is itself rather restrictive. A further important advantage of the composite approach is that it explicitly takes account of any heterogeneity in the data, including those that are related to particular respondent characteristics. Moreover, the error structure is crucial to the choice of model. In the decomposed approach, on the other hand, the stochastic part of the function is ignored, and thus much of the detail regarding the dispersion of values is lost.

At the conceptual level, the decision about which approach to adopt will depend largely on the importance that is given to an underlying theoretical model (i.e. MAUT in the decomposed approach) as compared to the ability of statistical inference to estimate the interactions between attributes. At the practical level, the approach that is chosen will be greatly determined by the number of health states generated by the descriptive system. The appeal of the decomposed approach is that a MAUF can be fitted to a relatively small number of values in order to generate values for an almost infinite number of health states. The composite approach, on the other hand, is best suited to situations where the ratio of direct values to estimated values is relatively high.

RESEARCH QUESTIONS

WHICH HEALTH STATES SHOULD BE VALUED?

The decomposed approach requires the valuation of all single-attribute health states; that is, all states for which one attribute is at less than its best level while all other attributes are fixed at their best level (or, alternatively, all states for which one attribute is at better than its worst level while all other attributes are fixed at their worst level). In addition to a value for the state with each item at its worst level, direct values for these states allow an additive model to be estimated. Since this is the most restrictive of the MAUF models, values for a subset of multi-attribute health states are usually elicited so that a multiplicative model, and possibly even a (partial) multilinear model, can also be estimated.

An important consideration when using the composite approach is that the directly valued health states should be widely spread over the valuation space so as to include as many combinations of items across the attributes as possible. This is subject to the constraint that the states are likely to be considered plausible by respondents. As with the decomposed approach, the less restrictive the models that are to be estimated, the more states that direct valuations will be required for. Given resource constraints which will place limits on the overall sample size, there will be an inevitable trade-off here between the twin objectives of eliciting direct valuations for as many states as possible and having as many observations on each state as possible. There is no consensus regarding the optimal trade-off.

In addition, it is necessary at the design stage of any valuation study to consider the maximum number of health states that any one respondent could reasonably be asked to value in any one elicitation exercise. There is also no consensus regarding this issue, but generally speaking there will be an optimal number of valuations per respondent, below which the valuation task may not be so well understood, and above which fatigue may result in less considered responses. The optimum is likely to vary across descriptive systems and will also depend on the characteristics of the sample and on the complexity of the valuation task.

WHICH VALUATION METHOD SHOULD BE USED?

There are essentially two main ways in which a set of health state valuations can be generated. First, respondents can be asked to rank different health states or asked to make a series of pairwise comparisons between them. This ordinal data can then be used to generate weights for items within attributes that are assumed to have interval scale properties. This approach has not been widely used to value health states although it is increasingly being used to value the benefits from health care more generally (see Ryan 1999). Second, respondents can be asked to value health states directly using one of three methods which purport to generate values that lie on an interval scale. These are the visual analog scale (VAS), the standard gamble (SG) and the time trade-off (TTO) (for detailed descriptions of these methods, see Torrance [1986]).

There has been considerable debate in the literature about the relative merits of each of these methods (Dolan et al. 1996a). Because the VAS method does not require people to make trade-offs between different arguments in their utility function, it is commonly regarded by economists as theoretically inferior to the SG and TTO methods which assume that improvements in HRQoL are a negative function of risk and a positive function of longevity, respectively. However, the VAS does have the practical advantages of being simpler to complete and cheaper to administer than both of the other methods. Therefore, if an algorithm can be found which maps VAS values onto SG and/or TTO ones, then it might be possible to "convert" valuations elicited via the VAS into theoretically superior SG and/or TTO values.

Since the SG is based upon the axioms of expected utility theory (EUT), it is regarded by many economists and decision theorists as the "gold standard" valuation method. However, there is evidence that people systematically violate the axioms of EUT (see Camerer 1995) and, more specifically, evidence that SG values cannot be automatically assumed to map directly onto utility (see Richardson 1994). The same can also be said of TTO values (see Dolan and Jones-Lee 1997). Therefore, it would seem that there is little to choose between the two methods although, as with the choice of modelling approach, much will depend on how much importance is attached to an underlying theoretical model. The important point in the context of this paper is that, in principle, any of the valuation methods can be used to value health states within either modelling approach.

How should the data be analysed?

There are two main ways in which MAUFs can be estimated using the decomposed approach. One way is to estimate MAUFs for each individual and then to combine the resultant utilities to determine aggregate item weights, the other is to aggregate the values for single-attribute health states and then produce a single aggregate MAUF (see Torrance 1982). The individual-based approach has the advantage that it allows the assumptions of the different functional forms to be tested on each individual, and, where appropriate, for different functions to be related to different respondent characteristics. However, since these assumptions are only ever likely to be satisfied approximately, it is a matter of judgement about when a particular functional form is considered a suitable approximation of a particular individual's preferences. The final weights attached to each item will then be sensitive to these judgements. The estimation of a single MAUF for the whole group mitigates against these problems but removes much of the information regarding the heterogeneity of preferences.

There are a number of issues relating to the nature of the data generated by studies which use the composite approach. Some concern the nature of the dependent variable i.e. the distribution of the health state values. If it is skewed (as is the case in a number of studies), it might be possible to transform the values so that they better approximate a standard normal distribution, and if it is censored or discrete, then the appropriate analytic technique(s) should be chosen. If analysis is to performed at the individual level (thus making the most efficient use of the data), then the fact that each respondent is likely to have been asked for a number of valuations also needs to be accounted for. Other issues relate to the how the independent variables (i.e. the items and possible interactions between them) are to be defined and coded, and how they are to be entered into the model.

Modelling in practice: HUI3 and EQ-5D

Recently, valuation tariffs have been generated for the HUI3 and EQ-5D descriptive systems. The former was estimated from the values of 256 respondents in Hamilton, Canada (see Furlong et al. 1998). The EQ-5D tariff was based upon the values of a representative sample of 2 997 members of the United Kingdom population (see Dolan 1997a). The studies were conducted in very different ways, and so a comparison between them will serve to highlight the implications of the choices outlined in parts 2 and 3.

The researchers involved in the HUI3 study appeared to give much greater weight to the normative appeal of MAUT than did their counterparts involved in the EQ-5D study. As a result, there was a predilection in favour of the decomposed approach among the former that did not exist among the latter. More importantly perhaps, the decomposed approach is suited to modelling valuations for a very large number of health states, and so it is not surprising that this approach was chosen to estimate a tariff for the 972 000 HUI3 health states. The composite approach was used to estimate a tariff for the 243 EQ-5D health states since statistical inference is better suited to estimating fewer valuations.

THE CHOICE OF HEALTH STATES

In order to estimate an additive MAUF, it was necessary to elicit values for the 37 single-attribute health states described by the HUI3. However, this functional form was found to be too restrictive when used to estimate a tariff for HUI1 (see Torrance et al. 1995). Therefore, three multi-attribute health states were also valued, thus enabling the tariff currently available to be based upon a multiplicative MAUF in which all attributes are complements for another (see part 2). Values for an additional 126 states were also elicited so that in principle a partial multilinear model could also be generated.

In the EQ-5D study, direct values were elicited for 42 health states. There were over 800 observations on each state and this enabled a 0.05 difference between the values of different states to be detected at the 0.05 level of significance (see Dolan et al. 1996b). With a sample of nearly 3 000 respondents, it would also have been possible to elicit direct values for every EQ-5D health state but the cost, in terms of the ability to detect small differences between states, was considered to be too great. In the event, it turned out that it would have been possible to estimate a very similar tariff from direct observations on about 30 health states but, of course, this was not known *ex ante*. And as noted above, there is no consensus regarding the optimal trade-off between eliciting direct valuations for as many states as possible and having as many observations on each state as possible.

With regards to the number of valuations per respondent, those in the HUI3 study were asked to value 23 health states using the VAS method plus three of these using the SG. In the EQ-5D study, respondents were asked to value the same 12 states using the VAS and TTO methods. While the methods and the balance between them differed, then, the total number of valuations elicited from each respondent was similar in the two studies. Therefore, whether HUI3 or EQ-5D is used, it would seem that somewhere around 25 valuations is the maximum number that any one respondent can be expected to give at any one time.

THE CHOICE OF VALUATION METHOD

As noted above, values in the HUI3 study were elicited using the VAS and the SG. The choice of SG appears to be further evidence that the researchers involved in the HUI3 study placed great emphasis on the axiomatic basis of their approach. The choice of VAS was more pragmatic, arising out of the fact that VAS values are easier and less time-consuming to elicit than SG ones. The VAS values were adjusted for an end-of-scale bias which describes the tendency for respondents to avoid using intervals at the extremes of the scale (Streiner and Norman 1995). The adjustment factor was estimated from an earlier study which had compared differences in VAS values with direct values for the differences between pairs of states (Torrance 1996).

The mean values of the three multi-attribute states for which there were both VAS and SG values were used to estimate a power function relationship between the two methods. This function was then used to convert all VAS values for single-attribute health states into implied SG values. A number of authors have estimated similar relationships between the methods (Torrance 1976 for the original model and Stiggelbout et al. 1996 for an overview). However, as in the HUI3 study, most analyses have been performed using aggregate-level data, thus making the choice between competing models more difficult. Analysis at the individual level confirms Torrance's original finding that the power function does not hold (Bleichrodt and Johannesson 1997), and possibly that no robust relationship exists at all (Dolan and Sutton 1997). This casts doubt on the robustness of any model that maps VAS onto SG or TTO values, particularly one that is estimated using only three data points.

The EQ-5D tariff was estimated directly from TTO valuations. The choice of TTO over SG was based on the results of an earlier study that had compared the two methods (Dolan et al. 1996a). Two variants of each method were tested, one using a specially designed board, the other using a self-completion booklet. According to standard psychometric criteria such as completion rates and reliability over time, the board-based variant of the TTO performed marginally better than both self-completion variants and significantly better than the board-based variant of the SG.

THE CHOICE OF ANALYSIS

In the HUI3 study, the values for single-attribute health states were first aggregated and then a single MAUF for the full sample was estimated. Given that each respondent valued only a subset of all single-attribute health states, it would not have been possible to estimate a MAUF for each individual separately. While the results of the aggregated model will not be sensitive to assumptions about the functional form of particular individuals preferences, it will not be possible to make any inferences about the variation in functional forms across individuals. The extent to which valuations for single-attribute health states can be related to particular respondent characteristics is also limited given the limited number of observations on each health state. The analyses to date suggest that the additive model is too restrictive a functional form for the aggregate data, and so the HUI3 tariff currently available is based upon a less restrictive multiplicative model. It remains to be seen whether a multilinear MAUF will perform better still.

The distribution of valuations in the EQ-5D study was highly non-normal, with clusters of values at the highest and lowest ends of the scale. However, it was not possible to find a suitable transformation of the data. That each respondent was asked for 12 valuations meant that the variance of the error term was likely to be partly determined by the individuals who valued the health states and hence was unlikely to be constant. To account for this, a random effects specification was used, thus enabling analysis to be performed at the individual level. A specific-to-general approach was adopted in which simple models were first estimated and then new variables were added if necessary. All the independent variables in the statistical analysis were dummies that derived from the ordinal nature of the EQ-5D descriptive system.

After testing numerous models with various combinations of interaction effects, the most parsimonious model to fit the data well (in terms of goodness-of-fit statistics) was based on an additive model, in which each of the five attributes was independent of one another. In addition to the ten main effects dummies, the model contained one interaction term which took account of the much greater disutility associated with being at the worst level on any of the attributes. The values generated by this model were found to differ widely according to the measure of central tendency (given the highly skewed nature of the data) and according to the age of the respondent (with values being much lower in the older age groups). As a result, EQ-5D tariffs have also been presented for the median values (see Dolan 1997b) and for respondents aged under and over 60 (see Dolan 2000b).

CONCLUDING REMARKS

This paper has attempted to set out some of the issues involved in deciding how best to model the relationship between health status domains and health state valuations. The issues in part 3 apply equally to all descriptive systems (with the possible exception of the Rosser Index, for which it might be possible to elicit direct values on all states from every respondent). However, the total number of health states that the chosen descriptive system generates might influence the choice of modelling approach. *Ceteris paribus*, as the total number of states increases, the robustness of the parameter estimates from the composite approach decrease, and so the axiomatic basis of the decomposed approach might become more attractive. This suggests that the greater the number of health states generated, the more restrictive the assumptions about the relationship between domains and valuations. As with most trade-offs, the most appropriate one here will depend on the decision context, determined largely by the extent to which *meaningful* changes in health status are being picked up by a more sensitive descriptive system and ignored by a less sensitive one.

The choice of modelling approach might also influence the choice of descriptive system. The axiomatic basis of MAUT, for example, might be so appealing that the attributes in a descriptive system could be described so as to make a particular functional form a more likely representation of the valuation data. For example, because the valuation of all single-attribute health states is central to the use of the decomposed approach, the attributes were designed to be orthogonal to one another; that is, being at any level on one attribute is consistent with being at any level on other attributes. If this is the case (which is of course an empirical question), then respondents would be able to imagine themselves at the worst level on one attribute at the same time as being at the best level on all other attributes.

Moreover, the HUI3 adopts a narrow "within-the-skin" conception of health which means that orthogonality is more likely to be satisfied. The attributes in the EQ-5D owe much to the wider definition health originally adopted by the World Health Organization. By including an attribute such as usual activities, orthogonality is much more likely to be violated but, since the composite approach does not require the valuation of all single-attribute health states, this is not a serious problem so far as modelling is concerned. While a philosophical debate about precisely what constitutes HRQoL is beyond the scope of this paper, the important point again is that the choice of modelling approach and the choice of descriptive system are linked.

Ultimately, the aim of any modelling procedure is to estimate a tariff of values for all the health states generated by a particular descriptive system, and so the ability of the model to predict observed values is one of the most important considerations. In the HUI3 study, the difference between the estimated and actual values for the three multi-attribute was 0.08 for the mildest state, 0.07 for the intermediate state and −0.04 for the most severe state. Whether differences of this magnitude are meaningful or not is open to question (O'Brien and Drummond 1994) but there appears to be a systematic relationship between the severity of the state and size of the difference. In the EQ-5D study, the mean absolute difference between the predicted and actual values for the 42 states valued in the study was 0.04 and for only three states did the difference exceed 0.10. Statistical tests showed that these errors were randomly distributed across health states.

It is difficult to directly compare the predictive ability of the different approaches to modelling because there have been very few direct comparisons to date. In the development of the HUI, a multiplicative MAUF has been found to perform significantly better than an additive model in terms of predictive ability and it remains to be seen whether the multilinear model performs better still. In one of the few head-to-head comparisons of the decomposed and composite approaches, (Currim and Sarin 1984) found that the latter performed much better than a multiplicative MAUT model in the context of job choice. There is certainly the need for such direct comparisons in the context of health state valuation. In this way, the precise trade-off that exists between the normative appeal of MAUT and the greater predictive ability of statistical inference will be better understood.

ACKNOWLEDGEMENTS

Many of the ideas contained within this paper came from a meeting with John Brazier and Jennifer Roberts, both of whom also provided comments on earlier versions. The author would also like to thank David Feeny for his helpful comments. The usual disclaimers apply.

REFERENCES

Bleichrodt H, Johannesson M (1997) An experimental test of a theoretical foundation for rating scale valuations. *Medical Decision Making,* 17(2):208–216.

Brazier J, Usherwood T, Harper R, Thomas K (1998) Deriving a preference based single index measure from the UK SF-36 health survey. *Journal of Clinical Epidemiology,* 51(11):1115–1128.

Brazier JE, Deverill M, Green C (1999) A review of the use of health status measures in economic evaluation. *Journal of Health Services Research and Policy,* 4(3):174–184.

Brooks R (1996) EuroQol: the current state of play. *Health Policy,* 37(1):53–72.

Camerer C (1995) Individual decision-making. In: *Handbook of experimental economics.* Kagel J, Roth A, eds. Princeton University Press, Princeton, NJ.

Currim IS, Sarin RK (1984) A comparative evaluation of multi-attribute consumer preference models. *Management Science,* 30(5):543–561.

Dolan P (1997b) Aggregating health state valuations. *Journal of Health Services Research and Policy,* 2(3):160–165.

Dolan P (1997a) Modelling valuations for EuroQol health states. *Medical Care,* 35(11):1095–1108.

Dolan P (2000b) The effect of age on health state valuations. *Journal of Health Services Research and Policy,* 5(1):17–21.

Dolan P (2000a) The measurement of health-related quality-of-life for use in resource allocation decisions in health care. In: *Handbook of health economics. Vol. 1B.* Culyer AJ, Newhouse J, eds. Elsevier, Amsterdam.

Dolan P, Gudex C, Kind P, Williams A (1996b) The time-trade-off method: results from a general population study. *Health Economics,* 5(2):141–154.

Dolan P, Gudex C, Kind P, Williams A (1996a) Valuing health states: a comparison of methods. *Journal of Health Economics,* **15**(2):209–231.

Dolan P, Jones-Lee M (1997) The time trade-off: a note on the effect of lifetime reallocation of consumption and discounting. *Journal of Health Economics,* **16**(6):731–739.

Dolan P, Sutton M (1997) Mapping visual analogue scale health state valuations onto standard gamble and time trade-off values. *Social Science and Medicine,* **44**(10):1519–1530.

Furlong W, Feeny D, Torrance GW, et al. (1998) *Multiplicative multi-attribute utility function for the health utilities index mark 3 (HUI3) system: a technical report.* (CHEPA working paper no 98/11.) McMaster University, Centre for Health Economics and Policy Analysis, Hamilton, Ontario. *http:// chepa.mcmaster.ca/*

Hawthorne G, Richardson J, Osborne R, McNeil H (1997) *The assessment of quality of life (AQoL) instrument: construction, initial validation and utility scaling.* (CHPE working paper no 76.) Monash University, Centre for Health Program Evaluation, Melbourne.

Keeney RL, Raiffa H (1993) *Decisions with multiple objectives: preferences and value tradeoffs.* 2nd edn. Cambridge University Press, New York.

Murray CJL (1996) Rethinking DALYs. In: *The global burden of disease: a comprehensive assessment of mortality and disability from diseases, injuries, and risk factors in 1990 and projected to 2020.* The Global Burden of Disease and Injury, Vol. 1. Murray CJL, Lopez AD, eds. Harvard School of Public Health on behalf of WHO, Cambridge, MA.

O'Brien BJ, Drummond MF (1994) Statistical versus quantitative significance in the socioeconomic evaluation of medicines. *PharmacoEconomics,* **5**(5):389–398.

Patrick DL, Bush JW, Chen MM (1973) Methods for measuring levels of well-being for a health status index. *Health Services Research,* **8**(3):228–245.

Richardson J (1994) Cost-utility analysis: what should be measured? *Social Science and Medicine,* **39**(1):7–21.

Rosser R, Kind P (1978) A scale of valuations of states of illness: is there a social consensus? *International Journal of Epidemiology,* **7**(4):347–358.

Ryan M (1999) A role for conjoint analysis in technology assessment in health care? *International Journal of Technology Assessment in Health Care,* **15**(3):443–457.

Sintonen H (1994) *The 15-D measure of HRQoL: reliability, validity and the sensitivity of its health state descriptive system.* (CHPE working paper no 41.) Monash University, Melbourne.

Stiggelbout AM, Eijkemans MJC, Kiebert GM, Kievit J, Leer JWH, Haes HJ (1996) The "utility" of the visual analog scale in medical decision making and technology assessment: is it an alternative to the time trade-off? *International Journal of Technology Assessment in Health Care,* **12**(2):291–298.

Streiner DL, Norman GR (1995) *Health measurement scales: a practical guide to their development and use.* 2nd edn. Oxford University Press, New York.

Torrance GW (1976) Social preferences for health states: an empirical evaluation of three measurement techniques. *Socio-Economic Planning Sciences*, 10(3):129–136.

Torrance GW (1982) Multi-attribute utility theory as a method of measuring social preferences for health states in long-term care. In: *Values in long-term care*. Kane RL, Kane RA, eds. Lexington Books, DC Health, Lexington, MA.

Torrance GW (1986) Measurement of health state utilities for economic appraisal: a review. *Journal of Health Economics*, 5(1):1–30.

Torrance GW (1996) *End of scale bias in feeling thermometer: technical notes for HUI3 preference modelling study.* McMaster University, Hamilton, Ontario.

Torrance GW, Feeny D, Furlong W, Barr R, Zhang Y, Wang Q (1996) Multi-attribute preference functions for a comprehensive health status classification system: health utilities index mark II. *Medical Care*, 34(7):702–722.

Weinstein MC, Stason WB (1977) Foundations of cost-effectiveness analysis for health and medical practices. *New England Journal of Medicine*, 296(13):716–721.

Chapter 10.2

THE UTILITY APPROACH TO ASSESSING POPULATION HEALTH

DAVID FEENY

INTRODUCTION

There are two key components to constructing summary measures of population health quality: a health-status classification system and a valuation function. The former was discussed in part 7. My remarks on that session are also relevant here (see chapter 7.2). The latter will be the focus of my brief remarks here. I will concentrate on three major topics: a conceptual foundation that supports a measure with interval-scale properties, key issues in the elicitation of preferences for health states, and the estimation of valuation functions, including the choice of functional form for preference functions and implications for the design of preference elicitation surveys. In a sense the first two topics are about getting the dependent variable, the left-hand side of the estimating equation, correct, while the third topic is about getting the independent variables, the right-hand side variables, correct.

CONCEPTUAL FOUNDATION THAT SUPPORTS A MEASURE WITH INTERVAL-SCALE PROPERTIES

Summary measures of population health quality are constructed by weighting the health states observed by some assessment of their value. The weights (utility scores) are thus being used as if they have interval-scale properties. It is therefore important to ground the construction of summary measures on an explicit foundation that supports interval-scale properties. It is important to appreciate the assumptions required.

There are a number of models of the underlying structure of preferences that support interval-scale properties. In economics and decision science, von Neumann and Morgenstern (vN-M) utility functions provide such a framework. Von Neumann-Morgenstern utility functions have frequently been employed as the conceptual foundation for health utility assessments for two major reasons. First, the vN-M framework is among the weakest set of assumptions sufficient to provide for a scale with interval-scale properties. Second, vN-M utilities deal with risk which is arguably inherent in virtually all health care and health policy decision-making contexts.

I will not provide a formal review of the relevant theory here (Feeny 2000; Feeny and Torrance 1989; Keeney 1988; 1992; Keeney and Raiffa 1993; Luce and Raiffa 1957; Torrance and Feeny 1989; von Neumann and Morgenstern 1944). The axioms of vN-M utility theory include transitivity and continuity. Thus, if A is strictly preferred to B and B is strictly preferred to C, then A must be strictly preferred to C. The continuity axiom states that there is a lottery comprizing probability p of outcome A and probability $(1 - p)$ of outcome C such that the subject would be indifferent between the lottery and outcome B for certain. This axiom is the conceptual foundation of the standard gamble approach for measuring utilities. The continuity axiom is also necessary for the interval-scale property of utility scores.

Other sets of assumptions may be sufficient for a scale to exhibit interval-scale properties. Advantages of the utility approach and its grounding in vN-M theory are that the assumptions are among the weakest required and are explicit.

Many authors will be point out, with considerable justification, that the axioms of vN-M utility theory are often violated in cognitive psychology experiments. Yet such results sometimes lead to premature dismissal of vN-M theory.

Some critics fall into the "nirvana" comparison trap. Yes, expected utility theory does not conform completely to the results of various studies. But do other models do any better?

Furthermore, empirical investigations indicate that the performance of expected utility models improves in studies in which experimental subjects participate repeatedly and have more time to learn (these issues are discussed briefly in Feeny 2000). Furthermore, it is useful to examine empirical evidence on which models of decision-making under risk are the most accurate predictors of the decisions that people actually make. The empirical evidence indicates that, in general, expected profit maximization and expected utility maximization outperform bounded rationality models (the type of models advocated by those who criticize expected utility maximization). This is especially the case when subjects have been faced repeatedly with similar decision-making problems. One interpretation is that expected utility maximization is an approximately accurate summary of the decision rules developed by well-informed, experienced decision-makers who have had the opportunity to engage in learning. In health applications in which individuals typically have relatively few opportunities to repeat similar decision-making situations and develop useful rules of thumb, we would therefore expect to observe less conformity with expected utility maximization. However, in applications with greater scope for repeated play and learning, expected utility maximization, in general, outperforms bounded rationality models. Furthermore, within health applications, there are a number of studies that support the predictive validity and construct validity of preference measurements.

Given that health-state descriptions specify the duration of the health state, responses to standard gamble (SG) questions reflect both the time and risk preferences of subjects. Some argue that SG scores are contaminated by risk preferences, that scores incorporating risk preferences are not appropriate in the context of constructing measures of population health quality. The argument is, however, not straightforward. In the context of cost-benefit analysis for resource allocation it is often suggested (Arrow and Lind 1994) that while individual agents are risk averse, society can be risk neutral. It is therefore argued, for instance, that the discount rate should not include a risk premium. Part of the rationale for this position is that cash transfers can compensate the losers of projects that fail. In the context of health, however, the scope for such transfers is severely limited (a similar argument is presented in Daniels 1998). Thus, it might be appropriate that utility weights used to construct measures of population health quality reflect the risk preferences of the community concerning health states.

Finally, vN-M utility theory endures as a widely accepted normative standard for decision-making under risk. Given that utility scores are often used in economic and other evaluative studies of health care and health policy, analyses which are inherently normative, the use of vN-M utilities would therefore seem appropriate.

In sum, any summary measure of population health quality needs to be based explicitly on a framework that provides scores (weights) with interval-scale properties. Von Neumann-Morgenstern's expected utility theory is one attractive foundation upon which to build such measures.

ELICITING PREFERENCES FOR HEALTH STATES

Economists are accustomed to studying market contexts in which consumers have a great deal of knowledge and experience and well-formulated preferences. In general, consumers have faced similar choices in the market on many previous occasions and are highly familiar with the products being offered, so are able to rank their bundles in order of preference.

The evaluation of preferences for health states is much more challenging. Typically, subjects do not know what their preferences for health states are off the top of their heads. As a result, elicitation interviews should provide a structured set of tasks that help subjects to make up their minds about what their preferences really are and to communicate them to the interviewer. Furlong et al. (1990) provides a detailed description of what should go into an elicitation interview. A common approach is to ask subjects first to rank order states. The second task is then to ask them to arrange states on a category scale (Feeling Thermometer, FT) with the most desirable state at the top and least desirable at the bottom. The third task, and the one that generates the interval-scale data that will be used, is the standard gamble (Chance Board).

In the standard gamble (based on the continuity axiom) the subject is presented with a choice between an intermediately ranked state for sure and a lottery with probability p of a more desirable outcome (often perfect health) and probability $1-p$ of a less desirable outcome (often dead, or in the context of multi-attribute systems, the pits—the state having the lowest level on all attributes of the health-status classification system being used). The process of choice in the lottery helps the subject to come to a judgement about just how good or bad the health state being evaluated is.

High quality preference elicitation studies rely on the use of choice-based techniques such as the standard gamble. Because the standard gamble (choice-based technique) is the final task, responses reflect the understanding which the subject has gained by being led through a series of tasks that have repeatedly asked the subject to think about preferences. High quality studies also carefully develop and pre-test the interview protocol and rely on the use of highly trained and carefully supervised interviewers.

Many investigators are tempted to rely entirely on category scaling (FT). Some believe that the FT is easier than the standard gamble (or time trade-off, TTO). The evidence for this assertion is mixed (Patrick et al. 1994). Second, as noted above, while the FT is an important step in helping the subject to construct and reveal preferences, it is still no more than an intermediate step. Third, unless the scale anchors are unambiguous, there are important aggregation problems. Fourth, there are well-documented end-of-scale problems with the FT: subjects avoid placing states close to the top and bottom anchors. Fifth, there are important context effects with the FT. Scores depend on the mix of states assessed at the same time. For these reasons, while the FT may be necessary, it is not sufficient for obtaining high quality preference scores with interval-scale properties.

As noted above, it is important to link the preference elicitation to a conceptual foundation. The standard gamble is based directly on vN-M theory. The time trade-off (Torrance et al. 1972) is another widely used choice-based technique. For TTO to provide utility scores (i.e. weights for population health quality) one must invoke not only the standard assumptions of vN-M theory but also the idea that people have utility functions which are linear in additional life years (Torrance and Feeny 1989). This extra assumption is not required when using the standard gamble.

Estimation of valuation functions

Multi-attribute health-status classification systems often describe more health states than can be easily scored directly. Even if reasonably precise direct utility scores could be obtained for all of the states described by a particular system, to achieve consistency across the entire preference space, it might still be desirable to estimate a multi-attribute utility function. In practice, direct utility scores are usually obtained for a set of states, and these are then used to estimate a multi-attribute function for the entire system. There are two popular basic approaches for estimation: the decomposed approach from decision science and various methods of statistical inference (Dolan refers to the latter as the composite approach). The two approaches are not mutually exclusive.

The decomposed approach, used in the estimation of multiplicative multi-attribute utility functions for the HUI1, HUI2 and HUI3 systems, and in the estimation of a number of specific multi-attribute systems (Revicki et al. 1998a; 1998b), relies on a multiplicative form for the function (from which the linear additive can emerge as a special case). One of its attractions is that it asks the minimum number of questions to obtain estimates for parameters of the multiplicative functional form (see below). Alternatively, preference scores for health states can be obtained and preference weights inferred through linear regression (or some other method of statistical inference). Because each assessor often provides scores for more than one state, random effects models are often employed.

The decomposed approach accommodates both linear additive and multiplicative forms. If there is evidence of the suitability of one of these underlying functional forms, the parsimony of the number of health states that must be evaluated to estimate the function is an attractive feature. If, however, one wants to explore richer functional forms, statistical inference techniques are more attractive. Both decomposed and statistical inference approaches were used for HUI3 as seen below. The issue in choosing between them is not, as Dolan (chapter 10.1) suggests, the number of health states described by the system. A carefully designed statistical inference approach permits identification of the parameters of a number of underlying functional forms. If potential compatibility with a variety of functional forms is not a priority in study design, a statistical inference approach may accommodate only a few alternatives. In such a case, the two approaches are not very different because the decomposed approach readily accommodates both linear additive and multiplicative functional forms.

Multi-attribute utility functions can be estimated at the individual level (one function for each respondent) or at the person-mean level, which employs mean observations from the entire sample as a representative respondent. It is also possible to use median or modal responses. If the goal is the acquisition of summary measures of population health quality, a person-mean approach that embodies average community values is appropriate.

Both individual-specific and person-mean approaches were used in the estimation of multi-attribute utility functions for the HUI2 system (Torrance et al. 1992). A total of 194 individual-specific functions was estimated along with a person-mean function. A collection of HUI2 health states was then scored using each of the 194 functions, then the mean score was computed and compared with the score derived from the person-mean function. The results were virtually identical, and it was this that prompted the choice of person-mean for estimation of the HUI3 scoring function (see below).

Estimating scores from preference-elicitation survey material can be quite demanding. Ideally each health state would be assessed using category scaling (FT) and the standard gamble (SG). What often happens in practice is that FT scores are obtained for all states and SG scores for a subset of states. Study-specific functions relating SG to FT scores are then estimated. For instance, for HUI2 the power function was used (Torrance et al. 1992; 1996). For HUI3 a number of functional forms were examined, including quadratic and cubic spline functions, and various non-linear techniques were used as well as the "traditional" power function (Furlong et al. 1998). Functions were estimated at the individual and person-mean levels. The power function did the best job of predicting directly measured SG scores and was therefore employed.

Whether a scoring function is obtained via the decomposed approach or statistical inference, the resulting function becomes available for "out-of-sample" prediction; it is likely to be used to generate scores for states that were not directly measured. Thus, it is very important to consider the choice of functional form carefully and to assess out-of-sample prediction performance of the estimated function thoroughly. The results of these exercises will strongly influence confidence in scores generated by the function.

Three basic functional forms have been used to estimate various multi-attribute preference functions: linear additive, multiplicative, and multi-linear. The functional forms for each appear below.

Notation: $u_j(x_j)$ is the single attribute utility function for attribute j.
              $u(x)$ is the utility for health state x represented by an n-element vector.
              k and k_j are model parameters.
              Σ is the summation sign with $j = 1$ through n.
              $\prod$ is the multiplication sign with $j = 1$ through n.

Additive

$$u(x) = \sum_{j=1}^{n} k_j u_j(x_j)$$

where $\sum_{j=1}^{n} k_j = 1$.

Multiplicative

$$u(x) = \left(\frac{1}{k}\right) \left[\prod_{j=1}^{n}(1 + k\, k_j\, u_j(x_j)) - 1 \right]$$

where $(1 + k) = \prod_{j=1}^{n}(1 + k\, k_j)$.

Multilinear

$$u(x) = k_1 u_1(x_1) + k_2 u_2(x_2) + \ldots$$
$$+ k_{12} u_1(x_1) u_2(x_2) + k_{13} u_1(x_1) u_3(x_3) + \ldots$$
$$+ k_{123} u_1(x_1) u_2(x_2) u_3(x_3) + \ldots$$
$$+ \ldots$$

where Σ all k's = 1.

The linear additive form makes the strongest assumptions about preference interactions among attributes (domains or dimensions of health status). The linear additive form assumes that there are no important preference interactions.

A simple thought experiment might help understanding of the concept of preference interactions. Assume that you start out in normal health (level one for each attribute in the HUI3 system; see Table 1). Now suppose that you suffer a loss in cognition and go from level one cognition to level five: you are very forgetful and have great difficulty thinking and in solving problems. On a scale in which normal health = 1.00 and dead (the lack of health status) = 0.00, please think about the disutility you would associate with being level five cognition but otherwise normal (that is the distance between normal health and being level five cognition: label this disutility as d_1). To continue the thought experiment, consider once again that you start from normal health and then suffer a loss in emotional health, going from level one emotion to level four emotion, being very unhappy (but otherwise healthy). What disutility would you associate with this loss? Label it as d_2. Now think about a third situation: you go from normal health to level five cognition *and* level four emotion. What disutility would you associate with this loss? Label this loss as d_3. Finally, please add d_1 and d_2. Is the sum greater than, less than, or equal to d_3? Most respondents will indicate that the sum of d_1 and d_2 is greater than d_3. Losing both cognition and emotion is worse than losing only one but not as bad as the sum of both losses.

If d_3 is greater than the sum of the individual losses, then emotion and cognition would be preference substitutes. The linear additive functional form would only be appropriate if the sum of the individual losses was equal to the loss of both—that is, there are no important preference interactions.

The bulk of the evidence on multi-attribute utility functions does not support the linear additive form, even though it has been frequently used. The multi-attribute preference function for the Quality of Well Being (QWB) scale is based on a linear additive function. It should be noted, however, that in the QWB if a subject has more than one symptom, only the worst symptom is scored (and for scoring purposes the existence of

Table 1   Multi-attribute health status classification system:
                      Health Utilities Index Mark 3 (HUI3)

Attribute	Level	Description
Vision	1.	Able to see well enough to read ordinary newsprint and recognize a friend on the other side of the street, without glasses or contact lenses.
	2.	Able to see well enough to read ordinary newsprint and recognize a friend on the other side of the street, but with glasses.
	3.	Able to read ordinary newsprint with or without glasses but unable to recognize a friend on the other side of the street, even with glasses.
	4.	Able to recognize a friend on the other side of the street with or without glasses but unable to read ordinary newsprint, even with glasses.
	5.	Unable to read ordinary newsprint and unable to recognize a friend on the other side of the street, even with glasses.
	6.	Unable to see at all.
Hearing	1.	Able to hear what is said in a group conversation with at least three other people, without a hearing aid.
	2.	Able to hear what is said in a conversation with one other person in a quiet room without a hearing aid, but requires a hearing aid to hear what is said in a group conversation with at least three other people.
	3.	Able to hear what is said in a conversation with one other person in a quiet room with a hearing aid, and able to hear what is said in a group conversation with at least three other people, with a hearing aid.
	4.	Able to hear what is said in a conversation with one other person in a quiet room, without a hearing aid, but unable to hearing what is said in a group conversation with at least three other people even with a hearing aid.
	5.	Able to hear what is said in a conversation with one other person in a quiet room with a hearing aid, but unable to hear what is said in a group conversation with at least three other people even with a hearing aid.
	6.	Unable to hear at all.
Speech	1.	Able to be understood completely when speaking with strangers or friends.
	2.	Able to be understood partially when speaking with strangers but able to be understood completely when speaking with people who know me well.
	3.	Able to be understood partially when speaking with strangers or people who know me well.
	4.	Unable to be understood when speaking with strangers but able to be understood partially by people who know me well.
	5.	Unable to be understood when speaking to other people (or unable to speak at all).
Ambulation	1.	Able to walk around the neighbourhood without difficulty, and without walking equipment.
	2.	Able to walk around the neighbourhood with difficulty; but does not require walking equipment or the help of another person.
	3.	Able to walk around the neighbourhood with walking equipment, but without the help of another person.
	4.	Able to walk only short distances with walking equipment, and requires a wheelchair to get around the neighbourhood.

continued

Table 1   Multi-attribute health status classification system:
Health Utilities Index Mark 3 (HUI3) *(continued)*

Attribute	Level	Description
	5.	Unable to walk alone, even with walking equipment. Able to walk short distances with the help of another person, and requires a wheelchair to get around the neighbourhood.
	6.	Cannot walk at all.
Dexterity	1.	Full use of two hands and ten fingers.
	2.	Limitations in the use of hands or fingers, but does not require special tools or help of another person.
	3.	Limitations in the use of hands or fingers, is independent with use of special tools (does not require the help of another person).
	4.	Limitations in the use of hands or fingers, requires the help of another person for some tasks (not independent even with use of special tools).
	5.	Limitations in use of hands or fingers, requires the help of another person for most tasks (not independent even with use of special tools).
	6.	Limitations in use of hands or fingers, requires the help of another person for all tasks (not independent even with use of special tools).
Emotion	1.	Happy and interested in life.
	2.	Somewhat happy.
	3.	Somewhat unhappy.
	4.	Very unhappy.
	5.	So unhappy that life is not worthwhile.
Cognition	1.	Able to remember most things, think clearly and solve day to day problems.
	2.	Able to remember most things, but have a little difficulty when trying to think and solve day to day problems.
	3.	Somewhat forgetful, but able to think clearly and solve day to day problems.
	4.	Somewhat forgetful, and have a little difficulty when trying to think or solve day to day problems.
	5.	Very forgetful, and have great difficulty when trying to think or solve day to day problems.
	6.	Unable to remember anything at all, and unable to think or solve day to day problems.
Pain	1.	Free of pain and discomfort.
	2.	Mild to moderate pain that prevents no activities.
	3.	Moderate pain that prevents a few activities.
	4.	Moderate to severe pain that prevents some activities.
	5.	Severe pain that prevents most activities.

Source: Feeny et al. (1995).

Note: Level descriptions are worded here exactly as presented to respondents in HUI3 preference measurement surveys.

another symptom is ignored). It is likely that the linear additive form would not have been a reasonable representation of the value of QWB health states if more than one symptom had been scored.

The UK multi-attribute preference function for the EuroQol EQ-5D system (Dolan 1997) relies on an ad hoc modified linear additive function. (The function is ad hoc in the sense that the underlying multi-attribute utility function to which the statistically estimated function corresponds is not specified explicitly.) The constant term for any dysfunction and the N3 term were included to enhance the fit. That these inclusions did improve the fit may well indicate important underlying preference interactions, but unfortunately, the design of the preference survey did not make it possible to identify them.

The linear additive function is a special case of the multiplicative function. In the estimation of multiplicative multi-attribute utility functions for the HUI1 (Torrance et al. 1982), HUI2 (Torrance et al. 1996), and HUI3 (Furlong et al. 1998) systems, the results firmly reject the linear additive form. Additional references on HUI are available at *http://www.fhs. mcmaster.ca/hug/index.htm*. Interestingly, results for scoring functions with several specific multi-attribute systems also reject the linear additive form (Revicki et al. 1998a; 1998b).

Preliminary results on the estimation of a multi-linear multi-attribute utility functions for the HUI3 system (Feeny et al. 1999) are instructive. Using a one-half 2^8 fractional factorial design, health states were selected so that 26 of 28 two-factor interactions (and four of 56 three-factor interactions) would be estimable (Feeny et al. 1994). Empirical results indicate that there are quantitatively important (regression coefficient ≥ 0.025; scores are on a 0.00 to 1.00 scale) and statistically significant ($p < 0.05$) two-way and three-way interaction terms. Interestingly, however, the signs of all of the two-way interactions are the same, indicating preference complementarity among the attributes in the HUI3 system. Preliminary results indicate that although the multi-linear form is less restrictive than the multiplicative and permits a richer set of interactions among attributes, the multiplicative form captures the important interactions. Further, the multiplicative function appears to out perform the multi-linear function in out of sample prediction.

Out of sample prediction evidence for the multiplicative HUI3 function is instructive (Furlong et al. 1998). Subjects were randomly allocated to a modelling survey (questions based on decomposed approach and fractional factorial design; responses used to estimate multiplicative and multilinear functions, $n = 256$) or a direct validation survey (used to assess predictive validity or agreement between directly measured scores and scores generated by the scoring function, $n = 248$). In the direct survey, subjects were asked to evaluate a collection of HUI3 health states spread across the space and including highly prevalent health states.

Agreement between these directly measured scores and scores generated by the multiplicative function is summarized in Table 2. The mean difference per health state between predicted scores and scores from the direct survey for 73 health states was –0.008. Results are similar if health states are weighted by their prevalence. In general, results are similar throughout the scale. The results for the 73 health states are more comprehensive than results for the three marker states. On average predicted and directly measured scores are very close. The intra-class correlation coefficient between directly measured scores and scores from the multiplicative function is 0.88. The multiplicative function performs well in out of sample prediction. This evidence and the superiority of the multiplicative with respect to the multi-linear function enhance confidence in the multiplicative HUI3 function. Indeed given that scores from the direct survey were not used in any way to estimate the multiplicative multi-attribute utility function for the HUI3 system these are very strong results in favour of the multiplicative function.

In sum, evidence to date indicates that there are quantitatively important and statistically significant interactions in preferences among attributes. In designing a preference-elicitation survey for estimating a scoring function it is therefore essential to anticipate relevant alternative functional forms and carefully select the health states upon which to obtain preference scores so that preference interaction terms can readily be identified. Furthermore, validation of scoring functions should include a rigorous assessment of out-of-sample prediction.

Table 2   Agreement between calculated and directly measured utility scores: external agreement

Survey	States	MD	MAD	Overall SD	ICC (95% CI)
HUI3	73 (not weighted by GP prevalence)	–0.008	0.087	0.1032	0.88 (0.49, 0.92)
HUI3	73 (weighted by GP prevalence, excluding PH)	+0.001	0.002	0.0061	—
HUI3	74 (weighted by GP prevalence, including PH)	+0.001	0.001	0.0040	—

CI = confidence interval

GP = general population (from 1991 General Social Survey)

ICC = intra-class correlation coefficient

MAD = mean absolute difference = $[\sum(|\text{predicted} - 10\% \text{ trimmed mean}|)/n]$

MD = mean difference = $[\sum(\text{predicted} - 10\% \text{ trimmed mean})/n]$

Overall SD = overall standard deviation = $[(\sum(\text{predicted} - 10\% \text{ trimmed mean})^2)/(n-1)]^{0.5}$

Source: Furlong et al. 1998, p. 79.

Conclusions

Summary measures of population health should involve the weighting of health states according to their quality or desirability. The utilitarian approach to assessing health-related quality of life, particularly von Neumann-Morgenstern utility functions, offers an explicit and rigorous conceptual foundation for work that generates scores with interval-scale properties. Techniques for eliciting utility scores for health states and the estimation of multi-attribute utility functions have improved substantially over the past three decades. As experience in Canada indicates, it is more than feasible to incorporate a multi-attribute health status classification system in population health surveys and use the resulting information to compute health adjusted life expectancy based on the preferences of members of the general population.

These estimates represent a substantial accomplishment but do have their limitations. Inherently any multi-attribute system embodies a less than fully comprehensive coverage of the potentially important dimensions of health status. The multi-attribute utility functions developed to date are based on preference measurements in which people were asked to think about experiencing various health states themselves and to place value on those health states. The resulting scores do not embody other potentially important characteristics. It may well be that the age, gender, or position in society of the recipients of health gains, and the magnitude of those gains, may also matter to members of the general population. Unfortunately, the methods for eliciting this type of preference information are much less developed than those for evaluating preferences for health states. Thus, the incorporation of age or equity weights is best done as a separate exercise (Field and Gold 1998; Williams 1999).

Nonetheless, widespread use of multi-attribute systems such as the Health Utilities Index can provide a firm foundation for constructing summary measures of population health quality. These multi-attribute systems can be readily incorporated in population health surveys. It is also possible to estimate multi-attribute preference functions based on preference measurements from random samples of the general population. These techniques provide an attractive and feasible approach to constructing summary measures of population health.

Acknowledgements

The author acknowledges the helpful comments of William Furlong and George W. Torrance on an earlier draft.

REFERENCES

Arrow KJ, Lind RC (1994) Uncertainty and the evaluation of public investment decisions. In: *Cost-benefit analysis.* 2nd edn. Layard R, Glaister S, eds. Cambridge University Press, Cambridge.

Daniels N (1998) Distributive justice and the use of summary measures of population health status, Appedix D in Committee on summary measures of population health. In: *Summarizing population health: directions for the development and application of population metrics.* Field MJ, Gold MR, eds. National Academy Press, Washington, DC.

Dolan P (1997) Modelling valuations for EuroQol health states. *Medical Care,* **35**(11):1095–1108.

Feeny D (2000) A utility approach to the assessment of health-related quality of life. *Medical Care,* **38**(9 Suppl.):II-151–II-154.

Feeny D, Furlong W, Boyle M, Torrance GW (1995) Multi-attribute health status classification systems: Health Utilities Index. *PharmacoEconomics,* **7**(6):490–502.

Feeny D, Torrance GW (1989) Incorporating utility-based quality-of-life assessments in clinical trials: two examples. *Medical Care,* **27**(3 Suppl.):S190–S204.

Feeny D, Torrance GW, Goldsmith CH, Furlong W, Boyle M (1994) *A multi-attribute approach to population health status.* (Proceedings of the 153rd annual meeting of the American Statistical Association.) American Statistical Association, Alexandria, VA.

Feeny D, Torrance GW, Goldsmith CH, Furlong W, Zhu Z (1999) Health utilities index mark III: multi-linear multi-attribute utility function. *Quality of Life Research,* **8**(7):600

Field MJ, Gold MR, eds. (1998) *Summarizing population health: directions for the development and application of population metrics.* National Academy Press, Washington, DC.

Furlong W, Feeny D, Torrance GW, Barr R, Horsman J (1990) *Guide to design and development of health-state utility instrumentation.* (CHEPA working paper no 90/9.) McMaster University, Centre for Health Economics and Policy, Hamilton, Ontario. *http://chepa.mcmaster.ca/*

Furlong W, Feeny D, Torrance GW, et al. (1998) *Multiplicative multi-attribute utility function for the health utilities index mark 3 (HUI3) system: a technical report.* (CHEPA working paper no 98/11.) McMaster University, Centre for Health Economics and Policy Analysis, Hamilton, Ontario. http://chepa.mcmaster.ca/

Keeney RL (1988) Building models of values. *European Journal of Operational Research,* **37**:149–157.

Keeney RL (1992) *Value-focused thinking: a path to creative decision-making.* Harvard University Press, Cambridge.

Keeney RL, Raiffa H (1993) *Decisions with multiple objectives: preferences and value tradeoffs.* 2nd edn. Cambridge University Press, New York.

Luce RD, Raiffa H (1957) *Games and decisions: introduction and critical survey.* Wiley, New York.

Patrick DL, Starks HE, Cain KC, Uhlmann RF, Pearlman RA (1994) Measuring preferences for health states worse than death. *Medical Decision Making,* 14(1):9–18.

Revicki DA, Leidy NK, Brennan-Deimer F, Sorensen S, Togias A (1998a) Integrating patient preferences into health outcomes assessment: the multi-attribute asthma symptom utility index. *Chest,* 114:998–1007.

Revicki DA, Leidy NK, Brennan-Deimer F, Thompson C, Togias A (1998b) Development and preliminary validation of a multi-attribute rhinitis symptom utility index. *Quality of Life Research,* 7(8):693–702.

Torrance GW (1986) Measurement of health state utilities for economic appraisal: a review. *Journal of Health Economics,* 5(1):1–30.

Torrance GW, Boyle MH, Horwood SP (1982) Application of multi-attribute utility theory to measure social preferences for health states. *Operations Research,* 30(6):1042–1069.

Torrance GW, Feeny D (1989) Utilities and quality-adjusted life years. *International Journal of Technology Assessment in Health Care,* 5(4):559–575.

Torrance GW, Feeny D, Furlong W, Barr R, Zhang Y, Wang Q (1996) Multi-attribute preference functions for a comprehensive health status classification system: health utilities index mark II. *Medical Care,* 34(7):702–722.

Torrance GW, Furlong W, Feeny D, Boyle M (1995) Multi-attribute preference functions: Health Utilities Index. *PharmacoEconomics,* 7(6):503–520.

Torrance GW, Thomas WH, Sackett DL (1972) A utility maximization model for evaluation of health care programs. *Health Services Research,* 7(2):118–133.

Torrance GW, Zhang Y, Feeny D, Furlong W, Barr R (1992) *Multi-attribute preference functions for a comprehensive health status classification system.* (CHEPA working paper no 92/18.) McMaster University, Centre for Health Economics and Policy Analysis, Hamilton, Ontario.

von Neumann J, Morgenstern O (1944) *Theory of games and economic behavior.* Princeton University Press, Princeton, NJ.

Williams A (1999) Calculating the global burden of disease: time for a strategic reappraisal? *Health Economics,* 8(1):1–8.

Chapter 10.3

Modelling health state valuation data

John Brazier, Nigel Rice and Jennifer Roberts

Abstract

An important task in deriving a summary measure of health is to incorporate stated preferences into health state classifications. This paper examines a range of alternative econometric models for dealing with a skewed, truncated, non-continuous and hierarchical (at the individual level) data set of standard gamble valuations of health states defined by the health state classification the SF-6D. Alternative specifications incorporating random effects for the individual level clustering, Tobit models to deal with skewness and truncation and ordered probit for the non-continuity did not produce models better than the simple mean model and were often worse in terms of inconsistency, fit and heterogeneity.

Introduction

There is a growing need to develop measures for summarizing the health of a population. A common approach has been to use preference-based measures of health that combine health state descriptive systems with a set of preference-weights usually obtained from the general population (Brazier and Deverill 1999). Commonly used examples of these preference-weighted health state classifications include the EQ-5D (Brooks 1996) and the HUI3 (Torrance et al. 1995). These classifications are typically too large for all the states defined by the classifications to be directly valued and so the approach has been to value a sample of states and then extrapolate to all states using econometric or mathematical means (Dolan 1997; Torrance 1982).

This paper examines the problems of estimating econometric models for a recently developed health state classification, the first version of the SF-6D, which has been derived from a larger generic measure of health, the SF-36 (Brazier et al. 1998). A sample of states defined by this classification have been valued using Standard Gamble (SG) by a convenience sample of patients, health professionals and students. The data generated by the valuation survey has a particularly complex structure, which poses many problems for econometric modelling. The distribution of the dependent variable is skewed, truncated and non-continuous. A further feature is the presence of individual heterogeneity and serial correlation since health state valuations may be due, in part, to unobserved individual characteristics rendering observations clustered within respondents. To our knowledge, there is no single, pre-canned estimation procedure that can deal satisfactorily with all of these features of the data. In this paper, our aim is to explore alternative models and estimation techniques that are readily available in commonly used econometric packages, in an attempt to provide a good predictor of health state valuations and thus derive a tariff. The problems of analysing these stated preference data have relevance beyond the confines of health to other areas of applied economics including transport and environment (Bates 1988), and applied econometrics in general.

The next section of this paper briefly describes the SF-6D health state classification. This section also outlines the survey in which health states were valued using standard gamble techniques. Section 3 discusses the complexity of the data generated by the valuation survey, and outlines a number of alternative model specifications that can be estimated in an attempt to predict the standard gamble scores. The results of the econometric analysis are reported in section 4, with discussion in section 5 and concluding remarks in section 6.

DERIVING AND VALUING HEALTH STATES VIA THE SF-6D

THE SF-6D

The first version of the SF-6D health state classification is shown in Table 1; it has the six dimensions of physical functioning, role limitation, social functioning, pain, mental health and vitality (δ = 1, 2, ..., 6), each with between two and six levels (λ) (Brazier et al. 1998). These dimensions and the wording of each level were taken from the SF-36 Health Survey, a profile measure of health widely used in clinical trials throughout the world (Ware, Sherbourne 1992). These dimensions were selected to represent the core aspects of health. This instrument has been found to perform well in psychometric terms at describing the health of people with a wide range of common medical conditions (e.g. Harper et al. 1997; Hollingsworth et al. 1995; McHorney et al. 1994). An SF-6D health state is defined by selecting one statement from each dimension, starting with physical functioning and ending with vitality. A total of 9 000 health states can be defined in this way. The structure of the SF-6D is similar to a number of other health state classifications used in economic evaluation of health care interventions, such as the EQ-5D which has 5 dimensions with 3 levels each (Brooks 1996), and the HUI3 with eight dimensions with between

Table I The SF-6D Health State Classification

Physical functioning (δ = 1)

λ

1. Your health does not limit you in <u>vigorous activities</u> (e.g. running, lifting heavy objects, participating in strenuous sports).

2. Your health limits you in <u>vigorous activities</u> (e.g. running lifting heavy objects, participating in strenuous sports).

3. Your health limits you in climbing <u>several</u> flights of stairs or in walking <u>more than a mile</u>.

4. Your health limits you in climbing one flight of stairs or in walking <u>half a mile</u>.

5. Your health limits you in walking <u>100 yards</u>.

6. Your health limits you in bathing and dressing yourself.

Role limitation (δ = 2)

λ

1. You have <u>no</u> problems with your work or other regular daily activities as a result of your physical health or any emotional problems.

2. You <u>have</u> problems with your work or other regular daily activities as a result of your physical health or any emotional problems.

Social functioning (δ = 3)

λ

1. Your physical health or emotional problems <u>do not</u> interfere at all with your normal social activities.

2. Your physical health or emotional problems interfere <u>slightly</u> with your normal social actvities.

3. Your physical health or emotional problems interfere <u>moderately</u> with your normal social activities.

4. Your physical health or emotional problems interfere <u>quite a bit</u> with your normal social activities.

5. Your physical health or emotional problems interfere <u>extremely</u> with your with your normal social activies.

Bodily pain (δ = 4)

λ

1. You have <u>no</u> bodily pain.

2. You have <u>very mild</u> bodily pain.

3. You have <u>mild</u> bodily pain.

4. You have <u>moderate</u> bodily pain.

5. You have <u>severe</u> bodily pain.

6. You have <u>very severe</u> bodily pain.

Mental health (δ = 5)

λ

1. You feel tense or downhearted and low <u>a little or none of the time</u>.

2. You feel tense or downhearted and low <u>some of the time</u>.

3. You feel tense or downhearted and low <u>a good bit of the time</u>.

4. You feel tense or downhearted and low <u>most of the time</u>.

5. You feel tense or downhearted and low <u>all of the time</u>.

Vitality (d = 6)

λ

1. You feel worn out or tired <u>a little or none of the time</u>.

2. You feel worn out or tired <u>some of the time</u>.

3. You feel worn out or tired <u>a good bit of the time</u>.

4. You feel worn out or tired <u>most of the time</u>.

5. You feel worn out or tired <u>all of the time</u>.

four and six levels each (Torrance et al. 1995). There is a more recently developed version of the SF-6D (Brazier et al. 2002) but this paper is concerned with the earlier version.

THE VALUATION SURVEY

A sample of 57 health states were chosen for valuation, from the 9 000 potential states available. These states were chosen to ensure that every level of each dimension appeared at least once. Health states included different combinations of attribute levels, including those with physical difficulty, those with mental problems, and those with some combination of the two.

The data reported here were elicited from a convenience sample recruited from a range of backgrounds including the health professions, health service managers and administrators, professional and technical staff at a large university Medical School, and students from health economics and medical courses. The respondents each valued 12 health states. These were selected from the sample of 57 states on the following basis: perfect health and two "core" states (i.e. those valued by most respondents); 16 "common" states (i.e. those valued by 1 in 5); and the remaining 50 states which were valued by 1 in 10. This selection of states was designed to enable the analyses to address a number of different issues, including an examination of the impact of background variables, internal consistency, a comparison of valuation methods, as well as the estimation of models.

The Standard Gamble (SG) technique was chosen as the main method for eliciting preferences since it has a strong theoretical foundation in expected utility theory; asking respondents to trade changes in health against risk. A self-completed version developed by Jones-Lee et al. (1993) was used, where the respondent is given a list of probabilities of success and failure for each question from which to select upper and lower bounds, as well as points of indifference. This version of SG has been found to perform better than a more conventional "ping-pong" approach using props (Dolan et al. 1996).

In the SG question, respondents are asked to choose between two alternatives. One is to live in a given SF-6D health state for 10 years. The second is to have a treatment, which may restore them to full health or fail and result in death. The question asked respondents to consider a range of chances of success from 100 in 100 (certain outcome) down to 10 in 100 (with a final box for immediate death preferred). Respondents were first asked to indicate with a tick all those chances of success where they would choose the risky treatment. Then they were asked to place a cross against cases where they would reject the treatment starting from 10 in 100. Finally, they were asked to indicate where it was most difficult to choose.[1] Respondents had the opportunity to indicate they would only choose the treatment if it had a lower than one in 100 chance of failure and to indicate at which level they would accept failure.

One hundred and sixteen people were approached to take part, and only 6 refused. Each respondent was given a booklet to complete, which contained questions on personal background and self-rated health, ranking and rating exercises (reported in Brazier et al. 1998), and the SG questions. The majority completed the questionnaire in supervised groups. The age of respondents ranged from 20–55, with a mean of 32 (SD = 8.9), and 49% were female. The majority had non-manual occupations. Out of a total of 1 320 possible SG questions, there were 1 037 usable observations across 106 individuals. No attempt has been made to filter the data by omitting "irrational" responses, though the proportion of responses logically inconsistent with the SF-6D was only 6% (Brazier et al. 1998).

Table 2 Descriptive statistics for the 57 health states

State	Count	Mean	Median	SD	State	Count	Mean	Median	SD
111311	44	98.76	99	1.62	523421	9	86.56	90	11.76
111323	9	98.42	99	1.57	323333	8	86.31	93.25	14.54
311211	29	97.14	97.5	2.33	311422	7	86.07	82.5	11.54
111122	8	96.81	98.5	4.28	323433	8	85.38	89.25	14.95
211111	21	96.61	99	7.78	223423	8	84.5	92.5	15.55
211211	9	96.5	99	3.86	422413	22	83.05	86.25	18.2
111212	20	96.22	99.25	6.14	424425	7	83	85	15.77
111312	18	95.69	97.5	5.54	624415	30	82.97	85	16.07
211212	7	95.21	97	4.95	521412	18	82.61	91.25	20.47
212222	8	95.07	96.5	5.14	424444	9	82.28	90	15.72
311222	22	92.18	96	8.90	313333	18	81.46	85	18.08
222432	31	91.98	95.5	9.42	423122	18	79.5	85	19.92
211223	8	91.95	97.5	13.43	423423	7	79.21	75	14.83
323422	30	90.98	95.5	9.61	323435	9	78.83	89.5	23.09
411412	8	90.81	96.75	10.61	623424	82	77.58	83.75	19.09
322323	22	90.73	90	8.62	324434	8	76.44	85	26.62
321412	8	90.56	94	7.64	624422	7	75	72.5	16.2
525112	40	90.39	95.75	12.51	623322	8	72.5	80	29.28
311212	7	90.29	96.5	17.80	422533	10	70.45	75	28.03
211442	8	90.06	96.5	11.88	624534	10	69.1	78.75	29.09
322313	9	89.72	95	15.54	623545	9	66.94	77.5	21.64
523111	22	88.81	93.75	11.94	624525	9	65.56	70	20.42
422434	22	88.68	94	12.66	624424	7	64.21	65	29.16
122424	10	88.45	96	11.8	424524	8	63.44	63.75	21.08
222222	10	88.45	97.75	15.34	624645	20	62.17	72.5	28.56
224244	50	88.14	92.75	13	625555	28	54.34	60	31.31
124143	127	88.13	95	12.82	525555	22	50.45	50	26.06
422334	9	88.11	92.5	12.26	625655	8	43.13	45	27.89
211222	7	87.33	90	14.98					

Descriptive statistics for the SG valuations of the 57 health states are reported in Table 2 (in descending order of mean valuation). Mean values range from 43.13 to 98.76 and are highly skewed towards the upper end of the scale suggesting that most respondents are not willing to take large risks to avoid the health state in question. There is clear heterogeneity reflected in the inverse relationship between the mean valuation and the standard deviation of these valuations. Median values are higher than means (in all but 5 cases) signifying the substantial skew in the data and this skew is also clearly shown by the distribution of 1 037 individual SG valuations shown in Figure 1.

METHODS

The data generated by the valuation survey described above has a complex structure which creates a number of problems for econometric estimation. Gravelle (1995) has pointed out that the derivation of a tariff for the full set of health states from individual valuations of a subset of states requires both estimation and aggregation and the data can be transformed or untransformed. Transformation, aggregation and estimation can occur in any order and different choices will produce different tariffs.

In the case of our SG valuations modelling can be done at the aggregate level using an appropriate measure of central tendency for the valuations of each of the 57 states, or at the individual level using all 1 037 responses with aggregation occurring via the regression model. Clearly using individual level data utilizes all of the information available and allows the estimation of the effects of respondent characteristics such as age and sex. It also avoids erroneous inference caused by wrongly infer-

Figure 1   Distribution of SG valuations

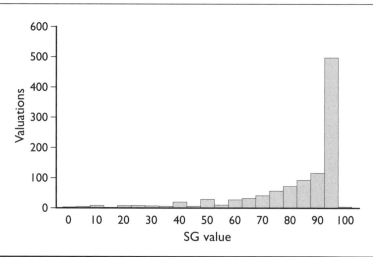

ring that aggregate level observed relationships hold at the individual level, a phenomenon referred to as the ecological fallacy. If individual response data is used it is important to recognize the variance structure of the data. Variation is both between respondent and within respondent (across health states). The latter is a direct consequence of within and between variability. Respondents did not value the same set of states and, although a balanced design was used in selecting health states for each individual, differences between health state values may be partly due to heterogeneity in the preferences of the respondents who valued them rather than the attributes of those states.

If modelling is done at the aggregate level the choice of the measure of central tendency is important since it represents a choice about which values are given greatest weight (Busschbach et al. 1999; Williams 1992). In the case of a highly skewed distribution like this one, the arithmetic mean gives a high weight to the upper end of the scale, whereas with the median equal weight is given to all responses. A common view has been that it is the mean that should be used regardless of the skewness of the data since this best reflects the individual's strength of preference. Another view would be that in the arena of public policy it is the median that should be used since in a voting context each person has an equal vote regardless of strength of preference. Strictly, neither is an ideal representation of the preferences of individuals, but rather than resolve the debate here we have estimated models using both measures of central tendency.

Before describing the models used in more detail, a third factor should also be considered. As well as being highly skewed, the distribution of SG scores is also truncated and non-continuous. SG scores are truncated at the upper limit since chance of treatment failure cannot be less than zero, giving a SG score of 100. In this data set the SG scores have a minimum of zero, indicating that the respondent would not accept any chance of failure for the treatment. However, SG scores of less than zero are theoretical possible in other data sets where health states are regarded as worse than dead. In addition the SG scores are discrete in that respondents can only specify a range of risk values within which they would accept treatment. These departures from normality and continuity warrant transformations of the dependent variable, and alternative estimation techniques. In combination with the complex form of heterogeneity, these issues present an interesting, and by no means straightforward, problem for econometric modelling.

MODELLING STANDARD GAMBLE SCORES

A number of alternative models can be formulated for predicting the SG gamble scores generated in the valuation survey. The general model is defined as:

$$y_{ij} = g(\beta' \mathbf{x}_{ij}) + \varepsilon_{ij} \qquad (1)$$

where $i = 1, 2, ..., n$ represents individual health state values and $j = 1, 2, ..., m$ represents respondents. The dependent variable, y_{ij}, is the SG score for health state i valued by respondent j.

x is a vector of dummy explanatory variables $(x_{\delta\lambda})$ for each level λ of dimension δ of the SF-6D. For example, x_{32} denotes dimension $\delta = 3$ (social functioning), level $\lambda = 2$ (...problems interfere *slightly*...). For any given health state, $x_{\delta\lambda}$ will be defined as

$x_{\delta\lambda} = 1$ if, for this state, dimension δ is at level λ
$x_{\delta\lambda} = 0$ if, for this state, dimension δ is *not* at level λ

In all there are 23 of these terms, with level $\lambda = 1$ acting as a baseline for each dimension. Hence for a simple linear model, the intercept represents state 111111 (full health), and the value of all other states is derived by summing the coefficients on the "on" dummies.

g is a function specifying the appropriate functional form. ε_{ij} is an error term whose autocorrelation structure and distributional properties depend on the assumptions underlying the particular model used.

This is an additive model, which, apart from additivity, imposes no restrictions on the relationship between dimension levels of the SF-6D. It does not enforce an interval scale between the levels of each dimension and neither does it impose ordinality on the levels. Hence it provides an opportunity to test the respondents' understanding of the scales.

In this specification each dimension level appears independently as an explanatory variable. However, there is the possibility of interactions between the levels of different attributes. Torrance et al. (1992) have suggested "...that the additional disutility added by a particular deficit is greater if it is the first and only deficit and less if it is the last of two or more deficits". Alternatively, for some states an interaction may increase the deficit over and above the sum of the two parts. The estimation of all possible interaction terms would have required a substantially larger proportion of the 9 000 health states of the SF-6D to be valued. There are, for example, 236 first order interactions alone. Given, the large number of possible interactions, and little evidence on which are likely to be important, there is a risk of finding significant interactions due to the play of chance. With this in mind, and given our primary aim of exploring alternative econometric modelling strategies, we have not considered interaction effects in this paper.[2]

ALTERNATIVE MODEL SPECIFICATION

The starting point is ordinary least squares (OLS) estimation of model (1), with g as a linear function. This simple specification assumes a standard zero mean, constant variance error structure, with independent error terms, that is $cov(\varepsilon_{ij} \, \varepsilon_{i'j}) = 0$, $i \neq i'$. This specification ignores the potential heterogeneity by assuming that each individual health state value is an independent observation, regardless of whether or not it was valued by the same respondent.

An improved specification, which takes account of variation both within and between respondents, is the one-way error components random effects (RE) model. This model explicitly recognizes that n observations on m individuals is not the same as $n \times m$ observations on different individuals. For the RE model the errors from model (1) are decomposed such that

$$\varepsilon_{ij} = u_j + e_{ij} \tag{2}$$

Here the error disturbance is represented by the components u_j and e_{ij}. The former specifies an unobserved individual specific random component and the latter an idiosyncratic observation-specific error component. Both are assumed to have zero mean and constant variance. Maximum likelihood estimation of the components additionally requires that they are random draws from Normal distributions. We also assume that the set of regressors, x_{ij} are exogenous in the sense that they are uncorrelated with the error components: $E(x_{ij}u_j) = 0$ and $E(x_{ij}e_{ij}) = 0$. We further assume that the allocation of health states to respondents is random, such that $cov(u_j,e_{ij}) = 0$.

The characteristic RE assumption, $E(x_{ij}u_j) = 0$, requires that the selection of respondents and the choice of health states is random. Violation of this assumption results in biased and inconsistent estimation of the parameters, β, of the RE model. The sampling of respondents and health states in this study was not random, as described above. In these circumstances a fixed effects estimator, such as least squares dummy variables (LSDV) may be preferable. Here consistency is obtained by conditioning on a set of $M - 1$ individual specific dummy variables. Here the respondent specific effects u_j are not assumed to be random, but are a set of fixed effects to be estimated, together with the vector of coefficients on the explanatory variables (β); hence the assumption $E(x_{ij}u_j) = 0$ is not required. Alternatively, the within-groups estimator may be used which sweeps out the individual effects by transforming the variables by subtracting their respective within individual group means. Again this ensures consistent estimation of the parameters, β. Note however, that fixed effects estimation cannot be more efficient than random effects estimation should the assumption $E(x_{ij}u_j) = 0$ hold and in practice may well be significantly less efficient.

The complex nature of variation in this data suggests a further class of models for consideration, those developed specifically to deal with hierarchical data structures often termed multilevel models (Goldstein 1995). The two-level variance components multilevel model is algebraically equivalent to the one-way error components RE model, denoted by the specification given in models (1) and (2) above. Estimation is by iterative GLS (IGLS), which offers a very flexible estimation routine allowing for the extension to many levels of a data hierarchy and more complex modelling of the variance components observed at any level of the hierarchy (see for example Goldstein, 1995). However, as with the more standard

RE estimator, the IGLS estimator is an unbiased and consistent estimator only when the assumption $E(x_{ij}u_j) = 0$ holds.

Finally we consider alternative functional forms (g in model (1)) to account for truncation and the discrete nature of the SG scores. Firstly, a RE Tobit specification is used in an attempt to account for the fact that the data are bounded between 0 and 100. Tobit specifications assume that the data are censored at a particular limit. This is different to truncation as we are assuming that some underlying latent variable can achieve a value greater than the limit observed.[3] However, as an approximation to truncated regression we fitted a RE Tobit model with censoring points at 0 and 100. Tobit models are also useful in this circumstance where scores are clustered at the upper end of the range. Secondly, we also tried two ordered Probit models in an effort to account for the discrete nature of the SG scores. These used an arbitrary ordering of 20 groups each of width 5, and also an ordering of 17 groups of varying widths to mirror the choices available to respondents.

As well as the core dummy variables describing each health state, it may also be that personal characteristics of the respondents have a significant influence on SG valuations of health states. Characteristics that are pertinent to the equity debate, such as age, sex, ethnicity and socioeconomic status will, if significant, point to the use of different social tariffs for different groups in order to ensure that preferences are treated in an equitable manner (Williams and Cookson 2000). The effect of respondent characteristics can only be investigated using models estimated at the individual level and the variables available to us in this study are age, sex, employment status, general health status and the presence of a chronic health problem.

RESULTS

Table 3 presents results for five alternative ways of estimating model (1) using the core set of dummy explanatory variables that represent the levels of each dimension of health that make up a health state as defined on the SF-6D. Estimation was carried out using STATA v6.0 and *MLwiN* (Goldstein et al. 1998). The first two columns use data at the aggregate level, so the dependent variable is the mean (or median) SG valuation for each of the 57 states. Columns (3) to (5) use data on individual responses, so the dependent variable is the individual SG valuations ($n = 1\ 037$).

A number of findings are robust across the models. Most coefficients have the expected negative sign representing detriments from the "full health" state 111111, but only the minority of coefficient estimates are significant at traditionally acceptable levels. The intercepts in all cases have the expected sign and size, and are not significantly different to 100 which represent the expected value of the "full health" state. The *role* dimension and lower levels of the *social functioning* and *pain* dimensions have no significant effect on the health state valuation in any of the models. In

Table 3 Core models

	(1) Mean	(2) Median	(3) OLS	(4) RE	(5) RE Tobit
C	101.086**	103.013**	99.819**	98.374**	99.710**
	(1.889)	(1.678)	(1.699)	(1.994)	(2.212)
PF2	–3.766*	–3.198	–2.904*	–1.563	–1.807
	(1.589)	(1.914)	(1.464)	(1.681)	(1.680)
PF3	–5.041**	–5.549*	–3.380*	–2.875	–3.199
	(1.685)	(2.178)	(1.529)	(1.694)	(1.688)
PF4	–7.214**	–9.063**	–7.540**	–6.350**	–6.541**
	(2.143)	(2.659)	(2.287)	(1.931)	(1.930)
PF5	–9.187**	–8.751*	–9.929**	–5.886*	–6.073*
	(3.212)	(3.836)	(3.223)	(2.456)	(2.472)
PF6	–11.212**	–11.108*	–10.165**	–9.980**	–10.233**
	(3.659)	(4.140)	(3.223)	(2.251)	(2.239)
ROLE2	–0.878	2.398	–0.105	–3.865	–3.995
	(2.577)	(2.832)	(2.917)	(2.289)	(2.282)
SF2	0.684	–0.736	1.394	1.885	1.936
	(2.755)	(2.693)	(2.955)	(2.587)	(2.573)
SF3	–4.311	–4.161	–3.476	0.325	0.537
	(3.153)	(3.389)	(2.781)	(2.401)	(2.383)
SF4	–5.484	–9.544**	–4.846	–1.456	–1.211
	(3.156)	(3.306)	(3.644)	(2.730)	(2.723)
SF5	4.528	1.411	5.452	–2.695	–2.828
	(3.158)	(3.177)	(4.151)	(3.544)	(3.594)
PAIN2	0.949	0.727	1.119	–1.365	–1.026
	(1.767)	(2.158)	(1.918)	(2.107)	(2.100)
PAIN3	–0.230	–1.860	–0.064	–1.365	–1.763
	(2.343)	(2.048)	(1.965)	(2.107)	(1.842)
PAIN4	–1.006	–2.956	–0.528	–1.569	–1.451
	(1.837)	(2.103)	(1.938)	(1.822)	(1.819)
PAIN5	–12.908**	–13.367**	–13.095**	–12.778**	–12.663**
	(3.533)	(4.156)	(4.065)	(2.601)	(2.589)
PAIN6	–19.457**	–18.857**	–20.161**	–17.157**	–17.032**
	(4.165)	(5.690)	(6.497)	(3.542)	(3.543)
MH2	–1.681	–3.492	–1.546	–3.741*	–3.903*
	(1.619)	(2.023)	(1.668)	(1.562)	(1.558)
MH3	–0.717	0.459	–1.356	–4.672*	–4.747*
	(2.461)	(2.788)	(2.503)	(2.102)	(2.094)
MH4	0.906	3.176	0.667	–3.456	–3.831
	(2.159)	(2.891)	(3.069)	(2.315)	(2.299)
MH5	–25.874**	–30.838**	–25.857**	–19.347**	–19.172**
	(3.532)	(5.351)	(6.002)	(3.865)	(3.895)
VIT2	–5.159**	–2.321	–4.849**	1.670	1.808
	(1.615)	(2.043)	(1.498)	(1.849)	(1.874)
VIT3	–5.890*	–3.679	–7.206**	–1.511	–1.393
	(2.414)	(2.919)	(2.137)	(2.173)	(2.221)

continued

Table 3   Core models *(continued)*

	(1) Mean	(2) Median	(3) OLS	(4) RE	(5) RE Tobit
VIT4	−7.049*	−1.926	−6.425*	−0.896	−0.851
	(2.919)	(3.539)	(2.963)	(2.666)	(2.700)
VIT5	−3.927	1.203	−3.843	−1.291	−1.341
	(3.711)	(3.947)	(3.945)	(2.919)	(2.931)
N	57	57	1 037	1 037	1 037
Adj R²	0.888	0.836	0.324	0.327	
RESET	0.025 [0.876]	1.199 [0.282]	1.560 [0.203]	4.710 [0.195]	6.410 [0.093]

PF is physical functioning, ROLE is role limitation, SF is social functioning, PAIN is bodily pain, MH is mental health and VIT is vitality.

* significant at $t_{0.05}$; ** significant at $t_{0.01}$.

contrast the more severe problems on the *physical functioning, pain* and *mental health* dimensions always attract statistically significant large negative coefficients. All the models have acceptable explanatory power and the Reset tests give no evidence of functional form misspecification.

Other results are more sensitive to model specification. Results are similar for the aggregate level mean and median models, except the *vitality* dimension attracts much larger coefficients if the mean is used as the measure of central tendency. The individual level OLS model gives very similar results to the mean model as expected. However a Cook-Weisberg test for heteroscedasticity indicates that the standard OLS assumption of homoscedastic errors is not applicable in these data ($\chi_1^2 = 338, p < 0.001$). Further, these data represent repeated observations on the 106 individuals sampled. A standard OLS assumption is that error terms are independent, $cov(e_{ij}, e_{i'j}) = 0$, $i \neq i'$, and again this is not appropriate here. OLS standard errors are biased when such assumptions are not realized and as such, the standard errors presented in Table 3 were corrected for intra-unit clustering and heteroscedasticity.

Column (4) shows the one-way error components RE model defined by models (1) and (2).[4] The coefficient estimates are generally smaller than those for the models which do not allow for individual respondent effects but the pattern of coefficients is largely similar. However, if the selection of either individuals or health states were not made entirely randomly, then the assumption $Corr(x_{ij}, u_j) = 0$ may be violated, resulting in biased and inconsistent estimates. In such circumstances, a fixed effects estimator may be preferable. Estimation of a fixed effects model produces results (Brazier at al. 1998), which are very similar to the RE specification. Also a Hausman test of fixed versus random effects specification (Hausman 1978) indicates that there is insufficient evidence to reject the assumption of individual effects being distributed randomly ($\chi_{23}^2 = 22$, $p = 0.51$). A Breusch-Pagan Lagrangian multiplier test of the significance of RE

(Breusch and Pagan 1980) confirms that the total variance is better treated as components of variation; both within and between individuals ($\chi^2_1 = 899$, $p = 0.001$). As a result we prefer the random to the fixed effects specification.

Standard variance components multilevel models were also estimated using iterative generalized least squares (IGLS) (see Goldstein, 1995). Again these results are not reported here since as expected they are extremely similar to the GLS RE results reported in column (4). The Tobit model presented in column (5) is an attempt to deal with the skew and truncation of the distribution of SG scores. The results are again very similar to the standard RE model reported in column (4).

An obvious criterion for assessing the different models is consistency of rankings of increasing health state valuations and intuitive signs attached to coefficient estimates. *A priori* we expect that all estimated coefficients have negative signs (with the exception of the constant which ought to be approximately 100). Further increasing severity of health state levels within a dimension should attract increasingly negative coefficient estimates creating a negative gradient across a dimension.

The mean, median and OLS models all have well behaved *physical functioning* scales, but for the linear RE and RE Tobit models the coefficient on PF5 is smaller than that on PF4 (although they are not significantly different). *Role limitation* and *social functioning* do not appear to be important in any of the models, with the exception of SF4 which attracts a very large coefficient in the median model. The *pain* dimension is well behaved in all models with the lower levels insignificant, and PAIN5 and PAIN6 attracting large coefficients. In the mean, median and OLS models only the highest level of the *mental health* dimension is significant, whereas in the RE and Tobit models MH2 and MH3 are significant but MH4 is not, resulting in a violation of the ordinality of the scales. The *vitality* dimension only has significant levels in the mean and OLS models and here the most severe level is not significant.

The ultimate aim of these models is to predict valuations for all states defined by the SF-6D. Table 4 presents diagnostic statistics for the within

Table 4   Diagnostic statistics for core models

Predictions	Mean	Median	OLS	RE	RE Tobit
JB	1.133[0.353]	0.851[0.791]	10.520[0.005]	1.999[0.368]	1.641 [0.440]
LB	8.874[0.567]	4.681[0.653]	11.607[0.170]	7.018[0.535]	6.461 [0.596]
MAE	2.579	2.934	2.539	3.124	3.469
No > |5|	5	9	7	15	14
No > |10|	0	1	1	1	1
$t (\bar{e} = 0)$	0^a	0^a	−0.965[0.339]	−1.596[0.116]	−3.872 [0.000]

a. zero by definition.

sample predictive ability of the models. These statistics reflect the models' ability to predict the actual mean (or median) valuation given to each state by our sample of 106 people. All of the models produce random prediction errors as reflected in the insignificance of the Ljung-Box (LB) statistic. The OLS model results in the smallest mean absolute error (MAE) but the distribution of errors in this case is not normal (Jarque-Bera (JB) statistic). In terms of overall error size the mean model performs the best with only 5 errors greater than |5| and none greater than |10|. These large prediction errors are made on states with a relatively small number of valuations (10 or less). Despite the support for the RE model from the Hausman and Breusch-Pagan tests, it does not predict well in comparison to the mean model. The tobit model is clearly the worst performer with large prediction errors that are also biased as reflected in the *t*-test of the null hypothesis that the mean prediction error is zero.

The ordered probit models using 20 and 17 groups did not perform well and the results are not reported here. The 17 group model was superior but still resulted in coefficient ordering that contravened the ordinality of the scales and only predicted 21 out of 57 health state valuations correctly.[5] Transforming the response to an ordered scale has some appeal since in reality respondents were presented with a finite set of options chose from when valuing a given health state. However, re-ordering in this manner does involve the loss of information, and for this reason the method may not be desirable. In addition the failure to fully account for residual heterogeneity may contribute to the poor performance of this model.

Given the large number of insignificant coefficient estimates presented in Table 3, it seemed worth pursuing the mean, OLS and linear RE models to see whether their predictive ability suffered as a result of making the models more parsimonious.[6] Omitting insignificant variables results in little change in the coefficients on the included variables. In terms of predictions the mean model is still superior but there is some reduction in predictive ability compared with the full model. The MAE is 2.926 with 7 errors greater than |5| and 1 greater than |10|. All the models also have a number of inconsistent results in relation to the ordinality of the dimension scales. A further problem is that for the mean and RE models the intercept is significantly lower than 100.

Based on the above results, full models are preferred both in terms of coefficient estimates and predictive ability. Of the alternative models presented here the aggregate mean model (Table 3, column (1)) is the best. White's test and an ARCH test suggest no remaining heteroscedasticity with this model ($F = 0.628$, $p = 0.876$; $F = 0.691$, $p = 0.409$ respectively). The model has good inside sample predictive ability; prediction errors are random and 52/57 valuations are predicted correctly to within 5 of the actual mean valuation. The outside sample predictions are not quite so good. The model was estimated on 29 randomly chosen health states and these estimates were used to predict valuations for the remaining 28 health states. The prediction errors are random ($LB = 4.165$, $p = 0.654$), but the

MAE is 5.724 with 13 errors greater than |5| and 4 greater than |10|. These results are not surprising given the relatively small sample of health states included here.

One disadvantage of a model estimated at this aggregate level is that it does not allow us to investigate the influence of respondent characteristics on SG valuations of health states. If respondent characteristics are important the aggregate mean model may not be appropriate. The effect of respondent characteristics is investigated here via the linear RE model. Characteristics such as age, sex and educational status were not statistically significant. The only significant respondent effect is a NON-WORK dummy variable that takes the value of 1 if the respondent is a student or a retired person. This dummy attracts a coefficient of 5.727 (s.e. = 2.864), implying that students and retired people give higher valuations to the health states than the other respondents. The coefficients on the core dummy variables are very robust to the inclusion of this respondent characteristic, and as such the full results for this model are not reported here. There is a slight increase in the adjusted R^2 compared to the core linear RE model presented in Table 3 (from 0.327 to 0.339). However, the Reset test suggests there may be a misspecification problem, $F = 6.250$, $p = 0.012$.

In order to investigate the effect of retired people and students on the tariff derived from our preferred mean model, we estimated this aggregate model excluding the valuations of this subset of respondents.[7] The results (not reported here) are virtually identical to the mean model presented in column (1) of Table 3 in terms of coefficient estimates, standard errors and the predictive ability of the model.

DISCUSSION

The econometric modelling of stated preference data presents a range of problems, which in the case of SG health state valuation data include skewness, truncation, non-continuity and a hierarchical structure at the individual level. There is no single estimation procedure for handling these problems simultaneously and therefore this paper has examined a number of alternative specifications. Previous work with these types of data have limited their analyses to mean models (Kaplan and Bush 1982) or used fixed effects models (Brazier et al. 1998) or random effects models (Dolan 1997) to deal with the clustering around individuals, but these studies have not reported the consequences of attempting to deal with skewness, truncation or non-continuity.

Alternative specifications have been attempted to model SG valuations of health states from a sample of 106 people valuing 12 states each. We acknowledge that these models have been estimated on an unrepresentative United Kingdom sample and do not provide a definitive tariff for valuing the SF-6D,[8] but it provides an opportunity to examine the methods for analysing such data. A number of findings are robust across these models and these suggest that *physical functioning, pain* and *mental health* are the most important dimensions of health determining valuations of health states as defined by the SF-6D. The results broadly support the ordinality of the SF-6D scales, with the mean model being the most consistent. However, even for the mean model there is an exception in relation to the vitality dimension of health. The lower levels are significant and the coefficients increase in absolute value with the severity of impairment up to VIT4, but the most severe level, VIT5, attracts a coefficient half the size of that on VIT4. This may have resulted from the selection of health states valued in the study. The results do not support the assumption of equal intervals between levels on each dimension, so the models were correctly specified in not constraining the estimates in this way.

The surprising finding was that the mean model was as good if not better than the more complex model specifications on this data set. Attempts to deal with the skewed and truncated nature of the distribution of SG valuations were largely unsuccessful. The RE Tobit model resulted in large, biased prediction errors suggesting that this is not an appropriate transformation of the dependent variable. While this model allows for both censoring (as an attempt to mimic truncation) and decomposition of the variance components, there are problems associated with this specification in that censoring is not the same as truncation and we have not fully adjusted for the heteroscedastic error terms at the bottom level. The latter leads to inconsistent parameter estimates and biased standard errors.

The ordered Probit models predicted badly and this may be a result of the inability to account for individual respondent effects in these models. Empirical support for the linear RE model shows that individual effects are important as the valuations are clustered by respondent. Nevertheless, despite the intuitive appeal of the RE specification given the study design, the aggregate mean model performs the best both in terms of coefficient expectations and predictive ability.

A potential disadvantage of the mean model is its inability to model the effect of respondent characteristics but in this study most respondent characteristics had no significant effect on health state valuation. This finding is in contrast to other empirical work that has found that age is generally positively related to valuation health states (Dolan 2000). The contradictory result may be due to our convenience sample which only included respondents from a relatively narrow age range (20 to 55 years). The finding that students and retired people value health states more highly than the other respondents may also be peculiar to our sample, as these groups formed a significant proportion of respondents (20/106).

CONCLUSION

The modelling of stated preference data is becoming increasingly important for helping policy-makers in the health sector. This chapter has examined for the first time a number of alternative specifications for dealing with the complexities found in an SG health state valuation data set. The results indicate that it is feasible to undertake modelling of these types of data and that a mean model is as good and often better than the more complex specifications. This has important implications for modelling health state valuations and related stated preference data sets.

We have raised a number of issues that must be addressed in the analysis of these types of data, the alternative specifications to address these features and some evidence on their importance in the models. Care should be taken in concluding that a simple mean specification is sufficient for all attempts to model health state classifications and other descriptive systems onto stated preference data, nonetheless this work can assist others seeking to identify the appropriate strategy for modelling stated preference data sets.

Notes

1 Respondents did not always indicate where it was most difficult to choose and in these cases the recommended procedure was adopted of taking the mid-point between the upper and lower values as a proxy (Jones-Lee et al. 1993).

2 Discussion and estimation of interaction effects in this data set can be seen in Brazier et al. (1998), see *http://www.shef.ac.uk/~sheg/publications.htm*

3 Truncated regression procedures are available to model such processes but were found to be unstable for these data.

4 The results presented here were estimated by GLS but MLE and GEE (available from the authors) produce extremely similar results, both for the estimated parameters and standard errors.

5 Predictive ability was judged in relation to whether the model placed the valuation in the correct group of the 17 groups defined.

6 Results are not reported here but are available from the authors.

7 Sample sizes did not allow us to estimate a separate model for students and retired people.

8 A tariff has been estimated for a revised version of the SF-6D using a representative sample of 611 members of the UK general population (Brazier et al. 2002).

References

Bates J (1988) Papers on stated preference methods in transport research. *Journal of Transport Economics and Policy,* **22**(1):7–9.

Brazier JE (1995) The SF-36 health survey and its use in pharmacoeconomic evaluation. *PharmacoEconomics,* **7**(5):403–415.

Brazier JE, Deverill M (1999) *Obtaining the "Q" in QALYs: a comparison of five multi-attribute utility scales. Sheffield Health Economics group* . (Discussion paper no 99/1.) School of Health and Related Research, University of Sheffield, Sheffield.

Brazier JE, Roberts J, Deverill M (2002) The estimation of a preference-based measure of health from the SF-36. *Journal of Health Economics,* 21(2):271–292.

Brazier JE, Usherwood T, Harper R, Thomas K (1998) Deriving a preference based single index measure from the UK SF-36 health survey. *Journal of Clinical Epidemiology,* 51(11):1115–1128.

Breusch T, Pagan A (1980) The Lagrange multiplier test and its applications to model specification in econometrics. *Review of Economic Studies,* 47(1):239–253.

Brooks R (1996) EuroQol: the current state of play. *Health Policy,* 37(1):53–72.

Busschbach JV, McDonnell J, Essink-Bot ML, van Hout BA (1999) Estimating parametric relationships between health state description and health valuation with an application to the EuroQol EQ-5D. *Journal of Health Economics,* 18(5):551–571.

Dolan P (1997) Modelling valuations for EuroQol health states. *Medical Care,* 35(11):1095–1108.

Dolan P (2000) The measurement of health-related quality-of-life for use in resource allocation decisions in health care. In: *Handbook of health economics. Vol. 1B.* Culyer AJ, Newhouse J, eds. Elsevier, Amsterdam.

Dolan P, Gudex C, Kind P, Williams A (1996) Valuing health states: a comparison of methods. *Journal of Health Economics,* 15(2):209–231.

Drummond MF, O'Brien BJ, Stoddart GL, Torrance GW (1997) *Methods for the economic evaluation of health care programmes.* 2nd edn. Oxford University Press, Oxford.

Goldstein H (1995) *Multilevel statistical models.* 2nd edn. Edward Arnold, London.

Goldstein H, Rasbash J, Plewis I, et al. (1998) *A user's guide to MLwiN, version 1.0.* University of London, Institute of Education, London.

Gravelle H (1995) *Valuations of EuroQol health states: comments and suggestions.* (Paper presented at the ESRC/SHHD workshop on quality of life.) Edinburgh.

Harper R, Brazier JE, Waterhouse JC, Walters SJ, Jones NMB, Howard P (1997) A comparison of outcome measures for patients with chronic obstructive pulmonary disease (COPD) in an output setting. *Thorax,* 52(10):879–887.

Hausman JA (1978) Specification tests in econometrics. *Econometrica,* 46(6):1251–1271.

Hollingsworth W, Mackenzie R, Todd CJ, Dixon AK (1995) Measuring changes in quality-of-life following magnetic-resonance-imaging of the knee – SF-36, EuroQol ((c)) or Rosser index. *Quality of Life Research,* 4(4):325–334.

Jones-Lee M, Loomes G, O'Reilly D, Philips P (1993) *The value of preventing non-fatal road injuries: findings of a willingness-to-pay national sample survey.* (HMSO 1993;70.) Transport Research Laboratory, London.

Kaplan RM, Bush JW (1982) Health-related quality of life measurement for evaluation of research and policy analysis. *Health Psychology,* 1:61–80.

McHorney CA, Ware JE, Lu JFR, et al. (1994) The MOS 36-item short form health survey (SF-36): III. Tests of data quality, scaling assumptions, and reliability across diverse patient groups. *Medical Care,* 32(1):40–66.

Torrance GW (1982) Multi-attribute utility theory as a method of measuring social preferences for health states in long-term care. In: *Values in long-term care.* Kane RL, Kane RA, eds. Lexington Books, DC Health, Lexington, MA.

Torrance GW (1986) Measurement of health state utilities for economic appraisal: a review. *Journal of Health Economics,* 5(1):1–30.

Torrance GW, Furlong W, Feeny D, Boyle M (1995) Multi-attribute preference functions: Health Utilities Index. *PharmacoEconomics,* 7(6):503–520.

Ware JE, Sherbourne CD (1992) The MOS 36-item short form health survey (SF-36): I. Conceptual framework and item selection. *Medical Care,* 30(6):473–483.

Williams A (1992) Measuring functioning and well-being, by Stewart and Ware. Review article. *Health Economics,* 1(4):255–258.

Williams A, Cookson R (2000) Equity in health. In: *Handbook of health economics.* Culyer AJ, Newhouse J, eds. Elsevier, Amsterdam.

Chapter 11.1

DETERMINANTS OF VARIANCE IN HEALTH STATE VALUATIONS

JOHANNES SOMMERFELD, ROB M.P.M. BALTUSSEN,
LAURIEN METZ, MAMADOU SANON AND RAINER
SAUERBORN

INTRODUCTION

In the past decade, there has been a rapidly growing interest in applying health-related metrics across population groups, societies, cultures and nations (e.g. Murray and Lopez 1996; Field and Gold 1998; Slottje et al. 1991; World Bank 1993). Such research, commonly termed cross-national or cross-cultural health research, has a long history, particularly of comparing perceptions of quality of life (QoL). In recent years, this type of research has been advocated and supported increasingly by the World Health Organization (WHO) (e.g. Murray and Lopez 1996; Gureje et al. 1997; Kessler 1999; Power et al. 1999; Room et al. 1996; WHOQOL Group 1998).

Summary measures of population health (SMPH) would need to be compatible across nations and cultures to serve as measures for making global health policy. Health state valuations on the basis of utility instruments such as rating scales (RS), e.g. the Visual Analogue Scale (VAS), or methods such as personal trade-off (PTO), time trade-off (TTO) and standard gamble (SG),[1] are one of the critical inputs that contribute to the calculation of SMPH. These methods are supposed to assess an individual's valuation of hypothetical health states in terms of a single number indicating the value placed on a health state relative to perfect health or death. They have been deemed feasible by many investigators to reflect health state preferences adequately, and are now being used in a large number of studies, mostly cost-utility analyses, across various countries.

To serve as inputs for global SMPH, for reasons of comparison in the context of policy, these instruments need to be cross-culturally relevant and sensitive to measuring comparable constructs across cultures. In other words, they are supposed to be cross-culturally valid, fulfilling validity criteria on various dimensions of equivalence (Guillemin et al. 1993; Herdman et al. 1997; 1998). Several scholars, however, have voiced doubts about the cross-cultural applicability of health profiles (e.g. Fox-Rushby and Parker 1995; Hunt 1986) as well as of utility measures (e.g. James and Foster 1999).

An individual's valuation of a certain health state to a large extent reflects values, assumptions and beliefs about health and illness in general, and "lived" experience with actual episodes of ill-health, impairment and handicap in particular. In valuation surveys, lay emphasis on qualitative features of illness and disability are neglected to the benefit of a numerical value. Social and cultural values and beliefs, on the other hand, are not "stable" cognitive phenomena; they reflect cultural orientation as well as social and socioeconomic positions within a society and can change over time.

It is well known that values and beliefs vary extensively among individuals, and between population groups, societies, cultures and nations (Hofstede 1980; 1998; Rokeach 1968). Much of this variation in beliefs is cultural in origin and due to different normative belief systems (Henrich and Boyd 1998; Landrine and Klonoff 1992). Evidence from research conducted in a variety of disciplines suggests that there is inter- and intra-cultural variation[2] in values related to a number of policy issues, e.g. the environment (Beckerman and Pasek 1997; Dunlap 1998; Nazarea et al. 1998), alcohol problems (Schmidt and Room 1999), the prevention of deaths (Mendeloff and Kaplan 1989) and, most importantly in the context of this book, the valuation of health states (cf. Patrick et al. 1985 for an earlier paper on this question).

This observation poses the fundamental question of how to understand and deal with variation in health state valuations. More than ten years ago, a number of scholars pointed out considerable problems with developing socio-medical indicators in one culture and transporting them into another. Hunt (1986) stressed the ambiguity inherent in the terms "health" and "illness" and underlined the considerable cross-cultural variability of meaning systems. Cautioning not to interpret variation in QoL measures solely in terms of variation in objective living conditions, Ostroot and Snyder (1985) suggested that systematic cross-national variation, or "cross-cultural bias", could be the root cause of variation. Similarly, Eyton and Neuwirth (1984) warned of "ethnocentrism" inherent in cross-cultural health studies.

Although universality would be a highly desirable asset for utility measures, such universally applied or applicable instruments may be regarded as cultural artifacts themselves as they transport Western values, notions of time, and concepts of science (Adam 1998; Bulmer 1998). Consequently, one has to weigh the inherent risk of imposing Western or universal notions of health and health states across cultures against the convenience and advantages of SMPH for public health policy. This weighing of advantages and disadvantages, rather than resulting in pure academic debate, should result in a clearer and more refined vision for appropriate research.

SMPH, by definition, aggregate large amounts of population-based data originally assessed at the individual level into global numerical figures. The variation of health state values, therefore, raises a number of fundamental concerns about SMPH. Aside from exclusively being a matter of methodological concern, i.e. limiting intra- and cross-cultural bias through epidemiological and psychometric "fine-tuning", the cross-cultural use of SMPH warrants answers on a variety of questions. Does variation simply reflect the fact that individuals and cultures differently value health states? Does it reflect health status associated with a given disease state or is the variation simply due to systematic variation, i.e. research bias? Can SMPH (also) accommodate cross-cultural and cross-national diversity? To what extent can and should that diversity be accepted and valued? Is there room for a qualification of valuations?

We address these questions by reviewing literature from a variety of social science disciplines, i.e. medical anthropology, epidemiology, psychometrics and econometrics. The chapter intends to contribute to the debate on cross-cultural applicability and sources of variation in SMPH by focusing on problems inherent in exporting utility measures on a worldwide scale, i.e. into a large variety of societal and cultural settings. We are focusing our interest less on simultaneous cross-national use of such methods in relatively cosmopolitan urban settings and among relatively well-educated citizens of, for example, London, Manila, Canberra, Santiago de Chile and Washington, DC. We are more interested in problems of applying these methodologies in culturally and socioeconomically heterogeneous settings, among "traditional" rural populations and population subgroups that may be socioeconomically or politically marginalized, not having had the opportunity to attain a certain level of formal education. We will illustrate the methodological challenges of investigating variation in health status valuations by presenting formative research from rural Burkina Faso.

SUMMARY OF PAST EMPIRICAL RESEARCH

Research addressing variation in health state valuations can be grouped into two major categories. First, research evaluating the applicability of SMPH in cross-national comparison and second, research elucidating methodological sources of variation.

RESEARCH EVALUATING THE APPLICABILITY OF SMPH IN CROSS-NATIONAL COMPARISONS

Research dealing with the applicability of SMPH in cross-national comparisons have dealt, in great detail, with issues of cross-cultural adaptation and equivalence of a variety of health profiles and, to a much smaller extent, with utility measures such as RS, SG, TTO, PTO and WTP in cross-national comparison. Since cross-cultural adaptation is a prerequisite for cross-national and cross-cultural comparison (Guillemin et al. 1993) only the latter can illuminate determinants of variation.

CROSS-NATIONAL ADAPTATION OF HEALTH PROFILES

In recent years, there has been considerable growth in the literature on the cross-national adaptation of instruments assessing health-related quality of life (HRQoL: for a review see Guillemin, Bombardier and Beaton 1993). Health profiles such as the IQOLA (Keller et al. 1998; Ware et al. 1995), the SF-36 (Perneger et al. 1999), the WHOQOL-100 (Power et al. 1999) and the Nottingham Health Profile (Hunt 1988; Hunt et al. 1991; Hunt and McEwen 1980) have been adapted to be applied in nations different from the country in which they were originally developed.

In addition, the literature abounds with research reports on cross-cultural adaptations of condition-specific QoL instruments, such as the Functional Assessment of Chronic Illness Therapy (FACIT; Lent et al. 1999), the Quality of Life in Epilepsy instrument (QOLIE-31; Cramer et al. 1998), the Recurrent Genital Herpes Quality of Life questionnaire (RGHQoL; Doward et al. 1998), the Quality of Life in Dermatology instrument (de Tiedra et al. 1998), the QoL with Onychomycosis instrument (Drake et al. 1999), the QoL for Urinary Incontinence (I-QoL) (Patrick et al. 1999), the QoL-MED for erection difficulties (Wagner et al. 1996), and the EuroQuality of Life (EQ-5D) in New Zealand (Devlin and Williams 1999). Culturally appropriate scales have also been developed for domains as different as perceived quality of care (Haddad et al. 1998) and depression (Sandermann et al. 1996).

Research into the cross-cultural adaptation of health-related measures aims at refuting the hypothesis that variation of an individual measure is due to non-equivalence or trans-cultural bias. Individual authors report varying degrees of cross-cultural equivalence.[3] However, this body of literature is still too diverse to result in generalizable statements. On the one hand, there is a wide diversity of instruments and cultures to which these instruments are adapted. On the other hand, most adaptation studies are about English-language instruments being translated into European languages or adapted to other Western, industrialized cultures. Consequently, the measures themselves can be considered culture-specific (Fox-Rushby and Parker 1995).

Adaptation of instruments between very heterogeneous cultures, for example, between cultures that are highly written and cultures that have strong oral traditions or between highly literate and illiterate population subgroups do not seem to exist. A review of the literature (Guillemin et al. 1993) suggests that there is a widespread variation in research methodologies to investigate and assure cross-cultural adaptation and a clear need to define common definitions of equivalence (cf. Herdman et al. 1997).

COMPARATIVE SMPH STUDIES

The disability-adjusted life years (DALY) measure is an important step forward in quantifying health changes in public health. However, there is an obvious scarcity of research on the feasibility of administrating PTO—and other health state valuation instruments such as SG, VAS and TTO—across cultures and nations. Murray and Lopez (2000) note that cognitively demanding techniques such as the SG, TTO and PTO are difficult to use with less educated individuals. If large scale empirical assessments in many different countries are to be achieved, the authors argue, instruments would need to be developed that are reliable and valid for populations with widely varying educational attainment. Murray and Lopez (2000) argue that self-reported health profiles like the EuroQol EQ5D or the SF-36 should be regarded with caution as the interpretation of these scales may differ across cultures or socioeconomic groups within cultures.

Murray (1996, p. 25) argues that health profiles—as a means to describe health states—should be interpreted with caution. He notes that the fundamental problem with current self-reported instruments is a lack of cross-cultural comparability. This should not be simply a question of language and the interpretation of the meaning of different categorical responses in different languages. The endpoints of scales for a given domain such as best or worst mobility may also have very different meanings across different cultures or across socioeconomic strata within a society.

A classic example is cited from Australia, where the aboriginal population with much higher mortality than the rest of the Australian population reports better health status on surveys. In response to the question how do you rate your overall health status, 2% report their health as poor and 10% report their health as fair, as compared with 4.5% in the rest of the Australian population reporting poor health and 16% reporting fair health. Therefore, Murray and Lopez (2000) argue that these self-reported health profiles must be interpreted with great care and that it is better to use observations where possible (however, there is a category of health outcomes which cannot be observed, namely pain and suffering).

Recently, research has been initiated in order to evaluate the universality of disability weights. Üstün et al. (1999) compared the rank correlations for a set of 17 health-related disabilities among health professionals in 14 countries, including Canada, China, Egypt, Greece, India, Japan, Luxembourg, the Netherlands, Nigeria, Romania, Spain, Tunisia, Turkey, and the United Kingdom of Great Britain and Northern Ireland. The study showed relatively consistent rankings and weights for disabling effects of 17 health conditions. However, there were statistically significant differences in rank between countries for 13 of the 17 health conditions. Physical disabilities showed the most uniform valuation. Overall, the authors concluded that "these differences are large enough to shed doubt on the assumption of universality of the disability rankings, and subsequently on the weights, and they are large enough to be investigated further in a systematic way."

To summarize, it is largely unknown, at this point, whether the above methodological approaches are applicable in developing country situations. The central question, therefore, is how cross-cultural variation in the relative importance individuals place on different domains of health can be explained and conceptualized.

SOURCES OF VARIATION

As the literature on the cross-cultural applicability of SMPH is limited and heterogeneous, evidence from research on sources of variation needs to be drawn from a larger set of literature, namely the more extensive body of literature on social science methodologies, with a focus on methods in cross-cultural application.

VARIATION AS THE RESULT AND SOURCE OF RESEARCH BIAS

Results from various studies suggest that variation of statistical summary measures may be the result of systematic variation of measurements, i.e. flaws in data collection, or flaws in study design or analysis, in other words: research bias. Biases are defined as presence of systematic variations in the measurement and can include:

- the incentive to misrepresent responses (strategic bias, compliance bias) implied value cues (starting point bias, range bias);

- scenario misspecification;

- hypothetical bias;

- information bias; and

- bias from sampling design, i.e. inference bias (Klose 1999).

Survey techniques and modes of administration of instruments

Social survey research, originating in England at the end of the 19th century, is a scientific approach with varying degrees of adaptation and acceptance across nations and societies (Bulmer 1998). The systematic elicitation of health status preferences can be considered a culture-specific process that cross-culturally is subject to acceptance issues.

More than twenty years ago, Chen and Murray (1976), based on a survey experience in Haiti, defined "a rural Third World survey...[as] the careful collection, tabulation, and analysis of wild guesses, half-truths, and outright lies meticulously recorded by gullible outsiders during interviews with suspicious, intimidated, but outwardly compliant villagers" (Chen and Murray 1976, p. 241). Twenty years of progress in cross-cultural health research have refined the discourse, though, not abolished the problems inherent in survey research, particularly in developing countries (Bulmer and Warwick 1993).

One definition of operational equivalence is whether certain methods in data collection and instrument administration are equally applicable in different cultures. Varying culture-specific norms of self-disclosure and respondent burden may affect the measurement and thus produce variation in response (Herdman et al. 1997). Another concern addresses the acceptability of methods to a particular culture under study. Of particular interest is the question of whether discrete choice instruments are acceptable in the respective culture and whether respondents are used to discrete choice responding.

Empirical evidence suggests that the mode of administration of a particular health state valuation method may affect the response. Intra-cultural as well as inter-cultural variations may be in force. In a study comparing health-related quality of life (HRQoL) assessments among US veterans, Weinberger et al. (1996) found large intra-cultural variations across methods of administration over short intervals for the SF-36. In cross-national research, country and gender differences in response styles may affect the measurement, probably reflecting educational attainment and varying ability to cope with the cognitive task of interpreting and responding to item choices (Watkins and Cheung 1995). In many cultures, acquiescence or courtesy bias may affect attitude statements (Bulmer and Warwick 1993; Javeline 1999). Knowledge and attitudinal surveys such as health valuation surveys appear to be particularly prone to a cultural reinterpretation of survey questions by respondents and thus to contextual bias (Stone and Campbell 1984).

In interviewer-administered scenarios, the relationship between interviewers and respondents in terms of social class, socioeconomic status, literacy, gender, and cultural background can have an important impact on response patterns. In male-dominated cultures, female interviewers may be unacceptable. Great social distance or discrepancy can affect the rapport or even inhibit valid responses. On the other hand, respondent-interviewer similarity, e.g. by using community members as interviewers, on the other hand, may increase the validity of responses (Chen and Murray 1976).

Eliciting health state valuations by lay persons implies they are translating subjectively experienced health states into linguistic terminologies. In other words, the value measurement task is "construed". In data collection efforts such as standardized health surveys, the central question is whether answer categories reflect the diversity of experience and the culture-specific understanding (perception) of the health state notion. Therefore, notions of self-perceived health, disability or ill-health need to be constructed in such a way as to take care of socio-linguistic norms of the sociocultural setting (Warnecke et al. 1997).

Valuation methodology

An important source of variation is due to identical descriptions of health producing different valuations (cf. Dolan and Sutton 1997). A number of investigators have reported discrepant weights for similar conditions when different measurement techniques were used. The typical pattern is that the SG yields the highest score, followed by the TTO and the RS (Nord 1992). A review by Revicki and Kaplan (1993) suggests that health status scales are poorly to moderately correlated with SG and TTO scores, and are more closely associated with RS preferences. Whether there is a "correct" method depends in the first instance on whether there are theoretical reasons for adopting a particular approach.

The approaches of utility measurement from expected utility theory, and the measurement of value by rating scales arising from psychometrics, represent rigorous systems. All of the techniques described above have been deemed feasible by some investigators for both general and patient populations. However, the method of rating scales appears simpler to administer than the tasks of SG or TTO. Krabbe et al. (1997) provide a review of the properties and practical implications of all instruments mentioned above.

Acceptability and construction of scales in cross-cultural comparison

RS methods are familiar to most people, at least in Western countries, from a variety of everyday experiences in which they are asked to provide information on an array of experiences (e.g. sporting events, movies). It is widely agreed that the cognitive burden of respondents with RS is less then with other techniques. However, empirical work has shown that people have difficulty directly assigning a number to feelings about health states (Patrick et al. 1994). Furthermore, difficulty in making absolute judgements should result in the avoidance of the extreme categories of a scale, resulting in a clustering of values that acts to reduce the range of possible responses (Streiner and Norman 1989). Other research suggests that RS provides valid and reliable results when the response continuum is made explicit to subjects (Kaplan and Ernst 1983). Richardson (1994) and Nord (1991) have challenged whether individuals' preferences using VAS report preferences that have interval scale properties.

When applying different health state valuations across various cultures, it is important to know whether questioning with scale response patterns are acceptable and known to a particular culture. Yu et al. (1993) showed great discrepancies in responses to different scales across various cultures and concluded that attitude measures such as the Likert and semantic differential scales are "culture-specific, emic instruments" which largely depend upon a subject's interpretation of the measures.

In Likert scales, the measure characteristics (number of items, number of scale points) can affect responses, as scale endpoints or midpoints may be avoided for cultural reasons or individuals choose extreme points for that same reason. In Asian cultures, for example, an even number of scale points appears more relevant than an uneven number. In semantic differential scales certain adjective pairs may be considered irrelevant by the respondent. A related issue is the number of scale points. If the choice of scale points is limited, respondents may be frustrated in trying to make fine distinctions. If there are too many response points, respondents may be equally unable to make fine distinctions.

Utility measures based on statistical or objective (aleatory) probability confront subjective or personal considerations of probability. In populations with low levels of formal education, another problem may arise from using numbers and thus translating lay knowledge, attitude and experience into a single numerical value. A quantified valuation is never a "value-free" act. It is based on lay or folk interpretations of numbers, statistics and probabilities (e.g. Adelswärd and Sachs 1996), in other words, a lay epidemiology. The question, therefore, is how far people are able to think in, and use, numbers, i.e. how far is a population's relative degree of numeracy developed? Does a population understand and accept a numerical expression of risk and uncertainty?

Types of scenarios and thinking in hypotheses

What illness scenarios and health domains the valuation instrument is composed of has an important effect on how respondents react to it. Research has shown that the type of case scenario (VAS versus category rating) has an important impact on results (Llewellyn-Thomas et al. 1984). There is, however, no agreement on the role of health profiles in the context of describing health states. The Global Burden of Disease (GBD) study only applied diagnostic labels, whereas the Dutch Study on Disability Weights has shown the importance of adding descriptions to ease the valuation task of respondents. The provision of health state descriptions is a necessity in case the respondents are lay people; whether these should be provided to health professionals should be a topic of research. Also the way these descriptions are formulated is not clear, e.g. by EuroQol profiles, or more elaborated profiles. A more conceptual question is whether these descriptions should be identical for the same health state across all countries, or whether these are allowed to vary across countries.

How the scenario is presented also has an impact (Johnson and Slovic 1995) upon response patterns. In case of SMPH methods that elaborate health scenarios, it is important to know whether the health and disease scenarios are acceptable in the culture under study. Studies suggest that inquiring about certain domains, for example, the life course (Ikels et al. 1992), may not be acceptable to every respondent. The same may hold true for questions relating to death and highly stigmatized diseases or impairments that may be considered shameful such as, for example, erectile dysfunction.

SOCIAL/ECONOMIC/DEMOGRAPHIC ATTRIBUTES OF RESPONDENTS
Type of respondent

Several authors suggest that knowledge of the condition to be evaluated can cause different valuations among different groups of respondents (Gold et al. 1996; Murray 1996). A distinction can, therefore, be made between respondents without a knowledge of the condition to be assessed (as many members of the general population tend to be), and those with a knowledge of the condition to be valued. This latter may further be broken down into those who have experienced the condition themselves or are still living in this state ("patients"); and those who have gained a knowledge of the health state through their work (professional health care providers).

If the respondent is the *patient*, the valuation will be restricted to his/her own health state. Health profiles like the SF36 or the EuroQol can be applied, as can utility measures. Many authors doubt the appropriateness of patients' responses. Various empirical studies have shown that patients and ex-patients adapt to their own health state and value this as less severe than non-patients. Furthermore, the knowledge of ex-patients and their family and friends extends to only a limited number of health states.

It is also argued that when a societal perspective is considered best for studies concerning health care resources in the public interest, the best articulation of society's preferences for particular health states should be gathered from a representative sample of fully informed members of the community. This also includes the argument that patient characteristics (age-sex distribution) do not necessarily follow that of the community. As a consequence, many authors (Gold et al. 1996) argue that patient preferences should not be used for valuing health states in the context of resource allocation decisions.

When the respondent is a *health professional*, the valuation may refer to a wide range of hypothetical health states. Health professionals have been seen as credible sources of preference scores because they have witnessed a particular condition or health state in hundreds of patients and are able to provide a considered judgement about the true long-term effect of the health state on a patient. They may be involved in the description of health profiles, as well as in valuing health states by utility measures. Gold et al. (1996), however, argue that health professionals may give too much weight to functional status and inadequately take into account more subtle and subjective influences of an illness (e.g. emotional problems, pain and discomfort) when attaching a value to a health state. In addition, health professionals do not constitute a representative cross section of the general public with regard to age, income and socioeconomic class, and therefore systematic bias may be built into these surrogate preferences. Many authors (Gold et al. 1996) find that using health professionals, then, to directly value health states is regarded as an unsatisfactory method of obtaining preferences.

If the respondent is a *community member*, the valuation may also refer to a wide range of hypothetical health states. As this involves lay people who are not knowledgeable enough to assess and classify the various physical, social and psychological domains related to a health state, they can only directly value health states based on existing health profiles. Researchers also question the appropriateness of this task. The level of understanding of the nature of particular health states by members of the general public or by others who are not experiencing the health state is not always accurate and can be heavily influenced by "cues" on how the assessment procedure is done (McNeil et al. 1982). Metaphorical non-equivalence, i.e. question and answer (non-) comprehension, can have an important effect on response patterns (Dunnigan et al. 1993).

Although efforts can be made to provide in-depth descriptions of health states, lengthy descriptions can result in cognitive overload, and the health states, even if described in detail, remain hypothetical. On the other hand, Llewellyn-Thomas et al. (1993) determined that subjects' pre-treatment ratings for the states produced by radiation for cancer did not change after they actually entered those states. This provides support for the view that people can visualize at least some specific health states relatively well. The use of community preferences coincides with the more theoretical point of view, as noted above, that the best articulation of society's preferences for particular health states should be gathered from a representative sample of fully informed members of the community.

Educational attainment

Formal education level has an important effect on an individual's ability to understand a specific value scaling task. Patrick et al. (1985), comparing health status values on a sickness-related dysfunction profile (the Sickness Impact Profile or SIP), found differences in understanding among consumer judges in Lambeth (UK) and in Seattle (USA) and hypothesized that these variations were due to educational differences. Watkins and Cheung (1995) showed that individuals with higher educational attainment are better able to cope with the cognitive task of interpreting and answering a SDQ-1 questionnaire. Cognitively demanding health valuation methods such as SG, PTO or TTO may, therefore, be difficult to employ with less educated respondents (Murray and Lopez 2000). In many developing countries with large illiterate population segments, their use among illiterate individuals would raise serious doubts about their validity and reliability.

Health status

For patient-based health status valuations it is important to consider that actual or perceived health status affects a patient's valuation. The current experience of illness has an impact on scale values (Rosser and Kind 1978). Variation was found in self-reported vision-related functional capacity in a comparative study among patients in Canada, Denmark, Spain, and the United States of America (Alonso et al. 1998). General health and vitality explained 50% of variation in Health Utility Index (HUI) scores among elderly disabled (Bartman et al. 1998).

Social and socioeconomic status

Social and socioeconomic status were found to have a significant effect on health state valuations with a EuroQol health state classification and a VAS in a study of 3 395 adults in Britain. Higher median valuations were given by lower class respondents and by respondents with intermediate and no educational qualifications (Gudex et al. 1996).

Age

The age of a respondent may contribute to variation, as older respondents may attach a higher value to health (Lau et al. 1986) or are less able to cognitively cope with the valuation procedure (Dolan and Kind 1996).

FORMATIVE RESEARCH IN BURKINA FASO

The Department of Tropical Hygiene and Public Health of Heidelberg University was, in 1999 and 2000, conceptualizing and conducting research in Burkina Faso in collaboration with the National Centre for Health Research in Nouna, Burkina Faso. Research on eliciting disability weights in Burkina Faso has a methodological character, i.e. it focuses merely on the choice of valuation instruments, rather than on the collection of weights on a comprehensive range of diseases.

Pilot research focuses on the feasibility of administering the instruments VAS, TTO, and SG, in the context of rural Burkina Faso. Respondents with a variety of disabilities were asked to value their own health state and two "marker" health states (blindness and hernia) (cf. Bakker and et al. 1994) using these instruments. The VAS was visualized by a feeling thermometer including arrows, while the SG was visualized by a probability wheel consisting of two circles (a red circle to represent probability/risk of dying, and a white circle representing probability of gaining full health) which overlap to indicate changing probabilities. Among other tools, a ranking exercise (to test consistency of responses), a two-week retest (to test reliability), and after-test interviews (to qualify the responses) were used to appraise the feasibility of the instruments.

The research led to the following first observations. Firstly, the response rates for the VAS, TTO and SG were 100%, 84% and 93%, respectively.

Second, the VAS scores of the own health state and the marker states corresponded in 73% of all exercises with the rank order of these states as expressed before by the respondent before the valuation exercises. For the TTO and SG, these figures were only 16% and 12%. Respondents also appear to rank, order, and qualify health states easily using the VAS, but tend to maintain identical proportions between the health states concerned. This questions the interval properties of the VAS in this context.

Third, the test-retest reliability of the valuation of the own health state was 0.64 for the VAS, 0.71 for the TTO and 0.70 for the SG. The relative high values of the latter two instruments might be explained by the large impact of destiny and social values on the responses which led to consequent valuations at both extremities. That is, the respondents had diffi-culties in understanding the concept of risk-taking in the SG exercise, and often related this to destiny: respondents are willing to take excessive risks or no risk at all, following their belief that their fate lies "in the hands of God". Furthermore, both in the SG and TTO, the respondent's behaviour was strongly influenced by family interests and social values. For example, in the TTO exercise, respondents were not willing to trade-off life years in case they still had family members to take care of, or were eager to trade-off life years in case they felt they were a burden on the family. These issues raise concern over the feasibility of applying SG and TTO for the purpose of valuing health state valuations in the context of rural Burkina Faso (cf. Baltussen et al. 2002).

Further research will include the valuation of hypothetical health states, involving the definition of health states of interest and framing and descriptions of these health states. The instruments will be administered to both health professionals and lay people to test variation.

Methodological strategies for investigating health state valuations and analysing determinants of variation

In light of the scarcity of formal cross-cultural comparisons, we see two major research strategies applicable to the investigation of variation in health state valuations. First, we believe that qualitative research is needed to precede and accompany quantitative research in health state valuations. Such qualitative research should aim at cross-national and cross-cultural comparisons. Second, we think it is self-evident that more quantitative research needs to be undertaken to compare health valuations formally with those from certain utility methods.

Qualitative research needs

Before deciding whether it is feasible to use standard utility measures across nations and cultures it will be crucial to conduct more in-depth qualita-tive research in a variety of cultural settings. Several scholars interested in the cross-national and cross-cultural application of SMPH have stressed the need to conduct preparatory qualitative research before developing SMPH. Qualitative research is particularly useful in elucidating and contextualizing determinants of variance in health state valuations in extremely diverse cultural settings. Such qualitative research can address a number of needs. It would complement or precede psychometric and econometric work by assisting the definition, understanding and develop-ment of conceptual domains and culturally appropriate scale items (Kessler and Mroczek 1996; Krause and Jay 1994); it would lead to contextually sensitive and culturally relevant indicators (Nazarea et al. 1998); and it would document and illuminate the large cross-cultural variability of attitudes and beliefs regarding health-related impairment and disability in a wide variety of settings.

A number of modern anthropological methods are available for this task, particularly those methods bridging qualitative and quantitative dichotomies (Bernard 1994; Trotter and Schensul 1998) and methods bridging anthropology and epidemiology (Trostle and Sommerfeld 1996). Qualitative and ethnographic research can be a valuable complement to comparative epidemiological research, as it sheds lights on the sociocultural and emotional context of health-related quality of life and the consequences of ill-health (Heggenhougen and Shore 1986; Marshall 1990). In addition, such qualitative research yields knowledge on the background of variations in health state valuations across individuals, e.g. potential sources of variation based on age, sex or income.

In addition to standard methods in qualitative research, a number of standardized qualitative research strategies would be applicable, e.g. Focused Ethnographic Study Guides (FES, cf. Gove and Pelto 1994), Rapid Anthropological Procedures (RAPs, Scrimshaw and Hurtado 1989), or Explanatory Model Interview Catalogues (Weiss 1997). Rapid Anthropological Procedures have been developed as tools for the collection of social and cultural data for policy-making. They use qualitative methods such as individual interviews, group interviews, focus group interviews, and observational techniques. Combining more standardized methods in cognitive anthropology, i.e. free listing, frame elicitation techniques, triad tests, pile sortings, ranking and ratings, could yield culture-specific notions of illness and impairment. This could be combined with multivariate data reduction techniques such as Multidimensional Scaling Analysis (MDS, Shepard et al. 1972) to represent how populations collectively perceive and value hypothesized disease states. Consensus panel discussions and Delphi methods can be used to assess community consensus around health states.

Qualitative research should not be limited, however, to preparatory or formative research. Such research could be a legitimate complement to SMPH research and its inherent "objectivist" epistemology (Kleinman 1994). Also, qualitative research does not need to be limited to producing only locally relevant information. Well-designed, qualitative research with similar questions and standardized instruments could yield important comparative data and thus contribute to comparative quantitative research. Effective comparative cross-cultural ethnographies on health values and the effect of values on valuations could thus remedy some of the methodological limitations of purely numerical SMPH-research, particularly in developing countries.

Advancing quantitative cross-national research

It is obvious that *well-designed* and rigorous quantitative cross-national research (Jowell 1998) needs to be advanced both in cross-cultural psychiatry (Kagitcibasi and Berry 1989) as well as in cross-cultural anthropology (Browner et al. 1988). Cross-cultural research should not be limited to overly similar societal settings, comparing, for example, neighbouring European countries or certain population groups in the United States, but should include heterogeneous cultures and population groups. A number of useful frameworks for structuring such cross-cultural research in the area have recently been published (e.g. McDaniels and Gregory 1991; Ostroot and Snyder 1985). In recent years, WHO-led research on cross-cultural applicability of SMPH has made important contributions to the methodology literature (e.g. Power et al. 1999).

IDENTIFICATION OF POTENTIAL DOMAINS OF FURTHER INQUIRY

In this section we outline some of the domains of inquiry that could be of further interest when investigating variation in health state valuations according to both methodological alternatives suggested above.

CROSS-CULTURAL VARIATION IN PERCEIVING AND INTERPRETING HEALTH, ILLNESS AND COPING WITH ILLNESS-RELATED DISABILITY

Health social scientists such as medical anthropologists, medical sociologists and health psychologists concerned with the social and cultural ramifications of illness and health from a cross-cultural perspective have dealt extensively with the cultural variation in the interpretation and experience of illness, and the social coping mechanisms around disease-related impairment. The field is so large and its different schools of thought so diverse, that it does not appear to be a worthwhile endeavour, in the context of this paper, to aim at a comprehensive review of the vast literature in these fields. However, for the purpose of identifying potential sources of variation in health state valuations and elaborating on potential methodological strategies, we are focusing on four major areas of cross-cultural variation that could trigger specific research:

a. variation in social, cultural and health values;

b. variation in the perception of illness and health risks;

c. variation in expectations of social consequences of illness; and

d. variation in concepts and notions of time.[4]

SOCIAL, CULTURAL AND HEALTH VALUES

A number of authors have aimed at investigating whether there are universal values (e.g. Schwartz 1994; Schwartz and Sagiv 1995) and how much cross-cultural diversity there is in human values, for example, work-related values (Hofstede 1980; 1998). Whereas universal value *types*, e.g. values of human life, good health, peace of mind and the importance of knowledge, do appear to exist (Bell 1994; Frenkel and Meller 1987), nations and cultures show considerable differences in value *patterns* (Schwartz 1994). In addition, social values are not stable. Their classification and rankings may change over time as a result of external changes (Fernandez et al. 1997).

The valuation of a (hypothetical) health state is shaped by individual values and attitudes towards health in general and his or her own health state in particular. To use Rokeach's (1968) well-known terminology on values,[5] health state valuations make reference to evaluative beliefs. These values may either reflect exclusively individual preferences or culture- or society-specific notions of good or ideal health.

Regarding its connotative dimensions, health appears to have a universally strong positive value (Chamberlain 1985; Diaz-Guerrero 1984; Frenkel and Meller 1987). However, in its indicative dimensions, health and its domains may be differently patterned or organized (e.g. Bice and Kalimo 1971; Pezza 1991). In other words, what meaning health has is highly culture-bound and what domains the construct, consequently, needs to be composed of (Patrick et al. 1973) requires cultural consideration. The cross-cultural variance in conceptualizing health and health states is, therefore, a serious threat to conceptual (or cultural) equivalence (Eyton and Neuwirth 1984). Recently published research from the WHOQoL group showed several basic facets of physical health, for example mobility, pain and discomfort, and work capacity, to be universally similar aspects of the quality of life concept. The authors interpret this as an indication of health being a universal domain of quality of life (Power et al. 1999). The authors, however, explicitly state that "this finding does not imply that quality of life *evaluations* are the same across cultures." (original authors' emphasis). In addition, the authors developed their instrument, the WHOQoL-100 quality of life assessment tool, by condensing an original global pool of 1 800 items to finally 100 items. A lot of cultural variation in health-related quality of life values will have been leveled out by this approach. For example, one of the cornerstones of health-related quality of life, cultural and social values attached to fertility, is known to vary tremendously across cultures and societies (cf. Snow 1997).

PERCEPTIONS OF ILLNESS AND RISK

Medical anthropological research has provided substantial empirical evidence about the variability of illness concepts[6] within and across human populations (e.g. Murdock 1980; Boster and Weller 1990; Weller 1984; Weller et al. 1993; Yoder 1991). Illness concepts or representations are constructs that, to a large extent, shape an individual's coping mechanisms, i.e. illness behaviour (Petrie and Weinman 1997). Research in a large variety of settings worldwide suggests that many biomedically defined diseases have no or only diffuse equivalents in local illness terminologies and taxonomies. Particularly in "traditional" societies, it is to be expected that biomedical sickness scenarios incorporated in health valuation instruments will be interpreted through the cultural lens of local illness concepts as well as previous illness experience. The recognition and perception of danger signs and symptoms (Bartman et al. 1998; Bletzer 1993) predicts treatment choice in a number of illnesses (Yoder and Hornik 1994; 1996). It can be hypothesized that underlying or assumed folk etiologic theories, i.e. lay attributions of causes of ill health to social or metaphysical origins, can affect the valuation of hypothetical health states. While holding spiritual-social explanations in many cultures depends on educational status (Edman and Kameoka 1997), further research would be needed to elaborate on how much of the variation in health state valuation is due to different underlying etiological theories. Health perception research (Petrie and Weinman 1997) has the potential to fertilize research on health state valuation. Both fields are interested in how patients evaluate actual or hypothetical health threats by constructing illness representations and thus develop coping strategies.

Health state valuations are built upon Western notions of risk and probability which may not be fully shared by respondents. Cross-cultural risk research looks at the variability of notions of risk and uncertainty within and across cultures and time (Babrow et al. 1998; Bontempo et al. 1997; Dake 1991; Dake and Wildavsky 1993; Douglas 1992; Krimsky and Golding 1992). Cultural anthropologists consider risk perception and risk behaviour as socially and culturally constructed in the sense of subjective or perceived risk, not merely as an objectively measurable phenomenon (Douglas 1992). The perception and assessment of risk is seen as a social process determined by specific cultural norms and values of a local community. Norms and values, grounded in the community's relationship towards its physical and social environment, guide the social construction of reality. Both influence the perception and assessment of what is considered dangerous or not and reflect cultural knowledge.

In cultures where beliefs in a human's predetermined fate or God's will are strong, risks can be seen as purely categorical, as interviewees will assume either a complete (100%) "risk" or no (0%) "risk". A related issue is an individual's perceived locus of control (Coreil and Marshall 1982; Wrightson and Wardle 1997) which may affect a health state valuation. More cross-culturally relevant research would be needed to assess the relative impact of perception of uncertainty and locus of control convictions on health state valuations.

EXPECTED AND HYPOTHESIZED SOCIAL CONSEQUENCES OF SICKNESS

Although disease and disability is a "human constant", the effects of disease and disability are highly variable across cultures (Scheer and Groce 1988). A society's understanding of disability or impairment due to illness and attitudes towards disabled persons are largely shaped by social and cultural values (Lane et al. 1993). Variation in health perception makes self-perceived morbidity surveys in developing countries highly problematic (Murray and Chen 1994).

Known, expected, and assumed ("hypothesized") social and economic consequences of an illness may have an important impact on an individual's health state valuation. Impairment, in certain cultures, may thus not be interpreted in (cost) utility terms, i.e. in terms of loss of working ability or time loss, but rather as a chronic or permanent loss of a person's ability to participate in community or household discourse and activity (e.g. Marshall 1996). When a disease is known to inflict social stigma, to disrupt social life, or results in the patient being a burden to his social environment, a disease state may be evaluated according to the societal and cultural consequences that the disease is believed to have. Consequently, the international nomenclature, standardized in the International Classification of Disease (ICD) or the International Classification of Impairment, Disabilities, and Handicaps (ICIDH), may not be able to capture the whole range of culture and society-specific coping mechanisms.

Concepts of time

The TTO presents the respondent with the task of determining what amount of time they would be willing to give up to be in a better versus poorer health state (Torrance et al. 1972). Concepts of time, however, are socioculturally constructed and vary widely across societies and cultures (Frankenburg 1992; Lash et al. 1998; Eickelman 1977). The Western concept of time as neutral, abstract and decontextualized emerged in industrializing Europe in the 19th and 20th centuries (Adam 1998; Goldman 1982). Neo-classical time-stream discounting has, therefore, been criticized in its assumptions as a cross-culturally valid method for the evaluation of social programmes (Hayden 1980). To our knowledge, there are no cross-cultural analyses of concepts of time and time preference with respect to an individual's health discounting.

Review of key hypotheses

In conclusion, several hypotheses have emerged and new hypotheses are emerging. First, cross-national research has addressed the question of whether psychometric instruments can be translated and adapted to other cultures. Whereas this adaptation process has been shown to be feasible for health profiles and certain disease-specific health state instruments as well as certain country clusters, there is a scarcity of evidence as to whether these instruments can be made applicable across culturally very heterogeneous societies or population subgroups. As stated earlier, successful adaptation precedes cross-cultural comparison. The evidence, therefore, cannot prove or refute the hypothesis of cross-cultural comparability or equivalence. As of now, the applicability of health state valuation methods such as RS, TTO or WTP has not been proven for developing country situations, particularly in population subgroups with little or no formal educational attainment.

Second, very few studies have compared SMPH across cultures and nations with a rigid quantitative methodology. This type of study hypothesizes that there may be universality in health status preferences. The little evidence available indicates that there is variance in health status rankings across nations and countries. The variation is still largely unexplained though a number of possible explanations emerge. Cross-cultural psychology and anthropology suggest that values about ill-health are created within culture-specific systems of meaning. As the valuation is the outcome of that cognitive, linguistic and emotional endeavour, researchers have hypothesized that variation is largely due to cultural differences in meaning systems. The qualitative evidence for this is large but needs to be substantiated by rigid comparative methodologies.

Third, some researchers have hypothesized that the disabilities resulting from certain health states described in the official nomenclature, e.g. the International Classification of Disease (ICD) or the International Classification of Impairment, Disabilities, and Handicaps (ICIDH), may not count as impairment in all cultures and that culture-specific manifestations of disablement are not reflected in the official nomenclature for disease and disability.

POLICY RELEVANCE

The above discussion suggests that the determinants of variation in health state valuations are not yet fully understood. Is there, as a consequence of different social and cultural value systems, a lack of universality in disability weights? Do these variations reflect an insufficient body of knowledge produced by, at times, "biased" research? A recent critical commentary argued that "health is so influenced by culture and economic differences that agreement on universal disability weights may prove impossible" (James and Foster 1999). The GBD study, however, warrants "that choices should be acceptable to as many people of as many different cultures as possible" (GBD summary, p. 8). It is still unclear whether and how such high level of global and cross-culturally valid acceptance can be produced through health state valuations.

In our opinion, more research is needed to support or refute this approach. In-depth qualitative research needs to accompany more and better structured cross-cultural comparisons. Such comparisons should go beyond comparing valuations by special subgroups such as health professionals, patient groups or population groups with higher levels of educational attainment or urban residency. If cultural representativeness is the goal, individuals from a large variety of population subgroups need to be included in national health valuation efforts. Excluding the general population means that their respective priorities are neglected.

Burden of disease assessments or cost-effectiveness studies as a tool for priority setting are not a value or end in itself but are only useful in as much as they are accepted and used by decision-makers. Value-laden measurements, however, tend to be received with scepticism, as seemingly objective numbers contain social preferences that are not based in the culture where the measure is to be a meaningful yardstick for policy-making. The use of data in general and research data in particular for policy-making is very precarious and there is very little hard evidence of proper use at all (Sauerborn et al. 1999). Those who provide data to decision-makers are, therefore, well advised to make sure that any cultural-bound assumptions (on health status and its valuation, and time and age preferences) are those of the population to whom the policy measures are finally attended to be applied. Studies are currently underway in rural Burkina Faso comparing the acceptance by policy makers at district and national level of "standard DALYs" with DALYs based on community data on health status preferences, time preference and age preference (cf. Sauerborn et al. 1996).

The acceptance and relevance of DALYs and other SMPH based on generic preferences may be particularly limited in regional and district settings. Making preferences local potentially increases the use of DALYs as one priority setting instrument (Sauerborn et al. 1998). Barker and Green (1996) argued that utility measures such as DALYs are valid only in specific cultural contexts and that they should be locally developed. To optimize the allocation of scarce health care resources at the district level there is a clear need for locally meaningful health state valuations adequately reflecting cultural beliefs and societal norms. DALYs could then be calculated incorporating community-based data on perceived and revealed disability and age and time preferences. This is not a plea for complete cultural relativity. However, the instruments should be such that they produce valid data and the valuations should be complemented or validated by qualitative research.

The question remains about which of the hypothesized determinants of variation should be respected when defining health policy and which determinants can possibly be neglected. This makes the issue of determinants of variation in health state valuation critical to SMPH-led makers of health policy. Variation due to methodological flaws in the design of cross-culturally comparative research obviously distorts policy-making and should be clearly avoided. Variation due to social/economic and demographic attributes of respondents, i.e. intra-cultural variation, should be interpreted with caution. Although allocative efficiency suggests that this variation should be respected to optimize health gains, equity concerns dictate a more careful consideration. That is, the direct translation of these preferences in health policy may lead to unwanted distributional effects, e.g. differences in health state valuations between male and female respondents would result in similar differences in the allocation of resources. Variations due to cross-cultural variation in perceiving and interpreting health, illness and coping with illness-related disability, should be respected in the definition of national health policies. Together with epidemiological variations, these variations in health state valuations constitute the sole determinant for optimal resource allocation. However, cross-cultural variations among countries, for equity reasons, will likely not be translated into health policy.

NOTES

1 Health state valuation instruments may aim to capture important health domains in one specific disease (disease-specific measures) or all health domains across a full range of diseases (generic measures). Only the latter category is considered relevant in this context as the nature of DALYs requires that disability weights are comparable across a full range of diseases. Generic measures can be subdivided into utility measures and health profiles. Among utility measures, the standard gamble (SG), the time trade-off (TTO) and the rating scale (RS) have been most often used. SG, TTO and RS are methods to measure preferences for health states on a scale from 0 (death) to 1 (full health). The standard gamble approach has been widely used to measure health state preferences (Torrance 1986). The SG is the classic method of eliciting utilities and is based directly on the axioms of the expected utility theory of von Neumann and Morgenstern. The technique asks the respondent to consider a hypothetical choice between the certainty of continued life in the health state of interest and a gamble between varying probabilities of death and full health. There is significant disagreement with respect to the feasibility of collecting preference weights using the standard gamble. Investigators favouring the approach have argued that when the standard gamble is collected properly, with appropriately designed visual aids and measurement props, it is feasible in general and patient populations (Torrance 1986). Others have found the approach cognitively demanding for patients and argue that the method is unnatural for many people who are unused to formulating their preferences in terms of gambles. The difficulty with the task is held by some to reduce the validity of the approach. Health profiles classify health states of individuals on the basis of their self-reported characteristics in various health domains in a comprehensive classification scheme (Torrance 1986). Well-known instruments are the SF-36, the Disability/Distress Index (DDI), the Health Utilities Index (HUI), the Quality of Well-Being Scale (QWBS), the 15-D Measure of Health Related Quality of Life, and the Quality of Life and Health Questionnaire. There is, however, little experience of using health profiles in developing countries (Shumaker and Berzon 1995). All generic measures include some combination of health perceptions—of physical, social, and psychological function and of impairment. A scoring system permits aggregation of information collected into an index score. The score of a health profile is an index that is sometimes a weighted aggregation of its specific domains. Health profile indexes are essentially arbitrary and lack the interval scale properties required to support resource allocation decisions (this requires that a change in health state weight from 0.1 to 0.2 should be equivalent to a change from 0.7 to 0.8). Although they are basically descriptive, health profiles can also be regarded as utility instruments in case the combinations of scores on all domains are valued by utility measures. Such an approach has been applied to the QWBS, HUI, DDI and the EuroQoL.

2 Instead of restricting our reflections to econometric or psychometric considerations for reducing sources of bias in assessing health valuations among diverse populations, in this paper, we are using rather wide conceptualizations of valuation and variation. By valuation we understand an appraisal or estimation of something in respect to excellence or merit. By variance or variation we mean the difference or divergence between individuals, population groups, societies,

and cultures in terms of their health-related values. Such variation can be either intra-cultural or intra-societal, addressing variation across different social strata or otherwise characterized population groups (e.g. Au 1997) or cross-cultural and cross-national in scope and origin.

3   A reasonable degree of cross-cultural equivalence was found for the Oral Health Impact Profile (OHIP; Allison et al. 1999). For the Nottingham Health Profile (NHP), little intercultural or interlinguistic variation was found comparing Britain and France (Bucquet et al. 1990). However, an earlier paper reported problems when translating the NHP into Arabic and Spanish (Hunt 1986). The Social Readjustment Rating questionnaire and the Cornell Medical Index were not useful among Vietnamese refugees in the United States (Eyton and Neuwirth 1984). However, the Chinese Values instrument was useful among University students in 22 countries (The Chinese Culture Connection 1987). A feasibility study of EuroQol in Japan (Hisashige et al. 1998) indicated to the authors a high degree of cross-national and cross-cultural applicability.

4   Compared to the literature reviewed in section 2, this more anthropological cluster of evidence and research is based on a different epistemological position and research paradigm. Cross-cultural and cross-national psycho- and econometrics imply an interest in discovering similarities in perceptions and attitudes, whereas most theory in anthropology focuses on difference and diversity rather than similarity. A more detailed discussion, not to speak of a reconciliation, of these different epistemologies and research paradigms is beyond the scope of this paper (see Kleinman 1994).

5   Rokeach (1969 p. 2) defines beliefs as "inferences made by an observer about underlying states of expectancy" and an attitude as "a relatively enduring organization of beliefs around an object or situation predisposing one to respond in some preferential manner," in other words a cluster or organization of underlying beliefs (cognitions, expectancies, or hypotheses)" (1969 p. 112). He differentiates between descriptive or existential beliefs (of the type "I believe that the sun rises in the east"), evaluative beliefs ("I believe this ice cream is good"), and prescriptive or exhortatory belief (of the type "I believe it is desirable that children should obey their parents").

6   Concepts of illness and disease concepts are determined by three related processes: a) signification, i.e. ideas, notions, concepts or properties implied by a term or expression, b) denotation, events, states and objects selected out and pointed to by virtue of what is signified by a term or expression, and c) connotation, non-criterial attributes, extrinsic aspects and secondary associations that sometimes accompany a form of suffering (Shweder 1991).

REFERENCES

Adam B (1998) Values in the cultural timescapes of science. *Cultural Values*, 2(2-3):385–402.

Adelswärd V, Sachs L (1996) The meaning of 6.8: numeracy and normality in health information talks. *Social Science and Medicine*, 43(8):1179–1187.

Allison P, Locker D, Jokovic A, Slade G (1999) A cross-cultural study of oral health values. *Journal of Dental Research*, 78(2):643–649.

Alonso J, Black C, Norregaard JC, et al. (1998) Cross-cultural differences in the reporting of global functional capacity: an example in cataract patients. *Medical Care*, 36(6):868–878.

Au K (1997) Another consequence of culture: intra-cultural variation. *The International Journal of Human Resource Management*, 8(5):743–755.

Babrow AS, Kasch CR, Ford LA (1998) The many meanings of uncertainty in illness: toward a systematic accounting. *Health Communication*, 10(1):1–23.

Bakker C, Rutten M, van Doorslaer E, Bennett K, van der Linden S (1994) Feasibility of utility assessment by rating scale and standard gamble in patients with ankylosing spondylitis or fibromyalgia. *Journal of Rheumatology*, 21(2):269–274.

Baltussen RMPM, Sanon M, Sommerfeld J, Würthwein R (2002) Obtaining disability weights in rural Burkina Faso using culturally adapted visual analogue scale. *Health Economics*, 11(2):155–163.

Barker C, Green A (1996) Opening the debate on DALYs. *Health Policy and Planning*, 11(2):179–183.

Bartman BA, Rosen MJ, Bradham DD, Weissman J, Hochberg J, Revicki DA (1998) Relationship between health status and utility measures in older claudicants. *Quality of Life Research*, 7(1):67–73.

Beckerman W, Pasek J (1997) Plural values and environmental valuation. *Environmental Values*, 6(1):65–86.

Bell W (1994) The world as a moral community. *Society*, 315:17–22.

Bernard BR (1994) *Research methods in anthropology: qualitative and quantitative approaches*. Alta Mira Press, Walnut Creek, CA.

Bice TW, Kalimo E (1971) Comparisons of health-related attitudes – a cross-national factor analytic study. *Social Science and Medicine*, 5:283–318.

Bletzer KV (1993) Perceived severity: do they experience illness severity as we conceive it? *Human Organization*, 52(1):68–75.

Bontempo RN, Bottom WP, Weber EU (1997) Cross-cultural differences in risk perception: a model-based approach. *Risk Analysis*, 17(4):479–488.

Boster JS, Weller SC (1990) Cognitive and contextual variation in hot-cold classification. *American Anthropologist*, 92:171–179.

Browner CH, de Montellano O, Bernard R, Rubel A (1988) A methodology for cross-cultural ethnomedical research. *Current Anthropology*, 29(5):681–689.

Bucquet D, Condon S, Ritchie K (1990) The French version of the Nottingham health profile. A comparison of items weights with those of the source version. *Social Science and Medicine*, 30(7):829–835.

Bulmer M (1998) Introduction: the problem of exporting social survey research. *American Behavioral Scientist*, 42(2):153–167.

Bulmer M, Warwick DP (1993) *Social research in developing countries: surveys and censuses in the third world*. UCL Press Limited, London.

Chamberlain K (1985) Value dimensions, cultural differences and the prediction of perceived quality of life. *Social Indicators Research,* **17**(4):345–401.

Chen KH, Murray GF (1976) Truths and untruths in village Haiti: an experiment in third world survey research. In: *Culture, natality and family planning.* Marshall JF, Polgar S, eds. University of North Carolina at Chapel Hill, Carolina Population Center, Chapel Hill, NC.

Coreil J, Marshall PA (1982) Locus of illness control: a cross-cultural study. *Human Organization,* **41**(2):131–138.

Cramer JA, Perrine K, Devinsky O, Bryant-Comstock L, Meador K, Hermann B (1998) Development and cross-cultural translations of a 31-item quality of life in epilepsy inventory. *Epilepsia,* **39**(1):81–88.

Dake K (1991) Orienting dispositions in the perception of risk: an analysis of contemporary worldviews and cultural biases. *Journal of Cross-Cultural Psychology,* **22**(1):61–82.

Dake K, Wildavsky A (1993) Theories of risk perception: who fears what and why? *Daedalus,* **119**(4):41–60.

de Tiedra AG, Mercadal J, Badia X, Mascarao JM, Lozano R (1998) A method to select an instrument for measurement of HR-QoL for cross-cultural adaptation applied to dermatology. *PharmacoEconomics,* **14**(4):405–422.

Devlin N, Williams A (1999) Valuing quality of life: results for New Zealand health professionals. *New Zealand Medical Journal,* **12**(112):68–71.

Dolan P, Green C (1998) Using the person trade-off approach to examine differences between individual and social values. *Health Economics,* **7**(4):307–312.

Dolan P, Kind P (1996) Inconsistency and health state valuations. *Social Science and Medicine,* **42**(4):609–615.

Dolan P, Sutton M (1997) Mapping visual analogue scale health state valuations onto standard gamble and time trade-off values. *Social Science and Medicine,* **44**(10):1519–1530.

Douglas M (1985) *Risk acceptability according to the social sciences.* Russel Sage Foundation, New York.

Douglas M (1992) Risk and blame. In: *Risk and blame: essays in cultural theory.* Douglas M, ed. Routledge, London.

Doward LC, McKenna SP, Kohlmann T, et al. (1998) The international development of the RGHQoL: a quality of life measure for recurrent genital herpes. *Quality of Life Research,* **7**(2):143–153.

Drake LA, Patrick DL, Fleckman P, et al. (1999) The impact of onychomycosis on quality of life: development of an international onychomycosis-specific questionnaire to measure patient quality of life. *Journal of the American Academy of Dermatology,* **41**(2 Pt. 1):189–196.

Dunlap RE (1998) Lay perceptions of global risk: views of global warming in cross-national context. *International Sociology,* **13**(4):473–498.

Dunnigan T, McNall M, Mortimer JT (1993) The problem of metaphorical nonequivalence in cross-cultural survey research: comparing the mental health statuses of Hmong refugee and general population adolescents. *Journal of Cross-Cultural Psychology*, 24(3):344–365.

Edman JL, Kameoka VA (1997) Cultural differences in illness schemas: an analysis of Filipino and American illness attributions. *Journal of Cross-Cultural Psychology*, 28(3):252–265.

Eickelman DF (1977) Time in a complex society: a Moroccan example. *Ethnology*, 16(1):39–55.

Eyton J, Neuwirth G (1984) Cross-cultural validity: ethnocentrism in health studies with special reference to the Vietnamese. *Social Science and Medicine*, 18(5):447–453.

Fernandez DR, Carlson DS, Stepina LP, Nicholson JJ (1997) Hofstede's country classfication 25 years later. *Journal of Social Psychology*, 137(1):43–54.

Field MJ, Gold MR, eds. (1998) *Summarizing population health: directions for the development and application of population metrics*. National Academy Press, Washington, DC.

Fox-Rushby J, Parker M (1995) Culture and the measurement of health-related quality of life. *Revue Européenne de Psychologie Appliquée*, 45(4):257–263.

Frankenburg R (1992) *Time, health and medicine*. Sage Publications, Newbury Park, CA.

Frenkel E, Meller Y (1987) Preferences for domains associated with quality of life. *Journal of International and Comparative Social Welfare*, 3(1-2):21–29.

Gold MR, Siegel JE, Russel LB, Weinstein MC, eds. (1996) *Cost-effectiveness in health and medicine*. Oxford University Press, New York.

Goldman SL (1982) Modern science and western culture: the issue of time. *History of European Ideas*, 3(4):371–401.

Gove S, Pelto GH (1994) Focused ethnographic studies in the WHO programme for the control of acute respiratory infections. *Medical Anthropology*, 15(4):409–424.

Groce NE (1999) Disability in cross-cultural perspective: rethinking disability. *Lancet*, 354(9180):756–757.

Gudex C, Dolan P, Kind P, Williams A (1996) Health state valuations from the general public, using the visual analogue scale. *Quality of Life Research*, 5(6):521–531.

Guillemin F, Bombardier C, Beaton D (1993) Cross-cultural adaptation of health related quality of life measures: literature review and proposed guidelines. *Journal of Clinical Epidemiology*, 46(12):1417–1432.

Gureje O, Simon GE, Üstün TB, Goldberg D (1997) Somatization in cross-cultural perspective: A World Health Organization study in primary care. *American Journal of Psychiatry*, 154(7):989–995.

Haddad S, Fournier P, Potvin L (1998) Measuring lay people's perceptions of quality of primary health care services in developing countries. Validation of a 20-item scale. *International Journal of Quality of Health Care*, 10(2):93–104.

Hayden FG (1980) A critical analysis of time stream discounting for social program evaluation. *Social Science Journal,* **17**(1):21–40.

Heggenhougen HK, Shore L (1986) Cultural components of behavioural epidemiology: implications for primary health care. *Social Science and Medicine,* **22**:1235–1245.

Henrich J, Boyd R (1998) The evolution of conformist transmission and the emergence of between-group differences. *Evolution and Human Behavior,* **19**(4):215–241.

Herdman M, Fox-Rushby J, Badia X (1997) "Equivalence" and the translation and adaptation of health-related quality of life questionnaires. *Quality of Life Research,* **6**(3):237–247.

Herdman M, Fox-Rushby J, Badia X (1998) A model of equivalence in the cultural adaptation of HRQoL instruments: the universalist approach. *Quality of Life Research,* **7**(4):323–335.

Hisashige A, Mikasa H, Katayama T (1998) Description and valuation of health related quality of life among the general public in Japan by the EuroQoL. *Journal of Medical Investigation,* **45**(1-4):123–129.

Hofstede G (1980) *Culture's consequences: international differences in work-related values.* Sage Publications, Beverly Hills, CA.

Hofstede G (1998) A case comparing apples with oranges: international differences in values. *International Journal of Comparative Sociology,* **39**(1):16–31.

Hunt SM (1986) Cross-cultural issues in the use of socio-medical indicators. *Health Policy,* **6**(2):149–158.

Hunt SM (1988) Subjective health indicators and health promotion. *Health Promotion,* **3**(1):23–34.

Hunt SM, Alonso J, Bucquet D, Niero M, Wiklund I, McKenna SP (1991) Cross-cultural adaptation of health measures: European group for health management and quality of life assessment. *Health Policy,* **19**(1):33–44.

Hunt SM, McEwen J (1980) The development of a subjective health indicator. *Sociology of Health and Illness,* **2**(3):231–246.

Ikels C, Keith J, Dickerson-Putman J, et al. (1992) Perceptions of the adult life course: a cross-cultural analysis. *Ageing and Society,* **12**(1):49–84.

James KC, Foster SD (1999) Weighing up disability. (Editorial). *Lancet,* **354**(9173):87–88.

Javeline D (1999) Response effects in polite cultures: a test of acquiescence in Kazakhstan. *Public Opinion Quarterly,* **63**(1):1–28.

Johnson BB, Slovic P (1995) Presenting uncertainty in health risk assessment: initial studies of its effects on risk perception and trust. *Risk Analysis,* **15**(4):485–494.

Jowell R (1998) How comparative is comparative research? *American Behavioral Scientist,* **42**(2):168–177.

Kagitcibasi C, Berry JW (1989) Cross-cultural psychology: current research and trends. *Annual Review of Psychology,* **40**:493–531.

Kaplan RM, Ernst JA (1983) Do category rating scales produce biased preferences weights for a health index. *Medical Care,* 21(2):193–207.

Keller SD, Ware JE, Gandek B (1998) Testing the equivalence of translations of widely used response choice labels: results from the IQOLA project, International Quality of Life Assessment. *Journal of Clinical Epidemiology,* 51(11):933–944.

Kessler RC (1999) The World Health Organization international consortium in psychiatric epidemiology (ICPE): initial work and future directions. *Acta Psychiatrica Scandinavica,* 99(1):2–9.

Kessler RC, Mroczek DK (1996) Some methodological issues in the development of quality of life measures for the evaluation of medical interventions. *Journal of Evaluation in Clinical Practice,* 2(3):181–191.

Kleinman A (1994) An anthropological perspective on objectivity: observation, categorization, and the assessment of suffering. In: *Health and social change in international perspective.* Chen LC, Kleinman A, Ware NC, eds. Harvard University Press, Boston, MA.

Klose T (1999) The contingent valuation method in health care. *Health Policy,* 47(2):97–123.

Krabbe PFM, Essink-Bot ML, Bonsel GJ (1997) The comparability and reliability of five health-state valuation methods. *Social Science and Medicine,* 45(11):1641–1652.

Krause NM, Jay GM (1994) What do global self-rated health items measure? *Medical Care,* 32(9):930–942.

Krimsky S, Golding D (1992) *Social theories of risk.* Praeger, Westport, CT.

Landrine H, Klonoff EA (1992) Culture and health-related schemas: a review and proposal for interdisciplinary integration. *Health Psychology,* 11(4):267–276.

Lane SD, Mikhail BI, Reizian A, Courtright P, Marx R, Dawson CR (1993) Sociocultural aspects of blindness in an Egyptian delta hamlet: visual impairment vs. visual disability. *Medical Anthropology,* 15(3):245–260.

Lau RR, Hartman KA, Ware JE (1986) Health as a value: methodological and theoretical considerations. *Health Psychology,* 5(1):25–43.

Lent L, Hahn E, Eremenco S, Webster K, Cella D (1999) Using cross-cultural input to adapt the functional assessment of chronic illness therapy (FACIT) scales. *Acta Oncologica,* 38(6):695–702.

Llewellyn-Thomas H, Sutherland HJ, Tibshirani R, Ciampi A, Till JE, Boyd NF (1984) Describing health states: methodologic issues in obtaining values for health states. *Medical Care,* 22(6):543–552.

Marshall M (1996) Problematizing impairment: cultural competence in the Carolines. *Ethnology,* 35(4):249–263.

Marshall PA (1990) Cultural influences on perceived quality of life. *Seminars in Oncology Nursing,* 6(4):278–284.

McDaniels TL, Gregory RS (1991) A framework for structuring cross-cultural research in risk and decision-making. *Journal of Cross-Cultural Psychology,* 22(1):103–128.

McNeil BJ, Pauker SG, Sox HC, Tversky A (1982) On the elicitation of preferences for alternative therapies. *New England Journal of Medicine*, 306(21):1259–1262.

Mendeloff JM, Kaplan RM (1989) Are large differences in "lifesaving" costs justified? A psychometric study of the relative value placed on preventing deaths. *Risk Analysis*, 9(3):349–363.

Murray CJL (1996) Rethinking DALYs. In: *The global burden of disease: a comprehensive assessment of mortality and disability from diseases, injuries, and risk factors in 1990 and projected to 2020*. The Global Burden of Disease and Injury, Vol. 1. Murray CJL, Lopez AD, eds. Harvard School of Public Health on behalf of WHO, Cambridge, MA.

Murray CJL, Lopez AD, eds. (1996) *The global burden of disease: a comprehensive assessment of mortality and disability from diseases, injuries and risk factors in 1990 and projected to 2020*. Global Burden of Disease and Injury, Vol. 1. Harvard School of Public Health on behalf of WHO, Cambridge, MA.

Murray CJL, Lopez AD (2000) Progress and directions in refining the global burden of disease approach: a response to Williams. *Health Economics*, 9(1):69–82.

Nazarea V, Rhoades RE, Bontoyan E, Flora G (1998) Defining indicators which make sense to local people: intra cultural variation in perceptions of natural resources. *Human Organization*, 57(2):159–170.

Nord E (1992) Methods for quality adjustment of life years. *Social Science and Medicine*, 34(5):559–569.

Ostroot NM, Snyder WW (1985) Measuring cultural bias in a cross-national study. *Social Indicators Research*, 17 (3):243–251.

Patrick DL, Bush JW, Chen MM (1973) Toward an operational definition of health. *Journal of Health and Social Behavior*, 14(1):6–23.

Patrick DL, Martin ML, Bushnell DM, Marquis P, Andrejasick CM, Buesching DP (1999) Cultural adaptation of a quality-of-life measure for urinary incontinence. *European Urology*, 36(5):427–435.

Patrick DL, Sittampalam Y, Somerville SM, Carter WB, Bergner M (1985) A cross-cultural comparison of health status values. *American Journal of Public Health*, 75(12):1402–1407.

Patrick DL, Starks HE, Cain KC, Uhlmann RF, Pearlman RA (1994) Measuring preferences for health states worse than death. *Medical Decision Making*, 14(1):9–18.

Perneger TV, Leplege A, Etter JF (1999) Cross-cultural adaptation of a psychometric instrument: two methods compared. *Journal of Clinical Epidemiology*, 52(11):1037–1046.

Petrie KJ, Weinman JA (1997) *Perceptions of health and illness: current research and applications*. Harwood Academic Publishers, Amsterdam.

Pezza PE (1991) Value concept and value change theory in health education: a conceptual empirical methodological review. *Health Values*, 15(4):3–12.

Power M, Harper A, Bullinger M, WHOQOL Group (1999) The World Health Organization WHOQOL-100: tests of the universality of quality of life in 15 different cultural groups worldwide. *Health Psychology,* 18(5):495–505.

Rokeach M (1968) *Beliefs, attitudes and values: a theory of organization and change.* Jossey-Bass, San Francisco, CA.

Room R, Janca A, Bennett LA, Schmidt L, Sartorius N (1996) WHO cross-cultural applicability research on diagnosis and assessment of substance use disorders: an overview of methods and selected results. *Addiction,* 91(2):199–220.

Rosser R, Kind P (1978) A scale of valuations of states of illness: is there a social consensus? *International Journal of Epidemiology,* 7(4):347–358.

Sandermann S, Dech H, Othieno CJ, Kathuki DM, Ndetei DM (1996) NOK-African Depression scale: the development of a culture-specific symptom scale to measure depression. *Curare,* 19(2):283–293.

Sauerborn R, Berman P, Nougtara A (1996) Age bias, but not gender bias, in the intra-household resource allocation for health care in rural Burkina Faso. *Health Transition Review,* 6(2):131–145.

Sauerborn R, Nittayaramphong S, Gerhardus A (1999) Strategies to enhance the use of health systems research for health sector reform. *Tropical Hygiene and International Health,* 4(12):827–835.

Sauerborn R, Schmidt CM, Baltussen R, et al. (1998) *Towards community-based assessment of the burden of illness.* (Discussion paper at the global forum on health research.) World Health Organization, Geneva.

Scheer J, Groce N (1988) Impairment as a human constant: cross-cultural and historical perspectives on variation. *Journal of Social Issues,* 44(1):23–37.

Schmidt L, Room R (1999) Cross-cultural applicability in international classifications and research on alcohol dependence. *Journal of Studies on Alcohol,* 60(4):448–462.

Schwartz SH (1994) Are there universal aspects in the structure and contents of human values? *Journal of Social Issues,* 50(4):19–45.

Schwartz SH, Sagiv L (1995) Identifying culture-specifics in the content and structure of values. *Journal of Cross-Cultural Psychology,* 26(1):92–116.

Shepard RN, Romney AK, Nerlove SB (1972) *Multidimensional scaling. Vol. 2.: Applications.* Seminar Press, New York.

Skevington SM, Mac Arthur P, Somerset M (1997) Developing items for the WHOQOL: an investigation of contemporary beliefs about quality of life related to health in Britain. *British Journal of Health Psychology,* 2(1):55–72.

Skevington SM, Tucker C (1999) Designing response scales for cross-cultural use in health care: data from the development of the UK WHOQOL. *British Journal of Medical Psychology,* 72(Pt1):51–61.

Slottje DJ, et al. (1991) *Measuring the quality of life across countries.* Westview, Boulder, CO.

Snow R (1997) *Monitoring the burden of reproductive ill-health in rural Bangladesh.* Consultancy report, International Centre for Diarrhoeal Disease Research, Bangladesh.

Stone L, Campbell JG (1984) The use and misuse of surveys in international development: an experiment from Nepal. *Human Organization,* **43**(1):27–37.

Sullivan M, Karlsson J (1998) The Swedish SF-36 health survey III: evaluation of criterion-based validity results from normative populations. *Journal of Clinical Epidemiology,* **51**(11):1105–1113.

The Chinese Culture Connection (1987) Chinese values and the search for culture-free dimensions of culture. *Journal of Cross-Cultural Psychology,* **18**(2):143–164.

Trostle J, Sommerfeld J (1996) Medical anthropology and epidemiology. *Annual Review of Anthropology,* **25**:253–274.

Trotter R, Schensul JJ (1998) Methods in applied anthropology. In: *Handbook of methods in cultural anthropology.* Bernard HR, ed. AltaMira Press, Walnut Creek, CA.

Tursz A (1997) Problems in conceptualizing adolescent risk behaviors: international comparison. *Journal of Adolescent Health,* **21**(2):116–127.

Üstün TB, Rehm J, Chatterji S, et al. (1999) Multiple-informant ranking of the disabling effects of different health conditions in 14 countries. WHO/NIH joint project CAR study group. *Lancet,* **354**(9173):111–115.

van de Vijver F (1997) Meta-analysis of cross-cultural comparisons of cognitive test performance. *Journal of Cross-Cultural Psychology,* **28**(6):678–709.

Wagner TH, Patrick DL, McKenna SP, Froese PS (1996) Cross-cultural development of a quality of life measure for men with erection difficulties. *Quality of Life Research,* **5**(4):443–449.

Ware JE, Keller SD, Gandek B, Brazier JE, Sullivan M (1995) Evaluating translations of health status questionnaires: methods from the IQOLA project. *International Journal of Technology Assessment in Health Care,* **11**(3):525–551.

Warnecke RB, Johnson TP, Chavez N, et al. (1997) Improving question wording in surveys of culturally diverse populations. *Annals of Epidemiology,* **7**(5):334–342.

Watkins D, Cheung S (1995) Culture, gender and response bias: an analysis of responses to the self-description questionnaire. *Journal of Cross-Cultural Psychology,* **26**(5):490–504.

Weinberger M, Oddone EZ, Samsa GP, Landsman PB (1996) Are health-related quality-of-life measures affected by the mode of administration? *Journal of Clinical Epidemiology,* **49**(2):135–140.

Weiss M (1997) Explanatory model interview catalogue (EMIC): framework for comparative study of illness. *Transcultural Psychiatry,* **34**(2):235–263.

Weller SC (1984) Cross-cultural concepts of illness: variation and validation. *American Anthropologist,* **86**:341–350.

Weller SC, Pachter LM, Trotter RT, Baer RD (1993) Empacho in four Latino groups: a study of intra- and inter-cultural variation in beliefs. *Medical Anthropology,* **15**(2):109–136.

WHOQOL Group (1998) The World Health Organization quality of life assessment: development and general psychometric properties. *Social Science and Medicine*, 46(12):1569–1585.

World Bank (1993) *World development report: investing in health*. Oxford University Press, New York.

Wrightson K, Wardle J (1997) Cultural variation in health locus of control. *Ethnicity and Health*, 2(1-2):13–20.

Yoder PS (1991) Cultural conceptions of illness and the measurement of changes in morbidity. In: *The health transition: methods and measures*. The proceedings of an international workshop, London, June 1989. Cleland J, Hill AG, eds. Health Transition Centre, Australian National University, Canberra.

Yoder PS, Hornik RC (1994) Perceptions of severity of diarrhoea and treatment choice: a comparative study of HealthCom sites. *Journal of Tropical Medicine and Hygiene*, 97(1):1–12.

Yoder PS, Hornik RC (1996) Symptoms and perceived severity of illness as predictive of treatment for diarrhoea in six Asian and African sites. *Social Science and Medicine*, 43(4):429–439.

Are disability weights universal? Ranking of the disabling effects of different health conditions in 14 countries by different informants[1]

Bedirhan Üstün, Juergen Rehm and Somnath Chatterji, on behalf of WHO/NIH Joint Project on Assessment and Classification of Disability[2]

Summary measures of population health (SMPH) provide a "common metric" for a wide range of health evaluations such as effectiveness of interventions or efficiency of health systems (WHO 1996). This metric adds "disability" (i.e. non-fatal health outcomes) to mortality, and thus results in a more realistic measure than what is obtained by measuring mortality alone (Murray and Lopez 1997). In the course of this book various attempts are made to develop composite health measures that combine information on mortality and non-fatal health outcomes to represent population health in a single number. However, the cross-cultural applicability of these methods as well as the equivalence of derived preferences has not been standardized globally, regionally and nationally.

Because of international comparability, great care must be taken in the construction of SMPH which involves value judgements in the calculation of the disability component in these measures captured in "disability weights" (also known as *preferences, valuations, or utilities*). A disability weight assigns a single numerical value to a given state that is worse than perfect health. We convert multiple aspects of disability (e.g. cognition, mobility, self-care, interpersonal relations, work or household activities, etc.) into a single number. The health status descriptions of some selected domains are transformed through a *"cognitive exercise"* to a value or preference that is usually elicited by the importance given to the condition, or by trading risks, time, money or personal lives. Usually a perfectly healthy state is given a weight of 0, and death is equivalent to a weight of 1. This disability weight, as a matter of fact, has the same anchor value for disability-adjusted life years (DALYs) or quality-adjusted life years (QALYs). The main difference is the sign. For DALYs the value is taken negatively (disability), for QALYs positively (quality of life).

In the original Global Burden of Disease (GBD) study these weights were determined with professional health care providers through the person trade-off (PTO) method (Nord 1995). Professional health care providers were chosen because they are thought to be familiar with health conditions and their outcomes, a familiarity that makes it easier to draw the often complex comparisons between the impacts of different disease states required by the PTO protocol.

These professionals were assumed to be representative of society as a whole. This theoretical assumption, however, requires empirical support. For empirical testing, preference measures should also be obtained from a variety of other groups such as policy-makers, persons with disabilities and others to see how these measures converge. Moreover, these disability weights are presumed to be universal, that is, equal across countries and cultures. There is a clear need for more systematic testing across different cultures, different informant groups, and alternative forms of measurement. The present study was in fact motivated by these concerns about the universality of the disability weights used in the construction of SMPH.

To obtain disability weights, a range of tools exist that measure the importance given to the condition (visual analog scales), or trading risks (standard gamble), time (time trade-off), money (willingness to pay) or groups of individuals (person trade-off). Of these methods none was perfectly suited to our needs for this study because we aimed to use the simplest possible method to test the invariance across various cultures and informants. Within a larger study on the cross-cultural applicability of a proposed revision of the *International Classification of Impairments, Disabilities and Handicaps* (WHO 1980; 1997), a sub-study examined whether expert ratings on the disabling effects of different health conditions were universal, in the sense of being stable across cultures and informant groups. Ranking was the chosen method rather than PTO because ranking requires less specialized participants, less time and no technical knowledge. The original GBD study protocol also used an ordinal ranking exercise in addition to a variant of the PTO protocol and required respondents to reconcile the discrepancies between the two during a deliberative phase (Murray and Lopez 1996).

The current study is the first independent attempt to replicate the results of the exercise carried out within the framework of the GBD study in different cultures with different informants. It should, however, be pointed out that because of the difference in methods, this study can only test the assumptions of the GBD study (e.g. stability of disability scores across cultures and informant groups). With the ranking exercise *disability weights cannot be derived* because no cardinal value was obtained with this method. Since the main aim of this present study is to test the underlying assumptions of the original GBD work, and since the alternative of using PTO requires much more time (two days per group compared to 10–15 minutes per person for rankings), the choice of method is justified because it was conceptually understandable, culturally meaningful and applicable in different cultures.

SPECIFIC AIMS OF THE STUDY

1. Are there statistically significant differences in the ranking of the disabling health conditions by key informants from different countries?

2. Are there statistically significant differences in the ranking of the disabling health conditions by respondents from different informant groups (medical professionals, allied health professionals, health policy-makers, consumers or caregivers)?

3. Could the ranking of the disability weights of the GBD study be replicated with a different methodology?

4. What are the underlying patterns in respondent ratings of disabling effects of health conditions?

METHODS

PARTICIPANTS

The ranking was part of the key informant interviews. Informants from a total of fourteen countries participated in this study: Canada, China, Egypt, Greece, India, Japan, Luxembourg, the Netherlands, Nigeria, Romania, Spain, Tunisia, Turkey, and the United Kingdom of Great Britain and Northern Ireland. Thus, all WHO regions were represented.

"Key Informants" were defined as those who by virtue of their position and knowledge have an understanding of disability that makes them representative spokespersons for their culture. For each site, 15 informants were to be selected, composed of three individuals from each of the following five groups:

• Medical professionals (e.g. MD, psychiatrist, psychologist, nurse)

• Allied health professionals (e.g. social worker, case worker)

• Policy-makers or opinion leaders in the area of disability services

• Individuals with a disabling physical health condition (or their caregivers)

• Individuals with a disabling health condition in the area of alcohol, drugs or mental health (or their carers).

The final number of participants included in this study ($N = 241$) varies slightly by country, but essentially, the quota of 15 was achieved in each country (see Table 2).

MATERIALS

Informants responded to a questionnaire including both open-ended and closed-ended items. In rank-ordering disability, key informants were presented with a deck of 17 cards listing different health conditions with short descriptions (see Table 1). They were instructed to rank them from the most disabling to the least disabling condition. The "most disabling condition" was described as that which would make daily activities such as dressing, feeding, moving around, and meeting basic day-to-day responsibilities very difficult; the least "disabling" as that which would not interfere with these daily activities. Codes were assigned to the 17 conditions, with 01 representing the most disabling, and 17 the least disabling. Thirteen of the 17 health conditions were adapted from the 22 indicator conditions of the GBD study (see Table 1) to measure the burden of disabilities and diseases within the DALY framework. The selection of the original indicator conditions was based on pre-tests showing that certain diseases were difficult to grasp by the respondents in certain cultures. Methodologically, ranking 22 conditions has also been shown to be too much of a burden on the respondent (Trotter et al. 2001). In addition to the original conditions, we had a special interest in including alcohol and drug use disorders and HIV infections, which were assumed to rank with "medium" disabling consequences and to show cultural differences (Mäkelä et al. 1981).

PROCEDURE

Each key informant was presented with a brief overview of the interview and its purpose. The interviewer then began by asking questions about demographic variables and their experience in the area of disabilities, followed by open-ended questions on language and disability, identification of and societal reactions to disability associated with selected conditions (e.g. difficulties with walking, psychotic symptoms, low intelligence, alcohol and drug related problems). The interview included the collection of demographic data, and questions about the language of disability in the culture, about existing compensation systems for disability, about the social stigma of disabilities, and about other societal reactions to disabling health conditions. This process served to frame the issue of the ranking exercise within the context of understanding the disabling consequences of health conditions. The assessment of social disapproval or stigma for different health and social conditions was identified using an 11-point rating scale with the endpoints labelled as none (= 0) and extreme (10). Once the open-ended portion of the interview was completed, the interviewer presented the respondent with the 17 different cards, and administered the instructions to rank the conditions in terms of their disabling effects. Finally, the respondent was asked to complete a self-administered questionnaire that addressed expected difficulties with everyday activities in a selection of health conditions and included the assessment of stigma related to various disabilities.

Non-parametric statistics for ordinal level variables were used to analyse the data. Overall ranking was established on the basis of median ranks. For conditions with the same median the arithmetic mean of rankings was taken as a second criterion.

To test for differences between countries or informant groups, the Kruskal-Wallis rank order analysis of variance for one factor was used. Kendall Tau-B correlations were computed to measure the association between different rank orders (Hays 1973). Statistical analyses were carried out with SYSTAT 8.0 and with StatXact 3.1 (exact calculations of Kendall Tau correlation and its confidence intervals).

RESULTS

Table 1 gives an overview of the relative rank order for the 17 different health conditions, ranked from most disabling to least disabling. Overall, quadriplegia was considered the most disabling condition, followed by dementia (rank 2), active psychosis (rank 3), and paraplegia (rank 4). At the opposite end of the spectrum, having vitiligo on the face (least disabling = rank 17), being infertile when a child is desired (rank 16), and having

Table I   Rank order of disabling effect of health conditions by severity

Health condition	Rank	Median	Mean	Standard deviation	N
Quadriplegia*	1	2	3.3	3.2	241
Dementia*	2	4	4.9	3.6	241
Active psychosis*	3	4	5.3	3.6	241
Paraplegia*	4	5	5.9	3.3	241
Blindness*	5	6	6.8	4.0	241
Major depression*	6	6	7.2	3.8	241
Drug dependence	7	8	7.8	3.9	222
HIV-positive	8	9	8.8	5.2	239
Alcoholism	9	9	9.2	3.6	241
Total deafness*	10	10	9.4	3.7	241
Mild mental retardation*	11	10	9.9	3.6	241
Incontinence	12	10	10.2	4.1	239
Below the knee amputation*	13	11	10.2	3.7	241
Rheumatoid arthritis*	14	12	11.5	3.6	241
Severe migraines*	15	12	11.6	3.8	240
Infertility*	16	16	14.6	3.6	238
Vitiligo on face*	17	16	15.0	2.4	238

* Adapted from the 22 conditions used in the GBD Study; the other 9 conditions were severe sore throat, fractured radius in a stiff cast, Down syndrome without cardiac malformation, severe anemia, recto-vaginal fistula, watery diarrhoea, 2 standard deviations below height/weight, erectile dysfunction, and angina.

severe migraines (rank 15) were deemed least disabling. Overall, the conditions at both ends of the spectrum, that is the most disabling and the least disabling conditions showed lower variability than the conditions in between.

There were, however, deviations from this order across countries. Table 2 shows that in the Netherlands, for instance, active psychosis is seen as more disabling compared to the overall sample rank. Interestingly, being HIV-positive is considered relatively less disabling in Japan, Luxembourg, Spain, Turkey and the United Kingdom, whereas it is considered the most disabling in Egypt and Tunisia. In general, HIV is the health condition with the most rank variation which may be due to relative frequency and special views about this particular disorder. In Egypt and Tunisia, HIV ranks as more disabling than quadriplegia. This is mainly because of the image of HIV as a stigmatizing illness in these countries.

Statistically, the differences between countries were significant for 13 out of 17 health conditions on the Kruskal-Wallis test. Only quadriplegia, paraplegia, below the knee amputation and mild mental retardation did not show rank differences between countries at the 0.05 significance level. It is interesting to note that three out of the four conditions that are judged uniformly across countries are prototypical physical disabilities. The fourth, mild mental retardation also shows little variation though it is less uniformly rated compared with the other three.

Although there are statistically significant differences of ranking between countries, the convergence of judgments is also quite evident. The Kendall Tau rank correlations between different countries averaged 0.61, which can be considered relatively high given the variability of cultures and experts participating. Within this average, there are, however, clear cultural differences for some comparisons, e.g. Turkey and the Netherlands have a Kendall Tau rank correlation of 0.41 (95% confidence intervals CI: 0.14–0.69), while the Netherlands and Tunisia correlate at 0.29 (CI: 0.03–0.56). On the high end, Luxembourg and Spain correlated at 0.87 (CI: 0.74–0.99), and Romania and India at 0.82 (CI: 0.72–0.92). The overwhelming majority of rank correlations ranged between 0.5 and 0.7 (typical confidence intervals: Kendall Tau: 0.50; CI: 0.27–0.73; Kendall Tau: 0.60; CI: 0.35–0.85. A table with all bivariate correlations between countries can be obtained from the first author).

The rank order ratings of different informant groups are summarized in Table 3. Only five out of 17 health conditions had significantly different rank orders between different informant groups: quadriplegia, HIV, total deafness, mild mental retardation, amputation below the knee. Interestingly, physical disorders are again the most prominent, but in this case as conditions with the most significant differences. The rank orders of Table 3 also reveal significant differences between some informant groups that might be expected to have convergent views. For example, the ratings between health professionals in the physical rehabilitation sector show the largest differences compared with consumers/caregivers in the

Table 2 Disability ranks associated with different health conditions by country

Health condition (Rank order in total sample)	Country													
	Canada	China	Egypt	Greece	India	Japan	Luxem-bourg	Nether-lands	Nigeria	Romania	Spain	Tunisia	Turkey	UK
Quadriplegia (1)[a]	2	1	2	1	1	2	1	3	1	1	1	2	1	2
Dementia (2)	3	8	3	3	2	1	2	2	6	2	2	3	2	1
Active psychosis (3)	1	5	4	2	5	3	3	1	3	3	4	6	4	4
Paraplegia (4)[a]	4	4	8	4	4	5	7	7	2	4	5	4	3	5
Total blindness (5)	8	3	5	9	3	4	4	9	5	5	6	5	5	8
Major depression (6)	5	6	7	7	6	8	6	4	4	7	3	7	11	3
Drug dependence (7)	7	2	6	6	11	7	5	6	10	11	8	11	7	M
HIV-positive (8)	10	9	1	5	7	13	15	12	8	8	13	1	14	14
Alcoholism (9)	9	10	11	8	10	10	8	5	13	13	7	12	10	6
Total deafness (10)	11	12	10	13	9	6	9	11	15	9	9	13	12	12
Mild mental retardation (11)[a]	6	11	9	12	12	15	10	13	11	10	10	9	8	7
Incontinence (12)	15	13	13	10	8	14	13	15	7	6	12	10	6	11
Below-the-knee amputation (13)[a]	12	7	12	11	14	9	11	14	12	12	11	8	9	13
Rheumatoid arthritis (14)	14	14	17	15	13	11	14	10	14	15	15	16	13	10
Severe migraines (15)	13	15	16	14	15	12	12	8	9	14	14	17	15	9
Infertility (16)	16	17	14	16	17	16	17	16	16	16	17	15	17	16
Vitiligo on face (17)	17	16	15	17	16	17	16	17	17	17	16	14	16	15
N	15	15	16	15	43	18	16	13	15	15	18	15	15	12

Note: Ranking ranges from 1 (most disabling) to 17 (least disabling). Most disabling condition defined as that which would make carrying out the activities of daily life very difficult; and the least disabling condition that which would not interfere with activities of everyday life. M=missing data; item not given.
a. no significant differences between countries on α = 0.05 level (Kruskal Wallis rank order analysis of variance).

Table 3   Disability ranks of different health conditions by informant group

| Health condition (Rank order of total sample) | Medical professionals | | | | | Allied health prof. (N=51) | Health policy-makers (N=35) | Consumers/ Caregivers | |
	Physical (N=14)	ADM (N=35)	Ph&ADM (N=14)	Other (N=11)	Total (N=74)			Physical (N=30)	Mental (N=45)
Quadriplegia	1	1	3	1	1	1	1	1	1
Dementia	2	2	1	2	2	3	2	4	2
Active psychosis	5	3	2	4	3	2	3	2	3
Paraplegia	3	4	4	3	4	5	4	6	4
Blindness	6	5	5	5	5	6	7	5	5
Major depression	4	6	6	6	6	4	5	8	6
Drug dependence	9	7	7	8	7	7	9	7	8
HIV-positive	10	11	15	11	11	12	6	3	7
Alcoholism	13	10	10	9	9	8	10	9	9
Total deafness	12	8	9	7	8	10	11	11	12
Mild mental retardation	14	13	8	12	13	9	8	10	13
Incontinence	7	12	14	13	12	11	12	12	11
Below the knee amputation	8	9	12	10	10	13	13	13	10
Rheumatoid arthritis	11	14	11	15	14	14	14	15	14
Severe migraines	15	15	13	14	15	15	15	14	15
Infertility	16	16	17	16	16	16	17	17	16
Vitiligo on face	17	17	16	17	17	17	16	16	17

same sector, with respect to rankings in the above conditions, and physical conditions in general. Overall, the rank orders between different informant groups had an average correlation of 0.76.

The research design allowed us to measure the influence of social disapproval or stigma on disability rankings for a subset of the conditions. There was a consistent effect for all tested relationships in the direction that higher stigma was associated with higher disability rankings, although the effect size was small (less than 0.10 on average for Kendall Tau correlations). In summary, stigma has a measurable but very small effect on disability rankings.

The resulting summary ranking across all judgments is very similar to the ranking of the experts in the GBD study (Murray 1996), derived with a different methodology (PTO). The respective rank order correlation is 0.77 for Kendall Tau (CI: 0.40–1.0; $z = 3.66$, $p < 0.01$). The only notable difference occurs for severe migraine, which ranked third in the GBD exercise, and eleventh in the present study. However, conditions varied in the way in which judgements were elicited for migraine in the two exercises. In the GBD exercise experts were continuously reminded that they should consider the artificial case of one continuous year of severe migraines with the consequence of staying in bed most of the time, in making their judgements. The failure to remind respondents repeatedly of this may have led to the comparability of the nominally same condition, severe migraine, being compromised. Without severe migraine, the respective correlations increase to 0.97 in the case of Kendall Tau (CI: 0.89–1.0; $z = 4.39$; $p < 0.01$). This level of convergence is so high that we can actually speak of almost identical rankings.

DISCUSSION

The main result of this study is that the rankings of the disabling effect of health conditions were found to be relatively stable across countries, informant groups, and methods, although there is some variation. The very high correlations between the GBD study and this study, as well as the fairly high level of agreement between the 14 countries in this study, and between eight informant groups, provide support for this statement. Thus, in the eyes of the respondents, the relative burden of different health conditions in terms of disability is fairly similar across the world. However, the results also indicate that there are sometimes quite pronounced differences between cultures and informant groups. These differences are large enough to be further explored in a systematic way.

From a theoretical point of view, there is no reason for disability weights to be universal. The actual burden of disability or activity limitations is modulated by many factors such as the environment, e.g. the burden of disability for individuals with paraplegia is likely to depend on the availability of helpful devices (wheelchairs, specialized cars, specialized workplaces) and social support. Clearly, in this respect there are differences between countries, and these differences should be reflected in the disability weights attached to certain health conditions. Thinking of differences of frequencies and interventions available to quadriplegic or blind persons in different cultures, it is tempting to think that disability weights would naturally vary from country to country. Since countries differ in providing treatments for different conditions (e.g. quadriplegia, HIV or depression), in our research we separated treated and untreated populations in order to evaluate the impact of interventions to reduce disability.

A secondly conclusion of this study is that valuation and description in the terminology of the GBD study may not be strongly related. The ranking exercise is directed exclusively at the extent of disabling conditions. All diseases have to be ranked solely on the basis of their disabling effects. On the other hand, the PTO methodology asks for a valuation (i.e. trade-off of persons with that disease). The basic comparisons are obtained through questions comparing the lives of 1 000 healthy people for one year versus 2 000 blind people dying. Thus, other aspects than just the disabling effects of health conditions (e.g. prognosis, pain, mood impact, public opinion) may drive the valuations.

In general, it can be said that the physical conditions are ranked more uniformly than the mental conditions across countries. This implies that though physical conditions such as quadriplegia, paraplegia and below-the-knee amputation are as a group viewed differently from conditions such as active psychosis, any differences are more likely to be a feature of individual respondent characteristics than of cultural differences. Also of note is the fact that the conditions with the most variation are mental conditions that lie in the mid-range of the rankings.

Any ordinal ranking can only indicate the relative effects of disability from different health conditions (e.g. active psychosis results in more disability than major depression), and not the absolute effects, which may vary tremendously between countries because of different formal and informal health and social support systems. Also, high agreement of health professionals or other key informants as experts does not necessarily mean that the real disability associated with the different health conditions is similarly uniform across countries. In different instances in the past, the consensus among experts has been shown to be at variance with actual behavior of subjects (Rehm and Gadenne 1990; Single 1997). Thus, the next step should be to conduct empirical studies to examine whether selected health conditions really have the same disabling effects in different countries and cultures across the world, and if they are stable with respect to different assessment methods and different informant groups.

It is indeed important to explore the methodology to elicit disability weights for cultural variation. Concepts of death, birth, time as well as valuation across these constructs may vary across cultures. While the use of disability weights assume an "etic" anthropological perspective, the "emic" qualities of these constructs may provide valuable insight and context such as framing of questions, and elicitation techniques. Our field experience has yielded important reactions from the subjects that their personal characteristics (e.g. risk aversion) or personal ethics may play an important role in determining how they rank these conditions. Therefore the elicitation technique, interview and tools provided for deliberation are of prime importance. Professionals may show a better understanding of different health conditions but they may also show professional prejudices towards the interventions and spontaneously relate them to resource allocation.

Finally, we would like to emphasize the importance of empirical data on disability and their universality. The valuation function is largely determined by the health status. We should objectify the components of health and study their interactions. The more these measures are based on empirical data, the more robust and universal will they become. An actual measurement of how subjects function with different health conditions in different cross-cultural contexts ought to be coupled with valuation exercises across cultures and respondent groups (Üstün and Chatterji 1998). This may then provide valuable insights into the determinants of values that people assign to disabling health conditions. If public policy decisions like resource allocation and priority setting are to be based on evidence, we need to make sure that they are formed by all parties concerned and based on "real life" data obtained by using the highest scientific standards.

NOTES

1 A more detailed version of this paper has been published previously in the *Lancet* (Üstün et al. 1999).

2 In collaboration with WHO/NIH Joint Project Advisors and Principal Investigators—Robert Battjes (NIDA, USA), Bridget Grant (NIAAA, USA), Cille Kennedy (NIMH, USA), Shen Yu Cun (China), V. Mavreas (Greece), R.S. Murthy (Bangalore, India), Hemraj Pal (Delhi, India), R. Thara (Chennai, India), M. Tazaki (Japan), C. Pull (Luxembourg), H. Hoek (the Netherlands), A. Odejide (Nigeria), R. Vrasti (Romania), J.L. Vazquez-Barquero (Spain), A. Chaker (Tunisia), A. Gogus (Ankara, Turkey), N. Dedeoglu (Antalya, Turkey), K. Ogel (Istanbul, Turkey), D. Mumford (United Kingdom).

REFERENCES

Hays WL (1973) *Statistics for the social sciences*. Holt, Rinehart & Winston, New York.

Mäkelä K, Room R, Single E, Sulkunen P, Walsh B, et al. (1981) A comparative study of alcohol control. In: *Alcohol, society, and the state. A report of the international study of alcohol control experiences, in collaboration with the WHO regional office for Europe*. Single E, Morgan P, de Lint J, eds. Addiction Research Foundation, Toronto.

Murray CJL (1996) Rethinking DALYs. In: *The global burden of disease: a comprehensive assessment of mortality and disability from diseases, injuries, and risk factors in 1990 and projected to 2020*. The Global Burden of Disease and Injury, Vol. 1. Murray CJL, Lopez AD, eds. Harvard School of Public Health on behalf of WHO, Cambridge, MA.

Murray CJL, Lopez AD (1996) Estimating cause-of-death: new methods and global and regional applications for 1990. In: *The global burden of disease: a comprehensive assessment of mortality and disability from diseases, injuries, and risk factors in 1990 and projected to 2020*. The Global Burden of Disease and Injury, Vol. 1. Murray CJL, Lopez AD, eds. Harvard School of Public Health on behalf of WHO, Cambridge, MA.

Murray CJL, Lopez AD (1997) Regional patterns of disability-free life expectany and disability-adjusted life expectancy: global burden of disease study. *Lancet*, 349(9062):1347-1352.

Nord E (1995) The person-trade off approach to valuing health care programs. *Medical Decision Making*, 15(3):201-208.

Rehm J, Gadenne V (1990) *Intuitive predictions and professional forecasts: cognitive processes and social consequences*. Pergamon Press, Oxford.

Single E (1997) The concept of harm reduction and its application to alcohol: the 6th Dorothy Black lecture. *Drugs - Education, Prevention and Policy*, 4:7-22.

Trotter R, Üstün TB, Chatterji S, Rehm J, Room R, Bickenbach J (2001) Cross-cultural applicability research on disablement: models and methods for the revision of an international classification. *Human Organization*, 60(1):13-27.

Üstün TB, Chatterji S (1998) Measuring functioning and disability - a common framework. *International Journal of Methods in Psychiatric Research*, 7(2):79-83. (Editorial)

Üstün TB, Rehm J, Chatterji S, et al. (1999) Multiple-informant ranking of the disabling effects of different health conditions in 14 countries. WHO/NIH joint project CAR study group. *Lancet*, 354(9173):111-115.

WHO (1980) *International classification of impairments, disabilities, and handicaps: a manual of classification relating to the consequences of disease*. World Health Organization, Geneva. (Reprint 1993)

WHO (1996) *Investing in health research and development*. (Report of the Ad Hoc Committee on Health Research Priorities.) World Health Organization, Geneva.

WHO (1997) *International classification of impairments, activities and participation, (ICIDH-2) beta-1 draft*. World Health Organization, Geneva.

Chapter 11.3

Measurement of variance in health state valuations in Phnom Penh, Cambodia

Ritu Sadana

Introduction

Initiated in 1992, the Global Burden of Disease (GBD) Study was conducted at the request of the World Bank and in collaboration with the World Health Organization (WHO) to develop a set of consistent estimates of disease and injury rates for 1990, as well as to develop a comparative index of the burden of each disease or injury, either from premature mortality or time lived with less than perfect health. This comparative index is the summary measure of population health, the disability-adjusted life year (DALY) (Murray and Lopez 1994; WHO 1996; World Bank 1993). By 1998, three volumes of the GBD Study's methodologies and final results were published on behalf of the World Health Organization and the World Bank (Murray and Lopez 1996a; 1996b; 1998), among other publications highlighting key findings or methods (Murray and Lopez 1996c; 1997a–d). The GBD Study's methods and findings have generated considerable discussion in the literature and international forums, as well as within the organizations collaborating on the study (for example Anand and Hanson 1997; Barker and Green 1996; Paalman et al. 1998; WHO 1998). The potential normative use of the GBD study's findings by WHO, the World Bank and national governments has raised concerns on the comparability and interpretation of findings across regions, cultures and socioeconomic groups, as well as on the policy relevance and implications for resource allocation in different health system contexts.

Much of the debate centres on the construction of DALY as a summary measure of population health, in particular the explicit social values incorporated within DALY. These include social values for severity weights for disability (e.g. disability weights for over 400 different health states partially based on valuations of 22 indicator health states), the discount rate for future health, age-weights across the life cycle, and target expectancy of life. This chapter reports on an empirical investigation of (i) whether the DALY protocol to elicit valuations for indicator health states may be replicated among non-health professionals in a developing country; (ii) whether differences exist between valuations of health states obtained from individuals with different demographic characteristics or health experiences; and (iii) whether differences exist between health and non-health professionals' valuations.

BACKGROUND

A severity weight is a quantified valuation of time lived in a less than perfect health state compared to time lived in perfect health. Measuring severity weights makes it technically possible to compare years of life lost due to premature mortality and years of life lived in health states worse than perfect or full health.[1] This comparison is necessary in the construction of summary measures of population health as morbidity and mortality are combined in a single index. Several approaches have been used to obtain severity weights for use within summary measures of population health or within cost-effectiveness studies: investigators may assign arbitrary weights; expert panels may estimate weights; studies may incorporate weights published in the literature; researchers may estimate the revealed (implicit) values based on policies or other social decisions such as current funding or resource allocations and then assign disability weights; or health state valuations may be elicited through primary data collection and severity weights subsequently assigned.

Several methodological issues arise in the literature reviewed elsewhere (see Sommerfeld et al. chapter 11.1 in this volume): a few relevant to this study are briefly noted. The first is whose values should be used in the construction of severity weights. Empirically there is growing evidence that different groups, such as health care professionals, patients experiencing health states to be valued, lay care givers and the general public, often provide different values for the same health state (Ashby et al. 1994; Nord 1992), akin to differences found in the measurement of health (Pierre et al. 1998). Few discuss why valuations may differ given different socioeconomic experiences, health status, asymmetry of information on health, and professional or political agency.

A second issue is what valuation method should be selected. A range of methods have been used to elicit valuations of health states, including the visual analogue rating scaling, magnitude estimation, individual trade-off methods such as the standard gamble or time trade-off, willingness-to-pay and social trade-off methods, including the person trade-off (see chapter 9.1 in this volume for details). Different approaches tend to reflect different disciplinary traditions and applications: for example, the standard gamble approach is preferred by economists as it is based on utility theory, supposedly provides valuations with interval scale properties, and underlines that risk is involved in the decision-making process, whereas the person trade-off method is favoured among those preferring to use a method that also simulates reality rather than a game, as this method directly asks individuals to allocate scarce resources among people. Although not necessarily providing valuations with interval scale properties, the visual analogue rating scale is the quickest method to obtain valuations and also the most commonly used (Krabbe et al. 1997). All methods assume individuals or groups may provide their preferences for time lived in a less than perfect health state—hypothetical or experienced health states—through a questionnaire, interview or exercise (Shibuya 1999) and that a single valuation exists for each health state. Those developing and applying methods to value health states have not conducted extensive qualitative investigations to provide greater insight on the actual meaning and interpretation of valuations obtained. Not surprisingly, research documents that different methods produce different valuations for the same health state (Dolan et al. 1996; Krabbe et al. 1997).

The third issue is how to describe a health state and communicate it to those who will value the health states. Conceptually, what is to be valued needs to be specified. This not only includes the health state, but also what the severity weight should or should not reflect. Empirically, two broad approaches exist: (i) develop a label and short qualitative description specific to each health state; or (ii) develop a classification system based on a series of domains that can be used to describe a broad range of generic or specific health states in a systematic way (see Sadana, chapter 7.1). Table 1 provides examples of these different approaches. Again, not surprisingly, research shows that using different methods to describe and communicate health states may influence the valuations obtained (Llewellyn-Thomas et al. 1984).

A fourth issue is that in addition to the specific method[2] or description of health states selected, the approach taken may be subject to a wide range of significant biases due to (i) the framing of questions; (ii) heuristic devices used by individuals to simplify complex cognitive tasks; and (iii) other details concerning the protocol employed, including the number and range of health states selected to be valued (Tversky and Kahneman 1981). Yet most studies do not discuss if valuations for health states obtained are biased by the overall approach taken. Furthermore, as there is no gold standard for the valuation of health states, the reliability of methods is often tested in lieu of validity—except for convergent validity—similar to the measurement of health status (see Sadana, chapter 7.1).

Several have proposed different criteria for severity weights incorporated within summary measures of population health *for comparative use across populations*. These include that weights should be "non-arbitrary...scientifically measured values" (Richardson 1994); that they should be "invariant over time and invariant between countries" (chapter 9.1); and that given that information contained within summary measures of population health may be used towards the social allocation of scarce resources, severity weights should reflect population-based values (Nord 1995).

Table I　　Standardized health state description approaches and examples

Type	Example
Health state specific label; qualitative	Breast cancer, second stage, under radiotherapy, with moderate weakness.
Health state classification: holistic narrative description; generic, qualitative	I am in the age range of 40–60 years. I have been tired and weak. I walk slowly and travel outside the house is difficult. Much of the day I am alone, lying down in my bedroom. Social contact with my friends is reduced.
Health state classification: holistic taxonomic description; generic, qualitative	Age: 40–60 year old Main activity: employee or housekeeper Mobility: travel with difficulty Physical role: walk with limitation, perform self-care Social role: social contact reduced Symptom/problem: general tiredness, weakness, weight loss
Health state classification: decomposed taxonomic description; generic, quantitative	21322 [corresponding to a health state classification system of 5 domains with 3 levels within each domain, e.g. the EQ5D]

Mobility:	Level 2:	I have some problems walking about
Self care:	Level 1:	I have no problems with selfcare
Usual activities:	Level 3:	I am unable to perform my usual activities
Pain/discomfort:	Level 2:	I have moderate pain or discomfort
Anxiety/depression:	Level 2:	I am moderately anxious or depressed

Note: adapted from Llewellyn-Thomas (1984).

OBJECTIVES

In developing countries, the validity and reliability as well as the feasibility and acceptability of implementing different methods and approaches to obtain health state valuations, have neither been systematically investigated across representative samples of populations, nor simply among non-health professionals in any given population. This study therefore set out to provide some empirical evidence concerning the feasibility of applying methods to elicit health state valuations and the reliability of results across different groups of non-health professionals, for indicator conditions in a developing country.

Specifically, the objectives of this study are to test (i) whether the DALY protocol to elicit valuations for indicator health states may be replicated among non-health professional women in Phnom Penh, Cambodia; (ii) whether differences exist between valuations of health states obtained from women seeking health services or residing in the community, or by age or number of school years completed; and (iii) whether differences exist between international health professionals' valuations of health states obtained for the GBD study based on the DALY protocol for measuring severity weights and those obtained from Cambodian women participating in this study.

REVIEW OF THE GBD STUDY PROTOCOL TO MEASURE SEVERITY WEIGHTS INCORPORATED WITHIN DALYS

CONCEPTUAL FRAMEWORK

Disability incorporated within the GBD Study is based on the conceptual framework of impairments (conditions and sequelae), disability (with different levels of severity) and handicap (social and economic consequences) found within the 1980 draft of the *WHO International Classification of Impairments, Disability and Handicap* (ICIDH)[3] (WHO 1980). *Disability* is defined in terms of the impact on the performance of the individual, and *handicap* in terms of the context of the overall consequences which depend on the social environment. The *disability* in DALY is based on this definition, rather than *impairment or handicap* (Murray 1994; 1996; Murray and Acharya 1997). The GBD study justifies the conceptual emphasis on *disability* due to the need for international comparability requiring the treatment of "like outcomes as like" regardless of the particular context of disability or characteristics of the individual beyond age and sex. However, in practice, the approach implemented to obtain valuations for indicator health states used a construct "somewhere between disability and handicap" (Murray 1996) and the actual interpretation of the severity weight is described as the "average level of handicap stemming from each condition" that does not take into account age, sex or other characteristics (Murray 1996 pp. 38–39). Nevertheless, the term DALY reflecting disability, rather than HALY reflecting handicap (Evans and Ranson 1995/1996), is retained.

SELECTION AND DESCRIPTION OF HEALTH STATES

First, 22 indicator conditions were selected from the 483 disabling sequelae selected for incorporation in the GBD study, in order to cover a wide range of disabilities and severity including those related to physical, mental, social functioning or pain. Short qualitative health state specific labels for each of the 22 indicator conditions are standardized and described for one year duration. For example, *severe migraine* is described as "imagine a person with a continuous severe migraine for one year. This individual would effectively be bed-ridden and unable to undertake any organized physical or mental activity. This condition is intended to be the proxy indicator for severe pain" or *below-the-knee amputation*, described as "in an individual without a prosthesis but with the basic aids, such as crude crutches, that are available in all societies" (Murray 1996: p. 94).

SELECTION OF PARTICIPANTS

A group of 12 international health professionals (7 men and 5 women) representing each of the six WHO regions, were selected as participants for primary data collection at the World Health Organization. According to the GBD study, experts are selected in order to minimize efforts needed to describe and communicate each health state and maintain the focus on severity rather than the prevalence of each condition.

VALUATION METHOD AND APPROACH

A formal assessment method to elicit health state valuations for 22 indicator conditions using the person trade-off (PTO) method[4] was designed that took approximately eight hours to complete for all 22 indicator conditions. The specific variant of the PTO method developed was designed to obtain internally consistent valuations, to minimize framing effects, and to promote group consensus (Murray 1996; Murray and Acharya 1997). The PTO method developed, however, is conceptually and cognitively demanding, and requires stamina to sustain interest in completing the exercise for all 22 indicator conditions.[5] The facilitator's role is described as "critical", and must provide "constant encouragement" to complete the exercise and to "challenge individuals to search for their own valuations based on careful reflection" (Murray 1996). The study documents a high degree of correlation of health state valuations within the 12 member expert group in Geneva using the PTO protocol, as well as in comparison with the pooled results of nine other group exercises with health professionals from different regions of the world (e.g. using the same protocol and facilitators). Although highly consistent ordinal rankings and valuations of health states across groups are achieved for the 22 indicator conditions, potential differences by age, sex, professional specialization, nationality or other characteristics of the expert participants are not provided.

ASSIGNING SEVERITY WEIGHTS

Within the GBD study, DALY assigns a value of 1 to years of life lost due to premature mortality, and 0 to perfect health. Time spent in a less than perfect health state is assigned a severity weight between 0 and 1. Health states valued worse than death are not allowed. To assign severity weights to each of the 483 non-fatal health outcomes incorporated within the GBD study, weights were assigned using a two step process. First, severity weights for each of the 22 indicator conditions generated from the Geneva valuation exercise were arbitrarily divided along the spectrum from health to death, into seven classes of severity noted in Table 2. Second, for the 483 conditions and sequelae, magnitude estimation and group consensus are used to estimate their distribution across the seven classes of disability using the 22 indicator conditions allocated to each class as pegs on the

Table 2   Disability class, severity weights and 22 indicator conditions: DALY protocol

Disability class	Severity weight	Indicator condition
1	0.00–0.02	Vitiligo on face; weight for height less than 2 SDs
2	0.02–0.12	Watery diarrhoea; severe sore throat; severe anemia
3	0.12–0.24	Radius fracture in a stiff cast; infertility; erectile dysfunction; rheumatoid arthritis; angina
4	0.24–0.36	Below-the-knee amputation; deafness
5	0.36–0.50	Recto-vaginal fistual; mild mental retardation; Down syndrome
6	0.50–0.70	Unipolar major depression; blindness; paraplegia
7	0.70–1.00	Active psychosis; dementia; severe migraine; quadriplegia

Source: Murray (1996).

scale from perfect health to near death by the same 12 international health experts in Geneva. Age-specific severity weights for untreated and treated forms for each of the 483 sequelae were then estimated. No further details on the second step of the methodology are published.

DEVELOPING AND TESTING METHODS

CONCEPTUAL FRAMEWORK

One aspect of replicating the DALY protocol was to determine whether local conceptions of the severity of health states overlap with the GBD study's conceptual focus on *disability* or practical interpretation reflecting "somewhere between disability and handicap". Qualitative group discussions ($n = 10$, with over 100 participants) with women aged 15–54 selected from urban and rural communities, in-depth interviews ($n = 33$) with women aged 15–54 with reproductive health conditions, physical disabilities or psychiatric conditions, and key informant interviews ($n = 15$) with male and female modern and traditional health care providers and community leaders, informed the development of a local conceptual framework for the burden of illness and disease (Sadana 2001).

Based on these qualitative investigations, the severity of health states (i.e. morbidity[6] and associated disability) included notions of social or economic consequences and other contextual factors, such as personal attributes, social status, previous illness history, household circumstances and community context, not only pain or physical or cognitive disability. Clearly, this local conceptual framework is broader than *disability* as conceptually defined within the GBD Study, as it explicitly incorporates notions of *handicap*. In this study, the conceptual understanding of what is to be valued concerning each health state (and the meaning of the severity weight), explicitly incorporates both *disability* and *handicap*.

SELECTION OF INDICATOR CONDITIONS AND DESCRIPTION OF HEALTH STATES

The original goal was to use all 22 indicator conditions from the DALY protocol and some 5 additional reproductive health state indicators[7], identified by individuals participating in the qualitative phase of the study. Through pretest group and individual exercises with women aged 15–45, all 22 indicator health state conditions and some 20 additional reproductive health states were tested. The selection of indicator conditions for this study in Cambodia was guided by the following criteria: (i) whether standardized qualitative health state specific labels as developed for the DALY protocol were understood easily by non-health professional participants; (ii) if not all 22 indicator health state conditions from the DALY protocol are selected, at least one indicator condition from each of the seven classes of disability is selected; (iii) indicator conditions that represent a broad range of health states including a range of severity covering physical disability, cognitive function, mental health, pain and discomfort as well as conditions with complex social responses; (iv) inclusion of two anchor conditions, representing potentially the worst and best health states as defined locally; and (v) less than 30 total indicator conditions, considered the maximum number manageable for a group or individual valuation exercise.

Based on these criteria, 11 of the original 22 GBD indicator conditions were selected, along with an additional 15 reproductive health indicators, noted in Table 3. Twenty-six hypothetical health states plus the individual's own health state were therefore selected for valuation.

Identical health state descriptions are used for the 11 indicator conditions from the DALY protocol with the exception of also adding the Khmer lay term for each condition in an effort to improve communication of the health state to non-health professionals. Similar qualitative health state specific labels are used to describe the 15 reproductive health indicator conditions. For death, the potential worst state, most participants during the pretest asked what type of death.[8] In order to provide consistent responses by the facilitators, maternal death was noted as the cause of death. The qualitative label for the best health state anchor was "bright skin/regular period/good understanding within the family", which corresponded to the local definition of a woman in the best health state. The duration for each condition, except for death, is stressed as one year, although most women in the pretest found this difficult to believe or understand conceptually. This is especially problematic, not surprisingly, for mild conditions and relatively short events.

SELECTION OF VALUATION METHOD AND APPROACH

The original goal was to use the PTO method as described within the DALY protocol, to elicit health state valuations. Through pretest group and individual exercises with non-health professional women aged 18–45,

Table 3   Health state indicator conditions, Cambodian reproductive health study

Type of indicator condition	11 of the 22 indicator conditions from DALY protocol	15 reproductive health and illness indicator conditions specific to this study
Physical disability	Below-the-knee amputation; blindness; deafness; quadriplegia	
Cognitive function	Dementia	
Mental health	Active psychosis; unipolar major depression	Toas (post-partum chills/weakness/sadness)
Complex social problem	Infertility; recto-vaginal fistula; vitiligo on face	AIDS; severe pain during sexual intercourse
Pain/discomfort (continuous, from exertion, intermittent, debilitating)		Moderate pelvic cramps and low back pain during menstruation; moderate dizziness; prolapse; STD with foul discharge and extreme pain (PID)
Reproductive illness, events, situations	Severe anaemia	Abortion at 3 months with haemorrhage and sepsis; miscarriage at 3 months with no complications; fetal death at 7 months; no suitable contraceptive method available; severe eclampsia; unable to breastfeed
Potential best and worst anchors		Bright skin/regular period/good understanding in family; death (maternal)

the PTO method, as well as a version of the standard gamble method, were unsuccessfully implemented.

Person trade-off method. For the PTO, the DALY protocol specifying both PTO1 (quantity of life of healthy versus disabled individuals) and PTO2 (quantity of life of healthy versus improved quality of life for disabled individuals) frames were attempted both as group and individual exercises. Five of the 22 indicator conditions were attempted, including blindness, infertility, below-the-knee amputation, severe headache and unipolar major depression. Almost all women selected from the community were reluctant to conduct either PTO1 or PTO2 in the urban pretest group aged 25–38 (8 out of 10 women) or in the rural pretest group aged 18–27 (10 out of 11 women). Almost all women seeking care from urban health care facilities aged 36–45 were reluctant to conduct either PTO frames in individual interviews (10 out of 12 women). Locally appropriate visual aids, such as a balance commonly used to weigh goods in the market, facilitated the comprehension of the trade-off. However, most women were unwilling to trade off lives, as found in other studies (Fowler et al. 1995): several women noted "…the choice is up to Buddha." Even though most women seemed to understand the trade-off, it is the author's opinion that many simply stated "I don't know" or "I don't understand" in an effort to avoid being forced to give an answer.

Standard gamble method. Given the unsuccessful implementation of the PTO, an alternative method that supposedly provides valuations on an interval scale was attempted. For the standard gamble, three chronic health states were attempted: blindness, infertility and severe anaemia. The specific frame was a gamble between a certain choice A, of 100 people being blind, or an uncertain choice B, of 100 people with the probability $(1 - p)$ of dying immediately. Normally, the probability combinations are varied in a high/low fashion and the final valuation is achieved when the participant is indifferent between choice A and choice B. Although a commonly used visual aid, a board with a wheel for probability combinations for healthy (p) or dead $(1 - p)$ was used, and analogies to other forms of gambling and betting were described, no one in the pretest groups or individual interviews understood or completed a standard gamble. Although in Cambodia gambling is socially unacceptable for women to participate in, it is the author's opinion that this was not an obstacle in completing the standard gamble exercise.

Visual analogue scale method. In the pretest, the category rating scale using a visual analogue scale (VAS) was successfully implemented. In the pretest, all women in group discussions and individual interviews completed consistent ordinal rankings and category ratings for the five indicator conditions attempted: blindness, infertility, below-the-knee amputation, severe headache and unipolar major depression. The visual aids of a 100 mm horizontal VAS with 100 equal-appearing division lines, a pointer, and index cards with each health state label and standardized descriptions in Khmer, were used. The top anchor of the scale was labelled "the most desirable health state, only positive consequences and no burden" while the bottom anchor of the scale was labelled "death". Participants were instructed that the rating should "best reflect the value of the burden (e.g. conceptually understood as both disability and handicap) that an average person with that health state for one year in Cambodia will experience". Each step on the scale is described as an equal interval (i.e. the distance between 15 and 20 is the same as between 70 and 75). Participants are also instructed that ties, clusters and the unequal spacing of health states along the VAS is allowed, given other studies' findings on the use of the VAS. For hypothetical health states, lucky numbers, such as 40 or 70 in Cambodia, were not selected more often, although this was initially observed when women valued their own health. As many women wanted to value some hypothetical health states worse than death, the label for the bottom anchor of the scale was changed to "the least desirable health state, worst negative consequences and heaviest burden".

DELIBERATIVE APPROACH

Although the DALY protocol calls to challenge participants "with the implications of their valuations" within a deliberative approach of "a group exercise which allows for substantial exchange and revision", in practice, such a format was inappropriate among semi-literate and literate Cambodian women participating in the pretest. This was so as even in relatively homogenous groups, women with the highest social status or literally the strongest voice set the model for others to follow. Also, many semi-literate women relied on or simply copied others in order to keep up with the group's pace. By observation, several individuals' views were therefore marginalized in the pretest groups. Hence for this study, individual reflection was chosen in lieu of group deliberation.

FINAL STUDY METHODS

VALUATION METHOD AND APPROACH

As noted, local concepts of disability and handicap formed the conceptual basis of what should be valued or disvalued associated with each health state. Individual interviews were designed so that women valued their own health state in isolation early on in the interview using a visual analogue scale. Women participants then subsequently ranked 26 hypothetical health states, ranked their own health state within the 26 ranked states, and then values were elicited for all 27 health states using a visual analogue scale. Facilitators read the full description of each health state and gave each woman a set of printed cards in Khmer with 26 hypothetical health state labels and short description, plus one card stating in Khmer "your health today and its burden (disability and handicap)". The facilitators engaged in discussions with each woman on what she understood as each health state, her own health, the value or disvalue attached to these different health states, and the implications of her values given the potential use of the information to compare levels of health across or within populations or to distribute scarce social resources. Women were not forced to change "irrational values"—i.e. one individual ranked and valued death as the best state[9]—but were required to provide internally consistent valuations (between ordinal ranking and VAS valuation of health states). As noted, some women ranked and valued a few health states worse than death, as found in other studies (Patrick et al. 1994), and the revised VAS accommodated women's views even though this was not consistent with the DALY protocol where death has a severity weight equivalent to 1.0 and all other health states are less than 1.0. Overall, the deliberation process encouraged individuals to defend their views in a non-threatening way, rather than forcing agreement with the facilitator through debate or pressure.

Along with the author, the facilitators included two Cambodian female lecturers from the Department of Psychology, Royal University of Phnom Penh, with substantial experience in conducting interviews and group discussions with women in rural and urban communities and within health services facilities. All discussions, interviews and exercises were conducted in Khmer, with explicit informed consent obtained from all individuals.

SELECTION OF PARTICIPANTS

A sample of female non-health professionals ($n = 40$) aged 15–54 years were selected as participants within this study. Half of these women were randomly selected from three urban districts in Phnom Penh, while the other half were randomly selected from individuals seeking health services for either mild or serious reproductive health problems, or psychological/ psychiatric conditions from two private reproductive health clinics and two large public hospitals in Phnom Penh. Age quotas ensured that women were selected across age groups. Although this study represents a small number of participants, the sample size is more than three times the number of participants that were included within the Geneva exercise with international health experts. Table 4 details participants' background characteristics by sample group.

ANALYSIS OF DATA COLLECTED

Valuations using a 100 mm visual analogue scale with 100 equivalent to the best health state and 0 equivalent to the worst possible health state (as two states were valued worse than death), were transformed to a 1–0 severity scale, with 1 equivalent a valuation of 0 and 0 equivalent to a valuation of 100. For the 26 indicator conditions, Spearman's rank order correlation coefficients (for ordinal ranks) and Pearson's correlation co-efficients (for cardinal values) were calculated in order to estimate the similarity of each group's ranking and valuation of health states, by sampling design (community or seeking services and by type of health problem), age group (15–24; 25–34; 35–44; 45–54 years) and years of education (0–3; 4–6; 7–10; 11 or greater).

RESULTS

For the overall sample, the average VAS valuation, standard deviation, and severity weight associated with each of the 26 hypothetical health states are presented in Table 5. At the mild end, the best anchor "bright skin/

Table 4　　Sample characteristics by group selection, Phnom Penh, Females

Characteristic	Community (n = 20)	Seeking care (n = 20)
Mean age (range)	34 (17–54)	32.7 (19–51)
Currently married	65%	75%
Participating in income generating activities	60%	55%
Residing in female headed households	25%	25%
Mean household size	5.8	5.2
≤ 6 school years completed	25%	50%
Currently pregnant	10%	20%
Children ever born	2.3	2.6

regular period/good relations within the family" has a weight of .015. At the worst end, rather than "death", two states are on average valued worse than death, AIDS (.936) and psychosis (.909). Standard deviations are greater for health states in the middle to mild portion of the spectrum. As expected given the use of the VAS, the disability weights associated with the array of 26 health states are fairly evenly spaced across the range of possible values between 0 and 1, except for states at both ends of the spectrum, as noted in Figure 1.

Table 5   VAS valuations, standard deviation, and severity weights for 26 indicator conditions, Cambodia study and severity weights from GBD study for 11 overlapping indicator conditions[a]

Health state	Valuation (0–100)	SD	Severity weights (1–0)	
			Cambodia	GBD
AIDS	6.4	11.9	0.936	
Active psychosis	9.1	10.8	0.909	0.722
Maternal death	9.4	18.7	0.906	
Blindness	18.2	10.8	0.818	0.642
Quadriplegia	20.0	12.1	0.800	0.895
Dementia	24.3	19.7	0.757	0.762
Deaf	30.4	22.1	0.696	0.333
Infertility	35.0	26.7	0.650	0.191
Severe eclampsia	35.3	20.7	0.647	
Below-the-knee amputation	36.8	15.6	0.632	0.281
Prolapse	39.6	17.2	0.604	
Recto-vaginal fistula	42.3	21.1	0.577	0.373
Severe pain during sex	43.3	23.6	0.567	
Vitiligo on face	46.4	25.9	0.536	0.020
Fetal death at 7 months	51.3	17.2	0.487	
Severe anaemia	51.8	22.0	0.482	0.111
Unipolar depression	54.9	19.0	0.451	0.619
STD w/symptoms	56.3	22.4	0.437	
Abortion at 3 months w/hem/sepsis	58.1	19.6	0.419	
Sad/chills/weak post-natal	58.4	18.6	0.416	
No satisfactory contraception	61.0	23.9	0.390	
Miscarriage at 3 months	65.6	19.3	0.344	
Unable to breastfeed	71.6	19.7	0.284	
Moderate cramps/period	71.8	20.2	0.282	
Moderate dizziness	81.3	17.8	0.187	
Bright skin—regular period	98.5	6.5	0.015	

[a] overlapping indicator conditions in bold.

Final column: Murray (1996).

Figure 1   Severity weights associated with 26 hypothetical health states, based on VAS valuations, *n* = 40, Phnom Penh, Cambodia

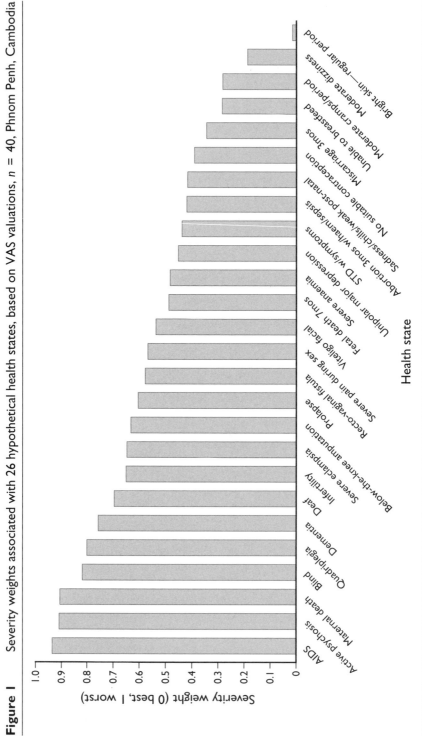

The similarity of ranking and valuation of health states for the 26 indicator conditions across sample groups and by age group or number of school years is remarkably high within this study. Table 6 notes that both the Spearman's rank order correlation and Pearson's correlation coefficients are .95 or higher between the community and seeking health services group, and between those seeking mild or serious reproductive health services. Across age and school year groups, these correlations are almost all above .90. The lowest correlations (.76/.81) are found between the group with the lowest number of school years completed (0–3) and highest number of school years completed (≥ 11).

Although numbers are small within each group, a closer look at the significant differences between the lowest and highest education group may generate some hypotheses concerning the source of variance. Table 7 notes health states with severity weights of at least .150 more or less severe based on the average valuations of the lowest versus highest education group.

Table 6   Correlations[a] of average health state valuations, 26 indicator conditions, across sample group, type of service, age and school years

Group			
Seeking services (n = 20)			
Community (n = 20)	.96/.98		

Type of service			
	Mild RH	Serious RH	Psych
Mild RH (n = 8)	—		
Serious RH (n = 7)	.95/.95	—	
Psych (n = 5)	.83/.87	.88/.90	—

Age				
	15–24	25–34	35–44	45–54
15–24 (n = 10)	—			
25–34 (n = 13)	.93/.93	—		
35–44 (n = 9)	.93/.93	.97/.96	—	
45–54 (n = 8)	.91/.92	.90/.93	.89/.94	—

School years				
	0–3	4–6	7–10	≥ 11
0–3 (n = 4)	—			
4–6 (n = 11)	.90/.88	—		
7–10 (n = 19)	.92/.93	.96/.97	—	
≥ 11 (n = 6)	.76/.81	.89/.90	.89/.91	—

a. Spearman's Rank Order Correlation Coefficient/Pearson's Correlation Coefficient.

Table 7   Health states with a difference in severity weights at least .150, based on health state valuations of individuals with 0–3 ($n = 4$) and ≥ 11 ($n = 6$) school years

Health state	0–3 years	≥ 11 years
A. Health states valued at least .150 points more severe by individuals with 0–3 school years than ≥ 11		
HIV+/AIDS	.982	.823
Quadriplegia	.920	.752
Infertility	.760	.580
Vitiligo on face	.715	.325
Severe pain during sexual intercourse	.635	.378
No suitable contraceptive	.445	.285
B. Health states valued at least .150 points more severe by individuals with ≥ 11 school years than 0–3		
Deafness	.557	.787
Fetal death at 7 months	.347	.598
Abortion w/ haemorrhage & sepsis at 3 months	.232	.510
Sad/chills/weak post-natal	.245	.478

Health states valued significantly more severe by the lowest education group include quadriplegia, infertility, vitiligo on the face, AIDS, severe pain during sexual intercourse and no suitable contraceptive. Health states valued significantly more severe by the highest education group include deafness, fetal death at 7 months, abortion with haemorrhage and sepsis at 3 months, and *toas*, a locally named post-natal condition where a women is sad, has chills and is weak.

Concerning the valuation of own health state, Table 8 lists the severity weight associated with the first trial when women valued their own health state in isolation, before being exposed to any of the indicator health conditions or discussing the meaning and implications of the valuation (ad hoc frame), and the second trial when women valued their own health state, after ranking the 26 indicator health states and discussed the implications of their valuations (deliberative frame). Women sampled from the community, with mild or serious reproductive health conditions, or in younger age groups, tend to value their health as more severe within the ad hoc frame, in comparison to the deliberative frame. The reverse is noted for women seeking services for psychological problems, in the oldest age group, or with least education, as these women tend to value their health less severe within the ad hoc frame, in comparison to the deliberative frame.

The severity weights for the 11 indicator conditions that overlap between the DALY protocol and this study are in bold in Table 5. Of these 11 health states, the severity weights based on the DALY protocol implemented in Geneva with international health experts are listed in the final

Table 8   Comparison of severity weight of own health state, based on first (ad hoc) and second (deliberative) valuation trial

	First	Second	p ≤ .05	Direction	Second severity weight similar to indicator health state
Group					
Community	0.305	0.256	•	Better	Moderate cramps/low back pain, moderate dizziness
Seeking care	0.401	0.397		Better	No suitable contraception
Type of service					
Mild RH	0.328	0.280	•	Better	Moderate cramps/low back pain/ period
Serious RH	0.507	0.474	•	Better	Severe anaemia, fetal death 7 mos
Psychological	0.370	0.476	•	Worse	Unipolar major depression
Age					
15–24	0.262	0.224	•	Better	Moderate dizziness
25–34	0.451	0.414	•	Better	*Toas* post–natal
35–44	0.331	0.279	•	Better	Moderate cramps/low back pain
45–54	0.331	0.366	•	Worse	No suitable contraception
School years					
0–3	0.462	0.600	•	Worse	Prolapse
4–6	0.452	0.333	•	Better	Miscarriage 3 mos
7–10	0.311	0.289		Better	Unable to breastfeed
≥ 11	0.233	0.250		Worse	Moderate cramps/low back pain, moderate dizziness

column and are generally much lower for eight conditions (particularly vitiligo on face, severe anaemia, infertility, below-the-knee amputation and deafness), higher for two conditions (depression and quadriplegia), and almost the same for one condition (dementia). Figure 2 is a scatter plot of the severity weights for health states common to both studies.

DISCUSSION

Given the objectives of the study, three areas are briefly discussed: (i) the feasibility and acceptability to replicate the DALY protocol to measure severity weights with non-health professionals among women in Phnom Penh, Cambodia and the potential validity of the approach taken instead; (ii) variation within Cambodia; and (iii) variation between international health experts' and Cambodian women's valuations for the same health states.

Figure 2   Comparison of severity weights for 11 overlapping indicator
conditions, person trade-off (PTO) with international
health experts in Geneva and Visual Analogue Scale (VAS)
with non-health professional women, Phnom Penh

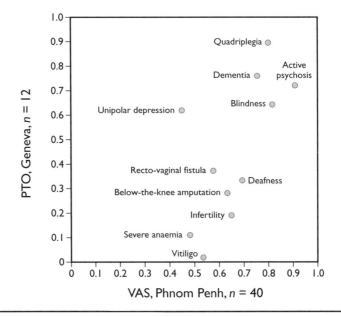

FEASIBILITY OF DALY PROTOCOL AND VALIDITY OF APPROACH
DEVELOPED

This study found that the DALY protocol to value health states and assign
severity weights to indicator conditions could not be replicated "as is"
among non-health professional women in Phnom Penh, Cambodia. Not
all women understood all 22 indicator conditions' labels or their qualitative descriptions. For a few indicator conditions, this was not surprising:
for example, the description of *angina* states that when assessing the severity of pain "do not take into consideration your clinical judgment that
someone with this degree of angina may have an increased risk of death",
or the label "*2 standard deviations below weight/height*". For a health state
to be understood by non-health professionals, how the state is described
using non-technical language seemed more important than familiarity with
the health state. Although not explicitly tested within this study, further
development of standardized health state descriptions that include labels
along with a classification system based on the conceptual understanding
of health (see Table 1 for examples) may improve description and communication to non-health professionals.

Concerning the valuation method, most individuals were reluctant to
conduct any variant of the person trade-off approach. Although not in the
DALY protocol, given the level of abstraction required, it is not surpris-

ing that no one completed a valuation based on the standard gamble. It is important to note that during the pretest, facilitators discussed that they could have "forced" women to use these methods and provide answers. However, it was their belief that the valuations obtained would neither reflect what women actually believed nor would they as researchers be able to defend the results. All women were able to complete valuations based on the VAS and facilitators believed that these values corresponded to the study participants' ideas reflected through in-depth discussions. This is so even if the VAS may be considered less "rigorous" in terms of achieving interval scale properties or theoretical grounding. This is not to argue that the valuation method selected and the deliberative process should necessarily be "easy" to implement, as making choices concerning scarce resources that will affect people's lives is a difficult process.

Critics of the VAS claim that the severity associated with mild states may be over-estimated, given the even spreading out of states across the full range of the scale. Given that individuals appear to place the available health states across the entire 100 mm scale, the inclusion of a sufficient range of health states in terms of severity that cover different types of health problems, as recommended within the DALY protocol, is good advice. Others have suggested using a log scale for the first ten points as one means to "deflate" the value attached to milder states.[10] However, valuations obtained from altered scales or from transformations of values based on estimated relationships to other valuation methods, should be evaluated for validity, i.e. do these still reflect the ideas of the people providing valuations?

Concerning the approach, individual interviews gave equal voice to each participant and ensured greater understanding of the valuation task, particularly for semi-literate women who generally required more time to complete the exercise. However, this choice placed all of the responsibility on the facilitator to raise questions in a non-threatening fashion with each participant, in order to resolve inconsistencies between ordinal rankings and VAS valuations, and discuss the implications of valuations made. Neutrality was very important: given the differences in power and agency between facilitators and participants, it was not uncommon that participants wanted to please the facilitator or avoid confrontation. Even with this understanding, differences in social status and authority between female participants and facilitators could not be removed, and may have nevertheless influenced the deliberative process and outcome of the exercise.

This and other factors concerning the validity of valuations obtained, raises the question of whether one can judge and defend one set of valuations based on in-depth deliberation and clarification of views versus another set of valuations that reflect a change from an individual's original views to fit potentially some target view, irrespective of the method used. If reflection on complex choices leads to shifts in values, evidence from this study suggests that despite simplifying the DALY protocol and conducting individual exercises, women shifted their valuations of their own health state in a defensible manner, as they incorporated information on the range of hypothetical health states over the course of the exercise. This finding bodes well for population-based surveys using simplified methods. Two pieces of evidence exist.

First, it appears that the ad hoc valuation of one's own health state may reflect some of the same biases associated with the self-report of morbidity or health that limit comparability across groups or populations status (see Sadana et al., chapter 8.1, and Murray et al., chapter 8.3). As Table 8 notes, the direction of change from the ad hoc to more deliberative valuation of one's own health state, for most subgroups suggests that by placing one's own health state in context of a range of health states, and discussing the meaning of the valuation, the direction of change indicates a greater understanding of the possible range of health states. For example, women in the community gave a better valuation of their health status, as did women with mild health problems or in younger age groups, during the second trial. It is possible that the ad hoc isolated valuation was an "over estimation" of the severity associated with their health state. The reverse is so for women with psychological problems, in the oldest age groups, or with the least amount of education, as their ad hoc valuations may have been an "under estimation" of the severity associated with their health state. Although these results are based on small numbers, similar "validity checks" may be useful to incorporate within population-based studies eliciting health state valuations. Given that clarification of values should occur from the ad hoc to deliberative trial, reliability in this case is not desirable.

Furthermore, values appear consistent between the valuation of one's own health state and the hypothetical health states included, given average severity weights for subgroups. The final column in Table 8 provides some guidelines on how to interpret the severity weights associated with valuations of one's own health state based on the second trial, in comparison with the severity weights generated for the hypothetical indicator conditions. For example, the average severity weight of their own health state associated with women seeking services for serious reproductive conditions (.474), is closest to the severity weights associated with the hypothetical health states of severe anaemia (.482) and fetal death at 7 months (.487). Developing similar approaches to improve the meaning and interpretation of valuations obtained in population based surveys may evaluate the validity of methods employed and enhance the credibility of results.

Variation within Cambodia

Based on the correlation coefficients reported in Table 6, variance of health state valuations within the sample is minimal for hypothetical states irrespective of demographic background or use of health services. For the subgroups where the correlation is weakest (among lowest and highest education groups), one hypothesis to explain the difference in severity weights of the same health state (see Table 7) is that for women with least education, states that were associated with stigma or shame were valued as more severe, while for the more educated group, avoidable or negative reproductive outcomes were valued as more severe. Although based on small numbers, these results suggest that population-based valuations of health states may be consistent, but that potential differences by socioeconomic level, particularly for the most vulnerable or marginalized populations, should be reported and discussed. This is important as the *means* to calculate summary measures should investigate and reflect different perspectives in a particular setting, even if population averages are ultimately used in the end.

VARIATION BETWEEN INTERNATIONAL HEALTH EXPERTS' AND
CAMBODIAN WOMEN'S VALUATIONS.

Not surprisingly, different conceptual basis, valuation method, range of health states, participants, deliberative approach and context, produce different severity weights for the 11 indicator conditions common to both protocols (see Table 9 summarizing differences in methods). Another limitation in the comparison is that men were excluded in the Cambodian sample. Nevertheless, a recognizable pattern exists: valuations for the more severe health states are more similar, while health states associated with stigma and shame, are much more severely disvalued by Cambodian women than by experts in Geneva. These differences may not simply be explained away by differences in methods, e.g. in particular, infertility (.650 in this study, .191 by Geneva experts).

These findings cannot determine whose values are more valid or more narrowly which valuation approach is more valid. The answers to these

Table 9   Differences in methods between Cambodian study and
GBD DALY protocol to elicit health state valuations

	Study	
	Quantifying Reproductive Health and Illness	Global Burden of Disease
Location	Cambodia: participants' homes & health services' locations	Geneva: World Health Organization
Participants	Cambodian women, non-health professionals, $n = 40$	International health professionals, 40% women, 60% men, $n = 12$
Valuation method	VAS	PTO
Facilitators	Cambodian female psychologists	GBD study team
Deliberative process	Individual reflection	Group discussion
Severity weight interpretation	Disability & handicap	Between disability & handicap
No. of indicator states	26	22
Average time	2 hours	8–10 hours

questions may vary depending on the intended use of the severity weights and more generally of summary measures of population health. However, if social values are to be explicitly incorporated within summary measures of population health, what does seem clear is that differences or similarities in health state valuations should be documented within and across populations and openly discussed.

CONCLUDING REMARKS

Further development and testing of methods to value health states should provide support for methods that are acceptable and reflect the way nonhealth experts think about health. Economist Jose-Luis Pinto Prades argues rationally that if participants in valuation exercises "cannot use the response mode most convenient to investigators, then investigators must find a response mode that works" for the participants (Pinto-Prades 1997, p. 78). It is also possible that no one magic question or approach exists to elicit health state valuations.

More generally, open discussion of the development and interpretation of health indicators that explicitly take into account social values is important, as social acceptance is not based solely on the technical soundness of a methodology—health policy is not simply a technocratic exercise. In fact the inclusion of population representative values may be as important as the technical debates on specific approaches to measurement. Concerning health state valuations, on one hand, improving the validity and reliability of severity weights should not be pursued at the expense of suppressing different perspectives. On the other hand, although efforts should be expended to improve valuation methods, researchers should not lose focus that the ultimate goal is to improve health, not the measurement of severity weights.

ACKNOWLEDGEMENTS

In addition to the individuals who consented to participate, I thank Kruy Kim Hourn and Sek Sisokhom, from the Department of Psychology, Royal University of Phnom Penh, for their persistence and insights during the field work in Cambodia; Carla AbouZahr, from the World Health Organization, Geneva, for being specifically interested in severity weights for reproductive health; and Christopher JL Murray, at the time of fieldwork, from the Department of Population and International Health, Harvard School of Public Health, for providing details of the GBD study protocol. Earlier versions of this chapter were presented in 1998 at the *Eighth Annual Public Health Forum: Reforming Health Sectors* held at the London School of Hygiene & Tropical Medicine, and at an *Informal Consultation on DALYs and Reproductive Health*, organized by the Reproductive Health Technical Support Unit, World Health Organization, Geneva.

NOTES

1   The need for a non-monetary value of a good did not originate within the health field, but environment sector. The disvalue associated with various types and levels of environmental pollution, in comparison with a clean environment led to the development of valuation methods. From a social perspective, a clean environment and a healthy population may be considered as public goods.

2   Biases specific to different methods, such as valuations of the severity of health states being confounded by time preference or risk aversion.

3   The draft ICIDH has now been recently finalized and renamed to the International Classification of Functioning, Disability and Health. The conceptual framework has also been modified (see WHO 2001).

4   Briefly, individuals completed two person trade-off (PTO) exercises. PTO1 is a trade between the life extension of healthy individuals versus the life extension of individuals in a given health state i. PTO2 is a trade between raising quality of life of those in health state i to perfect health for 1 year versus extending life for healthy individuals for one year. The exercise ends when individuals are indifferent between the trade-off. Both PTO exercises were conducted for each of the 22 indicator conditions, resulting usually in two health state valuations for each condition. Two PTOs are conducted to reveal to individuals their own inconsistencies. Individuals were then requested to resolve inconsistencies between the two valuations per condition, deliberate within the group, and revise in private. Each of the 22 indicator conditions were also ranked by severity and these ordinal rankings are compared with the rankings based on the final person trade-off valuation for each indicator condition.

5   Personal communication to the author by three of the participants in the Geneva expert group.

6   The range of morbidity was not limited to bio-medical disease labels or sequelae, but also indigenously named illnesses, conditions or events, that may be shaped by social norms and rituals, that depend on the individual's family or life cycle phase, or that reflect historical changes in social and political expectations for health. This knowledge informed the types of health states added as indicator conditions within this study.

7   Beyond the scope of this paper, these additional states were to include reproductive events or sequelae excluded from the estimation of disease burden within the GBD Study. For example, within the GBD study, by design many events or episodes are assigned a disability weight of .000 if it is assumed no subsequent disability results due to these problems. Within reproductive health—the focus of the larger study that this feasibility study was nested within—episodes of maternal haemorrhage, maternal sepsis and obstructed labour, among others, are assigned a disability weight of .000 within the GBD Study. Only selected sequelae resulting from one of these episodes, such as Sheehan's syndrome (.093) or severe anaemia (.065) following maternal haemorrhage; infertility (.180) following maternal sepsis; or stress incontinence (.025) or recto-vaginal fistula (.430) following obstructed labour, are given the indicated disability weights for the 15–44 year age group irrespective of treatment classification.

8   This may reflect that cause of death contributes to the valuation of death; however, this hypothesis was not tested within this study.

9   This participant explained that "if a woman died after giving birth, in her next life she will be a man and will then be much better off…she'll avoid a lot of misery".

10 Salomon J, personal communication.

REFERENCES

Anand S, Hanson K (1995) *Disability-adjusted life years: a critical review. Harvard Center for Population and Development Studies.* (Working paper no 95/06.) Harvard Center for Population and Development Studies, Cambridge, MA.

Ashby J, O'Hanlon M, Buxton MJ (1994) The time trade-off technique: how do the valuations of breast cancer patients compare to those of other groups? *Quality of Life Research,* 3(4):257–265.

Barker C, Green A (1996) Opening the debate on DALYs. *Health Policy and Planning,* 11(2):179–183.

Dolan P, Gudex C, Kind P, Williams A (1996) Valuing health states: a comparison of methods. *Journal of Health Economics,* 15(2):209–231.

Evans TG, Ranson MK (1995) The global burden of trachomatous visual impairment: II. Assessing burden. *International Ophtamology,* 19(5):271–280.

Fowler FJ, Cleary PD, Massagli MP, et al. (1995) The role of reluctance to give up life in the measurement of the values of health states. *Medical Decision-making,* 15(3):195–200.

Krabbe PFM, Essink-Bot ML, Bonsel GJ (1997) The comparability and reliability of five health-state valuation methods. *Social Science and Medicine,* 45(11):1641–1652.

Llewellyn-Thomas H, Sutherland HJ, Tibshirani R, Ciampi A, Till JE, Boyd NF (1984) Describing health states: methodologic issues in obtaining values for health states. *Medical Care,* 22(6):543–552.

Murray CJL (1994) Quantifying the burden of disease: the technical basis for disability-adjusted life years. In: *Global comparative assessments in the health sector.* Murray CJL, Lopez AD, eds. World Health Organization, Geneva.

Murray CJL (1996) Rethinking DALYs. In: *The global burden of disease: a comprehensive assessment of mortality and disability from diseases, injuries, and risk factors in 1990 and projected to 2020.* The Global Burden of Disease and Injury, Vol. 1. Murray CJL, Lopez AD, eds. Harvard School of Public Health on behalf of WHO, Cambridge, MA.

Murray CJL, Acharya AK (1997) Understanding DALYs. *Journal of Health Economics,* 16:703–730.

Murray CJL, Lopez AD, eds. (1994) *Global comparative assessments in the health sector: disease burden, expenditures and intervention packages: collected reprints from the Bulletin of the World Health Organization.* World Health Organization, Geneva.

Murray CJL, Lopez AD (1996c) Evidence-based health policy: lessons from the global burden of disease study. *Science,* **274**(5288):740–743.

Murray CJL, Lopez AD, eds. (1996b) *Global health statistics: a compendium of incidence, prevalence and mortality estimates for over 200 conditions.* Global Burden of Disease and Injury, Vol 2. Harvard School of Public Health on behalf of WHO, Cambridge, MA.

Murray CJL, Lopez AD, eds. (1996a) *The global burden of disease: a comprehensive assessment of mortality and disability from diseases, injuries and risk factors in 1990 and projected to 2020.* Global Burden of Disease and Injury, Vol. 1. Harvard School of Public Health on behalf of WHO, Cambridge, MA.

Murray CJL, Lopez AD (1997a) Alternative projections of mortality and disability by cause 1990–2020: global burden of disease study. *Lancet,* **349**(9064):1498–1504.

Murray CJL, Lopez AD (1997b) Global mortality, disability and the contribution of risk factors: global burden of disease study. *Lancet,* **349**(9063):1436–1442.

Murray CJL, Lopez AD (1997c) Mortality by cause for eight regions of the world: global burden of disease study. *Lancet,* **349**(9061):1269–1276.

Murray CJL, Lopez AD (1997d) Regional patterns of disability-free life expectany and disability-adjusted life expectancy: global burden of disease study. *Lancet,* **349**(9062):1347–1352.

Murray CJL, Lopez AD, eds. (1998) *Health dimensions of sex and reproduction: the global burden of sexually transmitted diseases, HIV, maternal conditions, perinatal disorders, and congenital anomalies.* Global Burden of Disease and Injury, Vol 3. Harvard School of Public Health on behalf of WHO, Cambridge, MA.

Nord E (1995) The person-trade off approach to valuing health care programs. *Medical Decision-making,* **15**(3):201–208.

Nord EM (1992) Methods for quality adjustment of life years. *Social Science and Medicine,* **34**(5):559–569.

Paalman M, Bekedam H, Hawken L, et al. (1998) A critical review of priority setting in the health sector: the methodology of the 1993 World Development Report. *Health Policy and Planning,* **13** (1):13–31.

Patrick DL, Starks HE, Cain KC, Uhlmann RF, Pearlman RA (1994) Measuring preferences for health states worse than death. *Medical Decision-making,* **14**(1):9–18.

Pierre U, Wood-Dauphinee S, Korner-Bitensky N, Gayton D, Hanley J (1998) Proxy use of the Canadian SF-36 in rating health status of the disabled elderly. *Journal of Clinical Epidemiology,* **51** (11):983–990.

Pinto-Prades JL (1997) Is the person trade-off a valid method for allocating health care resources. *Health Economics,* **6**(1):71–81.

Richardson J (1994) Cost-utility analysis: what should be measured? *Social Science and Medicine,* **39**(1):7–21.

Sadana R (2001) Social discourses and individual narratives: contexts, meanings and embodied experiences of reproductive health and illness in Cambodia. In: *Quantifying reproductive health and illness.* Doctoral dissertation. Harvard School of Public Health, Boston, MA.

Shibuya K (1999) *Quantifying the economic impact and health consequences of smoking.* Doctoral dissertation. Harvard School of Public Health, Boston, MA.

Tversky A, Kahneman D (1981) The framing of decisions and the psychology of choice. *Science,* **211**(4481):453–458.

WHO (1980) *International classification of impairments, disabilities, and handicaps: a manual of classification relating to the consequences of disease.* World Health Organization, Geneva. (Reprint 1993)

WHO (1996) *Investing in health research and development.* (Report of the Ad Hoc Committee on Health Research Priorities.) World Health Organization, Geneva.

WHO (1998) *DALYs and reproductive health: report of an informal consultation.* WHO/RHT/98.28. World Health Organizaton/Division of Reproductive Health, Geneva.

WHO (2001) *International classification of functioning, disability and health (ICF).* World Health Organization, Geneva.

World Bank (1993) *World development report: investing in health.* Oxford University Press, New York.

Chapter 11.4

A CONCEPTUAL FRAMEWORK FOR UNDERSTANDING ADAPTATION, COPING AND ADJUSTMENT IN HEALTH STATE VALUATIONS

JOSHUA A. SALOMON AND CHRISTOPHER J.L. MURRAY

INTRODUCTION

One of the most important controversies in the measurement of health state valuations revolves around the question of whose values should be used in constructing summary measures of population health (SMPH). Various types of respondents have been proposed, including individuals in the health states, families of these individuals, health care providers or the general public. A number of empirical studies have examined differences across these different groups (Balaban et al. 1986; Bennett et al. 1997; Boyd et al. 1990; Dolan 1999; Patrick et al. 1982; Revicki et al. 1996; Sackett and Torrance 1978; Saigal et al. 1999; Slevin et al. 1990).

In part, these controversies have been imported from related debates on health state valuations in other applications such as clinical decision analyses, which may have different requirements. For example, arguments that clinical cost-effectiveness studies should include valuations from patients in the actual health states under consideration do not necessarily imply that patients are the most appropriate respondents for valuations used in the construction of SMPH.

One key empirical finding that has emerged from a number of studies on valuations in different types of respondents is that individuals in a given health state often rate the state more favourably than those who are asked to consider the state hypothetically. One of the reasons that have been cited for this difference is that fact that individuals may adapt to their health condition over time. Thus far, however, there have been only a handful of longitudinal studies that included repeated valuations in the same patient groups in order to examine changes in valuations over time (Llewellyn-Thomas et al. 1984; Postulart and Adang 2000; Tsevat et al. 1995).

The goal of this paper is to provide a clear conceptual basis for understanding why individual assessments of their own health states may shift over time. We also aim to bring into clearer focus some of the reasons why the valuation of an individual's own state may differ from valuations of that state as a hypothetical. Although the word "adaptation" is often used generally to describe health changes over time, we will define three distinct types of changes, which we call adaptation, coping and adjustment, and present a formal framework for characterizing each of these three phenomena in the context of measuring health state valuations.

HEALTH STATE DESCRIPTION AND VALUATION

We begin with a brief explanation of the concepts and notation that we will use to describe adaptation, coping and adjustment.

REPRESENTATION OF HEALTH STATES

Assume that there are J domains that collectively constitute health. For example, domains of health might include mobility, vision, dexterity, cognition and affect, among others. Precise definition of the domains that constitute health is not required for this paper but is considered elsewhere in this volume in the description of the International Classification of Functioning, Disability and Health (see chapter 7.4).

Given that the J domains represent (by definition) an exhaustive catalogue of the relevant components of health, we may represent a specific state of health completely by indicating the levels on each of these domains. Defining y_j^* as the level on domain j, a particular health state may be represented as a vector of J elements:

$$(y_1^*, y_2^*, ..., y_J^*)$$

We use y_j^* to indicate the true level on a domain, which may not be measurable directly in practice for most domains.

INDIVIDUAL ASSESSMENT OF HEALTH STATES

When an individual is asked to assess her own health state, the way that she characterizes her level on a particular domain will depend not only on the actual level, but also on her own norms and expectations for health on that domain. On a categorical survey question, for example, the same true level of health may be considered "excellent" by some respondents and "good" or "fair" by others. Thus, an individual's assessment of the domain level associated with a particular health state may be represented as a function of the true domain level and a set of norms against which this true level is measured:

$$y_j = f_j(y_j^*, N_j)$$

where y_j is the assessed level on domain j, y_j^* is defined (as before) as the true level on domain j, and N_j represents the set of norms and expectations that an individual brings to bear on the assessment.

We postulate that norms and expectations will affect not only individual assessments of their own health states, but also the way that individuals characterize hypothetical states. For example, we might imagine that an individual who reports himself as having higher levels on a particular domain relative to others because of relatively lower expectations along that domain will similarly report relatively higher levels when considering hypothetical states, because this individual's entire scale of reference is shifted in relation to others'.

VALUATION OF HEALTH STATES

A valuation of a health state assigns a single number to a vector of levels on different domains of health. A valuation may be given by an individual either for his own health state or for some hypothetical health state. The mapping function by which levels on multiple domains are translated into a single valuation depends on the relative importance placed on different domains.

Broome argues in this volume (chapter 3.1) that such a valuation is impossible because domains of health are not separable from non-health domains of well-being, but we will not address this debate here. The framework we present applies even in the event that valuations of health are inextricably linked to the particular levels of non-health domains, but separability is assumed for the sake of clarity.

We may conceptualize valuations in either of two distinct ways:

1. as a function of the true domain levels associated with a given health state,

$$v(y_1^*, y_2^*, \ldots, y_J^*)$$

or

2. as a function of individual assessments of domain levels, which may depend on the individual's norms and expectations along these domains,

$$v(y_1, y_2, \ldots, y_J) = v(y_1^*, y_2^*, \ldots, y_J^*, N_1, N_2, \ldots, N_J).$$

It is possible that individual valuations of their own states will be affected by the norms against which they assess their own health on specific domains, but that these norms may be less influential in valuations of hypothetical states. If this hypothesis is correct, then self-valuations will take the form expressed in (2), while hypothetical valuations will take the form expressed in (1). In this paper, however, we will consider the implications of alternative modes of interpreting health state valuations for an individual's own health state and hypothetical states. Resolution of the uncertainty around the appropriate conceptualization will await further empirical study.

Adaptation, coping and adjustment

Adaptation

We define adaptation as change in the true health level on one or more domains over time.

As a simple example in which only one domain is affected, we may represent adaptation as a change from $(y_1^*, y_2^*, \ldots, y_J^*)$ to $(y_1^{*\prime}, y_2^*, \ldots, y_J^*)$.

For instance, imagine a right-handed person who suffers an injury that causes paralysis in his right hand. Immediately after the injury, his overall level of dexterity is lower than it was before the injury. After some time passes, however, he may develop greater proficiency in the use of his left hand. This improvement in his overall dexterity is an example of adaptation.

As we have defined it, adaptation refers strictly to changes in some y_j^*, and does not imply any change in the way true health levels are translated into individual assessments of these levels. While the individual who learns to use his left hand more effectively has a change in his actual health state, the norms against which he measures his own dexterity may remain the same. Thus, in the shift from $y_j = f_j(y_j^*, N_j)$ to $y_j' = f_j(y_j^{*\prime}, N_j)$ the individual's assessment of his health changes only via the change in actual health. If the individual's rating of his dexterity changes from "good" to "very good" over this time period, it is attributable to the actual improvement in his dexterity rather than a shift in the cut-points that define self-reported response categories.

Similarly, the difference in valuation depends only on the change in the true level of the affected domain. As we define adaptation, only self-valuations are affected, since neither the individual norms on the domain nor the relative importance of different domains is changed.

Coping

In contrast to adaptation, we define coping as a change in individual assessments of health levels along one or more domains that occurs without any change in the true level on those domains. In this case, the change in the individual's assessment occurs because of changing norms or expectations. Coping therefore applies to both assessments of domain levels in self-reports and descriptions of hypothetical health states.

Imagine an individual who suffers from hearing loss. At the onset of the disability, she may judge her hearing as "poor" in reference to the level to which she is accustomed. Over time, however, this reference point may shift as the individual's expectations for hearing decline. At the same level of hearing, the individual five years after the loss may judge this level to be higher than she did immediately after the loss. In this case, the actual level of hearing does not shift, but she may report it as "fair" rather than "poor". Similarly, if asked to assess the hearing of a hypothetical person who can only hear shouted words and loud music, she may characterize this state more favourably five years after her own hearing loss because of the shift in her norms.

Coping may be represented as a change from $y_j = f_j(y_j^*, N_j)$ to $y_j' = f_j(y_j^*, N_j')$. Because coping does not change the actual health level, the shift will only appear in the valuation function if valuation depends on assessed health levels rather than true health levels. For an individual valuing her own health state, we hypothesize that this valuation occurs through the filters of the individual's norms and expectations and will therefore reflect coping. Whether or not coping affects hypothetical valuations, on the other hand, is somewhat less clear.

ADJUSTMENT

Finally, we define adjustment as a change in the valuation of an identical health state at two different points in time, occurring without any change in either the true health levels or the norms that affect individual assessments of these levels.

Formally, adjustment is represented as a change in the valuation function, from $v(\cdot)$ to $v'(\cdot)$.

In the simplest terms, adjustment may be conceptualized as a shift in the relative importance of different domains. Assume, for the purpose of illustration, that individuals have additive valuation functions that depend on the true domain levels associated with a given health state:

$$v(y_1^*, y_2^*, \dots, y_j^*) = \beta_1 y_1^* + \beta_2 y_2^* + \dots + \beta_j y_j^*$$

This additive form is rather unlikely to provide an adequate representation of most individuals' valuation functions, but provides a convenient example without loss of generality.

Adjustment, in this case, may be represented as a change in the β parameters that act as weights on the different domains of health:

$$v'(y_1^*, y_2^*, \dots, y_j^*) = \beta_1' y_1^* + \beta_2' y_2^* + \dots + \beta_j' y_j^*$$

As a more concrete example, imagine an individual with an amputated leg. Prior to the amputation, her valuation of her own health state (and other states) may have depended strongly on the level of mobility. Several years after the amputation, however, she may place a greater emphasis on other domains such as cognition when she is valuing health states.

Adjustment, by altering the valuation function itself, will lead to different valuations of hypothetical health states in addition to changing the valuation of an individual's own health state. By contrast, adaptation works at the level of the health state, and will therefore affect only an individual's self-valuation; and coping modifies the assessment of a domain level relative to individual norms, and therefore may or may not affect valuations of hypothetical states.

DISCUSSION

In this paper, we have distinguished three different phenomena that may explain some of the variation over time in the health state descriptions and valuations of an individual considering his or her own state. We have presented a formal framework for characterizing each of these phenomena as changes in true health levels, changes in the norms that influence individual assessments of health levels, or changes in the way levels on multiple domains are translated into valuations.

Although the definitions of adaptation, coping and adjustment are framed in terms of shifts in individual descriptions and valuations of their own health states over time, some of their most important implications relate to debates about whose valuations to use in constructing SMPH, and about how to ensure comparability in health state descriptions and valuations within and across populations.

The notions of adaptation, coping and adjustment point to important considerations in developing data inputs for summary measures. One obvious question that follows from the distinction drawn here is: how should each of these phenomena be addressed in the construction of SMPH?

In the case of adaptation, it seems clear that real improvements in domain levels must be reflected in both descriptions and valuations of health states. In principle, since valuations are required for a continuum of health states, the process of adaptation simply leads to differentiation between what are in fact distinct health states.

Coping presents more of a dilemma because it represents a shift in individual assessments of domain levels attributable to varying norms and expectations that arguably should be irrelevant in assessing population health. Much of the current empirical and methodological agenda at the World Health Organization on the measurement of health is geared towards the development of instruments that allow for cross-population comparability (see chapter 8.3). In fact, what these efforts aim to adjust for at the population level is the same phenomenon which coping represents at the individual level, namely variation in assessments of equivalent levels of health in certain domains due to variation in norms and expectations. Coping explains this variation over time at the individual level; meanwhile, the analogous variation across different groups at the population level is one of the principal challenges to establishing cross-population comparability of health measures.

Finally, the notion of adjustment also lends itself to parallel interpretation in a larger population context. For example, the phenomenon of adjustment in a particular individual may be related easily to variation in valuation functions across individuals. This parallel suggests that adjustment is a phenomenon that should be included in the measurement of health state valuations for summary measures. Just as we might imagine that an individual's own health is one of many determinants of her valuation function, we can consider adjustment as a dynamic extension of this argument. If we allow that different individuals in a population may have different valuation functions that reflect real differences in how important domains are relative to each other, it seems logical to allow these valuation functions to change over time as these relative weights shift.

Clearly, many of the questions raised here point to a rich agenda for empirical research. By setting up a conceptual model for describing the phenomena of adaptation, coping and adjustment, we hope that this paper provides an explicit framework within which to address some of the important methodological and empirical challenges that remain. In particular, we believe that by distinguishing between these three phenomena, we may lend some clarity to the design of data collection efforts, and to continuing debates over whose values to use in the construction of SMPH and the analysis of variance and its determinants.

REFERENCES

Balaban DJ, Sagi PC, Goldfarb NI, Nettler S (1986) Weights for scoring the quality of well-being instrument among rheumathoid arthritics. A comparison to general population weights. *Medical Care*, 24:973–980.

Bennett CL, Chapman G, Elstein AS, et al. (1997) A comparison of perspectives on prostrate cancer: analysis of utility assessments of patients and physicians. *European Urology*, 32(S3):86–88.

Boyd NF, Sutherland HJ, Heasman KZ, Tritchler DL, Cummings BJ (1990) Whose utilities for decision analysis? *Medical Decision Making*, 10:58–67.

Dolan P (1999) Whose preferences count? *Medical Decision Making*, 19(482):486

Gabriel SE, Kneeland TS, Melton LJ3, Moncur MM, Ettinger B, Tosteson AN (1999) Health-related quality of life in economic evaluations for osteoporosis: whose values should we use? *Medical Decision Making*, 19(2):141–148.

Heckerling PS, Verp MS, Albert N (1999) Patient or physician preferences for decision analysis: the prenatal genetic testing decision. *Medical Decision Making*, 19:66–77.

Holmes MM, Rovner DR, Rothert ML, et al. (1987) Women's and physicians' utilities for health outcomes in estrogen replacement therapy. *Journal of General Internal Medicine*, 2(3):178–182.

Kind P (1995) Weighting life expectancy for quality: whose values count? *Quality of Life Research*, 4:447–448.

Llewellyn-Thomas H, Sutherland HJ, Tibshirani R, Ciampi A, Till JE, Boyd NF (1984) Describing health states: methodologic issues in obtaining values for health states. *Medical Care*, 22(6):543–552.

Otto RA, Dobie RA, Lawrence V, Sakai C (1997) Impact of a laryngectomy on quality of life: perspective of the patient versus that of the health care provider. *Annals of Otology, Rhinology and Laryngology*, 106(8):693–699.

Patrick DL, Peach H, Gregg I (1982) Disablement and care: a comparison of patient views and general practitioner knowledge. *Journal of the Royal College of General Practitioners,* **32**:429–434.

Postulart D, Adang EM (2000) Response shift and adaptation in chronically ill patients. *Medical Decision Making,* **20**:186–193.

Revicki DA, Shakespeare A, Kind P (1996) Preferences for schizophrenia-related health states: a comparison of patients, caregivers, and psychiatrists. *International Clinical Psychopharmacology,* **11**:101–108.

Sackett DL, Torrance GW (1978) The utility of different health states as perceived by the general public. *Journal of Chronic Diseases,* **31**(11):697–704.

Saigal S, Stoskopf BL, Feeny D, et al. (1999) Differences in preferences for neonatal outcomes among health care professionals, parents and adolescents. *Journal of the American Medical Association,* **281**(21):1991–1997.

Slevin ML, Stubbs L, Plant HJ, et al. (1990) Attitudes to chemotherapy: comparing views of patients with cancer with those of doctors, nurses and general public. *British Medical Journal,* **300** (6737):1458–1460.

Tsevat J, Cook EF, Green ML, et al. (1995) Health values of the seriously ill. *Annals of Internal Medicine,* **122**(7):514–520.

Chapter 12.1

THE POVERTY OF ETHICAL ANALYSES IN ECONOMICS AND THE UNWARRANTED DISREGARD OF EVIDENCE

JEFF RICHARDSON

Normative conclusions in economics are usually based upon a set of assumptions which are untenable in the health sector. Persistence with these assumptions highlights a more fundamental problem: the epistemology of normative economics—the methodology for drawing conclusions with respect to the improvement of social well-being—is itself flawed. Orthodox economics does not include a process for selecting relevant ethical assumptions or context specific ethical theories. Likewise, however, ethics as a discipline is flawed as judged by this same criterion, i.e. the ability to provide an ethical basis for economic and other analyses and which reflects defensible social values. Implicit criteria of universality and immunity from criticism, no matter how contrived the context, leaves ethical principles in an epistemological never-never land: never to be accepted because of empirical evidence about social values and never demonstrable from logical argument alone. It is suggested below that empiricism and ethical theory should be combined in a process described here as "empirical ethics". The endpoint of the suggested process would be, as in the physical sciences, the best currently available theory or hypothesis. The procedure cannot produce certainty and is itself an epistemological theory which cannot be conclusively "proved" by logic or empiricism. It is argued that, like old age, it is nevertheless the best of the available options.

INTRODUCTION

With limited resources there is a need for rules and institutions to ration resources including health services. The task of doing this in a way that maximizes social well-being is the defining task of economics, and economists have devised a theoretical schema and a set of procedures which, for the most part, provide a satisfactory indication of how best to use our resources. In the health sector both the theory and practice of orthodox economics are more problematical. Most fundamentally, the ethical basis of economic orthodoxy—welfarism, or a qualified form of libertarian utilitarianism—does not appear to represent the ethical views of the population. In every country where there is a functional government it has intervened, to a greater or lesser extent, to modify the outcome of the unregulated market, the mechanism which is commonly recommended by economists to achieve maximum social welfare. The rejection of the simple market implies the need for some other set of rules for allocating resources.

It is argued below in part 2 that, not only has orthodox economic theory failed to meet this challenge, but it has adopted a set of assumptions, definitions and conventions that impedes inquiry into social values and obscures the need for ethical enquiry. Ethical questions have been misrepresented as technical issues and as issues where economists have particular expertise and authority. In part 3 it is argued that when social objectives are imperfectly understood there should be an interactive "dialogue" between the public, economists and ethicists to identify widely held social values and that government decision-making should take these into account. It is suggested that the term "Empirical Ethics" would be a useful title for this process. In part 4 a number of the possible criticisms of this process are discussed and, in particular, the damaging assertion that the truth or otherwise of ethical, like physical, laws cannot be found by "voting". This criticism is evaluated in relation to the need for a methodology which bridges the chasm between "disembodied" ethical theories and acceptable policy action.

The chief focus of the paper is not upon the validity or otherwise of the assumptions of orthodox economics, although these are discussed. Rather, it is upon economic methodology or, more correctly, upon the epistemology of normative economics—the way in which economists justify normative conclusions and policy recommendations. It is argued that the almost total disregard of ethical theory is particularly damaging in the context of a value-impregnated field such as health and health care. However it is also argued that, as presently constituted, ethical discourse is flawed as a guide to useful policy. Propositions cannot be proven empirically: they cannot be proven by logic. At best they may help to highlight anomalies in other theories and demonstrate context specific conclusions which violate our moral intentions. Typically, however, the alternative theory is vulnerable to similar context-specific criticism. It is concluded that a useful two-way interaction between ethics and economics can only occur if there is agreement about the status of the knowledge which is achievable in the field of normative economics or applied ethics.

ETHICS AND THE CONCEPTUAL BASIS OF ECONOMICS

The assertion that one state of the world is better than another is always and unavoidably based upon an ethical judgement or belief. The distinction between the achievement of "economic efficiency" and a normative or equity objective such as a particular distribution of benefits does not arise from a fundamental difference in kind between economic "efficiency" and equity or normative objectives, but from the breadth of the acceptance of the ethical—normative—basis of "economic efficiency" and from linguistic convention. It is a convention which is misleading as it wrongly encourages economists to believe that their advocacy of "economic efficiency" is value free. Technical efficiency *per se*—the ability to do more with the same resources or to use fewer resources to do the same job—only results in an improved state of the world if the resources freed by technical efficiency produce more of something which is valued, and this judgement is necessarily "normative" or "ethical". "Pareto efficiency"—the assertion that social well-being is increased if no one is worse off and someone is better off—requires a normative judgement about what it means to be "better off".

Rather than seeking evidence regarding the determinants of individual and social well-being and analysing the ethical components, neoclassical economic orthodoxy adopts a set of assumptions and principles which very largely eliminates the need for ethical inquiry. The first of these is the assumption of "welfarism", the theory that social welfare is a function of individual utilities only. Secondly, utilities are defined by revealed preferences. Thirdly, preferences are determined by consequences and specifically consequences for the mix and volume of goods and services. In principle, processes may be conceptualized as consequences (Culyer 1998) but this seldom occurs and, with some exceptions, it would be difficult to incorporate "process utilities" in applied economic analyses.[1] Pope (2001) has also demonstrated that, in the context of risk, such a conceptualization is inconsistent with the axiomitization of behaviour which is of fundamental and defining importance for neoclassical economic orthodoxy.[2] Fourthly, efficiency is defined by the Pareto criterion noted above and it is assumed that the achievement of Pareto efficiency is self evidently desirable. Fifth, in order to overcome the problem of interpersonal comparisons, the "Kaldor-Hicks Potential Compensation" principle is usually assumed to be acceptable. This is the doctrine that one state should be considered better than another if losers in this second state could, *potentially*, be compensated by the winners while still leaving winners better off. Finally, and as the only concession to the existence of ethical preferences, it is conceded that there will be a social preference for certain distributions of well-being. However, in order to retain Pareto efficiency, it is generally argued that the redistribution of well-being should be achieved by a redistribution of wealth rather than by the provision of services or the regulation of trade.

The combined effect of these assumptions is to eliminate the need for an enquiry into social and ethical objectives other than the initial distribution of wealth. However, even a moment's reflection would convince most people that at least some of these assumptions are contestable. A policy aimed at maximizing utility, especially when it is defined by revealed preferences, requires the maximization of each person's choice (subject to non-interference with other individuals). But national health and health insurance policy have never had choice as their primary objective. Rather, these policies are primarily designed to maximize health *per se* or access to health services. These objectives may, theoretically, be a means or prerequisite to the ultimate end of utility maximization. But likewise they may be an end in themselves and would be widely regarded as being of greater importance than the satisfaction of preferences. Unsurprisingly, the available evidence suggests that "extra welfarism" (more correctly, notwelfarism) best describes the prevailing ethical objectives with respect to the provision of health services[3] (Hurley 2000; Olsen and Richardson 2001).[4]

The inadequacy of the orthodox economic framework in the health sector is also evident when the other pivotal assumptions are examined. Without consumer sovereignty and the revealed preference criterion for utility, debate would emerge over which, if any, of (at least) five concepts of utility was most useful for economic theory.[5] As noted by Hurley (2000), without the assumption of consequentialism the concept of efficiency embodied in economic orthodoxy would be questionable, as an outcome might be considered desirable or undesirable because of the process which led to the outcome and not because of the outcome *per se*. For example, and as argued by Mooney et al. (1991), "access" to health services, rather than health outcome, might be considered sufficient to meet social obligations in the health sector.

Consequentialism implies that patient history and context *per se* should not be of importance when health improvement is evaluated. In contrast, Ubel et al. (1999) found that survey respondents discriminate between previously healthy patients and long-term quadriplegics when priority is to be determined for a life-saving procedure which will leave both groups of patients with long-term quadriplegia.[6] As with procedural justice, respondents considered context and past history to be significant for assigning priority to health services.

As demonstrated in the theory of Welfare Economics, every competitive equilibrium in the idealized competitive model results in a Pareto efficient outcome and it is from this that the competitive model derives much of its appeal. However, the assumption that Pareto efficiency is self evidently desirable is aggressively counter-factual. It is not true that most of the population will remain neutral or pleased by the observation of a growing disparity in income, health status or access to services as long as they, personally, are not disadvantaged in absolute terms. To the contrary, there is little which will breed disharmony as quickly and surely as the granting of advantage to some members of a group while others are ignored.[7]

In practice, although virtually all policies have a redistributive affect which will disadvantage someone either implicitly or explicitly, these policies are justified by the Kaldor-Hicks potential compensation principle as a solution to the problem of interpersonal comparison. The acceptance of such a self-evidently defective principle is a testament to the strength of economists' desire to avoid ethical enquiry. At best, the application of the principle encourages the identification of *potentially* better states of the world. At worst, it redefines "better" to mean what, in the vernacular, is meant by "potentially better" and in so doing it permits advice to be based upon the covert and dubious ethical proposition that "potentially better" outcomes should be equated with outcomes which are truly "better".

A more benign interpretation of the Kaldor-Hicks principle is that economists leave the issue of whether or not to compensate to political decision-makers; and the fact that compensation seldom, if ever, occurs is outside the control of economists. The common disregard of distributional issues in economic analyses casts some doubt upon this interpretation and this is particularly true in the analysis of health and health programmes. When services are financed from flexible government revenue, healthy taxpayers are the losers. However there has never been a case of compensation for tax payers from those made better off because of health services. When health programmes are financed from a fixed budget, the inclusion of an additional set of services must be at the expense of a second set of services. Compensation for health services not received has also never occurred nor been contemplated and, in cases where life is lost, compensation is impossible. This indicates that the concept of "pure economic efficiency"—value free improvement—is misleading and it is hard to disagree with Williams' (1998) argument that, in practice, it is impossible to separate the analysis of efficiency and the analysis of distribution. It follows from this that ethical analyses should be of pivotal importance in establishing the normative foundations of policy analysis.

EMPIRICAL ETHICS

Rejection of the values embodied in economic orthodoxy implies the need for an enquiry into the values which should govern the allocation of health sector resources. The suggestion below seeks to circumvent two polar and unsatisfactory approaches. First, there is an empirical free ethics literature which reflects public values only incidentally or to the extent that ethicists' intuitions coincide with public values. Secondly, there is an empirical economics literature with limited or no ethical analysis. The assumption underlying the proposal below is that social values should be determined by the interaction of these two approaches: that ethical principles should be broadly consistent with community values but that community values should, in turn, be subjected to ethical scrutiny, debate, and revision.

In sum, it is suggested that ethical values should be elicited using an iterative process. Researchers should postulate population values (ethical principles) and then embark upon a series of empirical studies, both qualitative and quantitative. During these, the implications of population responses should be clarified by ethical analysis. For example, the implications of the "strong interval" property implicit in the use of QALYs or DALYs should be made explicit, viz, that a ten per cent drop in the utility index is of equal importance (value) as a ten per cent drop in the quantity of life (Richardson 1994); that a high rate of time preference means that a certain number of people will die prematurely whose lives could have been saved by the sacrifice of some short-term quality of life-enhancing programmes. Postulated ethical principles should be reformulated in view of population reaction to this information and then re-submitted for empirical testing. The process should continue until acceptable, stable (reliable and deliberated) ethical principles are identified: principles that withstand both *a priori* ethical criticism and the test of population support. The information obtained from this procedure should then be provided as input into the decision-making process.

Under some circumstances (which may also be the subject of empirically informed debate) it may be desirable to adopt the deliberative responses from the population as the appropriate indicator of social value and, therefore, policy should be directly based upon these responses. In other cases it may be more appropriate for decision-makers to be informed about population values, to exercise discretion, and trade-off population against other views. Finally, there may be a class of population values—hopefully small—where it would be hoped that decision-makers would override population values entirely (racism, sadism, etc.), a process referred to by Goodin (1986) as "laundering preferences".

As illustrated in chapter 13.3, it is possible to examine empirically the "meta issue" of whether or not the public believes that a particular moral issue should be decided by, or even influenced by, public opinion (the "Abdication Hypothesis"). At first, it may appear paradoxical to ask people if they have a preference for the sovereignty of their own preferences. There is, in fact, no inconsistency in a person expressing a preference when asked, but simultaneously favouring a decision process which does not depend upon this preference. The first and most obvious reason for this is a recognition of the inevitable asymmetry in information between an individual and a specialist. It is for this reason that Harsanyi (1996) argues that welfare economics should be reconstructed and based upon informed rather than actual preferences and that, in principle, decisions should be based upon surveys of individuals who have been exposed to a series of procedures which encourage deliberation. However, it is possible for individuals to reject the sovereignty of even well informed preferences. For example, Olsen and Richardson (2001) report surveys in both Norway and Australia in which respondents reject public preferences as the decision criterion and support the maximization of lives saved as an overriding principle. That is, paternalism is explicitly preferred to consumer sovereignty.

Even when there is no obvious alternative objective, such as life saving, individuals may prefer decisions to be made by the government. This may reflect a lack of confidence in the capacity of fellow citizens to make wise judgements and a belief that—at least in some contexts—governments have the capacity to ponder and assess a wider range of considerations than the individual and, further, that government may be less easily manipulated by particular interest groups. Indeed, it is a common view that this is precisely the role of government; viz, to make a series of difficult decisions on behalf of the population. This view was nicely expressed by a member of a focus group discussing the relevance of the social rate of time preference:

> I don't value public opinion…it is so easily manipulated, and people who represent us, you would assume, are competent. I don't have any faith in public opinion. If I have faith in anything, it is that the system is putting competent people in positions of power…. People are caught up with living their own life and they do not have time to go into every issue.

The belief that governments are elected to make decisions that the public do not wish to make or when people do not trust the wisdom of their fellow citizens has a long tradition extending back to Edmund Burke. It is not, of course, an unchallenged position and the belief that governments should be no more than the agent implementing the wishes of the majority was articulated by Rousseau.[8] Support for these two positions would be expected to vary by issue and between countries. It is likely, for example, that support for government decision-making would be significantly higher in European countries with their tradition of government intervention than in the USA where government appears to be less trusted. The general point, however, is that empirical ethics may include an inquiry into the extent of government interference and the circumstances and issues when this should occur.

OBJECTIONS TO EMPIRICAL ETHICS

For many ethicists and health economists the procedures suggested above might appear to be deeply flawed. The (lesser) concerns of the economist might be expressed as follows:

> Quantifying the strength of preferences for different ethical values will encounter significant measurement problems including inconsistency. People will not have considered many of the issues raised and their responses will be superficial. Revealed, not stated preferences, are the appropriate gold standard. The expectation that governments will process the ethical arguments provided to them and act as the idealized umpire when ethical issues conflict or when preferences need to be laundered is naive. Governments have short-term political objectives and, far from adjudicating contentious ethical issues, they normally seek the advice of economists and others. If government is the umpire there will be a circular process of decision shifting: economists seeking ethical guidelines from government which turns to economists for advice on precisely the same issues. Ethical input with respect to the allocation of health resources is, furthermore, superfluous. The objec-

tive of the health system is to provide health and this is something that needs technical, not ethical analysis.

These arguments do not alter the fundamental case for empirical ethics. It is not true that the objective of the health system is only to maximize health, defined in the narrow sense of mortality, morbidity, and health-related quality of life. Even with this narrow definition, there are ethical issues associated with the distribution of services, the right of some to purchase better services or to avoid queuing and thereby impose longer queues on others. Recent literature has also demonstrated the existence of ethical preferences relating to both procedural and distributive justice. For examples, see Nord (1999) and Menzel et al. (1999). Despite the common distrust of government among orthodox economists, there is little alternative to their assuming the role of ultimate arbiter over ethical issues, a role discussed further below.

The argument that the public will not have carefully considered many of the ethical issues and cannot therefore give consistent or sensible responses to ethical questions is an unproven assertion. A number of empirical studies of ethical preferences have now been undertaken and there are no obvious reasons for believing that they are all invalid. Further, shortcomings in present methodologies may simply reflect the fact that there has been remarkably little effort to devise methods for eliciting deliberative responses. A variety of options for achieving this exist: repeat interviews, group discussions, "triangulation" of issues by the use of multiple elicitation techniques, modified Delphi techniques, etc. It is the responsibility of researchers to devise both techniques and questions sufficiently simple that population values may be elicited. These have not been fully developed as orthodox economists have, as described earlier, circumvented the need for such evidence and ethical argument while ethicists have doubted the relevance of evidence altogether. This does not mean that methods cannot be devised which, to a greater or lesser extent, achieve the desired objectives.

The more fundamental objection to empirical ethics which is likely to be raised by ethicists may be summarized in the following way:

> It would be foolish to believe that ethical issues can be resolved simply by voting. Even with more sophisticated procedures designed to elicit deliberative responses, people might select immoral options. This is recognized by the need for the laundering of preferences; but laundering is simply a recognition of the fact that populations may be wrong in their ethical perceptions. They may vote for slavery, racist or other immoral policies. Ethics is immensely complex and it is no more sensible to elicit opinions from even well informed and intelligent amateurs than to vote on the laws of physics.

There are two implicit assumptions in this argument and both are unacceptable. First is the belief that ethical arguments must be fully consistent and applicable in all possible contexts. The immense complexity of ethics often arises only when ethicists seek the implications of an ethical theory in an unusual or abhorrent context. Thus, for example, simple utilitarianism may be criticized as it appears to permit torture if this generates more utility than it destroys. However, ethical issues may have broad application in uncontroversial areas. Welfarism, for example, is almost certainly a correct and defensible description of population values in markets less contentious than health care. More generally, and as noted earlier, there is ethical content in all normative advice and the ethical basis for much of this is simple and uncontroversial. There is no great complexity in the ethical principles which lead to the recommendation of technical efficiency. There is no ethical complexity in accepting that severity *per se* may be of independent importance in prioritizing health services or that we may wish to give priority care to individuals who have previously been disadvantaged, have not yet had their fair innings (life span), have been discriminated against, and so on. A significant part of empirical ethics has been, and should continue to be, the identification of such issues and the demonstration of their importance relative to more generally accepted goals.

The second implicit assumption in the passage is that an argument or procedure is flawed unless it achieves certainty and universality: that a procedure or ethical theory must be rejected if it might conceivably produce a wrong conclusion—one that is repugnant to our moral intuitions. However, ethical theory and normative economic analyses do not and cannot provide answers to ethical questions which are unambiguously true or immune from criticism. But this conclusion also applies to positive analyses. It is always possible that the current laws of physics, for example, may be falsified by new observations. A physical law is never unambiguously true, but represents the best current theory or hypothesis which may subsequently be corrected, generalized or rejected altogether. Analogously normative theories are tested for consistency and by comparing conclusion with well established ethical conclusions elsewhere. There is an unavoidable possibility that future analysis may demonstrate inconsistency in a previously unexplored context.

More generally, ethical theories must, themselves, be judged according to criteria which are not "objective" or demonstrably "true" or universal. For example, we may ask whether principles adopted are those which accord with moral intuition; which accord with a religious view; which are logically consistent with other commonly accepted ethical principles. However, to demonstrate that a particular set of criteria is appropriate or correct in some sense requires the application of a "meta-criterion," which itself needs justification and this justification requires a further (meta-meta) criterion. That is, any attempt at ultimate justification leads to an infinite regress. For the purpose of practical action, including the unavoidable need for economic and other policy, this is curtailed either by negotiation (and the acceptance of procedures rules) or by the referral of the issue to Parliament. In the intellectual market place, where such pragmatism may be eschewed, a moral theory or a set of criteria must eventually be sold by the persuasiveness of its supporting argument as discussed below. This is, essentially, what is done by Murray et al. (chapter 1.2) and Richardson (chapter 13.3) to establish minimal criteria for evaluating various summary measures of population health.

It may, of course, be argued that the successful marketing of an idea does not represent gold standard justification; that successfully marketed ideas may be wrong in some context, and that the procedure suggested here is, therefore, flawed. However, this rejoinder assumes that there must be certainty—that the theory must be universal and true in every context, no matter how contrived. But this implicit criterion will inevitably create disembodied theory which cannot help us identify best policy. It is disembodied in the sense that there is no criterion or justification for connecting theory to practical action as there will always be some context in which the theory is of doubtful validity as judged by the standard of another theory. Thus, if three ethical theories conflict with each other with respect to particular actions (for example, maximizing lives saved versus life years saved versus age and quality adjusted life years saved) then it is necessarily true that theory A will imply a (possibly extreme) event X which may appear unacceptable and which suggests the adoption of theory B. But theory B implies (extreme) event Y, which is also unacceptable and this suggests theory C. This, however, implies objectionable event Z which suggests theory A. Unless this circulatory can be ended and criteria established for the acceptance of a preferred theory—or minimally, its tentative acceptance in a defined context—then ethical theory will remain limited in its policy relevance.

As noted above, the possibility that a theory is wrong or inapplicable in a particular context is not unique to ethics. Physical laws may not fully explain empirical observations but this may not detract from their status of "best available theory" if this proves satisfactory over a sufficiently wide range of observations and there is no better, more general, explanation of events. Likewise when statistics and statistical theory are used to test hypotheses the result is subject to error and this is explicitly acknowledged. The response, however, is not to reject all hypotheses as fallible but to adopt a convention—usually the 95 per cent confidence criterion—and to regard null hypotheses as wrong and alternative hypotheses as supported when this conventional criterion is met. The criterion is necessarily somewhat arbitrary but makes possible the use of a powerful methodology in scientific research.

An integral part of empirical ethics should be an acceptance of the fact that argument and evidence are fallible and the conclusions are tentative and more or less strongly supported in some contexts than in others. It would be highly desirable for a convention to be adopted which indicated—as with the 95 per cent confidence criterion—that evidence and argument warranted tentative acceptance of a hypotheses or theory in a particular context.

The more serious criticism of a methodology based upon intellectual salesmanship as discussed above is that depending upon fashion and the rhetorical powers of the salesman virtually anything might be "sold". The challenging task will be to "sell" a convention in which an important element is the practical relevance of a theory and its capacity to endorse and defend particular policies. The chief obstacle to be overcome may well prove to be the greater appeal of elegant and abstract theory which purports to be independent of context and universal in scope. It is arguable that it is the appeal of such traits which derailed recent orthodox economic theory and increasingly replaced context specific empiricism with analytical, context free rationalism.

In sum, empirical ethics may be viewed as an attempt to connect ethical and economic analyses. The procedures described earlier do not bypass the need for ethical analyses by the adoption of convenient assumptions; nor do they become disembodied. Ethical views obtained empirically from the public must be subject to ethical scrutiny and debate. Reformulated ethical hypotheses may be further submitted to public scrutiny using deliberative methods. When options are identified consistent with a coherent and accepted ethical theory then this should be considered strong prima facie grounds for their adoption. In the event of outcomes where conflicting principles cannot be reconciled then for the purposes of economic policy government or a government endorsed authority must decide the issue. This is not a flaw in the suggested methodology but a recognition of the procedures that have been established by society for precisely this sort of problem solving. If theory and practice are to be connected, then the methodology must recognize and include the existence of these social institutions for conflict resolution.

CONCLUSIONS

The great strength of economics as a discipline is that it recognizes that, ultimately, its conclusions must be implemented in a real world society. As a consequence, it has adapted an explicit ethical theory—welfarism—and a set of value laden assumptions which bridge the gulf between abstract theory and the requirements for practical action. The great weakness, in the context of the health sector, is that the theory and assumptions do not describe community values. Further, the assumptions of orthodox economics has become so deeply embedded in economic theory and practice that it is often forgotten that welfarism is no more than a theory and that this theory may not be universally applicable. By contrast, while ethics is highly flexible in the range of issues it encompasses, it has failed to bridge the gap between theory and the requirements of practical action.

The suggested procedures described here as "Empirical Ethics" attempts to meld these two disciplines as they coincide in the health sector. The proposal entails, *inter alia*, the acceptance of some methodological convention or rule to indicate whether or not an ethical theory or hypothesis has sufficient empirical and ethical support for acceptance as the "best available theory" in a particular context. The convention would be the ethical counterpart to the five per cent criterion for tentative rejection of null hypotheses in statistical theory.

The present suggestion has the ontological status of a theory: it is hypothesized that these procedures will result in a better understanding of community preferences and an increased likelihood of aligning these preferences with the allocation of resources. That is, it is hypothesized that empirical ethics will assist with the maximization of social well-being which, as noted, is the defining problem of economic analysis.

Notes

1   Defining processes as part of the consequences of an action would imply that all of the considerations of *procedural* justice would be reconceptualized as consequences. The same consequence derived by two different processes would be seen as two different outcomes. This is clearly not intended by orthodox statements of theory in which the arguments of a utility function are conceived as goods, services and in some more general statements, may include utilities, or outcomes for other members of the society.

2   In Richardson (1999) I argue that axiomitization reflects the 2 500 year old methodological tradition of (philosophic) Rationalism—a tradition which was disregarded in the physical sciences and replaced by "Empiricism"—a tradition which was probably a prerequisite for the subsequent growth of scientific knowledge.

3   While loosely defined, "Extra Welfarism" refers to the existence of social objectives other than the maximization of utility. It usually includes health *per se* as an independent objective.

4   Empirical evidence indicates that when people are asked to select between the maximization of life and the maximization of utility as *social* objectives, the overwhelming majority select the former option (Olsen and Richardson 2001)

5   Richardson (1994) identifies four concepts: (i) psychological, pleasure/pain; (ii) psychological intensity of feeling; (iii) an ordinal ranking of preferences serving as an organizational framework in positive analyses; (iv) "N-M Utility," defined by the existence of behaviour consistent with the von Neumann-Morgenstern axioms of Expected Utility. A fifth concept corresponds with preferences which are intellectually determined (e.g. a preference for justice) even where there is no corresponding intensity of feeling or revealed behaviour.

6   Simple QALY or utility maximization implies that quadriplegics should receive lesser priority than ordinarily healthy people as they cannot be restored to full health. Ubel et al. (1999), however, found that survey respondents would not discriminate and would afford quadriplegics the same priority as patients who

could be returned to full health. Both groups would be given higher priority than previously normal patients who would become quadriplegics.

7   Interestingly, the Bible cites Jesus Christ as endorsing the Pareto criterion, but as a normative principle. In the same parable it is recognized that the common response to others' good fortune may be anger and envy (St Matthew 20).

8   It was believed, however, that with respect to significant issues and through an improbable mix of social behaviours, the public would reach a consensus on significant issues.

REFERENCES

Culyer A (1998) How ought health economists to treat value judgements in their analyses? In: *Health, health care and health economics*. Barer M, Getzen TE, Stoddart GL, eds. Wiley, Chichester.

Goodin RE (1986) Laundering preferences. In: *Foundations of social choice theory*. Elster J, Hylland A, eds. Cambridge University Press, Cambridge.

Harsanyi JC (1996) Utilities, preferences and substantive goods. *Social Choice and Welfare*, 14(1):129–145.

Hausman D (2000) *Why not just ask? Preferences, "empirical ethics" and the role of ethical reflection*. (Paper presented to WHO initiative on ethical issues in health resource allocation.) World Health Organization, Geneva. *www.who.int/whosis/fairness*.

Hurley J (2000) An overview of the normative economics of the health sector. In: *Handbook of health economics*. Culyer A, Newhouse J, eds. Elsevier, Amsterdam.

Menzel P, Gold MR, Nord E, Pinto JL, Richardson J, Ubel P (1999) Toward a broader view of values in cost-effectiveness analysis of health. *Hastings Center Report*, 29(3):7–15.

Mooney G, Hall J, Donaldson C, Gerard G (1991) Utilisation as a measure of equity: weighing heat. *Journal of Health Economics*, 10(4):475–480.

Nord E (1999) *Cost value analysis in health care: making sense out of QALYs*. Cambridge University Press, Cambridge.

Olsen J, Richardson J (2001) *Public preferences for the principles guiding health policy: does the public want a welfarist or a non welfarist government?* (CHPE working paper.) Monash University, Centre for Health Program Evaluation, Melbourne.

Pope R (2001) Reconciliation with the utility of chance by elaborated outcomes destroys the axiomatic basis of expected utility theory. *Theory and Decision*, 49:223–234.

Richardson J (1994) Cost-utility analysis: what should be measured? *Social Science and Medicine*, 39(1):7–21.

Richardson J (1999) *Rationalism, theoretical orthodoxy and their legacy in cost utility analysis*. (CHPE working paper no 93.) Monash University, Centre for Health Program Evaluation, Melbourne.

Ubel P, Richardson J, Pinto-Prades JL (1999) Lifesaving treatments and disabilities: are all QALYs created equal? *International Journal of Technology Assessment in Health Care*, 15(4):738–748.

Williams A (1998) If we are going to get a fair innings, someone will need to keep the score! In: *Health, health care and health economics*. Barer M, Getzen TE, Stoddart GL, eds. Wiley, Chichester.

Chapter 12.2

THE LIMITS TO EMPIRICAL ETHICS

DANIEL M. HAUSMAN

INTRODUCTION

Summary measures of population health are inevitably value laden. Different health states can only be compared in terms of their contribution to "quality of life", and quality of life is an evaluative notion. Additional questions concerning factors such as age-weighting and discounting raise further evaluative issues.

All of which creates difficulties, because evaluative questions are difficult and because values differ from country to country and group to group around the world. There seems something worrying in the prospect of some group of statisticians, economists, philosophers or theologians being called upon to determine the value of health states or whether future health states should be discounted. Given the difficulty and diversity of value judgements, would it not be better instead to rely on the values of the target population? Thus some argue for what Jeff Richardson calls "empirical ethics" (see chapter 12.1).

Richardson himself is cautious in championing empirical research concerning values, and indeed one of his empirically based arguments is, somewhat ironically, that people's time preferences should *not* be respected. In Richardson's view, research concerning population values should only affect decisions among alternatives that are ethically defensible. Certain issues and positions are thus off-limits. Racial discrimination and violations of fundamental rights are not to be tolerated, regardless of the values of the target population. Furthermore, even when several alternatives are ethically defensible, Richardson argues only for a prima facie deference to the values of the target population. If there are good reasons for rejecting the population's values, then those designing a summary measure of population health may do so.

In addressing the merits of empirical ethics, I shall not, however, limit my remarks to Richardson's cautious formulation. Even if no one would espouse a stronger version of empirical ethics, which holds that all ethical questions should be resolved by consulting the population's values, it is worth considering such a view. In highlighting its flaws, one sees both why Richardson's limits are necessary and why even his constrained empirical ethics is questionable.

THE CASE FOR EMPIRICAL ETHICS

It is worth distinguishing three arguments that could be given in defence of empirical ethics.[1] The first is a relativist argument that what is right or wrong, good or bad is simply a matter of social consensus. If the social consensus is that age weighting treats individuals unfairly, then age weighting (in that society) treats individuals unfairly.

Richardson rejects this relativist position, and he is wise to reject it, because relativism is implausible. It conflicts with the settled convictions of most people. Social approval of slavery, female infanticide, female genital mutilation, or ethnic cleansing does not make any of these practices right. Relativism also places an unjustified weight on how one draws the boundaries of societies, groups or populations. If the population is defined as the village, one answer may be correct. If it is the region, that answer may be wrong and a second answer correct. If it is the tribe, yet a third answer may be correct. Without principles for determining the relevant group, the answers to moral questions become arbitrary. Furthermore, when there is no consensus, how would the relativist decide moral questions? What does the relativist say about *reasons*? If the relativist maintains that it is possible to give good reasons criticizing or defending ethical statements, then the relativist must admit that a social consensus and the reasons that support it can both be mistaken. If, instead, the relativist denies that reasons have any role and holds that moral views are entirely matters of social convention, then the relativist cannot explain what people are disagreeing about when they argue about ethics. Surely they are not arguing about what the consensus in their society or societies in fact is. Denying that reasons have any role apparently implies that the social consensus is always right. But this too is implausible. Minority views and the views of social reformers are not always automatically mistaken—at least until the moment when they become majority views and become correct.

Relativism also makes little sociological sense. A social consensus on moral issues is not just a "given" to be measured, rather than to be queried. Which moral views are accepted today depends, as a matter of fact, on past arguments of moral reformers—often as part of religious movements. It is a matter of sociological fact that moral views depend on reasons. It is thus mistaken to suppose that today's consensus is no longer dependent on arguments. And if the consensus is subject to criticism, it cannot be automatically correct. Philosophical reflection should not be regarded as opposed to social determinations of what is right and wrong. Philosophical reflection instead plays a part within the social determination of what is right and wrong. For example, the consensus that once obtained in some areas in favour of female circumcision is crumbling in part because of rational criticism. Philosophical reflection and argument are a part of the process whereby groups of people resolve—and constantly reassess—moral issues.

This critique of relativism does not refute Richardson's case for empirical ethics, because he rejects relativism and relies on two different arguments that I have not yet discussed.[2] The first of these arguments is that ethical problems should be addressed by eliciting population values, because health priorities should conform to the wishes of those who are served by the health system. For example, one might argue that whether any of the health-care budget should go to fund cosmetic surgery depends on what people want and on what they believe to be just, not on some abstract moral theory. Just as members of a book club should read the books they choose to read, so members of some society or insurance group should be provided with the health measures and the health care that they choose. It is for this reason, not because of a commitment to moral relativism, that health measures and health policy should be based on the values of the target population. Those whose health is at stake and who are paying for the health care should be the ones to decide.

If health and its protection raised no moral questions, there would be no question that health policies should depend on the wishes of those they serve. But the measurement of health raises a myriad of moral questions. Funding cosmetic surgery rather than inoculations is not just a matter of social preferences. Age-weighting, discounting, and the weighting of different health states all matter ethically, and no reason has yet been given why the evident *interests* of the target population imply that their *values* should govern.

One might attempt a liberty argument. Just as consenting adults should be free to do as they please so long as their actions do not harm others, so should members of a society be free to make their own decisions, provided that there is unanimity, which is uncoerced and unmanipulated. But even if there were unanimity and no problems about the interests of current minorities, choices within a society have consequences for future generations and members of other societies and thus face ethical constraints. So the liberty argument fails.

One might instead make an argument for empirical ethics as a tiebreaker. If the alternatives are all morally permissible—that is, if all ethical constraints are satisfied by each of the alternatives under consideration (which may be the case that Richardson has in mind)—then surely the wishes of those who are immediately concerned should rule. But if the alternatives are all morally permissible, then the choice no longer raises moral questions, and it is misleading to describe those who defer to population values in such cases as committed to empirical *ethics*. The tiebreaking argument does not justify respecting population values in cases, which do raise moral questions, where population values may conflict with what is morally permissible.

Those who reject empirical ethics—who deny that ethical questions can be answered by taking a poll—do not (of course) deny that health systems should be responsive to the concerns of the populations they serve. There is no controversy about the need to find out what people want of their health systems. But finding out what people want of their health systems is not empirical ethics. What is at issue is whether moral questions should be resolved empirically, and the fact that the target population is most concerned with these questions does not imply that its answers are correct.

Richardson has a second argument in favour of empirical ethics. Just as one favours democracy, while recognizing that democratic procedures may lead to political mistakes, so one should favour permitting the values of the target population to govern the evaluation of health states, while recognizing that mistakes may result. Of course the argument for democracy has its limits, since almost all societies place limits on what can be decided by majority vote. But Richardson does, of course, place stringent limits on empirical ethics.

Do the reasons for favouring democracy carry over to the very different circumstances of defining a summary measure of population health? There are two main justifications for making decisions democratically: (1) the alternatives to democracy are too dangerous and (2) it is demeaning or unjust to deny competent adults an equal voice in social decision-making. In other words, democracy is both safer and more respectful or just than the alternatives. Similar reasons underlie the limitations on what majorities can decide. Fundamental rights and liberties and a regime that secures the self-respect of citizens cannot be abrogated by majority vote. Permitting democracy to extend to such questions would lessen security and would place justice and the equal moral status of adult citizens at risk.

These arguments apply to social decisions about what to *do* about health states. Although such decisions may be delegated, ultimately they should be responsive to the popular will. But this conclusion is irrelevant to the World Health Organization's (WHO) task. Even if WHO was attempting directly to guide health policy, rather than to measure health and the performance of health systems, its job would be to provide correct inputs into social decision-making, not to anticipate how those decisions (whether correct or incorrect) will be made. Whether to build a bridge or tunnel connecting midtown Manhattan and New Jersey should be decided democratically, but questions concerning the relative costs and benefits of the alternatives are not up for a vote. Furthermore, the attempt to establish a summary measure of population health is not directed immediately toward policy. Judgements concerning the severity of health states are no more political choices than are judgements concerning wealth or nutrition.

Although moral questions concerning what is right and wrong are very different from most scientific questions, there is no stronger case for deciding moral questions democratically than there is for deciding scientific questions democratically. The democracy argument applies only to political actions, and it thus does not apply to questions about how to evaluate health states. Those who support empirical ethics might complain that this disenfranchises the population. *Of course it does.* It disenfranchises *everyone*, because it maintains that the answers to evaluative questions, like the answers to factual questions, cannot be found by taking a vote. With respect to political decisions, on the other hand, there is, of course, no question of disenfranchising anyone.

A related case might be made that relies on the need for popular acceptance of health state measures. If WHO's evaluation of health states does not seem reasonable to members of the populations whose health WHO is attempting to measure, then WHO's measure will not be accepted. Whether or not depression is in fact much worse than paraplegia, a measure of health states will not be acceptable or influential unless the comparison of these health states seems right to the relevant populations. So, the argument concludes, evaluations of health states must be determined by empirical investigation rather than by philosophical argument.

There is something to this argument, though not enough to vindicate empirical ethics. What is right about the argument is that, for political reasons, WHO's valuations cannot conflict too flagrantly with the settled convictions of the world's populations. This constraint is however weak, because few people have settled convictions concerning the precise evaluation of different health states and improvements. There is a huge margin of uncertainty and reasonable disagreement, and thus a very large space for direct consideration of ethical questions. Furthermore, the need to justify the evaluations across populations undercuts the claims of empirical ethics, which aims to determine attitudes within a specific target population.

Although there is a great deal to be said for finding out what people value, there is little to be said for empirical ethics—even when it is as limited as Richardson wants it to be. The main problem is that the defender of empirical ethics poses a false dichotomy: either statisticians and health professionals decide, or the values of the target population rule. As Richardson himself emphasizes (see chapter 3.7), there should instead be a dialogue between the values of the target population and the moral arguments of those who have laboured long over these issues. If the moral arguments of the statistician or health analyst are conclusive, then they should transform the social consensus. If there is wisdom in the social consensus (and the experts are sensitive and open-minded enough to recognize it), then the values of the population will reveal narrowness or flaws in the arguments of the experts. If the values within a society are genuinely moral values, then they must be both sensitive to rational argument and rationally defensible. Nothing should prevent the analyst from influencing the population's values and being influenced by them. Those who study health should have no authority beyond that conveyed by their arguments. But on moral issues those concerned with health should defer only to arguments, not to mere consensus. Empirical ethics is not a kind of ethics, and it is not an acceptable replacement for ethics. Population values have an important place *within* ethical reflection; they should not compete with it.

NOTES

1   Economists who maintain that well-being is the satisfaction of preference are committed to the view that the value of a health state is determined by preferences. This view should not be confused with empirical ethics. Unlike the defender of empirical ethics, who counsels investigation of the values of a population in lieu of facing ethical questions directly, the economist's view implies that there are objectively correct or incorrect answers to questions about well-being, which depend on preferences. For an examination of this view of well-being and of the ethical commitments implicit in much of economics, see Hausman and McPherson (1996).

2   I am not sure to what extent Richardson endorses these arguments, because his essays (this volume) provide grounds to challenge both arguments. I do not know if he has other reasons for espousing empirical ethics.

REFERENCES

Hausman D, McPherson M (1996) *Economic analysis and moral philosophy.* Cambridge University Press, Cambridge.

Issues in comparing the health of two populations

Gavin Mooney

Key questions

In addressing questions surrounding the comparison of different populations' health, the first issue to be raised is whether devoting scarce analytical resources on attempting to answer them is worthwhile. A second issue is whether these questions are capable of being answered satisfactorily. Only after that does it seem important to try to address more direct questions of how best to do this.

It may seem unnecessary to examine the question of whether it is important to consider whether one population is healthier than another. Primarily the importance of trying to do so lies in any uses that might be made of this information. There would seem to be two. Whether, for example, one region of a country has higher health status than another might prompt investigation of why. Second, if one region has a lower health status than another, then depending on how equity is considered in policy terms, there may be a case for devoting more resources to that region.

To establish that population A is healthier than population B does not seem a worthwhile activity. It becomes so only on two counts. First, if there is a possibility of knowing why that is the case, the information might be used to alter the situation and improve things. There would seem to be a parallel here with a screening programme. To screen to determine that a subpopulation are at greater risk than the remainder of the population is normally considered to be justified only when there is some effective intervention for the higher risk group. It would not be enough simply to identify them as being at high risk. It is also the case that even when such a difference is established and some explanation provided, it may well be that the less well population might nonetheless opt for its lower level of health because of other advantages that it perceives it has. An issue here is that of the relative weight that is attached to some concept of the freedom of the individual, in particular with respect to freedom of choice.

Second, a resource allocation formula might be based on the notion of health need where the greater the health need the greater the resources allocated to that region.

Intra- and inter-country issues

The extent to which such issues might lead to these useful outcomes is likely to be greater within a single country than if comparisons of population health were extended across national and cultural boundaries. Even within countries, however, there would seem to be a case for caution in such an exercise. There are potential measurement problems here but, even before getting to these, some issues related to values arise. If the two (or more) populations are genuinely comparable in terms of their value bases, then comparing their health status might well be justified. The occasions on which such genuineness will be present, however, seem rather few and the larger the population groupings involved, the less likely that genuine homogeneity will apply. Different socioeconomic classes, for example, and different cultural groupings, even within the same society, may well have different constructs and different preferences for health.

Writing from Australia it is easy to make this point. This is very much a multi-cultural society to which different cultural groupings bring different preferences to the valuation of health. Additionally, the Aboriginal population also brings a different, much more holistic, concept of health than more Western-orientated Australians do. Comparability in such circumstances becomes at best difficult.

It is also the case that while these concerns can apply even to preferences for death, when health measures encompass quality of life as well, the prospects for homogeneity of values diminish. The greater the differences in culture and perhaps also in living standards, the less likely will it be that the construct, and the preferences for that construct, will be the same across the different cultures.

Also, if it could be shown with considerable certainty that the Irish have a higher health status than the Italians or the Iranians, in what context is this information valuable and to what extent would it be considered valuable to the Irish, Italians and Iranians, or indeed to anyone else? This is not a rhetorical question as the gathering of information to make this comparison in adequate detail and precision, assuming it can be done, is not a costless exercise. Given the relative lack of analytical skills in health care, especially in developing countries, and the need for these analytical skills to be used as well as possible, given the costs involved, it is important that the question of why it is to be done is thought through and it is established in advance that it will be useful.

Varying preferences for health and health care objectives

Preferences for health are notoriously difficult to pin down. To assume that they are uniform across different cultures seems difficult to justify. To attempt to impose a single set of values across different cultures appears at best unfortunate. To do so requires that there is or there is deemed to be a single set of universal preferences for health. This is doubtful in the reality; it is dubious as an ethical proposition to try to impose it. It may even be counter productive in the context of improving health (discussed below). Amartya Sen (1992) makes the point that a major criticism of utilitarianism (and much of the DALY literature and some of the other measures that the World Health Organization (WHO) is considering in this context are rooted in utilitarianism) is that for many people there is a truncated ability to manage to desire. This may be because of chronic deprivation or earlier (and perhaps also chronic) expectations being frustrated. Quite how best to handle these considerations is not immediately clear (also discussed below).

The concepts of universalism in preferences for health and for the construct of health certainly need to be thought through in some detail. It is unlikely to be the case that all cultures and all societies will subscribe to a common value system for health.

It is now the case (WHO 2000) that WHO seeks to encourage countries to consider issues beyond simply a health-based summary measure of population health and include other factors. This seems highly desirable. WHO has advocated extending summary measures of population health to include distribution of health, responsiveness and its distribution, and equity in financing. Unfortunately, as the summary measure of population health is extended to include other factors, no matter how desirable this might be in principle, the prospects of its applying with a common set of values across different cultures would seem to diminish.

Take equity in delivery of health care as an example. It is the case that equity can be viewed in various different ways. If, as this author has done, one lives in different countries then it becomes clear that the extent to which different cultures value equity varies. How they define it may well vary too.

There are thus two factors at work. There is the concept of equity; and there is the relative value attached to that, for example, as compared with the weight attached to efficiency or to freedom of choice or how financing is organized. There is also the question of whether all health services across the globe subscribe to the same set of goals and all the same attributes in their health social welfare function.

It has been argued that measuring population health in total in some summary measure across a whole country and comparing that with population health in another country is comparable with international comparisons of gross national product. There is some merit in that argument although given the difficulties involved in comparisons of GNP and the problems of interpretation in such comparisons, it is not clear that such an approach leaves comparison of summary measures of health in a good light. What makes such comparisons yet more problematical for health is that there would seem to be much greater hope for reaching a universal definition and concept of income than of health although income is not devoid of such problems. Valuing income is certainly more straightforward than valuing health. WHO, however, wants to go further, as indicated above, and introduce four other measures in such international comparisons, each defined in the same way and not allowing the concept (e.g. of equity) to vary according to local (i.e. national) preferences.

There is a need for greater recognition here of the variability of preferences across different countries. What is at stake is in essence three things. First, what are the objectives of each health care system? There is no reason to believe once we move beyond a rather vague goal of the promotion of the health of the population that all countries will adopt the same objectives. Second, what (and whose) values are to be used to determine the relative weights to be attached to the different components of the objectives of health care systems? Third, who is to determine whose preferences are to be used? There is no reason to believe that there will be universal answers to these three questions.

These are no easy matters to deal with and there are some considerable risks for WHO in "imposing" a single uniform system of values across all health care systems. There would seem to be risks for the individual countries as well. Whether it is a good thing or not, it is clear that some countries attach a greater weight to equity in health care than others. Some are more concerned with protecting individual patient choice, e.g. of being able to choose and change one's general practitioner more or less at will. Others are more concerned with considerations of community autonomy. Some see private health insurance as a way of taking the weight off the public system and more equitable for the rich to pay for private health insurance. Others argue for a more "social solidarity" type system as in Scandinavia where the extent of the private sector and private health insurance is small. Some countries see fee-for-service as being the way to pay general practitioners because it helps to preserve their market status. Others argue for greater weight to be attached to public and population health and thereby seek at least an element of capitation to encourage general practitioners into more public health orientated endeavours.

Not all of these variations in objectives point to the same outcomes for designing the universally perfect health care system. Opting for consumer choice, for example, tends to go with fee-for-service medicine, a mixed public and private system which relies more on competition. This, however, often means placing a lower value on (or attached to) equity. Competition, for example, is likely to lead to centralization geographically of services. Fee for service remuneration may make the pursuit of population health orientated goals more difficult.

A further concern about any attempt to establish some universal set of values for health and for health care is that there is some limited evidence and certainly much belief that self-esteem is important in the promotion of health status. In Aboriginal communities, for example, the question of being on their own land, participating in the decision-making processes, respecting community autonomy and self-determination more generally are all factors which appear to be relevant to both the health status of Aboriginal communities and how best to organize health services for Aboriginal people (McDermott et al. 1998). Indeed it can well be argued that much of the explanation of why Aboriginal people in Australia have such low health status, however measured, compared with white Australians, is that they have had health values and health system values imposed upon them. It is only recently, once white governments and white health services began to listen to the values being expressed by Aborigines, about their attitude to health, how they want their health services organized, that improvements in their health status have begun to occur.

A change in emphasis

What to do in these difficult circumstances seems clear. First, WHO needs to reflect much more than has been apparent to date on the uses to which summary measures of population health might be put and to ensure that the investment in such exercises is justified in some sort of global cost benefit framework. Especially is this true of any analytical resources used to construct such measures in developing countries because the opportunity costs there are so high.

Second, there is a need to recognize that the goals of individual countries' health care systems may well vary. To assume that all countries subscribe to the same five objectives of population health—equity in health, responsiveness, the distribution of responsiveness, and equity in financing—seems questionable. At best this assumption needs to be tested. It is also necessary to determine whether each is conceived in the same terms, even if in each country it is present. Equity in health may be the goal in some countries; equity of access the goal in others. This same word can thus have different meanings in different health care systems.

Third, while there are different sets of values that might be tapped to determine what both the objectives and the relative weights are that might be attached to these, there is a case for looking at each society's or each community's values upon which they as citizens want their health services based (Jan et al. 2000). This eliciting of preferences from whomever each country deems is relevant is something that WHO might encourage and promote. If the example of Aboriginal Australians is a useful guide then this would mean first that there will not be an imposition of external values, and also that being able to express these values may assist in building greater ownership both of the health care system as a social institution and of an agreed culturally determined notion of health.

That path is a more complex one than WHO is currently pursuing. It rests on the fundamental assumption that the task is to try to help countries to build better health care systems and a healthier population. To this point the goal that WHO has set and that implied in this paper are the same. The only difference is that here these goals are set according to the values of the local community as they themselves perceive these and are not set universally.

In some ways this relativistic path is more difficult. Fortunately, given the relationship between self-esteem and health status, if local values are respected, it is likely to be a more successful route for promoting the health of the population of each community.

REFERENCES

Jan S, Mooney G, Ryan M, Bruggemann K, Alexander K (2000) The use of conjoint analysis to elicit community preferences in public health research: a case study of hospital services in South Australia. *Australian and New Zealand Journal of Public Health*, **24**(1):64–70.

McDermott R, O'Dea K, Rowley K, Knight S, Burgess P (1998) Beneficial impact of the Homelands Movement on health outcomes in central Australian Aborigines. *Australian and New Zealand Journal of Public Health*, **22**(6):653–658.

Sen A (1992) *Inequality re-examined*. Russel Sage, New York.

WHO (2000) *The World Health Report 2000. Health systems: improving performance*. World Health Organization, Geneva.

Chapter 12.4

EMPIRICAL ETHICS, MORAL PHILOSOPHY, AND THE DEMOCRACY PROBLEM

DAN W. BROCK

A central issue for the development of summary measures of population health (SMPH), as well as for their use in the prioritization of health care resources, is the source of the value and ethical assumptions employed. Some, not surprisingly they are often social scientists, hold that any ethical premises should be empirically grounded, derived through empirical research on the actual values and ethical beliefs of real persons. Others, and again not surprisingly they are often philosophers and other normative theorists, hold that empirical research is irrelevant to establishing ethical and value judgements because they are normative not empirical claims and so require normative argument for their support. Neither of these polar positions is in my view correct.

Empirical research has been used to supply ethical and value premises in several different contexts. First, in developing weights for different states of disability. Once one delineates different domains and levels of function, as in a measure like the Health Utilities Index (Torrance et al. 1992), different relative values must be assigned to those different states of disability in order to make comparative judgments of the impact on health of different states of disability and to arrive at overall assessments of health where there are multiple functional limitations. Some of the early work derived disability weights on a scale from 1 representing perfect health and 0 representing death by simply asking individuals, using standard gambles, time trade-offs, or interval scales, their preferences for life with a particular disability. Second, for health care resource priorities and trade-offs: Erik Nord and many others have used the person trade-off method to enable people to express in a quantitative form specific normative concerns for fairness (Nord 1999). Since most people care both about aggregate health benefits and how they are distributed, this early work simply asked for preferences about trade-offs, such as between producing the greatest aggregate health benefit and treating the sickest, to assign quantitative weight to these distinct moral concerns. Finally, empirical research has been done on some explicit assumptions of SMPH such as whether people use discount rates or age-weight health benefits.

A variety of methodological concerns can be and were raised about these early empirical efforts, but ethical concerns were raised as well. One was simply the general scepticism of philosophers noted above about whether any ethical conclusions could possibly follow from this empirical research. But another was that this empirical ethics did not elicit reasoned, reflective and critical judgments, but instead only raw unreflective and unreasoned preferences (Daniels 1998). More recent work, for example, by Nord using the person trade-off method to elicit concerns of fairness and by Christopher Murray to determine disability weights, has attempted to employ a much more complex deliberative process; people are offered and/or asked to articulate reasons for their responses, to confront inconsistencies in their initial valuations, to consider the different responses of others and the reasons for them, and sometimes to try to reach a consensus with others (Murray 1996; Nord 1999). This is still an empirical process, but one that attempts to map moral reasoning about the relevance and content of concerns for fairness or of the value of health with different disabilities. This more sophisticated recent work represents in my view a clear advance over the earlier elicitation of raw preferences.

Since the issues in each of the three contexts noted above concern well-being and fairness, they have also been the subject of work by moral philosophers. While work in moral philosophy has not provided precise quantitative measures for well-being or quality of life, it has developed frameworks for general accounts of well-being (Brock 1993; Griffin 1986). Likewise, philosophical analysis has addressed such issues as what priority to give the worst off in health care resource prioritization (Brock 2002). And the possible moral bases for discounting and age weighting have been the subject of analysis and debate in moral philosophy (Daniels 1988; Parfit 1984).

There ought, in my view, to be an interplay between this empirical ethics and moral philosophy. Both are addressing the same substantive issues. From the empirical work we do not want people's raw preferences on the moral or value questions, but rather their considered and critical judgements which are only available after a process of moral reasoning that reflects the moral complexities and controversies involved. The more sophisticated recent empirical work represents an attempt to have real people confront the results of more theoretical and philosophical work on these moral questions, though it is in my view still at an early stage and much empirical and philosophical work remains to be done. We need the best work in moral philosophy to be done in parallel with, but also integrated into empirical ethics.

An important and difficult problem is that there is no reason to think that even at the end of the day there will be a complete convergence between moral philosophy and empirical ethics on these ethical and value questions. We then face what has been called the democracy problem

(Daniels 1993). The problem is what health policy should be when what people want conflicts with our best ethical and value standards. These ethical questions cannot just be left to experts, but neither should we deny that people can be mistaken about them. Let me just indicate two of the complexities of the democracy problem in the context of SMPH and health care resource prioritization. First, the role of empirical ethics varies depending on the ethical or value issues in question, though I believe it is never fully authoritative. For example, if philosophical accounts of well-being or health related quality of life are too general to yield disability weights, there may be a strong case for the common practice of employing preference-based values, though important ethical and methodological issues remain about exactly how that should be done. On the other hand, there may be less of a role for empirical ethics on whether health benefits should be age weighted or discounted, if moral reasons can be brought directly and perhaps decisively to bear on these questions.

Second, the democracy problem is a deep problem in political philosophy concerning the legitimate bases of political authority and the role of political decision-makers. Who is making SMPH or resource prioritization decisions, as well as how they will be used, affects how the democracy problem should be resolved in particular cases. For the World Health Organization's purposes in the Global Programme on Evidence for Health Policy it is probably best to use the ethical assumptions judged to be most reasonable, making those assumptions explicit together with their supporting reasons and/or the process by which they were derived (such as the process for deriving disability weights). Where the ethical assumptions are especially controversial, as in the case of discounting and age weighting, sensitivity analyses for differences in them are appropriate. This will allow different countries or organizations who make use of the data independently to evaluate the ethical assumptions, the reasons for them, and the sensitivity of the data to them. For resource prioritization I believe the problem is more complex and difficult. It is in significant part the longstanding problem in democratic theory of whether the role of decision-makers and representatives is to exercise their own best judgment or instead simply to reflect their constituents' wishes; the issue is of course highly controversial, but most agree that neither simple answer is adequate for all contexts and a more complex view that combines both the exercise by decision-makers of their own best judgment while also taking account of their constituents' wishes is necessary. If this is correct for health care resource prioritization, empirical ethics will have a role, but a limited and not decisive role, in informing the ethical and value judgments that are inevitably a part of that process.

REFERENCES

Brock DW (1993) Quality of life measures in health care and medical ethics. In: *The quality of life*. Nussbaum M, Sen A, eds. Clarendon Press, Oxford.

Brock DW (2002) Priority to the worst off in health care resource prioritization. In: *Medicine and social justice*. Rhodes R, Battin MP, Silvers A, eds. Oxford University Press, New York.

Daniels N (1988) *Am I my parents' keeper? An essay on justice between the young and the old*. Oxford University Press, New York.

Daniels N (1993) Rationing fairly: programmatic considerations. *Bioethics*, 7:224–233.

Daniels N (1998) Distributive justice and the use of summary measures of population health status. In: *Summarizing population health: directions for the development and application of population metrics*. Field MJ, Gold MR, eds. National Academic Press, Washington, DC.

Griffin J (1986) *Well-being: its meaning, measurement, and moral importance*. Clarendon Press, Oxford.

Murray CJL (1996) Rethinking DALYs. In: *The global burden of disease: a comprehensive assessment of mortality and disability from diseases, injuries, and risk factors in 1990 and projected to 2020*. The Global Burden of Disease and Injury, Vol. 1. Murray CJL, Lopez AD, eds. Harvard School of Public Health on behalf of WHO, Cambridge, MA.

Nord E (1999) *Cost value analysis in health care: making sense out of QALYs*. Cambridge University Press, Cambridge.

Parfit D (1984) *Reasons and persons*. Clarendon Press, Oxford.

Torrance GW, Zhang Y, Feeny D, Furlong W, Barr R (1992) *Multi-attribute preference functions for a comprehensive health status classification system*. (CHEPA working paper no 92/18.) McMaster University, Centre for Health Economics and Policy Analysis, Hamilton, Ontario.

Chapter 13.1

ACCOUNTING FOR TIME AND AGE IN SUMMARY MEASURES OF POPULATION HEALTH

Aki Tsuchiya

The issue addressed in this section is whether or not summary measures of population health (SMPH), designed to answer the question "Is population A healthier than population B?", should be subject to temporal discounting and/or age weighting.

The type of SMPH of interest here is of a *descriptive* nature: this tries to capture the volume of health *per se* among a specified population at a given point in time. The crucial question to ask to see whether or not temporal discounting is of relevance is therefore the following:

(1)   Population A in 20 years' time will have one 40-year-old in condition x for a month.

Population B in 10 years' time will have one 40-year-old in condition x for a month.

The two populations are exactly the same in all other relevant aspects.

Is population A healthier than population B?

To apply temporal discounting in descriptive SMPH means to answer "yes" to this question, which is not right. The only difference between population A and B is when an identical (ill-)health event occurs, and differential points in time itself cannot alter the amount of health within a population. Note that temporal discounting is an economic technique that brings to "present value" and makes directly comparable the value of things that take place at different points in time, or over a stretch of time. The logical necessity of temporal discounting arises from the requirement to compare *values* in an *inter-temporal* context. In other words, (a) when we are comparing crude numbers or quantities of things as opposed to their values to individuals or to society, then it is inappropriate to discount, and (b) when the context is entirely contemporal, or cross-sectional, it is also inappropriate to discount.[1] What question (1) does in essence is to compare the level of health at two different points in time: it does not refer to the value of a population being healthy. Therefore, the answer to question (1) is "no, the two populations are equally healthy", and temporal discounting does not apply to descriptive SMPH.

However, there is a similar but different kind of SMPH that looks at health as a social desideratum, and reports the desirableness of the level and distribution of this among a specific population. Let us refer to this kind of measure as *prescriptive* SMPH. In this case, the relevant question to ask becomes:

(2) Population *A* in 20 years' time will have one 40-year-old in condition *x* for a month.

Population *B* in 10 years' time will have one 40-year-old in condition *x* for a month.

The two populations are exactly the same in all other relevant aspects.

Suppose there is a certain resource that can be used now in two alternative ways: project *a* will prevent the 40-year-old in population *A* to develop condition *x*, and project *b* will prevent the 40-year-old in population *B* to develop condition *x*: the costs of the two projects are equal.

Is project *b* more desirable than project *a*, in other words, in the absence of this intervention, is the present value of the health of population *A* larger than that for population *B*?

Note that it is now the *present value* of the state a given population is in with respect to their health rather than the sheer volume of health that is the issue. Because a given resource (typically, money) will generate capital interests by investment, this generates opportunity costs with the passage of time, and therefore resources are subject to temporal discounting. Question (2) is equivalent to comparing an offer of a given size return in 10 years and the same size return in 20 years, for a fixed amount of investment today. In other words, it is about converting present resources into the future health. Since future resources are subject to a positive temporal discount rate, so should be future goods which resources are transformed into. The implication of this is that the present value of a good at a closer point in time is larger than the present value of the same good at a farther point in time: i.e. the present value of preventing condition *x* in 10 years' time is larger than doing the same in 20 years' time. Thus it is project *b* that is more desirable. The actual discount rate depends on the market discount rate for secure capital investments in the relevant time period (e.g. government bonds), whether or not the exchange rate between money and health is assumed to stay constant over time,[2] and whether SMPH are designed for the so-called "stationary population" interpretation,[3] or the "cohort interpretation (of period life tables)".[4] However, it is important to remember that none of these affect the level of health *per se* between populations *A* and *B*.

Let us move on to the issue of age weighting and descriptive SMPH. The question to ask is as follows:

(3) Population *A* this year has one 60-year-old in condition *x* for a month.

Population *B* this year has one 20-year-old in condition *x* for a month.

The two populations are exactly the same in all other relevant aspects.

Is population *A* healthier than population *B*?

Here, the only difference between the two populations is the distribution of (ill-)health in terms of patient age. To apply age weighting to descriptive SMPH implies that the answer to this question is "yes". One case where this is appropriate is where the same condition *x* (e.g. "being bedridden and depressed but without pain") is assumed to imply a different degree of loss in health, with reference to full health and death, depending on patient age. Although this is a theoretical possibility, this is presently not the standard assumption in the prevailing literature. Existing methods that quantify the degree of health loss due to a given condition *x* do so under the assumption that this is independent from patient age. The only other case where this is appropriate is where being in full health at different ages imply different degrees of healthiness so that a 20-year-old in full health now is "healthier" now than a 60-year-old in full health now, which is highly confusing if not nonsensical. Therefore, the answer to question (3) again is "no, the two populations are equally healthy".

Let us compare this with the case of age weighting and prescriptive SMPH:

(4) Population *A* this year will have one 60-year-old in condition *x* for a month.

Population *B* this year will have one 20-year-old in condition *x* for a month.

The two populations are exactly the same in all other relevant aspects.

Suppose there is a certain resource that can be used now in two alternative ways: project *a* will prevent the 60-year-old to develop condition *x*, and project *b* will prevent the 20-year-old to develop condition *x*: the costs of the two projects are equal.

Is project *b* more desirable than project *a*, in other words, in the absence of this intervention, is the value of the health of population *A* lager than that for *B*?

Again, it is the desirableness of health, and not health itself, that is the issue. To the extent that society values a single healthy year of life differently according to people's age, one of the two populations in question (4) is in a more desirable state than the other with respect to health. Society may chose to employ weights in prescriptive SMPH for efficiency reasons and/or equity reasons. For example, if people of certain ages or those at certain life stages are seen to contribute more to social welfare than others, then keeping these people in good health is more desirable than keeping others in good health, and this will lead to age weights based on an efficiency criterion.[5] Or, if there is an inequality aversion regarding the distribution of overall health within a population, so that an additional unit of health is valued more if given to an individual with poorer health than to an individual with richer health, then this, under certain conditions, will lead to age weights based on an equity criterion.[6] Note that this does not preclude the possibility that a society may value all healthy years equivalently regardless of age *and* be neutral to the distribution of health within the population, in which case there will be no age weights. Moreover, these cannot be applied to descriptive SMPH, which objective is to report the level of health as such, independently of its effects on social welfare.

Therefore, if the context involves values and decisions at some specific point in time, then temporal discounting and age weighting become relevant to SMPH, but not otherwise. For contexts where the objective is simply to report the levels of health of different populations, then neither of these is relevant. However, there is a possible criticism. The process by which different health states are given weights to reflect the degree by which they differ from full health and/or death is typically referred to as "valuation" exercises, and involves values. Is it appropriate that SMPH that include these weights should be referred to as "descriptive" despite the incorporation of these valuations?

To address this, let us first look at the evaluation task. The objective of an evaluation exercise, be it standard gamble or time trade-off, etc., is to place a given adverse health state on an interval scale with full health and death as two reference points. The idea is to weigh the years of life lived in adverse health and to link this to a lesser number of years of life lived in full health so that the two will be equivalent.[7] In this respect, a summary measure that accounts for less than full levels of health does have some values incorporated. However, what the procedure does is to convert ill-health into full-health-equivalents, where the value of a life-year spent in full health itself is still not accounted for. In other words, the *value* of an adverse health state is compared with the *value* of full health, but once this is done, it is the *number* (and not the value) of total full-health-equivalent life years that is reported in a prescriptive summary measure. And it is when this number of life years is converted to the value of life years that the summary measure becomes a prescriptive measure for which temporal discounting and age weighting are potential issues. The term descriptive does not imply that there are no values involved: it is perfectly possible to *describe* the value of something. In this section, the terms denote whether the summary measure simply reflects health itself or incorporates different social (present) values of being healthy.

To conclude briefly, the answer to the main question set for this section is that neither temporal discounting nor age weighting is relevant to descriptive SMPH, designed to answer the question: "Is population *A* healthier than population *B*?"

ACKNOWLEDGEMENTS

At the time of writing, the author was a post-doctoral research fellow of the Japan Society for the Promotion of Science, and a visiting research fellow at the Centre for Health Economics, University of York, UK. A very much earlier version of this paper was presented to the WHO conference on Summary Measures of Population Health, held at Marrakech, 6–9 Dec. 1999. Valuable comments were offered by many, and special thanks are due to Jan Barendregt and Alan Williams. The usual disclaimer applies.

NOTES

1   Further, note that temporal discounting itself does not imply that the future good (as opposed to a present good) is of less value in any inherent way. All it means is that the future good has less value *seen from a given reference point* (present), due to the temporal distance between the two points.

2   If the value of health relative to money increases (decreases) over time, then the discount rate for health should be smaller (larger) than that for money.

3   Imagine a complete period life table. The stationary population interpretation holds that each row of the life table represents what happens to people at different ages, during a single year. For example, row 10 concerns those presently at age 10, and row 40 concerns those presently 40 years old. Since there are no inter-temporal elements under this interpretation, SMPH designed for this interpretation should not include temporal discounting at the aggregation stage *within* the measure. However, to compare the present value of a stationary prescriptive SMPH for, say 2010 with that for 2020, then discounting is relevant.

4   Imagine, again, a complete period life table. The cohort interpretation holds that each row represents the best estimate of what is expected to happen to a newly born cohort through the future years. Under this interpretation, the row for age 0 corresponds to year 0, the row for age 10 corresponds to year 10, and so on for a particular cohort. In other words, each row of the life table will be representing events that are expected to arise at different points in time. Therefore discounting is relevant at the aggregation phase *within* the measure, as well as for comparing present values for SMPH for different years.

5   An example of this is the age weight function in DALYs (disability-adjusted life years), based on welfare interdependence (Murray 1994; 1996).

6   An example of this is the fair innings weights, based on a health-related social welfare function with positive aversion to inequalities in health (Williams 1997).

7   The exposition is given with health expectancies in mind. However, the same applies for health gaps, where loss of health is reported by converting ill-health into death-equivalents.

REFERENCES

Murray CJL (1994) Quantifying the burden of disease: the technical basis for disability-adjusted life years. In: *Global comparative assessments in the health sector*. Murray CJL, Lopez AD, eds. World Health Organization, Geneva.

Murray CJL (1996) Rethinking DALYs. In: *The global burden of disease: a comprehensive assessment of mortality and disability from diseases, injuries, and risk factors in 1990 and projected to 2020*. The Global Burden of Disease and Injury, Vol. 1. Murray CJL, Lopez AD, eds. Harvard School of Public Health on behalf of WHO, Cambridge, MA.

Williams A (1997) Intergenerational equity: an exploration of the "fair innings" argument. *Health Economics*, 6 (2):117–132.

AGE WEIGHTING AND TIME DISCOUNTING: TECHNICAL IMPERATIVE VERSUS SOCIAL CHOICE

JEFF RICHARDSON

INTRODUCTION

Four propositions are discussed below. The first is that both age weighting and time discounting of future years of life represent ethical/social judgements about the value of life. They are not related to the usual conception of "health" or the healthiness of the population and for this reason should not be included in indices of population health. Secondly, the methodology for obtaining valid age weights is still in its experimental stage and the weights published to date should be treated with great caution. Thirdly, while discounting is likely to be included in the ideal protocol for the economic evaluation of health programmes, this reflects an ethical judgement and not a technical imperative. The use of undiscounted future benefits is defensible if this is implied by social values. Finally, while both time and age discount factors should reflect social values, the elicitation of these values is problematical. It is concluded that the ethical nature of these and similar decisions should be the subject of the form of analysis described in chapter 12.1 as "Empirical Ethics".

HEALTH-RELATED UTILITY VERSUS SOCIAL VALUE

The present (social) value of a life year may be expressed as equation (1).

$$\text{Present value} = A \cdot D \cdot (X_i ...) \, (LY)(QoL) ... \qquad (1)$$
$$= A \cdot D \cdot (X_i ...)(QALY \text{ or } DALY)$$

where A = an age weight; D = discount factor; LY = a life year; QoL = Quality of Life (utility) index; X_i = other indices of social value.

There is a fundamental distinction between the first two and the last two concepts captured in equation (1). The QALY/DALY (unweighted) is time-based. A life year represents duration—time—and QoL represents the quality of that time. For this reason the QALY/DALY (unweighted) is something "felt" or experienced in "real time": a person will experience different sensations when their QoL changes and this will occur whether or not they explicitly conceptualize what is happening. By contrast, an age weight and discount factor are not experienced or felt in this way; they are not based upon duration of time but upon a particular attitude or belief with respect to the treatment of the QALY/DALY or, more commonly, the QALY/DALY of another person. Over-simplifying somewhat, they are cerebral concepts concerning the appropriate distribution of QALYs/DALYs between groups of individuals who are differentiated by age or time. Restated, QALYs/DALYs may be conceptualized as "litres" of "utility" which, in a real sense, exist. A change in the number of QALYs arising from a health programme which increases either the number of life years or the quality of those years indicates a change in the flow of sensations experienced by beneficiaries of the health programme. A change in the age or time weight or a change in the distribution of beneficiaries between the different (time and age) groups has no such effect. However the same flow of sensations is now deemed to have a different social value and, as usually conceptualized, this arises from the social preferences/utilities of the society as a whole—primarily non-beneficiaries—and not from the preferences/utilities, beliefs or experience of those receiving the new services who, in aggregate, continue to experience the same flow of sensations. For the non-beneficiaries the satisfaction of social preferences will have little effect upon what is "felt" or upon the flow of sensations other than a transitory satisfaction or irritation if they learn that their preferences have or have not been respected. In the limiting case, (as with foreign aid) the individuals whose preferences are embodied in the preference weights may have no idea whether their preferences have been respected.

A possible response to this line of argument is that each of the four elements—age, time, quality weights and life years—are simply different dimensions of social value and that each independently exists in "preference space": a 10% change in the numerical value of any of the four elements has an identical impact upon social preference or utility. While the arithmetic of this rejoinder is correct it misses the essential point of the argument. As with the various goods and services which constitute the GDP, the four elements of social preference/utility can be combined but they may also remain separate. The argument here has been that two of the four elements share an important defining characteristic—they reflect the magnitude of sensations that are experienced. The remaining two likewise share a defining characteristic—their numerical value has no relationship to the sensations experienced but reflect these abstract, cerebral beliefs or intellectualized preferences of a group which does not experience the flow of real time sensations which define the QALY/DALY.

Whether or not it is useful to separate these four elements is a different issue from their separability.[1] If separation serves no purpose for either theory or policy then it is a pointless exercise. It is argued below, however, that the suggested distinction is useful for both theory and for an appreciation of the implications of various policy options.

A second possible objection to the distinction is that in practice it is blurred by the techniques used to measure the DALY and, to a lesser extent, the QALY. In the former case a group of experts is asked to assign values to health states using the person trade-off (PTO) technique. This, in turn asks respondents to adopt a social perspective and to alter the number of beneficiaries in two health programmes until the value of the two programmes is equal. This is, conceptually, a different task from the QALY procedure which asks survey respondents to imagine themselves as patients experiencing the health state; a procedure which is closer to the usual gold standard for utility measurement, namely the revealed preference of the person experiencing the utility. Despite this, there is widespread, but not universal support for the view that QoL should be assessed by a representative cross section of the community and not by the patient. When this occurs, not for reasons of survey convenience, but because it is believed that community values are the gold standard, then the resulting index number will, indeed, be a conceptual hybrid which, like the DALY, has elements of both individual utility and social value. This does not, however, imply that the use of a one step hybrid is superior to a conceptually simpler statistic and it was partly to avoid this lack of conceptual clarity, that Nord et al. (1999) recommended the use of patient values to assess QALYs and, subsequently, to assess "social value" from a community survey which is appropriately obtained from the community.

While there is no coercion in the way in which we construct concepts, it is coherent and potentially useful to conceptualize and define the burden of disease in units corresponding with what is (or may have been) experienced or "felt", and "social value" as reflecting the importance which society places upon this latter quantity. The distinction is particularly useful if there are problems or policies where it is helpful to know the extent of the suffering or the aggregate loss of sentiency arising from a disease as distinct from the average social valuation of this.[2] The distinction would, for example, be valuable if the health of different communities with different values is to be compared. This suggests that the distinction between health-related utility and its social value is, in fact, useful and should be explicit in the literature. If the "burden of disease" is intended to primarily reflect the "health" of a community and the loss of sensations/utility arising from disease then there is an additional reason for adopting the distinction.

Given the common meaning of the word, it would, additionally, be misleading to include age and time weights in the definition of "health" and in the calculation of a numerical index of healthiness. This may be simply illustrated. Consider two populations with an identical age distribution and an identical life expectancy of 90 for each healthy individual. In population A there are 2 unhealthy children of 10 who will die in 30 years at the age of 40. In population B there is 1 unhealthy individual who is about to die at age 75. The years of life lost for the two populations are therefore $2 \times (90 - 40) = 100$ and $1 \times (90 - 75) = 15$. If future life years are discounted at 5% per annum the present value of YLL arising from the premature death of the two children and the person aged 75 will be 9.4 years and 10.9 years respectively. While 10.9 exceeds 9.4 it would be misleading to describe population A as being healthier than population B.

A similar example indicates the inappropriateness of including age weights in the definition of health. Population A and B now have life expectancies of 80. In population A a 20 year old is about to die. In population B 20 people are about to die at the age of 70. Thus the YLL in the two populations are 60 and 200 respectively. With age weights of 1.5 and 0.4 at ages 20 and 70 the weighted YLL would equal 90 and 80 respectively. While this case is less clear, it appears improbable that most would regard the death of a single youth aged 20 as indicating greater unhealthiness than the death of 20 people aged 70. It would not, however, be particularly surprising if the judgement was made that the age weights were correct and the death of a 20 year old was of greater social concern than the death of 20 people aged 70.

Definitions are a matter of linguistic convention and it is time consuming and unhelpful to debate questions of the form "What is meant by *healthiness?*" There is, however, a strong argument for clarity of expression and for the alignment of definitions with common usage and, as illustrated above, this implies the separation of the concepts of health and the value of health. This should apply not simply to time and age discounting but to the various other dimensions of social value which might be included in "cost value analysis" as discussed by Nord (1999) and Nord et al. (1999).

AGE WEIGHTS

In principle, there is no fixed list of attributes which may or may not affect social value and the variables and their importance will almost certainly vary between countries. Elsewhere it has been suggested that this list should include severity (Nord et al. 1999); context (the Rule of Rescue), health potential (non-discrimination against the disabled), maintenance of hope, certainty of treatment, previous health benefits received (Menzel et al. 1999) and the achievement of a "fair innings" or life expectancy (Williams 1997). There is a large research agenda to determine which of these or which other factors are of importance and of social relevance. To date, the enquiry has been largely empirical: those suggesting the relevance of variables have supported their argument with population surveys. There are two limitations with this approach. First, various psychometric problems arise. In particular, the framing of questions may bias respondents and, for this reason, results need to be replicated using different methodologies. Secondly, and as discussed below, the results of such surveys should be exposed to ethical criticism and, if necessary, reformulated and retested before being considered as options for policy. Thus, as a minimum, the implications of survey results should be thoroughly explored.

The second problem is the possibility of double counting. The legitimate ethical reasons for age weights have been discussed by Tsuchiya (chapter 13.2) who also reviews the various empirical studies. The latter are clearly intended to capture a social value associated with age but not included elsewhere. The first and most obvious possible overlap arises if the age weight simply reflects the respondent's correct expectation that the quality of life will decline with age, a factor already taken into account in QALY based studies. A further possible reason for age weights is a recognition of the additional social value of people in their middle years arising from their contribution to both their family and to the economy. Double counting would occur if age weights were used to capture this added value if the contribution to the GDP was separately included as a benefit in the study as commonly occurs.

It is also doubtful whether the age weights reported to date are valid in the context of economic evaluations of life saving interventions for people at different ages. In this context a smaller number of lives, life years or QALYs may be preferred to a large number because of the age weights. This implies that age weights are, in effect, an "exchange rate" between the number of people whose lives will or will not be saved at different ages. This in turn implies that they must possess a "strong interval" property, i.e. imply a trade-off between lives which truly reflects social values. More specifically, a 10% increase in the value of an age weight will have exactly the same effect upon the measured value of life years as a 10% increase in the number of life years and this relationship may be used as a test of reflective equilibrium.[3]

Results to date would almost certainly fail this test. The study by Cropper et al. (1994) implied that, on average, the value of remaining life years to someone at age 20 is 2.66 times greater than the average value of remaining years to someone aged 60. Similarly, the average value of remaining years at age 30 is 4.4 times more valuable than the average value at age 60.[4] Johannesson and Johansson report results that imply an average value after the age of 30 which is three times greater than the average value after an age of 50 despite there only being a 20 year difference in these ages.[5] The mathematical function estimated by Cropper et al. implies that the value of each remaining year at age 50 is, on average, almost 7 times greater than the value of each remaining year at age 70. Such results are highly implausible. Even less plausible is the implication by Cropper that the value of years between the ages of 20 and 30 is negative—30 year olds having a higher value than 20 year olds. This implies that as the 20 year old ages the total value of the smaller number of remaining years increases. The results are not necessarily wrong as a sufficiently large discount rate could produce this outcome.[6] (Of course there would be double counting if such age and time discount rate were both included in a study.) However it is probable that survey respondents would not persist with this pattern of responses if these implications were drawn to their attention.

In sum, these results are possible but not probable. It is likely that surveys of this sort must, as a minimum, include procedures to encourage deliberation and reflection upon the implications of the numerical values that are elicited.

DISCOUNTING

Discounting the future is justified, broadly, by the existence of a positive rate of time preference (RTP) and by the social opportunity cost of capital. The latter justification is based upon two assumptions; first, that on the margin, spending on current health can be reduced, funds invested in the capital market and spent on the production of future health; and, secondly, that we have enough information to calculate the present loss and the future gain in health status resulting from this re-allocation of resources. Neither assumption is true. Our knowledge of the health production function for the present is very limited and the function for future health—and the relation between future marginal inputs and benefits—almost totally unknown. There is probably no example in any country of a government reducing current funding and investing in order to increase future health expenditures. Almost precisely the opposition occurs. Most budgets are determined historically. Consequently, a reduction in present spending will generally reduce, not increase, future budgets and government spending.

Murray (1996) presents a similar argument, namely, the "health research paradox", and concludes that at least some discounting must occur. There is, he argues, a finite probability that additional research expenditure will find a way of eradicating a disease which has a stable (or increasing) incidence through time. The expected undiscounted benefits are therefore infinite and, no matter how small the probability of discovering a cure, all possible resources should be devoted to this research programme.

If benefits were equated with "expected benefits", i.e. the size times the probability of benefits, then the argument would be compelling. However, the "Expected Utility Hypothesis" has been exhaustively tested and the empirical evidence clearly indicates that it is systematically violated and that the hypotheses does not describe behaviour (Schoemaker 1982). There is also no compelling reason for accepting the common argument that the hypothesis should be regarded as a normative theory which describes rational decision-making. To the contrary, there are contexts where adherence to the rule is irrational as it disregards factors which are relevant to decision-making, viz, the wide range of emotions which may be experienced in the pre-outcome period (see Pope 2000). Keynes and Allais are among those who have disputed the belief that conformity with the Expected Utility Hypothesis and the associated axioms represent the hallmark of rational behaviour and that alternative behavioural algorithms such as the maxi-min principle are necessarily irrational.

The more compelling arguments for time discounting are associated with the RTP. The three standard theoretical explanations for this are based upon a diminishing marginal utility of income, risk aversion and "myopia". Corresponding with these three arguments for an individual RTP, there are similar arguments for a social RTP. First, it is assumed that income per capita will rise through time depressing the marginal utility of income and the desirability of income transfers from the present. Murray (1996) counter argues that there is no reason to presume that a declining marginal utility of income implies a similar decrease in the marginal utility of life *per se*. The rejoinder may or may not be true. The availability of "new experiences" certainly declines with age and this may, in fact, reduce the marginal utility of latter years. The more persuasive argument is that there will be a decreasing marginal "social" value. The "fair innings" argument and the argument for egalitarian outcomes both imply a lesser social value of additional life years as life expectancy increases and it is widely believed that this will happen in the future.

Secondly, each individual faces a probability of death which increases with age. Postponement of present benefits is therefore risky as the future benefits may never be experienced. For society as a whole this risk does not exist or is significantly reduced as the risk of societal extinction is fairly remote (Murray 1996). It is unlikely, however, that a representative group of the population, acting as citizens and contemplating the appropriate social rate of time preference would focus upon the likelihood of species extinction. Rather, it is likely that they would focus upon the undeniable risk facing each individual.

Thirdly, there is an undeniable "time myopia"—an impatience to experience pleasure. An ice cream today is generally preferred to an ice cream in a week's time even when the intervening risk of death is very small. While many, including Sen (1992), have argued that society may have a different RTP from the individual the arguments are not persuasive and individual myopia therefore appears to be the quantitatively most significant reason for a personal and social RTP.

One superficially attractive approach to this theoretically vexed question is to approach the public directly and, using a variety of techniques, elicit the actual rate of time preference and bypass the need to determine reasons. Thus, for example, Olsen (1993) argues that the discount rate for health programmes should be based upon the time preference for health which, in Olsen (1995), is estimated to be about 10%. By contrast, Dolan and Gudex (1995) infer an RTP of zero from the results of their time trade-off surveys. Most recent authors have assumed that the appropriate social RTP should be determined from the individual RTP and, in empirical surveys, the appropriate discount rate has usually been set equal to the average rate of survey respondents. This implies the ethical judgement that the public's intertemporal preferences should be respected.

This ethical judgement was not universally accepted in the past. For example, Hume argued that there was no quality in human nature which "causes more fatal errors in our conduct, than that which leads us to prefer whatever is present to the distant and remote". Pigou described pure time preference as "wholly irrational" and attributed it to a "faulty telescopic faculty" and Harrod believed that pure RTP represents the "conquest of reason by passion". Alfred Marshall, the founder of modern micro-economics, was particularly scathing on this subject when he argued that a high rate of time preference indicated that people had "less power of realising the future, less patience and self control...they are impatient and greedy for present enjoyment...like the children who pick the plums out of their pudding to eat them at once". (Quotations cited from Robinson 1990; Tong 1998 and Ng 1999). These were the early statements of "extra-welfarism", the rejection of private preferences as the sole and over-riding criterion for the allocation of resources (see Richardson 2001 and Hurley 2000).[7]

There is, in fact, a sound basis for rejecting private intertemporal preferences. The choice of discount rate will redistribute health services through time: a low or zero rate will favour those expecting sickness in the future. High rates will favour the currently ill. This indisputable conclusion indicates that the social RTP is not solely or even primarily about the (Pareto) efficient allocation of resources through time. Current losers cannot, even in principle, be compensated by future beneficiaries if they die because of the intertemporal mix of services which results from the chosen discount rate. It is almost as improbable that those who are currently suffering but survive could receive compensation from the future group of people who will benefit.

When time discounting is viewed as a distributional issue there is a further reason why social decision-makers may discount the future, namely self interest. It is likely that decision-makers regard their task as primarily representing the interests of a particular constituency—those currently alive and living in a particular nation. The constituency clearly has some interest in future generations and an interest in the well-being of people in other countries. But the importance weight attached to the well-being of those other groups does not arise solely or even primarily from self interested myopia, diminishing marginal utility of income or the likelihood of species extinction. Concern for children may be described as "self interest" but even here there is a likely discontinuity in the treatment of future benefits when the beneficiary switches from parent to child. The present value of the child's future benefits will depend, in large part, upon the desired parents' distribution of utility between parent and child. Outside this context the social discount rate will almost entirely reflect distributional preferences and the various personal and ethical considerations which determine these preferences.[8]

THE ABDICATION HYPOTHESIS

In chapter 12.1 it was suggested that citizens might elect to abdicate responsibility for certain decisions and prefer for them to be taken by governments. This possibility was labelled the "Abdication hypothesis". Its validity was empirically tested in the context of a survey of health related rates of time preference.

Four sets of postal questionnaires were distributed to residents of Victoria, Australia. In each of these, respondents were asked to imagine that they were a member of a government committee with responsibility for allocating a limited budget. In the first two versions, respondents were told that Programme 1 would save the lives of "a large number of people". Further, "a large and very accurate survey...shows that nearly all people would support the programme if the benefits occurred immediately..." (if they did) the programme would be "good value for money". However the lives are saved in the future and the survey indicates that people "do not want to pay taxes now for a programme that will help people only after X years". In version 1 and version 2, X was 10 and 20 years respectively. In the remaining two versions respondents were again asked to imagine themselves as a member of a government committee. But this time they were asked to choose between a programme that will detect cancer and save the life of 100 people immediately and a programme which will detect cancer and save 250 lives in X years. The value of X was again 10 and 20 in the two versions respectively.

In all four versions respondents were asked to consider two sets of arguments; viz:

- The large majority of the population wants Programme A. The democratically elected government should follow the wishes of the population. Therefore you should vote for this programme.

- The government should not always follow public opinion if it considers that people are being short sighted. The government should do what it believes to be best and, if the cost is reasonable, introduce policies which it believes will be best for the community. Therefore you should vote for Programme B.

Results summarized in Table 1 indicate the following:

- A significant majority of the respondents (a weighted average of 66% across the four versions) were prepared to override public preferences when larger benefits could be obtained in 10 years.

- Only a minority—35%—were prepared to override public opinion when the benefits were in 20 years. This indicates the existence of a positive "social rate of time preference". The benefit of the future programme clearly declined with time and, with it, the willingness to override public opinion.

Table I   Should governments override public preferences with
respect to the allocation of resources over time?
Results of a pilot study (*n* = 78)

	Per cent			
	Yes	No	Total	*n*
Governments should override public opinion when the programme:				
a) *Is a good buy now. Public rejection is because:*				
benefits are in 10 years	69	31	100	16
benefits are in 20 years	39	61	100	23
beneficiaries themselves voted against the programme and				
benefits are in 10 years	75	25	100	16
benefits are in 20 years	36	64	100	22
beneficiaries voted for the programme and				
benefits are in 10 years	75	25	100	16
benefits are in 20 years	39	61	100	23
b) *The public prefers cancer cure now for 100 rather than*				
250 cancer cures in 10 years	44	54	100	16
250 cancer cures in 20 years	25	75	100	20
Overall weighted average				
10 years	66	34	100	
20 years	35	65	100	

- Respondents did not change their answers when they were informed that beneficiaries did or did not vote against the programme which would subsequently benefit them. This suggests that among our respondents there was no strong belief that individuals should be held accountable for their earlier decisions (at least when this was expressed in the form of a vote).

- There was only minority support for overriding public opinion when present and future benefits were for cancer patients. This suggests the possibility of context specific judgements although the format of the questions differed sufficiently for this to have affected the results.

The general principle underlying this first set of questions was directly tested by asking respondents to indicate which of three general statements about government decision-making they most supported. Results, in Table 2, reveal that only 22–26% of respondents believe that, as a general principle, the government should always follow public opinion even when it believed the public was being short sighted. The remainder believed that, to a greater or lesser extent, governments should override public preferences with about the same number supporting the adoption by the government of a compromise position between their beliefs and those of the public, and the hard line position that the government should entirely ignore public preferences.

Table 2   In general, should governments override public opinion?

	Benefits received in:	
General principle	10 years (% yes)	20 years (% yes)
a) Even if the government believes the public is being short sighted, it should follow public opinion and spend exactly what the public wants on saving lives in the future.	26	22
b) If the government believes the public is being short sighted, it should compromise and spend more than the public wants but less than they believe to be right, on saving lives in the future.	36	40
c) If the government believes the public is being short sighted, it should take no notice of public opinion and do what it believes is right.	38	38
Total	100	100
N	50	45

If the results of this pilot survey correctly reflects public opinion then it is clear that, at least in Australia, the population believes that governments, not the community, should make certain decisions. As discussed in chapter 12.1, this might reflect a belief that governments have a greater capacity to assess issues carefully. Alternatively, respondents may mistrust the acumen and wisdom of their fellow citizens and have greater confidence in the decision procedures adopted by government. Finally, it is at least possible that individuals have been socialized to believe that certain classes of decisions are the business of government and not the citizenry. While inconsistent with the self determining, empowered and self reliant individual implicit in orthodox economic theory the real world citizen may elect to delegate certain decisions.

This latter possibility may well reflect a recognition of the fact, noted above, that discounting in the context of health is not, primarily, a technical question concerning the efficient allocation of resources through time but rather, a distributional issue. Low discount rates advantage a different group of people than high discount rates. Detailed normative judgements concerning the distribution of income are commonly left to the government and are not made the subject of binding social surveys.

CONCLUSIONS

With respect to the use of age weights and time discounting the following conclusions have been reached:

1. There is a persuasive argument for excluding both of these forms of weighting from summary measures of population health designed to measure the burden of disease. Neither of these variables specifically relate to the consequences of disease nor to the associated "burden"

when this is conceptualized in terms of the loss of duration and quality of time—the flow of sensations—which might otherwise have been
experienced. Rather, both time discounting and age weights reflect the
value that is placed upon this burden. While the social valuation of this
concept of disease burden is clearly of interest, there are reasons for
separating the burden and the social valuation of the burden. The
magnitude of both the time discount and age weights are presently
contestable. Further, the meaning of the composite SMPH combining
life years, quality of life, time discounting and age weights is necessarily somewhat unclear and consequently less accessible to decision-
makers.

2. Secondly, the age weights reported in the literature have not been validated. The published magnitudes have highly implausible implications
   for the relative worth of the remaining life years of different age cohorts.
   It is likely that these implications would be widely rejected and also
   rejected by those who were initially questioned. This highlights the need
   for the use of "deliberative weights": weights that are constructed from
   the responses of people who have been encouraged to deliberate upon
   the issues and their implications. There is also a possibility that the use
   of age weights will result in double counting if they reflect not only a
   "pure age effect", but also the changing quality of life and the social
   contribution of individuals at different stages of their life.

3. Time discounting alters the relative importance of the burden of disease borne by *different individuals:* changing the discount rate will
   redistribute the well-being that will be experienced. Consequently, there
   are prima facie grounds for government intervention as it is an accepted
   role of the government to ensure equity in the distribution of benefits,
   and the legitimacy of the government's redistributive function is well
   established.

4. There is empirical support for the argument that governments should
   not simply accept the rate of time preference of the community but to
   interfere with the inter-temporal distribution of health benefits when
   it believes that the community is being short sighted.

More generally, this chapter illustrates the need for further empirical
research and ethical criticism. The rate of time preference, in particular,
is universally treated by economists as a technical issue and the sole province of economists. However decisions which redistribute well-being between individuals at a given time or between individuals through time are
quintessentially ethical. Economists can only clarify the nature of these
choices and employ various methods to assist with decision-making. They
have no mandate to usurp the usual processes for social decision-making.

NOTES

1 More generally distinctions are based upon differences and not upon similarities!

2 Likewise it is sometimes valuable to measure the physical value of output as distinct from its market value as recorded in the GDP.

3 The property is, essentially, identical to the requirement of a "strong interval" property in the calculation of QALYs suggested by Richardson (1994; see also chapter 3.7 of this volume). In this context, a 10% increase in the index of QoL will have the same impact as a 10% increase in life years and, consequently, the QoL index must be constructed so that its value reflects the desired exchange rate between the quality and quantity of life.

4 It is reported that life saving of one individual aged 30 is equivalent to saving the life of 11 people at age 60. Assuming a life expectancy of 80:

$$
\begin{array}{rcl}
11 \times 60 \text{ year old} & = & 1 \times 30 \text{ year old} \\
11 \times \text{life expectancy of } 20 & = & 1 \times \text{life expectancy of } 50 \\
220 \text{ years after age } 60 & = & 50 \text{ years after age } 30 \\
4.4 \text{ years (average) after age } 60 & = & 1 \text{ year or after age } 30
\end{array}
$$

5 Assuming a life expectancy of 80, people aged 50 and 30 have life expectancies of 30 and 50 respectively. Johannesson and Johansson (1997 p. 596) report that 5 lives at age 50 were equivalent to one life at 30. Hence:

$$
\begin{array}{rcl}
5 \times 50 \text{ year old} & = & 1 \times 30 \text{ year old} \\
5 \times \text{LE of } 30 & = & 1 \times \text{LE of } 50 \\
150 \text{ years after age } 50 & = & 50 \text{ years after age } 30 \\
3 \text{ years after age } 50 & = & 1 \text{ year after age } 30
\end{array}
$$

6 If the value of life years following age 30 was sufficiently high relative to the (lower) value of years following age 20 then there is a discount rate which is sufficiently high to effectively eliminate the importance of other years and thereby make the discounted value of future life at age 30 greater than at age 20.

7 There is explicit recognition in the environmental literature that the imposition of present preferences upon the future generations may be unacceptable. (Robinson 1990).

8 It is possible to argue that ethical or distributional preferences are simply a reflection of "utility": that we support ethical behaviour only because it increases our utility. The argument is not compelling. It implies that every action must maximize utility "or why else would it have been taken?" At best the argument blurs otherwise clear and separate concepts. The argument implies that the entire subject matter of ethics and social justice is a subset of utilitarianism and it would be necessary to adopt a cumbersome terminology to distinguish utility arising from personal pleasure/pain from utility arising from duty, from obeying religious laws, etc. At worst the argument is tautological. Actions maximize utility or they would not have been taken. But the reason they were taken, and their significance is that they maximize utility (and are therefore appropriate actions!).

References

Cropper ML, Aydede SK, Portney PR (1994) Preferences for life saving programmes: how the public discounts time and age. *Journal of Risk and Uncertainty,* 8(3):243–265.

Dolan P, Gudex C (1995) Time preference, duration and health state valuations. *Journal of Health Economics,* 4(4):289–299.

Menzel P, Gold MR, Nord E, Pinto JL, Richardson J, Ubel P (1999) Toward a broader view of values in cost-effectiveness analysis of health. *Hastings Center Report,* 29(3):7–15.

Murray CJL (1996) Rethinking DALYs. In: *The global burden of disease: a comprehensive assessment of mortality and disability from diseases, injuries, and risk factors in 1990 and projected to 2020.* The Global Burden of Disease and Injury, Vol. 1. Murray CJL, Lopez AD, eds. Harvard School of Public Health on behalf of WHO, Cambridge, MA.

Ng Y (1999) Efficiency, equality and happiness: on the ethical foundations of public policy. *International Journal of Development Planning Literature,* 1(14):1–16.

Nord E (1999) *Cost value analysis in health care: making sense out of QALYs.* Cambridge University Press, Cambridge.

Nord EM, Pinto JL, Richardson J, Menzel P, Ubel P (1999) Incorporating societal concerns for fairness in numerical valuations of health programmemes. *Health Economics,* 8(1):25–39.

Olsen J (1993) On what basis should health be discounted? *Journal of Health Economics,* 12(1):39–53.

Olsen J (1995) *Should we discount health? If so at what rate?* (Paper presented to the Economics Working Party of the Pharmaceutical Benefits Advisory Committee, February 14.) Sydney.

Olsen J, Richardson J (2001) *Public preferences for the principles guiding health policy: does the public want a welfarist or a non welfarist government?* (CHPE working paper.) Monash University, Centre for Health Programme Evaluation, Melbourne.

Pope R (2001) Reconciliation with the utility of chance by elaborated outcomes destroys the axiomatic basis of expected utility theory. *Theory and Decision,* 49:223–234.

Richardson J (1994) Cost-utility analysis: what should be measured? *Social Science and Medicine,* 39(1):7–21.

Robinson JC (1990) Philosophical origins of the social rate of discount in cost-benefit analysis. *Milbank Quarterly,* 68(2):245–265.

Sen A (1992) *Inequality re-examined.* Russel Sage, New York.

Tong F (1998) *Discount and health: a conceptual perspective.* (Masters research paper.) Monash University, Department of Economics, Clayton.

Tsuchiya A (1999) *Age-related preferences and age weighting health benefits.* Kyoto University, Department of Economics, Japan.

Williams A (1997) Intergenerational equity: an exploration of the "fair innings" argument. *Health Economics,* 6 (2):117–132.

Chapter 13.3

AGE WEIGHTS AND DISCOUNTING IN HEALTH GAPS RECONSIDERED

CHRISTOPHER J.L. MURRAY AND ARNAB ACHARYA

INTRODUCTION

Disability-adjusted life years (DALYs) were developed as a health gap measure to quantify the burden of disease and injury on human populations for the Global Burden of Disease Study (Murray 1996). Murray and Acharya (1997) have reviewed the specific formulation of DALYs and the arguments underpinning the social values explicitly incorporated into DALYs. This paper summarizes the arguments supporting the use of age weights and time discounting in health gaps. It draws on the previous paper by Murray and Acharya (1997).

AGE-WEIGHTING

Imagine the situation where there is only one course of antibiotics available and two individuals with meningitis arrive simultaneously at the emergency room. The only difference between the two that we know about is their age: one is 2 years old and the other is 22. Their prognosis is identical. Which patient would we choose to treat? According to the principle of reducing the duration of life lost, we should always prefer to save the younger patient who has the prospect of more years of life to be saved. Several studies, however, including some population surveys have found that individuals prefer to save the lives of young adults over young children (Institute of medicine 1986; Lewis and Charny 1989; Johannesson and Johansson 1996).

Should this apparently widely held preference be reflected in DALYs? The answer depends on two questions. Why do individuals hold this preference? And, once these reasons are identified, do they justify using these preferences in calculating the burden of disease? A preference for preventing a young adult death over a newborn death cannot be explained by the duration of expected life lost, even when these durations are discounted.

Such preferences imply some other age-dependent preference whereby life years lived at different ages are valued differentially. These age-dependent preferences that explain the difference between preferences for saving lives at different ages and those predicted on the basis of duration of expected life lost with or without discounting are defined as age-weights.[1] Johannesson and Johansson (1996) surveyed population preferences for saving life years at different ages and found strong non-uniform age-weighting, such that one QALY for a 30-year-old was equivalent to three QALYs at age 50 and nine QALYs at age 70.

While age-weighting may reflect nearly ubiquitous preferences, the reasons for age-weighting may well vary. At least three types of arguments have been advanced to explain preferences for years of life lived at different ages. Individuals may value their own health at different ages as more or less important. Wright (1985) found that individuals in the population assigned greater importance to being healthy during "infancy" and the "period of raising children". Busschbach et al. (1993) used a form of trade-off to investigate preferences of student and elderly respondents for healthy time lived at different ages. Both groups attached the greatest importance to years of life lived at age 10 and lower weights to ages 5 followed by 35, 60 and 70 in descending order. Even if every year of life has the same intrinsic value to the individual, we may be "induced" to attach greater importance to years of productive adult life. All consumers in society depend on producers for food and other items of consumption. Net producers, therefore, have a magnified role in contributing to social welfare. Such human capital type arguments could be extended not only to distinguish years lived by different age groups but also years lived by individuals with different incomes or educational levels. Such a fully elaborated human capital approach would not be consistent with the principles on restricted information proposed for the formulation of DALYs.

Some individuals play a critical role in providing for the well-being of others—consider parents and their young children. A more general notion of interdependence would also generate age-weights of some form. In such a framework, the greatest contributors to the well-being of others would not necessarily be those who earn the most. Some net contributors to the well-being of others may earn no dollars but may work within the household. *A priori*, we would not expect rich individuals or more educated individuals to contribute more to the welfare of others than poor or less educated individuals. This broader concept of flows between individuals contributing to the well-being of others provides a much more convincing argument for age weights if these flows are a function of age. The empirical evidence reviewed above on population preferences for age-weighting suggests that these flows are a function of age with years of life lived as a young or middle-aged adult being valued more.

As with net dollar transfers between individuals, age does not explain all of the variation in net flows contributing to the well-being of others. There must be individuals of the same age who contribute more to the well-being of others than similarly aged individuals. Should the life years of these altruists be assigned a greater relative value? If such individuals could reliably be identified, some may sympathize with this argument. Age, however, is a variable which does not discriminate between the lives of different individuals but simply differentiates periods of the life cycle for a cohort. Taking into consideration altruism, or some other factor that predicted net flows to the well-being of others, would lead to discrimination between different people's lives. Based on the proposition to restrict the information used to establish relative values to age (and sex), it seems reasonable to consider age-weighting because of different roles and contributions of different age groups but to reject proposals to pursue this logic to identify other variables predicting net flows.

Another perspective on age-weighting can be seen in light of the Hampshire (1989) principle that "first among the shared potentialities is the recognition of justice, which is necessary to all human associations: of the obligations of love and friendship and of families and kinship; of the duties of benevolence, or at least of restraints against harm and destruction of life" (p. 32). Those to whom the society assigns clear responsibility of caring directly for the most vulnerable will be valued. By recourse to this minimalist assignment of responsibilities we avoid particularities of any given society.[2] It is important to admit this instrumentalist view and see its limit. The age weighting does not depend on the social contingencies; a social welfare system that cared for all children and for the very old would not entail removing this condition, given our accepted knowledge of human psychology and human productivity. The well-being of some age groups, we argue, is instrumental in making society flourish; therefore collectively we may be more concerned with improving health status for individuals in these age groups.

DISCOUNTING FUTURE DALYS

The extensive literature on discounting future health and the wide array of arguments for and against discounting is discussed more completely in Murray (1996). Acharya and Murray (forthcoming) have shown that utility maximizing individuals may possibly not discount their own future health especially if they suspect that their material life is likely to be better in the future. We are somewhat in agreement with Anand and Hanson (1997) when they argue that even if individuals have high discount rates for their own health or for social health benefits because of individual or social pure time preference, this may not be a convincing argument for discounting future health for the purposes of social decision-making. Likewise, we concur that the discount rate implied by the uncertainty that the world will exist in the future would be a small but non-zero positive number—nowhere in the vicinity of 3% or even 0.1% year.

Many economists have argued that there is a great deal of theoretical and empirical support for discounting future health in the context of designing health polices.[3] We are convinced that the only strong argument for discounting is the disease eradication/health research paradox.

The eradication/research paradox can be seen through an example. Imagine that the population is constant over time and the disease incidence rate is stable. If the policy-maker is interested in a longer time-period, say, T, then following the usual functional form as an intertemporal value function, the policy-maker would have the following minimization problem subject to some budget constraint:

$$U = \sum_{t=1}^{T} \rho^t \Delta_t$$

where Δ_t is the sum of all DALYs lost at time t, and

$$\rho = \frac{1}{1 + r}$$

where r is the time discount rate.

One of the features of equation U is that DALYs lost for large t are approximately zero due to the first term in the right hand side. Since DALYs lost in the future count less through ρ, policy-makers would minimize equation U by favouring the reduction of DALYs in the periods nearer to the current period, even if the technology improves. If $r = 0$, then future DALYs lost would count as much as current DALYs lost. If technology can be improved significantly to either eradicate or cure a great number of diseases in the future by shifting current dollars toward research then significant sacrifices of current DALYs would be justified. Essentially, without discounting, the possibility of improved technology entails that treatment and prevention of health care be postponed to a time when Δ can be driven to zero.

A solution proposed by Anand and Hanson (1997) to avoid this problem is to impose convexity from the loss of Δ_i^t, the DALYs lost by individual i at time t. But this is inadequate to save us from the research paradox. We show this below. From their formulation, we surmise that each evaluation of personal loss of DALYs (arising out of onset of some medical condition at time t) is made into a convex function by $(\Delta_i^t)^\alpha$, where $\alpha > 1$. Anand and Hanson propose the following optimization problem. Subject to some budget constraint, minimize:

$$B = \sum_{t}^{T} \sum_{i}^{N} (\Delta_i^t)^\alpha$$

where $\alpha > 1$.

We would presume that this is added across people (N) and then added across time for a fairly large T, the end of the planning horizon. Then it is plausible that there is a t_1, a large number, by which time most disease can be completely eradicated or cured as result of good research. All that is needed is that research progresses at a rapid rate sometime into the future. Since for t_1 and for all subsequent periods Δ_i^t can be driven towards zero at t_1 for nearly all persons, we postpone all savings of DALYs to these periods.[4] That convexity is not enough to save us from the research paradox. Conditions which would save us from the research paradox may be possible—for example, a version of the Inada condition or the von Weizsäcker's *overtaking criterion*; however, Anand and Hanson (1997) do not elaborate on them. Further it is not clear how these conditions should be interpreted in this situation.

Our argument that $r > 0$ should not be taken as a purely mathematical argument. Improving technology makes future generations better off than the present generation. Since the payoff is greater in the future we postpone all interventions. This seems to be an excessive sacrifice borne by the present generation. Anand and Hanson (1997), by referring to a paper by Anand and Sen (1994), seem to view future generations' health as analogous to their enjoyment of the environment. The analogy is not altogether justified. The present generation by using resources to better its own health does not deprive future generations of resources in the same sense, say, as strip mining would. In the latter case there is an act of depriving the future generation of something that is irreplaceable. In the case of favouring the health of the present generation, we deprive future generations in the same way as we do when the present generation dissaves.[5] Also not favouring their own health over the others might induce excessive sacrifices in light of technological progress. The formulation in Anand and Hanson (1997) does not preclude excessive sacrifice by the present generation.

As noted by Parfit (1984), an excessive sacrifice argument may lead to a different form of discounting of the future than would a classical exponential decay discounting function, where more distal generations are discounted more than proximal generations. Based purely on the argument of excessive sacrifice, life years for generation $n + k$ are no more or less important than life years for generation n. We simply cannot call upon the current generation to sacrifice so much of currently available health resources to improve the health of future generations. Each future generation, however, would have an equal claim on current resources. Of course, the small but non-zero probability of global disaster and the extinction of mankind means that we would slightly discount the claims of generation $n + k$ compared with generation n.

A declining discount rate perhaps similar to an exponential decay may be used for proximal generations for two reasons. First, there is substantial but steadily decreasing generation overlap for the next two to four generations. Beneficiaries of an intervention purchased today which prevents burden in 50 years would be a mix of currently living and future generations. Second, the current generations may have some legitimate special concern for specific members of the next generation such as their children and grand-children above and beyond their concern for all future generations. We could, therefore, conclude that a discount function which approximates the classical exponential decay function for 100 to 150 years and is thereafter flat may adequately reflect concerns over excessive sacrifice brought about by the eradication and research paradoxes. The empirical findings of Cropper et al. (1994) are consistent with the notion that individuals may have a much lower marginal discount rate for distant events than for proximal events.

Precisely because the issue of discounting is not easily resolved, in *The Global Burden of Disease* (Murray and Lopez 1996), DALYs by age, sex, cause and region have been published with and without discounting. The standard DALY incorporates a 3% discount rate. The choice of 3%, however, is entirely arbitrary. The value 3% is a low positive rate that is probably at the lower limit of acceptability for those economists who are persuaded by opportunity cost arguments and is at the upper limit for those who are willing to accept a positive discount rate for the reasons of excessive sacrifice.

CONCLUSIONS

We have given specific arguments for age-weighting and discounting future health to avoid excessive sacrifice. For those like Anand and Hanson (1997) who are not convinced by such arguments, however, we recommend that they use DALYs[0,0], i.e. DALYs with no age-weighting and no discounting—results of which have been published in detail for 1990 by Murray and Lopez (1996). Those undertaking cost-effectiveness studies should consider publishing results for standard DALYs and DALYs[0,0], as well as specific variants as required.

Even though DALYs[0,0] are available, it is important to recognize that variations in the discount rate or age-weighting factor have little effect on the broad results for burden of disease (Murray and Lopez 1996; Murray and Acharya 1997). In its standard form, using 3% discount rate and age weights, the DALY provides a convenient tool for comparative burden of disease and cost-effectiveness analyses and provides useful input into debates on allocation of resources for health research and health interventions. For national or local studies of allocative efficiency, the value choices in the standard DALY can be easily modified to inform health policy debates in different social and cultural settings.

NOTES

1   Two functional forms of age-weighting would meet this definition. One would simply be a multiplier that would be the ratio of the value of preventing a death at each age divided by the relative value expected on the basis of discounted duration. An intuitive interpretation of such age-weights, however, is hard to establish. Alternatively, we can define the relative value of each year of life lived at each age. There are a number of reasons discussed in the text as to why the value of each year of life lived may differ. Because the functional form in which the age weight appears in the usual DALY equation has a more direct

interpretation, we have exclusively examined age-weights of the form that attach a value to each year of life lived at each age.

2   Hampshire (1989) argues that there are common needs that may be character-ized as constituting a tolerable life, though they are recognizable through diverse specific satisfaction. Without answering to these needs, human life becomes nasty and brutish, less than human. See also Walzer (1992) on this point.

3   This literature is vast. See Viscusi and Moore (1989) and Cropper et al. (1994) for the empirical reasoning; for opposing evidence see Redelmeir and Heller (1993) on what has become known as the "time paradox"; see Murray (1996) for an opposite view on theoretical grounds. See Hammit (1993) for the continuing debate on this.

4   Murray and Acharya (1997) develop the mathematical argument. They show that even if the natural burden of disease (burden without any interventions) is constant every year with steady technological development, without discount-ing an egalitarian intervention plan will not prevent a suboptimal amount of loss of DALYs. Hence, under the formulation B, fairness may not be preserved without a positive discount rate.

5   Ramsey (1928) and other economists have opposed discounting in this case. Anand and Hanson's claims against discounting do not seem this strong. Something such as environment can be seen as owned by all generations; and here Coase's theory is completely inapplicable as most future generations cannot interact with the present one and pay us not to pollute. Sen (1984) points out that the future generations may have certain rights and discounting the well-being of future generations may lead to violation of those rights. He writes (p. 347):

> Suppose (an) investment project...will eliminate some pollution that the present generation will otherwise impose on the future. Even if the future generation may be richer and may enjoy a higher welfare level, and even if its marginal utility from the consumption gain is accepted to be less than the marginal loss of the present generation, this may still not be accepted to be decisive for rejecting the investment when the alternative implies long term effects of the environmental pollution. The avoidance of oppression has to be given value of its own.

There may be some obligation to the present generation which if not taken into account may violate the rights of the present generation. It does not seem that the future generations have a right to the present generations' savings.

REFERENCES

Acharya A, Murray CJL (forthcoming) Discounting future health states. In: *Fairness and Goodness: Ethical issues in health resource allocation.* Wikler D, Murray CJL, eds. World Health Organization, Geneva.

Anand S, Hanson K (1997) Disability-adjusted life years: a critical review. *Journal of Health Economics,* **16**(6):685–702.

Anand S, Sen AK (1994) *Sustainable human development: concepts and priorities.* (Working paper no 90.04.) Harvard Center for Population and Development Studies, Cambridge, MA.

Busschbach JJV, Jessing DJ, de Charro FT (1993) The utility of health at different stages of life: a quantitative approach. *Social Science and Medicine,* 37(2):153–158.

Cropper ML, Aydede SK, Portney PR (1994) Preferences for life saving programs: how the public discounts time and age. *Journal of Risk and Uncertainty,* 8(3):243–265.

Hammit JK (1993) Discounting health increments. Editorial. *Journal of Health Economics,* 12:117–120.

Hampshire S (1989) *Innocence and experience.* Harvard University Press, Cambridge, MA.

Institute of Medicine (1986) *New vaccine development. Establishing priorities. Disease of importance in developing countries.* National Academy Press, Washington, DC.

Johannesson M, Johansson PO (1996) *Is the valuation of a QALY gained independent of age? Some empirical evidence. (Mimeo).*

Lewis PA, Charny M (1989) Which of two individuals do you treat when only their ages are different and you can't treat them both? *Journal of Medical Ethics,* 15(1):28–32.

Murray CJL (1996) Rethinking DALYs. In: *The global burden of disease: a comprehensive assessment of mortality and disability from diseases, injuries, and risk factors in 1990 and projected to 2020.* The Global Burden of Disease and Injury, Vol. 1. Murray CJL, Lopez AD, eds. Harvard School of Public Health on behalf of WHO, Cambridge, MA.

Murray CJL, Acharya AK (1997) Understanding DALYs. *Journal of Health Economics,* 16:703–730.

Murray CJL, Lopez AD, eds. (1996) *The global burden of disease: a comprehensive assessment of mortality and disability from diseases, injuries and risk factors in 1990 and projected to 2020.* Global Burden of Disease and Injury, Vol. 1. Harvard School of Public Health on behalf of WHO, Cambridge, MA.

Parfit D (1984) *Reasons and persons.* Clarendon Press, Oxford.

Ramsey FP (1928) A mathematical theory of savings. *Economic Journal,* 38: 543–559.

Redelmeier DA, Heller DM (1993) Time preference in medical decision making and cost-effectiveness analysis. *Medical Decision Making,* 13(3):212–217.

Sen A (1984) Approaches to the choice of discount rates for social benefit-cost analysis. In: *Discounting for time and risk in energy policy.* Lind RC, ed. John Hopkins University Press, Baltimore, MA.

Viscusi WK, Moore MJ (1989) Rates of time preference and valuations of the duration of life. *Journal of Public Economics,* 38(3):297–317.

Walzer M (1992) Moral minimalism. In: *From the twilight of probability: ethics and politics.* Shea WR, Spadafora A, eds. Science History Publication, Canton, MA.

Wright S (1985) Subjective evaluation of health: a theoretical review. *Social Indicator Research,* 16:169–179.

Chapter 14.1

HEALTH AND EQUITY

FRANCES P. KAMM

In this article, I shall consider some principles for rationing and resource prioritization in health.[1] I shall also try to provide philosophical foundations for these principles, beginning at the most basic level. These issues arise at both a micro and macro level. At the micro level, some can fall under what is described as the *responsiveness* of a health care system, for example, is it procedurally fair between competitors for health care and just in what it gives to each? ("Responsiveness", in the World Health Organization health system performance framework, is used to refer to respect for autonomy, dignity, and confidentiality and allows for the measurement of the distribution of health care.) To apply what I say about fairness and justice to the macro level, *often* all we have to do is think of cases where how we allocate resources will affect large numbers of people instead of a few. Sometimes, as I shall indicate, there is more to moving from micro to macro.

I shall distinguish between goodness, fairness and justice. To make one distinction clearer, consider the following case: A doctor must decide whether to stop a big pain in person A or a small pain in person B. She thinks, correctly, that she will do more good if she helps A. But she also remembers that yesterday B suffered a much *bigger* pain than A will suffer and no one helped B (A suffered nothing in the past). So she thinks it would be unfair to let B suffer again, even though she will do less good if she helps him. If it is overall right to do this, this means she does the morally better thing in helping him and the state of affairs in which B is helped rather than A is morally better than one in which A is helped. But this is not because it produces more good.

I distinguish justice from fairness as follows: considerations of fairness are essentially relational, that is, how is A treated relative to B? Justice is concerned with someone getting his due. I can make a situation more just but less fair by giving only one of two people his due when otherwise neither would be given his due. A particular relation between people is equality; sometimes it is fair, but other times, fairness demands inequality—

as when one person has morally relevant characteristics in virtue of which he should be treated differently.

Justice and fairness are typically thought to function as "side constraints" on the maximization of the good. That is, unlike the good, they are not treated as factors that we are also treating as goals to be maximized. If they were only goals, it might be morally right to treat someone unfairly in order to maximize fairness overall (or to minimize unfairness). But if fairness is a side constraint, this would account for why such behaviour is often ruled out. This distinction may be important to keep in mind when constructing a measure for the health of populations. Some would like to have a measure that assigns grades to end-states of population health that includes considerations of how fairly health is distributed. But this involves treating fairness as a characteristic of an end-state (i.e. as part of a state which it is our goal to achieve) rather than as a side constraint on bringing about end-states. If we aim to maximize the grade, this may incorrectly lead us to deliberately act unfairly in order to maximize fairness. This is one reason to think of fairness and goodness as separate considerations.

EQUALITY, PRIORITY AND THE VEIL OF IGNORANCE

Some think that providing equal health or health expectations for all persons is a requirement of fairness. This might be denied for several reasons. The first is that if the only way to produce equality of health between people were to *reduce* the health of some without improving that of anyone, then (all other things equal) this would be morally wrong. (This is known as the "leveling down" objection to equality.) The second reason is that it may be morally most important to raise the health of the worst-off people, even if the route to doing this required us to introduce inequality. For example, suppose the Blues are relatively worse off healthwise and in bad health in absolute terms. The Reds are better off healthwise. If the *only* way to help the Blues raise up in absolute terms involved introducing a system that helped the Reds even more than the Blues, it might still be morally desirable. Giving priority to helping the worst off might be justified because we thus produce more good. That is, on account of diminishing marginal utility, each unit of resource devoted to the worst off produces more good than if it were given to those already better off. But even holding the amount of good we produce constant, it can be morally more important to help those who are worst off because (other things equal) it is morally more important that a good go to someone who has less. In giving priority to the worst off, we do *first compare* people to see who is worse off, but then we know whether we are satisfying the priority principle just by seeing if the worst off is getting better off; we need not compare him to someone else, except to know when to stop focusing on him because he is no longer worse off than others. The principles I shall be discussing in the rest of this article are consistent with giving *significant priority* to those who are the worst off in health care but not necessarily consistent with achieving equality or with always helping the worst off at no matter what cost in improved health to those already better off.

Of course, it is an empirical question whether doing what creates inequality in health leads to those worst off in health having better health than they would otherwise have. Empirical data may show that what produces inequality in health also makes those with the worst health worse off *in absolute terms* than they would be were there equality of health. (I shall return to this issue below.)

One ground for requiring equal prospects for health (understood as normal species functioning [NSF]) is that it is necessary for equal opportunity to develop and use one's talents and abilities. Norman Daniels argues in this way. The first part of Rawls's second principle of justice requires equal opportunity, and so as a Rawlsian, Daniels argues for equal normal species functioning (Daniels 1985). If all anyone could want in the way of opportunity were equality with others, there would be no point in introducing inequality of opportunity as a means to making the absolute level of opportunity each person had greater, and hence no justification (within a Rawlsian framework) for such inequality. However, suppose everyone were *equally sick*; then everyone could still have equal opportunity, for everyone would be working under an equal burden in exercising their talents and abilities. I assume we think that this is not yet an ideal condition even from the point of view of opportunity. Hence we really want *more* than equal opportunity; we want the degree to which people can use their talents not to be negatively affected by sickness (even if this were to occur equally). If this is so, then it is again at least possible that unequal health could increase the absolute degree to which sickness does not interfere with people's using their talents and abilities. (An easy-to-imagine case is one where doctors are kept healthier than others because this is necessary to maximize the health of other members of the population.)[2] This criticism reminds us that equality is only a comparative notion; but we want a certain absolute level of health to be insured as well.

The argument for equal NSF as a precondition for equal opportunity may also face the problem of instability. Suppose talents and abilities are unequal among people and fair incentives result in some being better off economically than others. If health varies with social class (as some data suggest) (Marmot 1999), then equal NSF will be short-lived; it will undo itself. But those worse off in health may still do better overall (on other dimensions of well-being) as a result of the inequality. (It is even logically possible for them to do better in absolute terms healthwise than with equality, though in fact this may not be true.)

That we think leveling down to achieve equality is morally problematic may bear in an interesting way on a claim made by Christopher Murray and his coauthors (Murray et al. 2000). They say, "We propose that the relation 'is healthier than' can be defined such that population A is healthier than population B *if and only if* an individual behind a veil of ignorance would prefer to be one of the existing individuals in population

A rather than an existing individual in population B, holding all non-health characteristics of the two populations to be the same." They also say, "Imagine two populations, A and B, with identical mortality, incidence, and remission for all non-fatal health states, but with a higher prevalence of paraplegia in population A. Behind a veil of ignorance, an individual will prefer to be a member of population B" (p. 987). As Murray and coauthors note, it is important whether we use a thick veil, as Rawls does, or rather a thin veil. A veil is thin if it allows people to know a great deal about the different populations, including the differential rates of conditions such as paraplegia. People do not know only who they would be in a community—the person with or without paraplegia. Given knowledge of different rates of illness, they can make probability calculations of getting an illness. Thin veils are involved when people say that the results one gets from using a veil of ignorance can depend on one's risk aversiveness. Rawls uses a thick veil—one doesn't know about the distribution of various conditions in a society or between societies; one is deliberately hindered by Rawls from using subjective probabilities in decision-making. Rawls gets his maximin results—make the worst off as well off as possible—not by assuming that people are very risk averse. He denies he needs this assumption. Rather, if one lacks the data to reasonably formulate subjective probabilities, one is deciding on principles that will determine the whole life prospects of people, and one is a head of family, one need not be risk averse to favour maximin, he thinks. Why does Rawls *use* a thick veil instead of a thin veil? I shall return to this question at the very end of this article. For now, let us consider the use of the thin veil in the paraplegia case and its relevance to leveling down.

The higher incidence of paraplegia in population A might result in *greater equality* of health in population A than in B by leveling down. Hence, if one cared about equality from behind a veil of ignorance, one might prefer to be a member of population B. One could avoid this result by insisting that those behind the veil must not care about relational goods such as equality or by insisting that equality not be achieved by leveling down. Without such restrictions on the decision-making of those behind the veil, what a person would choose from behind a thin veil of ignorance will not be an adequate test for which is the healthier society. This problem for the criterion of the healthier society using choice-behind-a-veil arises because a worsening of health might unavoidably produce a characteristic (e.g. equality) of potential interest to choosers behind a thin veil.

CONFLICTS WITH DIFFERENT NUMBERS OF PEOPLE

Suppose we are dealing with two-way micro conflict cases between potential recipients of a scarce resource. When there are an equal number of people in conflict who stand to be as badly off if not aided and gain the same if aided (and all other morally relevant factors are the same), fairness dictates giving each side an equal chance for the resource by using a random decision procedure. This is so even though the health outcome would be the same even if we were unfair.

But there may be a conflict situation in which *different numbers of* relevantly similar people are on either side and they stand to be as badly off and gain the same thing. (In micro situations, there will be few on either side, in macro many.) The following Aggregative Argument applied in a micro context tells us that it is a better outcome if more are helped: (1) It is worse for both B and C to die than for only B to die; (2) A world in which A dies and B survives is just as bad, from an impartial point of view, as a world in which B dies and A survives. Given (2), we can substitute A for B on one side of the moral equation in (1) and get that it is worse if B and C die than if A dies.

But even if it would be a worse outcome from an impartial perspective that B and C die than that A dies, that does not necessarily mean that it is right for us to save B and C rather than A. We cannot automatically assume it is morally permissible to maximize the good, for doing so may violate justice or fairness. (In other cases, seeking the greater good may be correctly constrained by justice. For example, we should not kill one innocent bystander to save five people from death.)

Here is an argument against its being unjust or unfair to save the greater number in the case of A, B and C. The Balancing Argument (I) claims that in this conflict, justice demands that each person on one side should have her interests balanced against those of one person on the opposing side; those that are not balanced out in the larger group help determine that the larger group should be saved. If we instead toss a coin between one person and any number on the other side, thereby giving each person an equal chance, we would behave no differently than if it were a contest between one and one. If the presence of each additional person would make no difference, this seems to deny the equal significance of each person. Thus, justice does not here conflict with producing the most good.

How might we extend these principles to conflicts when the individuals are *not* equally needy? Consider a case where the interests of two people conflict with the interests of one. The position to which one person would fall (death) and his potential gain (10 years of life) is matched by one of the tandem (D). The potential loss of the second person of the pair (E) is very small, for example, a sore throat. To take away C's 50 per cent chance of having 10 years of life rather than death in order to increase the overall good produced by the marginal benefit of a sore throat cure fails to show adequate respect for the single person who could avoid death and gain the 10 years. This is because from her *personal point of view*, she is not indifferent between her being the one who gets the 10 years and someone else getting it. The form of reasoning I am here using to justify *not* maximizing the good gives equal consideration from an impartial point of view to each individual's partial point of view, so it combines objective and subjective perspectives. Hence, I call it *Sobjectivity*. It accounts for why we should give fair chances. It also implies that certain extra goods (like the throat cure) can be morally irrelevant; I call this the Principle of Irrelevant Goods. Whether a good is irrelevant is context-dependent. Curing a sore throat is morally irrelevant when others' lives are at stake, but not when others' ear aches are. This Sore Throat Case shows that we must refine the claim that what we owe each person is to balance her interests against the equal interests of an opposing person and let the remainder help determine the outcome. Sometimes the remainder is not determinative. Further, so long as what is at stake for C or D is large, *no number of the small losses occurring in each of many people should be aggregated on D's side* so as to outweigh giving C and equal chance of avoiding the large loss.

The Sore Throat Case also raises the possibility that self-interested reasoning ex ante behind a veil of ignorance cannot be relied on to give morally correct answers. For using such reasoning, each person would consider that he maximizes his expected good by there being a procedure, ex post, which saves the one and also allows us to provide the sore throat cure. Yet this seems the wrong conclusion.

But suppose the additional lesser loss in one of the tandem is losing a leg. We should save a person's life for ten years rather than save someone from losing a leg when all else is equal and these are the *only* morally relevant choices. However, perhaps it is correct to together save one person's life for ten years and a second person's leg than to give a third person an equal chance at having his life saved. This might be because one and only one life will be saved no matter what we do and the loss of a leg is a large loss. This would be evidence that giving someone *his equal chance for life* should not receive as much weight from the impartial point of view as saving a life when we would otherwise save no one. (Perhaps we can be more precise: giving each side a 50 per cent chance in the Sore Throat Case is closer to what each side deserves—if the sore throat should raise one side's proportional chance slightly—than giving one side 100 per cent. By contrast, the addition of a leg may raise the proportional chance owed to one side enough that 100 per cent is closer to that figure than 50 per cent.)

So far, I have been discussing decision procedures that are consistent with what philosophers call "pairwise comparison". That is, we check to see that for everyone who will fall to a certain level on one side that there is someone who will fall to a very similar level on the other side before we consider weighing in those who will not fall to levels anywhere as bad to determine which side gets aided. This is one way of being sure we help the worst-off people first. However, I have also attended to how great a gain someone could receive if he is helped. For it is possible that if we cannot give the worst-off person very much, we should give more to those who would not be as badly off if not helped. This approach gives some priority to the worst off but not lexical priority. Furthermore, it is possible that principles which involve pairwise comparison to see who will be worse off are requirements of fairness in choosing whom to aid only in micro situations (e.g. in the emergency room). To make macro decisions, for example, whether to invest in research to cure a disease that will kill a few people, depriving them of ten years of life, or in research to cure a disease that will only wither an arm in many, we might have another principle. It permits aggregation of significant (though not insignificant) lesser losses (which can be corrected) to many people to outweigh even greater losses to a few, even though no individual person in the larger group would have as bad a fate as each individual in the smaller group would have. As such, it does not give absolute priority to helping the worst off (even greatly). As the Principle of Irrelevant Goods emphasized, whether a lesser loss is significant and hence aggregatable over people is judged relative to the nature of the greater loss, and so determining if a lesser loss is aggregatable is context-dependent. On this view, the important point is that whether a lesser loss should be aggregated over people to weigh against a greater loss in others is *not* merely a function of how many people suffer it, but also of its size relative to the size of the greater loss. There are no number of headaches such that we should prevent them rather than certainly save a few lives.

Notice that this may raise a problem of intransitivity: suppose that relative to n, y is a significant lesser loss. So at the macro level, it may be better to prevent many people from losing y than to save a few from n. But relative to y, z is a significant lesser loss, and so it would be better to save a great many suffering z than a few suffering n. Yet, it may be that relative to y, z is not a significant loss, since "significant" is context relative and so is not transitive.

My suggestion for dealing with this problem is as follows: if we can save a few suffering from n, we may save many from suffering y instead, but we should not go so far as to save a great many from suffering z. (This is so on the continuing assumption that the people are alike in all morally relevant respects besides the size of these losses.) This is true, even though if some suffering n were not present, we should save a great many from z rather than save many from y. This is because which act is correct can depend on the alternatives we can bring about.

Finally, in the micro level cases involving different numbers of people, suppose we have a choice between helping one person (A), who will be very badly off and much benefited by our aid, or helping a couple of people (B and C), each of whom will be as badly off as A but not benefited as much by our aid. So long as the lesser benefit is significant, it is morally more important, I think, to distribute our efforts over more people, each of whom will be as badly off as the single person rather than provide a bigger benefit concentrated in one person (other things equal). One way to analyse this situation employs what I shall call Balancing Argument (II): find the part of the potential large gain to A (part 1) that is balanced by the smaller gain to B. Now we must decide how to break that tie between them. If we care about giving priority to those who are worst off, we will care more about benefiting the next person in the group, C, rather than giving an additional benefit (part 2) to A who, having received part 1 would already have more than C. This means that instead of breaking the tie between A-with-part-1 and B by giving A a greater benefit, we break the tie by helping two people, each to a lesser degree.[3]

SAME NUMBERS OF PEOPLE WITH DIFFERENT RELEVANT FEATURES

A theory of the fair distribution of scarce resources should also tell us if certain characteristics that one candidate for the resources has to a greater degree than another are morally relevant to deciding who gets the resource. I call this the problem of allocation when there is *intra-personal aggregation*, because one candidate has characteristics the other has *plus* more that make possible greater goods. We have already considered principles that apply when the additional goods we can achieve, if we help one rather than another of the worst-off people, are distributed over several people. The question arises whether we can revise these principles to apply when additional goods we can achieve are *concentrated* in one person rather than another.

A system I suggest for evaluating candidates for a resource who differ intra-personally starts off with only three factors—need, urgency, and outcome—but it could add other factors later. Urgency is defined as how badly off someone's life will go if he is not helped. "Need" is defined as how badly someone's life *will have gone* if he is not helped. "Outcome" is defined as the difference in expected outcome produced by the resource relative to the expected outcome if one is not helped; that is, the benefit someone will get from the resource. The neediest people may not be the most urgent. Suppose C will die in a month at age 65 unless helped *now* and D will die in a year at age 20 unless helped *now*. I suggest that often this will mean that D is less urgent but needier, since one's life *will often have gone* much worse if one dies at 20 rather than at 65. (This does not mean we should always help the neediest; for example, if we could only extend the younger life to age 22 but could give the 65-year-old ten years more, this would be a reason to help the 65-year-old).[4]

Notice that there is an ordinary sense of urgency in which both C and D are equally urgent, namely they require care just as soon—*now*—in order to be helped.[5] I have chosen to use "urgent" to refer to how bad one's prospects are; I shall use "urgent-C" (short for "urgent care") if necessary to refer to how soon treatment is needed.

COMPARISON OF *WHAT*?

In thinking about how urgent or needy someone is, or how good an outcome is, we must think how badly or well will life go, or have gone, *in what ways*? In microallocation of health services, I believe we should be concerned with the *health*-way rather than overall well-being (including economic and cultural factors). This means that at the micro level, health is treated as a separate sphere of justice.[6] So, if E would be in worse health than F, the fact that F would be economically much worse off than E is not a reason to say F is more urgent than E is and treat F with the health care resource. But suppose E's health overall has been painlessly much worse than F's in his life (e.g. limited mobility), but F now faces a lot of pain and E just a little. It is possible that we should consider all *dissimilar* aspects of ill health and help E, so that he will not have had to lead a much worse life healthwise than F. On the other hand, since we can only help E's future in a small way and can do nothing to undo his past, the much greater good we can do for F's future may be determinative. (Some may find the judgment that we should help E more convincing when we ignore E's past but decide based on the fact that he but not F *will* also have limited mobility *in the future*. Some may think it correct to consider only how much pain each will have in the future or will have had overall, since some part of this pain is the aspect of well-being we can affect now. I shall not here choose between these conflicting ways of deciding. For more on this, see Kamm (2002) and Scanlon (1998).

By contrast, at the macro level, when deciding whether to invest in providing one health service or another, it might be that we should make an *all-things-considered judgment* about how well off people have been or will be. That is, the way in which people have and will fare in health may be considered together with the way they have or will fare economically and culturally. This means health would not be treated as a *separate sphere of justice* at the macro level. This has important implications for the very idea of "health equity". Suppose, for example, that we can invest in curing a disease that causes the poor to die at age 70 or a disease that causes the rich to die at age 60. If we care about equality, we might chose to invest in the former, since having a nicer life might compensate the rich for having a shorter one; things will be overall more equal if the poor at least live longer, so long as their lives are worth living. *So, equity of health—getting the just or fair amount of it—is not inconsistent with inequality of (prospect) for it.* (We already knew this as a result of the discussion in section 1, for there the possibility was raised that helping the worst off might, theoretically, require inequality of prospects for health.) Even those who care about equality may not care about equality of (prospects for) health *per se* but rather equality of a bundle of goods, including health as one good. It is when those who have less on one dimension (e.g. health) *also* have less on other important dimensions of value (e.g. wealth) that egalitarians should be most concerned about equality on a particular dimension.

Notice that if this is so, it alters how we look at such empirical results as the Whitehall Study.[7] Researchers found a perfect correlation between class and health in the positive direction, that is, as class went up, health went up; as class went down, health went down. Concern with the data should not be merely that there is correlation between wealth and health; presumably, it is the causal direction that is crucial. We should not be disturbed if greater health *causes* greater wealth, for that just means that when people are healthier, they are more productive, and that is one of the things we expect and even hope for. (Of course, if this were the direction of causality, we may still be concerned that some are healthy and others are not.) We should (plausibly) be disturbed if the direction of causality is such that greater wealth causes greater health so that the poor are not only short on money but also on health. If we are disturbed by this data, assuming the second causal direction, is this best described as concern over inequality of health, that is, concern that all classes do not have the same level of health? Suppose the data showed a perfect correlation, only negative, that is, as class goes up, health goes *down*; as class goes down, health goes *up*. I hypothesize that we would not be as concerned with this second result as we are with the first, yet there is just as much lack of equality in health on the basis of class in this second, hypothetical, result as in the first, actual result. I venture that we would be less concerned because we think that the goods of high social class may compensate for the poorer health. When there is such compensation, there may be *overall* equality between classes.

But, of course, it may be that overall equality is not the right goal, if we can increase the absolute position of some further with overall inequality. So, if wealthier people had better health but the inequalities of wealth were fair (for example, because they improved the absolute condition of the worst off overall, even including their relatively lower health), then the resulting inequality of health might be fair, too. On this view, we should be disturbed by the Whitehall results only because we think the distribution of wealth is unfair (perhaps, in part, because it results in lower *absolute* health for the worst off with no adequate compensations, by comparison with a different distribution of wealth).

An alternative to an all-things-considered judgment is to treat health as a separate sphere, even at the macro level, in the way we treat liberal freedoms. We would not consider a person who lacked a right to free speech that others had to be adequately compensated by the fact that he has more money than they have. This should also be the position of those who think equal health is a precondition for equal opportunity and equal opportunity has priority over improving the economic or cultural condition of the worst off. If health is a separate sphere, we would have to compare how people are doing just along the health dimension separately, even at the macro level. But notice that if those who have more economic wealth or power than is just are helped to achieve the correct and equal level of health, we may increase the *overall* unjust inequality between them and others. For this reason we might make getting the correct level of health conditional on the overall better-off people ceding some of the other (admittedly) non-compensating goods they have in greater abundance than others. (One way to do this is require them to pay for their health care.) There is an asymmetry here: we cannot deny them their right to certain health prospects because they have other things; but we could deny them other things because they get correct health prospects. Of course, if inequality in wealth always causes inequality in health (let alone lower levels of health in absolute terms), we may have to decide whether equalizing health (to the extent this is under our control) is worth the requirement of equality in other areas. Alternatively, if there is an intervening mechanism through which inequality in wealth produces differential health, we may be able to just interfere with that mechanism directly.

WEIGHTING OF FACTORS

Let us return to need in the microallocation context. To consider how much weight to give to need, we hold the two other factors of outcome and urgency constant and imagine two candidates who differ only in neediness. Often those who will have had the worse life healthwise are those who will have had fewer healthy years if not helped. Then one argument for taking differential need into account is fairness: give to those who, if not helped, will have had less of the good (e.g. life) that our resource can provide (at least if they are equal on other health dimensions) before giving to those who will have had more of it even if they are not helped. Fairness is a value that depends on comparisons between people. But even if we do not compare candidates, it can often be of greater moral value to give a certain unit of life to a person who has had less of life, i.e. the younger.

But need will matter more the more absolutely and comparatively needy a candidate is, and some differences in need may be governed by a Principle of Irrelevant Need, which implies that relative to a context, some differences in need are morally irrelevant. This is especially so when each candidate is absolutely needy, a big gain for each is at stake, and if the needier person is helped he will wind up having more of the good (e.g. a longer life) than the person who was originally less needy than he. Need may also play a different role depending on whether life is at stake or quality of life is at stake, for a low quality of life can be less bad for someone than his dying. When it is, we deprive the needy of less if we do not give them priority when quality of life is at stake, and of more if we do not give them priority when life is at stake. For a different view, see endnote 4.

Suppose there is conflict between helping the neediest person and helping the most urgent person (when we can give each the same benefit). I claim that when there is true scarcity, it can be more important to help the neediest than the urgent. If scarcity is only temporary, the urgent-C should be helped first, since the others will be helped eventually anyway.[8]

Still, there are constraints on the relevance of need (one concept of the worst off) in a correct theory of distribution. For example, it may be impermissible to give a resource to the person who will have had a worse life healthwise because he will have less overall of the good we can provide, if it fails to respect the rights of each person. Consider another context: If two people have a human right to free speech, how long someone's right has already been respected may be irrelevant in deciding whom to help retain free speech. If having health or life for a number of years were a human right, it might not be appropriate to ration resources on the basis of the degree to which people's rights have already been met (or on the basis of whether they have had more of other goods). On this view, how much life one had already would not be a reason to ration life-saving resources on the basis of age, so long as one had not reached the age guaranteed by right.

An additional consideration that militates against helping on the basis of need where this is linked to rationing according to age relates to the risks it may be rational for each individual to take. Suppose the probability of conditions arising that cause loss of life is low in youth but high in old age, and there is a fixed total health resource budget/per person to be distributed over the course of her life. Assume also that (for the most part) if one dies in youth, one will lose out in a longer future than if one dies in old age and one will also have had a worse life. Even on the latter assumptions, it would not necessarily make most sense to invest resources so as to insure against the smaller probability of death in youth (when the procedures funded by these resources will probably not be used) and ignore much higher probabilities of death in older age (when procedures would be useful). Suppose it turned out to be rational for people to accept some risk of death when young to ensure care when old. Then each person who is old now will have accepted (and survived) the risk he takes when young. It would be unfair to now deny him treatment to help the young person for whom it too was rational to accept the small risk of death through absence of resources (Daniels 1988).[9]

Now we come to outcome. Some might think it appropriate to take into account all the effects of a resource in determining the outcome it produces. By contrast, at least in micro contexts, I suggest:

(1) Effects on third parties whom a resource helps only indirectly should be given less weight than its direct effects, even though these are indirect effects on health. For example, if we face a choice between saving a doctor and a teacher, the fact that the doctor will be irreplaceable in saving lives should not mean that all the lives he will save (an indirect effect of the resource he gets) are counted on his side against the teacher. (Hence, this goes beyond the view that only health effects should count.)[10]

(2) Some differences in outcome between candidates may be irrelevant because achieving them is not the goal of the particular "health sphere" which controls the resource (e.g. that only one potential recipient in the health care sphere will write a novel if he receives a scarce drug should not count in favour of his getting it. The health care system is not the National Endowment for the Arts).

(3) Other differences in expected outcome between candidates may be covered by the Principle of Irrelevant Good, even if they are part of the health sphere. For example, relative to the fact that each person stands to avoid death and live for ten years, that one person can get a somewhat better quality of life or an additional year of life should not determine who is helped, given that each wants what she can get. One explanation for this is that *what both are capable of achieving (ten years) is the part of the outcome about which each reasonably cares most in the context*, and each wants to be the one to survive. The extra good is frosting on the cake. The fact that someone might accept an additional risk of death (as in surgery) to achieve the "cake plus frosting" for herself does not necessarily imply that it is correct to impose an additional risk of death on one person so that another person, who stands to get the greater good, has a greater chance to live.[11]

However, it might be suggested that, in life and death decisions, any *significant* difference between two people in expected life years should play a role in selecting whom to help. This result would be analogous to the claim that if we could save x's life or else y's plus z's leg, we should do the latter. Still, because the large additional benefit would be concentrated in the same person who would already be benefited by having her life saved for at least the same period as the other candidate, I think, it should count for less in determining who gets the resource than it does when the additional benefit is distributed to a third person. This is on account of the greater moral importance of first helping to some significant degree either person avoid the bad fate faced by each, and the diminishing moral value of providing an additional benefit to someone who would already be greatly benefited. (The same issue arises for large differences in expected quality of life among candidates for a resource in situations where improving quality of life is the point of the resource.)[12]

Between the irrelevant differences in goods and those that are large enough to outweigh other factors might be differences in outcome that should be treated by giving people chances in proportion to the good of the differential outcome.

What if taking care of the neediest or most urgent conflicts with producing the best relevant difference in outcome? Rather than always favouring the worst off, we might assign multiplicative factors in accord with need and urgency by which we multiply the expected outcome of the neediest and urgent. These factors represent the greater moral significance of a given outcome going to the neediest (or most urgent), but the non-neediest could still get a resource if her expected differential outcome was very large. Furthermore, doing a significant amount to raise those who are very badly off in absolute terms to an appropriate minimal level of well-being might have lexical priority over even an enormous improvement in those already much better off.

My views on outcome, need and urgency can be summarized in an *outcome modification procedure for allocation*. We first assign points for each candidate's differential expected outcome. We then check the absolute level of need and urgency of candidates. If some are below a certain minimal level of well-being and the good we can do would significantly raise them toward the minimal level, these receive the resource. For those above this minimal level of well-being, we assign multiplicative factors for their need and urgency in accordance with the moral importance of those factors relative to each other and relative to outcome. We multiply the outcome points by these factors. The candidate with a sufficiently high point score gets the resource. If the difference is too small to be morally relevant, we give equal chances. If it is in between, chances in proportion to the score might be suitable.[13]

QALYs AND DALYs

QALYs and DALYs are used to measure the impact illness has on someone in terms of both morbidity and mortality; they also measure the impact of care on someone in terms of reducing both morbidity and mortality. The theory of outcomes is that we can do more than merely count the number of years that will (we expect) be gained as a result of health intervention—note that even this is a step beyond merely considering whether a life has been saved but not considering *for how long it will be saved*. We also count how good these years will be. So we may multiply the number of years of life by the quality of each year. Alternatively, we may determine how effective aid is by considering how badly someone's life would have gone—or as it is said how disabled he would have been—without the intervention. In this way, we see how much reduction in such disabled years we produce by the intervention. We aim to increase QALYs and decrease DALYs, though not by eliminating the life.

How do we measure the quality of a life or the degree to which it is disabled? Philosophers have tried to offer hedonistic, desire-satisfaction, and objective list theories of good and bad lives to answer such questions. That is, they have suggested that a life is of higher or lower quality, depending on how much pleasure/pain there is in it, how many of one's desires (regardless of the object of desire) are satisfied, or how much of certain objective goods (including but not limited to pleasure/no pain) there are in it. But those who use QALYs and DALYs do not use such philosophical theories. They either take surveys of ordinary people (in QALYs) or experts (in DALYs), asking them to rate the quality of various lives with or without various limitations on them. The aim is to assign numbers to the effects of aid. Two tests are often used in achieving this goal: the trade-off within one life test and the standard gamble test. (I shall deal separately with the test dealing with trade-offs between people.) In the first, we are asked how many years with disability x we would trade for how many years of perfect health. So if ten years of life as a paralysed person would be exchanged for five years as a healthy person (ranked at 1), we know that being paralysed is to be assigned a .5 value. The trade-off test also makes clear that people would exchange some length of life for some increased quality of life (or disability reduction). The standard gamble test asks one to imagine what risk of death one would take (e.g. in surgery) to exchange some length of life at one level of quality/disability for the same length at a higher quality. For example, is a 40 per cent chance of death and a 60 per cent chance of perfect health equivalent to a 100 per cent chance of life with paralysis? The greater the chance of death one would take to achieve perfect health, the worse is the state from which one is escaping, presumably.[14]

Let us consider the DALY, in particular. Suppose perfect health is rated at 1; wearing glasses reduces the quality of the life to .999 (and so one is disabled to .001); paralysis brings one down to .5. Having this information can be important in deciding not only how much good we can do if we aid or how much badness will occur if we do not. It can also help us decide whom to aid when we cannot aid everyone, it is claimed. For example, if we think it just to give priority to helping the worst off (not necessarily overall worst, but perhaps only healthwise worst), it is important to know that paralysis is worse than wearing eyeglasses. If we ranked paralysis no lower than wearing eyeglasses, we could not argue in favour of investing in cures or preventions for paralysis rather than nearsightedness (a macro decision) or treating a person to cure or prevent paralysis in an emergency room rather than cure or prevent nearsightedness (a micro decision). Of course, even if we would reduce more DALYs if we treated paralysis rather than nearsightedness, the cost of doing so may be much greater, and hence the DALYs reduced per dollar (cost effectiveness of allocating) might be greater if we instead treated nearsightedness. (If this were so, it also implies that for every one paralysis we cure or prevent we could cure or prevent hundreds of cases of nearsightedness. I shall return to this issue below.)

Notice that I have mentioned both curing and preventing a disability. It would seem reasonable to think that one would want to avoid (and hence prevent a disability) in accordance with how bad it would be to have the disability and hence how much one would want to be cured of it if one had it. If one knew that if one fell into a state x, there would be no good reason to try to leave it, would it be reasonable to want to avoid it? Surprisingly, the answer might be yes as going into the state might be disruptive of one's current plans, but once in it one alters one's plan so that there is no more reason to leave it (Brock forthcoming). Avoiding disruption of current plans might be the only reason to avoid state x. Brock has suggested that this is why nonparalysed people rank paralysis as worse than people who are already paralysed. If avoiding disruption of current plans were the only reason, or at least a contributing reason, to avoid paralysis, it would not be unjust for society to put a higher value on preventing a nonparalysed person from becoming paralysed and a lower value on curing a paralysed person. (Another less normative and more purely psychological finding might be pointed to in this connection. Psychologists Daniel Kahnemann and Amos Tversky (Kahneman 1994) report that subjects ask higher compensation ex ante than ex post for an injury. That is, when asked how much they would want in order to go through some loss, they ask for more than they ask as compensation once they have suffered the loss.)

However, if those with disabilities must engage in less intrinsically valuable activities, and/or have diminished freedom to choose whether to do something or not (even if their remaining options are good ones), these might be reasons, I believe, to rate curing a disability as highly as preventing it. In any case, in what follows, I shall assume this is so.[15]

THE WORST OFF

Let us now consider some particular allocation problems. Some who recommend employing DALYs also believe that in allocating, we should help those who are worst off first, at least when expense per DALY is the same as it would be if we helped those who were not worst off. Hence, lowering DALYs and helping the worst off are not incompatible. But, even when the choice is between helping two people, helping the worst off need not follow *just* from trying to minimize DALYs. This is because in helping the worst off, we might not reduce as many DALYs as in helping someone who is not as badly off. If we must choose between helping a greater number of people each avoid a small disability and one person avoid a large disability (when the people are otherwise relevantly similar), total DALYs reduced could be the same. Yet those who think it is right to favour the worst off might still prefer to help that person. Dan Brock (forthcoming) points out that if we just consider people's rankings of various health conditions, and 1 represents perfect health for one year while wearing eyeglasses reduced health by .001 per year, then we could produce as much good by relieving one thousand people of the need to wear eyeglasses for twenty years as if we save someone's life who would go on to live in perfect health for twenty years. But if we should try to help the worst off person (still assuming same cost/per DALY reduced), we should save the life nevertheless.

I agree with Brock about this last case, but notice that preventing the aggregate of small disabilities may not always be the morally wrong answer. For example, suppose that having a sprain for a year reduced one's health to .9. Might saving the life of an eighty-year-old for one additional year really be morally the equivalent of providing (a) ten people with a drug that relieved their sprain for a year, or (b) one person with a drug that relieved his sprain for ten years? (Eighty-Year-Old Case.) The possibility of option (b) should remind us that aggregation can occur intra-personally—within one life—and that many small losses or gains (in the sense of avoidance of these losses) occurring to one person can have more moral significance than many small losses (or avoidance of these) occurring to many people. For example, twenty small headaches occurring in one life can be much worse than twenty small headaches occurring in the life of twenty people. Notice also that the moral difference between alternatives (a) and (b) decreases depending on whether we conceive of each of the ten people in (a) as either facing one year in their lives in which they suffer from a sprain (a year we can improve) or, by contrast, facing the same ten years of sprain as the person in (b) but having only one year of relief from that greater burden.

Finally, we have been considering a case in which we might save one person's life for a year, and we probably imagine this as rescuing someone from death. But we might put the choice differently: we have to decide when someone is 50 whether to give him medical treatment that is good enough to help him live to age 81 or only good enough to help him live to age 80. If we give him the medical care that only helps him live to age 80, we will be able to help someone not suffer from a sprain for ten years. This case compares intra-personal aggregation in the latter person and long-term prospects for life (rather than rescue efforts) in the former. In such a case, it may be less clear that we should favour extending the life over avoiding aggregate smaller losses than it is in Brock's original case.

What if more DALYs could be reduced if we aid 1 001 people so that they no longer need eyeglasses for twenty years, at less cost per DALY reduction, than if we save someone's life for twenty years? We might still think it right to help the worst off person have his life saved. We could use a method like that embodied in the Outcome Modification Procedure I described above to represent favouring the worst off in a DALY system: multiply the number of DALYs reduced when we help the person who would be worst off if not helped by a multiplicative factor that represents the greater moral value of aiding him. This will also lower the cost/per DALY reduction in her case.

But now consider the following scenario: One person is on island A, and another person is on island B. They share all the same properties, except that one just recently lost a hand and the other did not. We can save the life of either one but not both. Each will be as badly off as the other if we do not help him (dead). But if we help the person without the hand, we cannot reduce DALYs as much. (Call this the Islands Case.) I think it is morally wrong to decide to aid on this ground. We cannot rely on the principle of giving weight to the worst off to account for this conclusion, since each would, by hypothesis, be as badly off as the other if not aided. However, the Principle of Irrelevant Good, which I described above, can account for the right decision.

The point in the Islands Case is that the part of what is most important to each person can be had by either—long life saved with good quality of life. Furthermore, we should take seriously from an *objective* point of view the fact that each person, from his *subjective* perspective, wants to be the one to survive. We should, therefore, not deprive either of his equal chance for the great good of extended survival for the sake of producing the additional benefit to one person. This benefit is irrelevant in this context, though perhaps not in another. This is especially true when that one person is someone who would already be getting the other great benefit of additional life. (That is, it is a case of concentrated rather than dispersed additional good.)

Now consider the Islands Case (2), exactly like the Islands Case, except that there are six people on each island and each on island A will have lost his hand while all on island B will be perfectly formed. The additional claim of the Principle of Irrelevant Good is that if any individual's having a benefit that is an irrelevant good is not a reason to deprive someone else of an equal chance for a major good, then no number of these benefits aggregated across many people (possibly yielding a large total) should deprive other people of their equal chances for a major good.

On the basis of these cases, we can see that it is compatible with recognizing that not having a hand makes a life worse to think that, relative to the question of whose life we should save, it could be a morally irrelevant consideration. Hence, targeting funds to replace a missing hand is not inconsistent with giving equal weight to saving the lives of the disabled and the non-disabled.[16]

EX ANTE OBJECTIONS

Here are two objections that may be raised to giving two people equal chances to have their lives saved when one will yield a larger benefit or reduction in disability: (1) The paralysed person would himself accept some additional risk of death if the treatment we used on him would insure his not only living but being cured of paralysis. (People do, after all, undergo surgery with risk of death in order to remove their disabilities.) Does this not mean we should be allowed to impose that greater risk of death on him in order that someone else live in a nonparalysed state? (2) Ex ante, behind a veil of ignorance, before we know whether we are paralysed or not, we would assume that we had an equal probability of being the paralysed or nonparalysed person. Hence, we increase our own chances of living a nonparalysed life—which we prefer—if we agree, ex ante, to a policy which always saves the nonparalysed person's life. (The conclusions of (1) and (2) differ slightly, since (1) may only require us to give a greater proportional chance of survival to the person who will not be handicapped; (2) requires complete preference.)

My response to (1) is that being willing to take a risk of death in order to achieve a benefit for oneself is morally different from risking death in order to benefit someone else. The response to (2) is related to the response to (1), since a similar use of ex ante reasoning in (1) could suggest that one is, in a sense, taking the risk for oneself. This is because behind a veil of ignorance, one should think that for all one knows, it is oneself who will be benefited if the odds favour the non-handicapped person. My response to this extension of (1), as well as to (2), is that this form of ex ante reasoning is a moral mistake. As Thomas Scanlon has pointed out (Scanlon 1982), it is a mistake to think of people behind the veil of ignorance deciding what is morally correct by each imagining that he might possibly occupy any one of various positions in real life, though, of course, he can occupy only one. Someone who reasons in this way might, for example, maximize his average expected good by allowing some positions to be very much worse than others, if he is taking the small risk of falling into a bad position for the sake of a greater probability of falling into the good ones. An alternative is to view the veil of ignorance as a device that forces each person to identify with each of the separate individuals who will actually occupy the various outcome positions. When different people will actually occupy the different possible positions, some person will definitely (not just possibly) be abandoned, while others will benefit. Deciding how it is appropriate to treat these people in relation to each other is not answered either by one person imagining that he might be in the worst position (for this is comparable with no one actually being in it) or by saying that how we treat a person is acceptable so long as he stood to maximize his expected outcome by taking the risk of being treated in that way.

This analysis of ex-ante reasoning brings one to the final major point I wish to make in response to some of those who wish to employ QALYs and DALYs. They note that the data on trade-offs and gambles shows that individuals are willing to trade life years for improved quality of life or reduced disabilities. So, for example, suppose someone is willing to take a 5 per cent risk of death (thereby risking losing, let us say, twenty years of life) in order to have a 95 per cent chance of being cured of paraplegia. From such data—which we can refer to as an individual welfare function—they would like to derive implications for society as a whole—deriving a social welfare function. Apparently, they think the above data from the individual case would validate the conclusion that as a society, we can allow five people to die of one disease so that 95 people can be cured of paralysis when the one hundred are otherwise relevantly similar for moral purposes. (This presumably would be true in a microallocation scheme, where the one hundred people came into the emergency room at the same time, as well as in a macro decision about how to invest our research funds. Recall that I considered distinguishing the micro from the macro decision.)

But is this a correct argument for trade-offs between people? When an individual takes a chance, no one may die and he may benefit. Indeed, he takes the risk hoping this is so. And when each person in the society thinks of the gamble in his case, he may also imagine that he will not die and hope to benefit. But *in the group, some people will certainly die* (given that it is large enough) and others will be benefited. Further, each person hopes that this certain death will be someone else's. Perhaps this is a morally significant reason not to derive the social welfare function from the combination of individual welfare functions. To repeat, it can be argued that we will get the morally wrong principle of social justice, if we think that ex ante reasoning behind a veil of ignorance involves each person thinking of what probability he has for occupying each outcome-position—for example, 95 chances to be one of the cured, and five to be one of the dead. Rather, the veil of ignorance should lead each person to take seriously the fates of the separate persons who will actually occupy each of the outcome-positions, including the ones involving death.

Indeed, to return to an issue raised at the beginning of this chapter, Scanlon believes that forcing people to identify in this way with each person is why Rawls uses a thick veil (excluding probability calculations). If we engage in policies that we know will leave some to die to achieve lesser goods for a greater number of people, we must be able to give a justification to those who will die. Scanlon implies that saying to them either "you would have chosen to run the risk of being someone who will be left to die" or "you would have chosen to run the risk of being left to die" are not sufficient justifications. Though there may be others.

NOTES

1 I dealt with this issue at length in *Morality, Mortality, Vol. 1* (Kamm 1993).

2 Rawls' first principle of justice calls for *maximal* equal liberty. This too means that it is possible that unequal liberty could increase the absolute level of liberty of some from what it would be under non-maximal equal liberty.

3 I developed this additional balancing procedure in responding to Derek Parfit's discussion of cases of this sort in an unpublished manuscript.

4 It is interesting to note that most ordinary people surveyed by Erik Nord disagree that being older makes someone less needy of more life than a younger person. Furthermore, they think that where life is at stake there should be less distinction between helping young and old, while when quality of life is at stake one might favour the young. Their (unconscious) reasoning seems to be the opposite of the one I would suggest for these two cases, i.e. when something very important (life) is at stake, they think we should not distinguish between people; when something less important (quality) is at stake, we may distinguish between young and old. I get the opposite result by taking seriously that having had more life can make one less needy of that very important thing, other things equal. See Nord et al. (1995).

5 As pointed out to me by Derek Parfit.

6 For the idea of separate spheres of justice, see Walzer (1983).

7 Cited in Marmot (1999).

8 In *Morality, Mortality, Vol. I*, I did not distinguish urgency from urgent-C and hence mistakenly claimed that in temporary scarcity, the urgent should be treated before the needier.

9 I take this to be the main point of the view Norman Daniels defends in *Am I My Parents' Keeper?* (Daniels 1988).

10 It might be suggested that this is true because the person who would *not* be selected for aid is being inappropriately evaluated from only an instrumental point of view, and not also as an end-in-himself. That is, because he is not useful to others, he is rejected. But consider the following case: we have a scarce resource to distribute and if we give it to A, he can then also carry it to another person, C, who needs our resource. B cannot do this. In this case, it is permissible, I think, to select A over B, excluding B since he cannot be instrumentally useful. Doing this helps us to better serve those who directly need our resource. Hence (surprisingly), it seems it is not essentially distinguishing persons on the basis of their instrumental role that determines if our behaviour is objectionable, but whether we are using our resource for its best *direct* health effects.

11 Again, this conclusion conflicts with the choice that would be made if each person behind a veil of ignorance were trying to maximize his expected good.

12 Erik Nord claims that most of the people he surveyed do not care about the length of life that someone will live in deciding whom to help (above a significant outcome), but they do care about the probability of someone achieving any significant outcome. Presumably, this means they would favour giving a resource to someone who will almost certainly achieve a good outcome, rather than to someone who would have a much lower chance of a good outcome. But if one is offered certainty of getting two years of extra life with one treatment or a 50 per cent chance of twenty years with another treatment, and one is young, it is not unreasonable to think one is doing better to take the latter option. But, if we combine people's surveyed tendency to discount degree of good outcome with the relevance in their mind of probability of good outcome, we conclude that they would favour giving the resource to the person when he chooses the first treatment, but not the second, if it is scarce. This favours the conservative over the maximizers inappropriately, it would seem. See Nord (1995).

13 This can still be only a rough guide where more than two candidates are present. Since what we ought to do is a function of what the alternatives are, it may not always be right to produce what gives the higher score. For example, in the case I discussed on p. 690 involving one person who will lose n, many who will lose x and yet more who will lose z, I argue that we should help prevent z rather than x if it were only a choice between x and z, but should help x if it were a choice between all three.

14 Is it possible that state A could be worse than B and yet we would take a greater risk of death to avoid B than A? Yes, if there were some reason why it would be inappropriate to risk death to avoid A in particular (e.g. because one deserved A), Certainly, we could take an equal risk of death to avoid state A and state B, and yet one of the states is worse than the other, since the less bad one is already bad enough to make a maximal risk worthwhile. The validity of the gamble test is threatened by these possibilities.

15 Wanting a cure for a longstanding condition could be an indication that the cured life is thought to be better even by the disabled person, though it might just indicate a desire to be like the majority. If the majority were disabled and they desired a cure, however, this would be stronger evidence that the condition is worse than the non-disabled one.

16   I do not claim that this is a complete analysis. There is much more to be said about disabilities and the equitable distribution of resources. For more on this, see my "Deciding whom to help, health-adjusted life years, and disabilities" (Kamm forthcoming), and "Disabilities, discrimination, and irrelevant goods" (Kamm forthcoming).

References

Brock DW (Forthcoming) Ethical issues in the use of cost effectiveness analysis for the prioritization of health care resources. In: *Bioethics: A philosophical overview*. Khusfh G, Englehardt Jr. HT, eds. Kluwer Publishers, Dordrecht.

Daniels N (1985) *Just health care*. Cambridge University Press, Cambridge, MA.

Daniels N (1988) *Am I my parents' keeper? An essay on justice between the young and the old*. Oxford University Press, New York.

Kahneman D (1994) *The cognitive psychology of consequences and moral intuition. The Tanner lectures in human values (Unpublished work)*. University of Michigan, MI.

Kamm FM (Forthcoming) *Deciding whom to help, health-adjusted life years, and disabilities*.

Kamm FM (Forthcoming) *Disabilities, discrimination, and irrelevant goods*.

Kamm FM (1993) *Morality, mortality. Vol 1: Death and whom to save from it*. Oxford University Press, Oxford.

Kamm FM (2002) Owing, justifying and rejecting. *Mind*, **111**(442):323–354.

Marmot M (1999) *Social causes of social inequalities in health*. (Working paper no 99/01.) Harvard Center for Population and Development Studies, Cambridge, MA.

Murray CJL, Salomon JA, Mathers CD (2000) A critical examination of summary measures of population health. *Bulletin of the World Health Organization*, 78(8):981–994.

Nord E, Richardson J, Street A, Kuhse H, Singer P (1995) Maximizing health benefits vs. egalitarianism: an Australian survey of health issues. *Social Science and Medicine*, **41**(10):1429–1437.

Rawls J (1971) *A theory of justice*. Harvard University Press, Cambridge, MA.

Scanlon T (1982) Contractualism and utilitarianism. In: *Utilitarianism and beyond*. Sen A, Williams B, eds. Cambridge University Press, Cambridge.

Scanlon TM (1998) *What we owe to each other*. Harvard University Press, Cambridge, MA.

Walzer M (1983) *Spheres of justice*. Basic Books, New York.

Chapter 14.2

FAIRNESS IN EVALUATING HEALTH SYSTEMS

ERIK NORD

INTRODUCTION

The World Health Organization (WHO) has contructed a set of main indices by which countries' performance in the health domain may be evaluated. The indices are as follows:

a. *Average population health.* This is to be measured in terms of disability adjusted life years (DALYs), which—like quality-adjusted life years (QALYs)—is an index that purports to capture both longevity and levels of symptoms and functioning.

b. *Equity in population health.* This can mean equality between individuals as well as equality between socioeconomic groups.

c. *Responsiveness* of the health care system to legitimate expectations in the population as to how nicely and respectfully patients are treated. This refers to such qualities of health care as respect for dignity, autonomy and confidentiality, promptness in attention, access to social support networks for individuals receiving care, adequacy of "hotel functions" (food, furniture, toilet facilities), and freedom of choice between care providers.

d. *Equity in responsiveness* across social subgroups. The more subgroups that are treated with less responsiveness than the majority, and the greater these subgroups are, the lower is the country's score on equity in responsiveness.

e. *Fairness in financing* of the health care system. This has to do with the shares of out-of-pocket payment, private insurance and public insurance respectively in total health care financing.

WHO has further introduced a global index based on these five main indices that summarizes in one single number the overall performance of a country in matters of health.

I have elsewhere expressed doubts regarding the meaningfulness of compressing information on so many different aspects of health system performance into a small set of numerical indices (Nord 2002, see also: *http://www.eriknord.no/engelsk/WELCOME.htm*). In the present paper, I argue that the issue of fairness in health care does not seem to be covered adequately by the proposed set of indices. As an example, I particularly look at the issue of prioritizing according to capacity to benefit. I summarize results from various studies of public preferences that shed light on this issue and discuss the significance of such preference measurements for health policy.

CONCERNS FOR FAIRNESS IN RESOURCE ALLOCATION

I define a fair resource allocation in health care as one that accords with some accepted set of views about the strength of claims of different patient groups (Broome 1988; Lockwood 1988). Whose views should count, and how they should be established, is a matter of debate. According to one definition, resource allocation is fair when it is consistent with observed values, preferences and expectations in the general public. According to another definition, however, resource allocation is fair when it is consistent with a logically stringent theory of justice. Judgements of fairness then depend on which theory of justice is applied. I personally believe criteria for judging fairness must derive from both public preference measurements and theoretical ethical analysis. I return to this below.

Many countries have developed guidelines for priority setting in health care that aim at securing fairness. The guidelines are based partly on ethical reflection in academics and policy-makers (e.g. Daniels 1985; Dutch Committee on Choices in Health Care 1992; Menzel 1990; Norwegian Commission for Prioritising in Health Care 1987; Swedish Health Care and Medical Priorities Commission 1993), partly on measurements of values, attitudes and preferences in samples of the general population (e.g. Campbell and Gillett 1993; Charny et al. 1989; Dolan and Cookson 1998; Nord et al. 1995; Olsen 1994; Oregon Health Services Commission 1991; Pinto-Prades 1997; Ubel and Loewenstein 1995).

A review of existing literature in industrialized countries such as Australia, England, Holland, New Zealand, Norway, Spain, Sweden and the US suggests that ethicists' and policy-makers' reflections, and results from public preference measurements, converge on the following points regarding fairness (assuming "all else equal" in each case):

a. It is unfair to discriminate on the basis of sex, race, education, income or social status.

b. It is fair to allocate resources to those who have substantial capacity to benefit rather than to those who have little capacity to benefit.

c. It is fair to give priority to those with severe symptoms and dysfunctions over those with less severe problems—even if the former may not have as high a capacity to benefit as the latter.

On a number of other issues there is considerable disagreement. These include prioritizing between the following groups (still assuming "all else being equal"):

d. The young versus the elderly

e. Low-cost patients versus high-cost patients

f. The productive versus the non-productive

g. Those with a healthy life style versus those with an unhealthy life style

h. People with responsibility for others versus people without such responsibility

i. Those who are in need now versus those who will be in need in the future

j. Those who are well adapted to their health problems versus those who are ill adapted to the same problems

This overview of issues tells us at least two things. One is that, although fairness partly has to do with treating people on an equal basis, the notion of fairness in resource allocation is quite different from the notion of equality in population health. Many choices in health care that may be judged in terms of fairness do not affect equality in health at the population level, compare, for instance, items g–j above. At the same time we know that inequalities in health at the population level derive to a considerable extent from population variance in genes and living conditions. These have little to do with resource allocation decisions in health care. An index of equality in population health can therefore not serve as a measure of health system performance with respect to fairness.

The other thing the overview tells us is that the concept of fairness is multifaceted. I doubt that the way to include concerns for fairness in performance evaluation of health systems is to construct one global index for it.

Possibly one could construct some *indicators* of fairness. One could, for example, compare average waiting times for various kinds of elective surgery in men and women, young and old, productive and non-productive, etc. and use ratios between such waiting times as indicators of fairness.

But how much of the issue of fairness can be covered in ways like this? Selecting and queuing individual patients for treatment is perhaps the easiest decision context to study. At the same time fairness is a concern also at higher levels of decision-making, for instance, in distributing money across technologies (including pharmaceuticals), departments and hospitals that serve different diagnostic groups. In these contexts, quantification of standards of fairness and deviations from these seems a much more difficult task.

I would also think that judgements of fairness vary across cultures and that a set of indicators of fairness therefore would have to be composed differently in different countries.

I do not go deeper into these practical problems here. But the need to take into account concerns for fairness in system performance assessment is not to be shirked. In the following I take a closer look at one aspect of fairness on the list above that I deem to be particularly important. That is the weight that should be assigned to "capacity to benefit".

CAPACITY TO BENEFIT FROM TREATMENT

The concept of capacity to benefit from treatment has four dimensions. One is the degree of functional improvement and/or symptom reduction obtained if treatment is successful. Another is the probability that the treatment will be successful. A third is the number of years that the patient gets to enjoy the benefit. A fourth is the amount of resources required to obtain the benefit: if A and B are equally ill and both can be cured, but A at a lower cost than B, then A has a greater capacity to benefit per dollar than B. The statistically expected number of gained QALYs or DALYs per dollar are summary measures of capacity to benefit that incoporate all these four dimensions.

Few will argue that people with little capacity to benefit can claim resources that others would be helped much by, compare point b on the above list of fairness issues. What is less clear is how one should prioritize between two patients or patient groups when they both have substantial capacity to benefit, but one has greater capacity than the other. A utilitarian will say that the group with the greater capacity to benefit should come first, while an egalitarian will say that there should be no discrimination as long as capacity to benefit is substantial in both groups.

If performance is measured in terms of average population health and equality in population health—as currently proposed by WHO—a system will tend to score well if it gives priority to those who have the highest capacity to benefit. The reason is that the effect of such a policy on average population health is always positive, while equality is not necessarily compromised.

To develop this, consider a situation where everybody is healthy except for four people who are at disability level 0.5 on a scale from zero (dead) to unity (healthy). There are resources to treat only two of the four. A and B can be completely cured, while C and D can be helped to an intermediate level 0.8. If A and B are given priority, then the resulting distribution of health will be two people (C and D) remaining at level 0.5, while everybody else will be at level 1.0. If A/B and C/D are given equal priority, then statistically one from each pair will be treated. The resulting distribution of health will be two people remaining at level 0.5 (for instance A and C), one person at level 0.8 (D) and all others (including B) at level 1.0. So the two distributions would be as follows:

1. (1.0, 1.0, 0.5, 0.5, 1.0, 1.0,..........1.0)

2. (0.5, 1.0, 0.5, 0.8, 1.0, 1.0,..........1.0)

The former distribution implies higher average population health than the latter. At the same time it is not clear that the former distribution is less equal than the latter.

In other words, a system that favours A/B over C/D might score better as judged by WHO's performance criteria than a system that gives equal priority to the two groups. The question is: Should WHO be happy with that? Or could it be argued that the latter system is more fair and should be given credit for that?

ETHICAL THEORY AND PUBLIC PREFERENCES

Ethical theory gives no clear answer to these questions. Harris (1987) argues strongly against setting priorities according to capacity to benefit, while Daniels (1993), when reviewing the work of Scanlon (1982), Broome (1987), Brock (1988), Kamm (1989; 1993), and Menzel (1990), concludes that neither at the clinical level nor at the budget level is it clear what would be a fair allocation rule. He reaches this conclusion even after considering arguments invoking people's self-interest behind a veil of ignorance.

In a response to Harris, health economist Alan Williams (1987) seems to concede that the issue has no clear logical answer, which leads him to conclude that "at the end of the day, we simply have to stand up and be counted as to which set of principles we wish to have underpin the way the health care system works."

A number of such counts have been undertaken in the last decade by, among others, Paul Dolan in England, José-Luis Pinto in Spain, Jeff Richardson in Australia, Peter Ubel and colleagues in the US and Jan Abel Olsen and myself in Norway. The studies are reviewed elsewhere (Nord 1999a; 2001a).

Although results to some extent vary, the overall impression from the empirical studies is that the general public in countries like Australia, England, Norway, Spain and the US would find it unfair for their health care systems to prioritize strictly according to patients' capacity to benefit. There is a tendency for people to think that as long as capacity to benefit is substantial, patients' claims on resources should not depend too strongly on whether they will benefit moderately, considerably or very much. People express these preferences whether the benefit is in terms of improved functioning or increased life expectancy, and whether they are asked to imagine themselves as health administrators making decisions on behalf of others or asked to think of their own self interests behind a veil of ignorance.

The value of such preference measurements is debatable. In particular, one needs to look carefully at the ways in which the preferences were elicited, in order to judge how reflective and unbiased they are and how robust they therefore would be to counter-arguments and other ways of asking about the same issues.

The quality of the studies is highly variable in this respect. For instance, in studies by Patrick et al. (1973), Nord et al. (1995a), Ubel and Loewenstein (1995) and Ubel et al. (1999), subjects were just asked to fill in forms without any prior discussion of ethical issues and little time for or encouragement of reflection. On the other hand, in a study by Nord (1993), subjects gave explanations of their choices that were perfectly reasonable, and studies by Nord (1994), Murray, Lopez (1996) and Dolan and Cookson (1998) were all conducted in focus groups where subjects had ample time for debate. Cost studies of Nord et al. (1995b) and Abellan-Perpiñan and Pinto-Prades (1999) go quite far in testing for robustness to counter-arguments and changes in framing respectively. In other studies, robustness to changes from the caring-for-others to the self-interest perspective has been indicated (Nord 1994; Nord et al. 1995b; Richardson and Nord 1997).

In summary, I submit that the degree to which people emphasize capacity to benefit varies. More high quality, deliberative empirical work is needed to draw a more accurate picture of public values and preferences in this area. At present it does, however, seem that in countries like Australia, England, Norway, Spain and the US, the societal valuation of health outcomes is much less tightly related to their size than what is suggested in conventional health economics theory and what is perhaps assumed in the set of health system performance indicators currently proposed by WHO. This message from public preference measurements is not incompatible with ethical theory, inasmuch as debate among utilitarians and egalitarians has been unable to show that one position is more logically sound or more consistent with intuitions than the other.

POLICY IMPLICATIONS

I and others have elsewhere suggested various ways of incorporating the above egalitarian views in models for economic evaluation of health programmes (Menzel et al. 1999; Nord 1999; 2001b; Nord et al. 1999). Suffice it here to say that, in the light of the above data, it would seem inappropriate for WHO to construct a system for assessing health system performance that includes indices for average population health and equality in population health, but gives no account of the extent to which resources are allocated fairly across patients with different characteristics, including different capacities to benefit from treatment.

REFERENCES

Abellan-Perpiñan JM, Pinto-Prades JL (1999) Health state after treatment: a reason for discrimination. *Health Economics*, 8(8):701–707.

Brock DW (1998) Ethical issues in the development of summary measures of population health states. In: *Summarizing population health: directions for the development and application of population metrics*. Field MJ, Gold MR, eds. National Academy Press, Washington, DC.

Broome J (1987) *Fairness and random distribution of goods.* (Mimeo).

Broome J (1988) Goodness, fairness and QALYs. In: *Philosophy and medical welfare.* Bell JM, Mendus S, eds. Cambridge University Press, Cambridge.

Campbell A, Gillett G (1993) Justice and the right to health care. In: *Ethical issues in defining core services.* The National Advisory Committee on Core Health and Disability Support Services, Wellington.

Charny MC, Lewis PA, Farrow SC (1989) Choosing who shall not be treated in the NHS. *Social Science and Medicine*, 28(12):1331–1338.

Daniels N (1985) *Just health care.* Cambridge University Press, Cambridge, MA.

Daniels N (1993) Rationing fairly: programmatic considerations. *Bioethics*, 7:224–233.

Dolan P, Cookson R (1998) *Measuring preferences over the distribution of health benefits. (Mimeo).* University of York, Centre for Health Economics, York.

Dutch Committee on Choices in Health Care (1992) *Choices in health care.* Rijswijk: Ministry of Welfare, Health and Cultural Affairs, The Netherlands.

Harris J (1987) QALYfying the value of life. *Journal of Medical Ethics*, 13(3):117–123.

Kamm FM (1989) The report of the US Task Force on organ transplantation: criticism and alternatives. *Mount Sinai Journal of Medicine*, 56:207–220.

Kamm FM (1993) *Morality, mortality. Vol 1: Death and whom to save from it.* Oxford University Press, Oxford.

Lockwood M (1988) Quality of life and resource allocation. In: *Philosophy and medical welfare.* Bell JM, Mendus S, eds. Cambridge University Press, Cambridge.

Menzel P (1990) *Strong medicine: the ethical rationing of health care.* Oxford University Press, New York.

Menzel P, Gold MR, Nord E, Pinto JL, Richardson J, Ubel P (1999) Toward a broader view of values in cost-effectiveness analysis of health. *Hastings Center Report*, 29(3):7–15.

Murray CJL, Lopez AD, eds. (1996) *The global burden of disease: a comprehensive assessment of mortality and disability from diseases, injuries and risk factors in 1990 and projected to 2020.* Global Burden of Disease and Injury, Vol. 1. Harvard School of Public Health on behalf of WHO, Cambridge, MA.

Nord E (1993) The relevance of health state after treatment in prioritizing between patients. *Journal of Medical Ethics*, 19(1):37–42.

Nord E (1994) *Seminarserie om veiledende verditall for prioritering i helsevesenet. [Workshops on a value table for prioritizing in health care].* (Working paper no 1/1994.) National Institute of Public Health, Oslo.

Nord E (1999) *Cost value analysis in health care: making sense out of QALYs.* Cambridge University Press, Cambridge.

Nord E (2001b) Health state values from multiattribute utility instruments need correction. *Annals of Medicine,* 33(5):371–374.

Nord E (2001a) Severity of illness versus expected benefit in societal evaluation of health care interventions. *Expert Review of Pharmacoeconomics and Outcomes Research,* 1(1):85–92.

Nord E (2002) Measures of goal attainment and performance in the World Health Report 2000. A brief, critical consumer guide. *Health Policy,* 59(3):183–191.

Nord E, Richardson J, Street A, Kuhse H, Singer P (1995a) Maximizing health benefits vs. egalitarianism: an Australian survey of health issues. *Social Science and Medicine,* 41(10):1429–1437.

Nord E, Richardson J, Street A, Kuhse H, Singer P (1995b) Who cares about cost? Does economic analysis impose or reflect social values? *Health Policy,* 34(2):79–94.

Nord EM, Pinto JL, Richardson J, Menzel P, Ubel P (1999) Incorporating societal concerns for fairness in numerical valuations of health programmes. *Health Economics,* 8(1):25–39.

Norwegian Commission for Prioritising in Health Care (1987) *Retningslinjer for prioritering innen helsevesenet. [Guidelines for prioritising in health care.]* Universitetsforlaget, Oslo.

Olsen JA (1994) Persons vs years: two ways of eliciting implicit weights. *Health Economics,* 3(1):39–46.

Oregon Health Services Commission (1991) *Prioritization of health services. A report to the Governor and Legislature.* Salem, OR.

Patrick DL, Bush JW, Chen MM (1973) Methods for measuring levels of well-being for a health status index. *Health Services Research,* 8(3):228–245.

Pinto-Prades JL (1997) Is the person trade-off a valid method for allocating health care resources. *Health Economics,* 6(1):71–81.

Richardson J, Nord E (1997) The importance of perspective in the measurement of quality adjusted life years. *Medical Decision-making,* 17(1):33–41.

Scanlon T (1982) Contractualism and utilitarianism. In: *Utilitarianism and beyond.* Sen A, Williams B, eds. Cambridge University Press, Cambridge.

Swedish Health Care and Medical Priorities Commission (1993) *No easy choices – the difficulties of health care. SOU 1993:93.* Ministry of Health and Social Affairs, Stockholm.

Ubel P, Loewenstein G (1995) The efficacy and equity of retransplantation: an experimental survey of public attitudes. *Health Policy,* 34(2):145–151.

Ubel P, Richardson J, Pinto-Prades JL (1999) Lifesaving treatments and disabilities: are all QALYs created equal? *International Journal of Technology Assessment in Health Care,* 15(4):738–748.

Williams A (1987) Qualifying the value of life. Response. *Journal of Medical Ethics*, **13**(3):123

Chapter 14.3

FAIRNESS AND HEALTH

DAN W. BROCK

Fairness concerns the comparative treatment or conditions of different individuals. We can wrong someone by lying to them, but if we treat them unfairly, or their condition is unfair, it must be relative to how we treat, or to the condition of, others. Consequentialism is the moral view that actions and institutions should seek to maximize aggregate good without regard to its distribution, except in so far as its distribution affects the aggregate; cost-effectiveness analysis is the natural analytic tool for pursuing this aggregative goal in health. Consequentialism thus ignores concerns about fairness. The concern for fairness takes seriously the separateness of persons and seeks treatment of individuals that they can reasonably accept from their own subjective point of view.

I am in agreement with Kamm on most major points in her account of the constraints of fairness on promoting best outcomes in health and health care (chapter 14.1). She is correct that fairness or justice does not require equality, but instead special concern or priority to the worse off. She is correct as well that the main factors relevant to selection of candidates for health interventions are need, outcomes, and urgency, though I believe that in circumstances of persistent scarcity urgency should receive little weight.

I think it is useful to distinguish four main questions of fairness or justice in the health sector to appreciate the full scope of the issues since Kamm's discussion focuses on only one of them. First, how much of a societies overall resources should be devoted to health as opposed to other goals or goods? Second, how should health resources be allocated to different health programmes or interventions? Third, which individuals should be selected to receive scarce health interventions? Fourth, what is a fair distribution of the costs of providing health interventions? These questions are of course not completely independent—how much overall resources are devoted to health will determine what is available for allocation to different health programmes, which will in turn determine which interventions are available to distribute to individuals. Kamm's discussion, as have most discussions of fairness or justice in the distribution of health care, focuses on the third of these questions, though it has some implications at least for the second. She is principally concerned with micro choices between different patients for a scarce resource.

It is important to distinguish these different questions for a number of reasons: first, the kind of information available for them is often different, which will put different constraints on the considerations that can be used to answer them; second, because the questions themselves are different there is reason to believe that the considerations relevant for answering them may be different; and third, the social roles and responsibilities of decision-makers for them will be different, also affecting how they should be answered. All but the third question on which Kamm focuses of selecting patients for scarce health interventions are primarily what she calls macro choices and I want to discuss briefly how the issues may change at the macro level; Kamm says very little about this and does not explain her few remarks about why macro standards should be different than micro standards. But first, I want to make a few remarks about her treatment of the micro patient selection choices.

KAMM ON MICRO ALLOCATION

It is standard to distinguish three rationing problems, all of which at their core raise issues of fairness—priority to the worst off, aggregation, and fair chances versus best outcomes (Daniels 1993; Brock 1998). Kamm's account of priority to the worst off is complex, but it rests in large part on the relevance of need and urgency to patient selection: need, as she uses it, is a global, largely backward looking consideration, asking how badly healthwise a person's life will have gone if she is not helped; urgency is forward looking asking how badly off someone will be healthwise if she is not helped. As Kamm points out, need and urgency can conflict (A will die in a month at age 65 if not helped now, and B will die in a year at age 20 unless helped now—A is more urgent, B more needy), but each captures a sense in which individuals can be worse off than others. Need has full temporal scope—how badly will a person's entire life have gone if she is not helped; urgency focuses on how badly off a person will become looking forward if she is not helped. Since need, as I understand Kamm's use of it, includes consideration of what urgency considers, but takes a more inclusive temporal perspective, why should urgency be given separate weight? My own view is that it should be given little if any weight in comparison with need, but in any case we need more justification for giving it separate moral weight apart from need. There are many additional complexities in the priority to the worse off problem that Kamm did not have time to take up here, but the view she sketches does address that problem.

The aggregation problem concerns primarily when benefits to some individuals can be aggregated together so as to receive higher priority than producing lesser aggregate benefits to fewer different individuals—the

problem takes many forms. When different numbers of persons compete
for a life saving resource, Kamm presents an aggregative argument to show
that it is worse if B and C die than if A dies. She then presents a balancing
argument to show that it is not unfair to save the greater number: in a
conflict justice demands that each person on one side should have her
interests balanced against those of one person on the opposing side; those
that are not balanced out in the larger group determine that the larger
group should be saved. But I think this is not what fairness requires. Fairness requires that each party in the conflict receive a fair chance to have
her needs met and to be saved. Kamm grants that when we can save only
one of two people who need saving, fairness requires random selection
between them. When it is one versus two, we can assume that if need and
urgency are the same, no one of the three has any greater claim to be saved
than the others, and this suggests that fairness still requires that we give
no one of the three a greater chance to be saved; we could do so by toss-
ing a coin between the one and the two. Kamm argues that this denies the
equal significance of each person since the addition of a second person on
one side makes no difference. Some would conclude from this that fairness requires chances proportional to the numbers, but whether one supports equal chances or proportional chances many would reject Kamm's
argument that there is no conflict between fairness and saving the greater
number in these conflict cases (Brock 1988). If the difference in numbers
is great enough, we might decide straightaway to save the greater number without giving all equal or proportional chances, but this should be
understood as utility or best outcomes overriding fairness. I agree with
much of the rest of Kamm's treatment of the aggregation problem, and
her treatment elsewhere of its complexities is the best that we have, though
there are other variants of the aggregation problem that have not been
adequately explored (Kamm 1993).

The third rationing problem is called the fair chances versus best outcomes problem and Kamm does not address it explicitly, though she takes
up some instances of it. One is the conflict case just discussed—the conflict between saving B and C or saving A. As already noted, I believe fairness requires giving A either an equal or proportional chance of being
saved even though this means we may not produce the best outcome;
Kamm rejects that fairness conflicts with best outcomes here. The other
principal place she addresses this problem is with her principle of irrelevant
good, though this principle obviously bears on permissible aggregation as
well. For example, in the conflict case of saving A or saving B plus curing
C's sore throat she argues that the additional benefit to C is an irrelevant
good for the choice of whether to save A or B; we must still give each a
fair, presumably equal, chance to be saved, although saving B plus curing C's sore throat is the better outcome. The fair chances—best outcomes
problem is perhaps most clear in a case like the following—we can save
50 year old A for 25 years or 50 year old B for 26 years (of course, in reality
we could never make precise predictions of this sort); we produce more

QALYs, or prevent more DALYs, by saving B. Kamm would call this an irrelevant good because each stands to get the major part of what they could get and so the additional benefit to B should be irrelevant to the choice. A different way of thinking about this case is to imagine A arguing that he needs saving just as much as B, will lose everything just like B if he is not saved, and so deserves a fair chance to have his need met when we cannot save both. I think the most natural way of putting the objection to choosing between A and B on the basis of which choice will produce the best outcome is that the very small gain in benefits produced if we save B is too small to justify morally the very great difference in how we would treat the two—saving one and letting the other die (Brock 1988). The fair chances-best outcomes problem is another aspect of giving a full account of equity in health.

I should add that some have argued for giving those who will benefit less a chance to receive the treatment they need on different grounds than fairness. If one has some chance of getting the treatment one needs, even in conditions of severe resource scarcity which make the chance small, one does not take away all hope of having one's needs met; hope may be especially important in the case of effective, but scarce, life-sustaining treatment (Menzel et al. 1999).

MACRO ALLOCATION

Let me turn now briefly to a few ways in which problems of equity may be different at the macro level, in particular for the first two questions I noted above of how much overall resources should go to health, and how those resources should be devoted to different health programmes. It might be thought that the first question is not a matter of justice, but should be settled simply by societal preferences for health versus other goods, but this would be a mistake. As many have argued, providing access to some level of health care to all members of a society is a requirement of justice because of the importance of health care to people's opportunity, well-being, life itself, and ability to plan their lives. Suppose one follows Norman Daniels in focusing on the impact of disease on people's opportunity, and specifically on fair equality of opportunity; this is why providing health care to prevent or treat disease is a matter of justice (Daniels 1985). One implication of this view for summary measures of population health which are to be used to help inform us about justice in the distribution of health and of health care is that they should focus on measuring health-related effects on opportunity, which may be different than the health-related effects on people's overall well-being. This is only one example of the general point that given the quite different uses of summary measures of population health, for example to monitor the health of a population and to help determine just distributions of health resources, no single measure may be best suited for these disparate uses.

Another point about this macro question is that those making decisions about the allocation of resources to health versus other aims and goods should arguably not ignore the indirect non-health effects of different resource allocations to health, for example the economic benefits of reducing many health problems. These decision-makers have responsibilities for the overall justice and well-being of the society when they allocate resources to different social goals and should take account of their decisions on that overall well-being. This is very different than the choice of patients to receive a scarce resource at the micro or clinical level, where the usual view is that fairness requires physicians to ignore whether greater economic benefit may come from treating some rather than other patients.

Consider now the second broad macro level question, how should health resources be allocated to different health programmes and needs? Some health conditions, such as Alzheimer's dementia, are concentrated in a particular age group, but many other conditions, such as some mental illnesses, are distributed across quite heterogeneous populations in terms of age and baseline health status. This means that in the latter kinds of cases treatment or prevention programmes will be directed to patients with widely varying need in Kamm's sense—that is, how badly their lives will have gone if they do not receive treatment. It is not clear how decision-makers could give weight to need in prioritizing resources for health programmes of the latter sort—if the interventions are life saving they may be directed to people across a broad age spectrum, and if they are quality of life protecting or enhancing they may be directed to people whose quality of life if not treated may vary greatly because of differences in baseline health status apart from the condition to be treated. In addition, of course, there is a wide variation in the seriousness of outcomes without treatment for a particular condition from wide differences in the severity of different patients' condition with the same disease to be treated. Need (in Kamm's sense) will be in many if not most cases too heterogeneous to be given meaningful content and weight in prioritizing different treatment programmes at the macro level, and so this interpretation of who is worst off—those with greatest need—will be difficult if not impossible to apply there.

The same problem will often exist for urgency—how badly off will a person be if not helped—when applied at this macro level; if a particular treatment or prevention intervention would be given to patients with widely varying baseline health status, then how badly off healthwise they would be without the intervention will likewise vary widely. Urgency too looks too heterogeneous to be effectively employed for these macro prioritization choices.

Much empirical work, such as Erik Nord's studies, that seeks to assess to what degree people will sacrifice aggregate health benefits in order to treat the worst off interprets the worst off as those who are sickest, roughly understood as having the disease with the greatest adverse effect on length and/or quality of life (Nord 1993). This is a different interpretation of the worst off than either need or urgency as Kamm uses them, but it may be the main feasible interpretation for these macro prioritization choices. Interestingly, it may also be what ordinary people have in mind when they express a desire to give priority to the worst off in health resource prioritization, despite the fact that moral reasons may favour using the broader notion of need, and perhaps as well urgency.

The micro level choices on which Kamm focuses are which patients will receive a treatment and which patients will not, in effect an all or nothing choice for each patient in need of treatment. At the macro level, however, the resources to be allocated are typically money to fund different treatment programmes. Money is divisible in a way that one heart needed by two patients for transplantation is not, and so macro level allocation is usually a matter of the relative priority for funding to be given to different health programmes or interventions. That one health programme A promises a small gain in aggregate health benefits over a competing programme B need not mean that A is fully funded and B receives no funding, but only that A should receive higher priority for, or a higher level of, funding than B. In conditions of resource scarcity, persons with the disease that A treats will have a somewhat higher probability of being successfully treated than will those who have the disease that B treats; in the case of prevention, those at risk of A will have a somewhat higher probability of successful prevention than will those at risk of B. When there is significant resource scarcity this form of allocation proportional to benefit can involve a significant sacrifice in aggregate health benefits that could have been produced by preferring the more cost-effective alternative. But doing so will mitigate significantly the fair chances-best outcomes conflict; individuals who are served by B will have no complaint that the small difference in expected benefits between programmes A and B unfairly forecloses all chance of their having their health needs met. Instead, the small difference in expected benefits between programmes A and B need only result in a comparably small difference in the resources devoted to A and B; it is not obvious that this is unfair to those patients served by B, whose needs would be somewhat less well served than patients in programme A. The fair chances-best outcomes conflict may be mitigated as well when the scarce health interventions to be prioritized are not life-saving, but instead only impact individuals' quality of life. In those cases, the difference in outcomes for individuals who receive a needed health intervention that is given a higher priority and individuals who do not because their condition is given lower priority, is much less; no one can argue that if they are not treated they will lose everything, as in the scarce organ transplantation case. This will make any unfairness in treating one but not the other arguably less compelling.

Another difference that arises at the macro level of prioritization of different health programmes by policy-makers, as opposed to different patients by physicians, concerns one part of the separate spheres issue—should the non-health benefits, such as indirect economic benefits in reducing lost work time from treating a condition like substance abuse, as well as the health benefits of different health programmes, be relevant to their prioritization. The traditional understanding of the physician-patient relationship and the physician's commitment to the patient's health related well-being excludes consideration of these indirect, non-health benefits, and a variety of considerations could be offered in support of that understanding, including specific concerns about fairness. Kamm herself comments in passing that at the macro level the separate spheres limitation may not hold, and I think she is correct, but an account of health care equity will require exploring how the specific roles and responsibilities of decision-makers should affect the resource allocations they make.

SOME ADDITIONAL ISSUES FOR AN ACCOUNT OF EQUITY AND HEALTH

I will conclude these comments by simply mentioning several of the more important additional complexities or problems for giving a full account of equity in the health sector. First, nearly all the work by philosophers and bioethicists on distributive justice and fairness in the health sector has focused on the distribution of health care resources. But health care and inequalities in access to health care are of concern certainly primarily because of their effects on health and health inequalities. But as the accumulating evidence concerning the social determinants of health makes increasingly clear, the effects of social determinants such as socioeconomic inequality and education have a much greater impact on health and health inequality than does health care (Wilkinson 1996). This means that an account of health equity is at least as pressing as an account of health care equity, and an account of health equity will not be independent of an account of the equity of socioeconomic inequalities more generally; for example, other things equal we might assume that the health inequalities caused by morally justified socioeconomic inequalities would not be *per se* unjust, but if we have an independent account of health equity it might instead call into question the justification of otherwise equitable socioeconomic inequalities. The general point is that work on accounts of equity in the health sector needs to distinguish more clearly between equity in health and equity in health care, and to remedy the tendency to focus on the latter while ignoring the former.

Second, much of the work on equity in health and health care, such as Kamm's both in her paper and elsewhere, largely ignores that a person's health without treatment as well as the benefit from treatment are typically matters of probabilities. Of course, for many purposes we then simply estimate expected health and expected health benefits, but that is not always adequate; to take two examples, I believe that we cannot simply assume that the worst off can be determined by a person's expected health without treatment without regard to the range of alternative possible outcomes, especially when one outcome with a significant probability is death, nor can we assume that acceptable aggregation in the face of certain outcomes transfers straightforwardly to aggregation in the face of uncertain outcomes.

A third important issue is when, in what way, and for what reason, the age of potential benefit recipients can fairly affect resource prioritization. Put in terms of QALYs or DALYs, is a QALY or DALY of equal value independent of the age at which it is received; QALYs are typically not age weighted whereas DALYs have been, but even if some age weighting is not unjust age discrimination, the reasons for age weighting will determine both whether it is just as well as what particular age weights are morally justified.

A fourth issue that has received considerable attention in the United States is whether giving weight to differences in outcomes in priority setting, for example as measured either by QALYs or DALYs, constitutes unjust discrimination against the disabled when their disabilities result in their benefiting less from interventions than otherwise similar patients (Brock 1995; 2000). To give just one example, if we adjust years of life extension from health interventions for the quality of life or disability level of the persons whose lives are extended, we will give less value to saving or extending the lives of persons with disabilities than of persons without them. While some have accepted this as an acceptable implication of any prioritization process that is sensitive to the different benefits of different health interventions (Hadorn 1992), it has seemed to many to be unjust and some have suggested that so long as a person considers his or her quality of life to be acceptable and worth living, no adjustment to the value of extending it should be made based on the relative level of his or her quality of life (Kamm 1993). Potential discrimination against the disabled in resource prioritization can take a number of forms, and I believe the problem of disability discrimination represents a deep and unresolved problem for resource prioritization.

Fifth, on most accounts of equity, there are multiple considerations relevant to assessing the equity of health resource prioritization; this requires assigning specific weights to the different considerations in order to determine an equitable and complete overall prioritization of different programmes. Even if priority to the worst off were the only consideration relevant to equity besides best outcomes, it would be irrational to give absolute weight to the worst off without regard either to how worse but not worst off groups may be affected or to the cost in overall health benefits forgone. It is an open question how far moral reasoning can take us in developing principled bases for these trade-offs, but too little work has been devoted to developing them to conclude that none are possible. However, for now and in the foreseeable future we face both significant indeterminacy and disagreement in what considerations should be given what weight in an equitable prioritization of health resources. How to determine fairly an overall prioritization in the face of this indeterminacy and disagreement is in part a political matter, but it is a matter of procedural justice or fairness as well. Some limited work has been done on the nature of fair procedures for health resource prioritization, but the quite different contexts in which resource prioritization and allocation takes place requires the development of fair procedures sensitive to those different contexts and the different social roles and responsibilities of participants in them (Daniels and Sabin 1997).

Sixth, I have said nothing here about the fourth question I distinguished at the outset—what is a fair distribution of the costs of health interventions? For example, in the United States there is considerable controversy about whether fairness requires some form of community rating in health insurance, or whether instead some forms of risk rating are fair. Some make a special case for limited risk rating when individuals are responsible for unhealthy behaviours that are the cause of their health needs. There is disagreement as well about the extent to which the costs to individuals of services or insurance should be scaled to incomes or ability to pay. There has been very little systematic work applying theories of justice or fairness to fair funding of the health care system.

Finally, it should be mentioned that there are serious consequentialist challenges to fairness itself, as opposed to particular interpretations of fairness. Perhaps the most interesting challenge appeals to ex ante or Veil of Ignorance reasoning and argues that from a position of ignorance about what particular position one will occupy in a distribution of health or health care, it is reasonable to assume one has an equal chance of being anyone (Menzel 1990). It is then claimed to be rational for all to prefer the distribution that produces the greatest overall health benefit because that will give each the greatest expected health benefit. Consequentialists then argue that this choice standpoint satisfies the moral requirement of impartiality, and that maximization of overall expected health benefits would only be rejected from a partial standpoint from which one can favour one's own known position. Since Rawls' use of the Veil of Ignorance in *A Theory of Justice* there has been much discussion of this form of reasoning in political philosophy, in particular within work on contractualist theories of justice, and both the use of ex ante reasoning, as well as what distributive principles would be agreed to from an ex ante position, are controversial; the use of ex ante reasoning for selecting distributive principles for health care needs more critical assessment (Rawls 1971; Scanlon 1998).

I have not been able to do more here than simply point to some of the additional problems and complexities for developing a full account of health and health care equity. I have done so, nevertheless, in order to give some sense of the scope of the agenda of unfinished work on equity in health and health care.

REFERENCES

Brock D (1988) Ethical issues in recipient selection for organ transplantation. In: *Organ substitution technology: ethical, legal and public policy issues*. Mathieu D, ed. Westview Press, Boulder, CO.

Brock DW (1995) Justice and the ADA: does prioritizing and rationing health care discriminate against the disabled? *Social Philosophy and Policy*, **12**(2):159–184.

Brock DW (1998) Ethical issues in the development of summary measures of population health states. In: *Summarizing population health: directions for the development and application of population metrics*. Field MJ, Gold MR, eds. National Academy Press, Washington, DC.

Brock DW (2000) Health care resource prioritization and discrimination against persons with disabilities. In: *Americans with disabilities: exploring implications of the law for individuals and institutions*. Francis L, Silvers A, eds. Routledge, New York.

Daniels N (1985) *Just health care*. Cambridge University Press, Cambridge, MA.

Daniels N (1993) Rationing fairly: programmematic considerations. *Bioethics*, 7:224–233.

Daniels N, Sabin J (1997) Limits to health care: fair procedures, democratic deliberation, and the legitimacy problem for insurers. *Philosophy and Public Affairs*, **26**:303–350.

Hadorn D (1992) The problem of discrimination in health care priority setting. *Journal of the American Medical Association*, **268**(11):1454–1459.

Kamm FM (1993) *Morality, mortality. Vol 1: Death and whom to save from it*. Oxford University Press, Oxford.

Menzel P (1990) *Strong medicine: the ethical rationing of health care*. Oxford University Press, New York.

Menzel P, Gold MR, Nord E, Pinto JL, Richardson J, Ubel P (1999) Toward a broader view of values in cost-effectiveness analysis of health. *Hastings Center Report*, **29**(3):7–15.

Nord E (1993) The trade-off between severity of illness and treatment effect in cost-value analysis of health care. *Health Policy*, **24**:227–238.

Rawls J (1971) *A theory of justice*. Harvard University Press, Cambridge, MA.

Scanlon TM (1998) *What we owe to each other*. Harvard University Press, Cambridge, MA.

Wilkinson R (1996) *Unhealthy societies: the afflictions of inequality*. Routledge, London.

Chapter 14.4

ALL GOODS ARE RELEVANT

JOHN BROOME

Frances Kamm's investigation of fairness is immensely detailed and impressive (see chapter 14.1). I agree with a great deal of her paper, but in this comment I am sorry to say I am going to take up one point that I do not agree with. This particular point is important because it has some direct practical consequences for the rationing of resources in health. It is the idea of irrelevant goods. Kamm argues that some goods in some circumstances count for nothing. But I believe that all goods always count for something.

Kamm's argument uses this example: two people, A and B, are mortally sick. We have enough serum to save only one of them. If we save B, that is all we can do. But if we save A, there will be enough serum left over to cure C's sore throat. What ought we to do?

Kamm points out that, if there were no sore throat to worry about, we would have no grounds for discriminating between A and B. We ought to treat them in some way that does not involve discrimination. Holding a fair lottery to decide between them would be the best way. Kamm next points out that the mere presence of a sore throat makes no difference to this conclusion. It is still wrong to discriminate, even though by choosing to save A we can also cure a sore throat. The sore throat is not important enough to justify us in giving A precedence over B.

From this, Kamm argues that a sore throat is so unimportant that it counts for nothing at all when saving life is in question. Her argument is that if it counted for anything at all, it would be enough to determine that we ought to save A rather than B. In the absence of the sore throat, there is a perfect balance between saving A and saving B. So if the sore throat counted for anything at all, it would tip the balance. But it does not tip the balance; it is not the case that we ought to save A rather than B. Therefore, the sore throat must count for nothing in the context.

Kamm goes on to draw the inference that any number of sore throats must be irrelevant whenever there is a question of saving life. We should never choose to cure sore throats, however many we can cure, in preference to saving a life.

I agree with Kamm that we ought not to give A precedence over B in her example; we should hold a lottery to choose between the two. I explain it by a different calculation from hers.

The choice before us is either (1) to hold a lottery between A and B, save whichever person wins the lottery, and also cure C's sore throat if A wins, or alternatively (2) to decide directly to save A and also cure C's sore throat. What benefits can we expect from each of these options?

First, the benefits of (1). If we choose by means of a lottery, we act fairly. A and B both have equal claims on us to be saved, and fairness requires us to respect their claims equally (see Broome 1990). We would respect them equally if we were equally to save both people, but we are not able to do that. The next best way of giving equal respect to the equal claims is to give both people an equal chance of being saved. This we can do, and therefore fairness is best served by doing it. We give each person an equal chance by holding a lottery. So holding a lottery achieves the value of fairness.

What further benefit does (1) bring? We do not know exactly, because if we hold a lottery, we do not know whether we shall eventually save A or B. We can only calculate the expected benefit. (1) certainly saves one life, and it has a one-half chance of curing a sore throat. So the expected benefit is one life plus one half a sore throat cured. Adding this to the fairness makes the total expected benefit of (1): fairness and one life saved and half a sore throat cured.

What is the benefit of the option (2)? This option does not give proper respect to B's claim to be saved. It therefore achieves no fairness. On the other hand, it certainly saves one life and cures one sore throat. So its total expected benefit is: one life saved and one sore throat cured.

Which options should we choose? When we compare their expected benefits, we see that (1) is better if and only if fairness, in the context, is worth more than half a sore throat cured. The value of fairness certainly depends on the context, and in the context of determining whose life to save, it is obviously very important. It is certainly worth more than half a sore throat. So (1) is the better option, and we ought to hold a lottery.

Given my way of calculating, from the fact that we ought to hold a lottery, it does not follow that curing a sore throat counts for nothing in the context. It only follows that it counts for less than twice as much as fairness in the context. So Kamm's conclusion does not follow.

I believe that a lot of small benefits can add up to be as important as one large benefit. When a patient in a United Kingdom hospital gets a headache, he or she is given an analgesic. Over a few years, the UK Health Service gives out a few million analgesics to cure headaches. The cost of all these pills adds up, and eventually it will amount to more than enough to save someone's life. Evidently, the Health Service thinks that curing all those headaches is as valuable as saving a life. I agree.

REFERENCES

Broome J (1990) Fairness. *Proceedings of the Aristotelian Society*, **91**(1):87–102.

Chapter 15.1

SUMMARY MEASURES OF POPULATION HEALTH: CONCLUSIONS AND RECOMMENDATIONS

CHRISTOPHER J.L. MURRAY, JOSHUA A. SALOMON,
COLIN D. MATHERS AND ALAN D. LOPEZ

INTRODUCTION

The regular assessment of population health is a key component of the public policy process to improve health levels and reduce health inequalities in the World Health Organization (WHO) Member States. Population-level estimates of mortality, morbidity and health states in countries by age, sex and cause, are useful for numerous public health purposes, ranging from the monitoring of new epidemics to measuring progress in reducing old ones for which disease control programmemes are in place. To describe health patterns adequately in almost 200 Member States according to age, sex and cause, a vast array of estimates need to be generated. It then becomes a major challenge to interpret the key findings of such a review or to compare levels of population health across countries unless the data are summarized in some fashion.

The simplest and most widely used method for producing population health statistics is to aggregate data on individuals in order to generate statistics such as the proportion of the population (or of a particular population subgroup) suffering from a given health problem or living in a particular health state, or the number of individuals who die from a particular cause during a specified interval. This approach rapidly becomes unwieldy when a number of problems are being monitored and we want to make comparisons over time, across population groups, or before and after some health intervention.

Summary measures of population health (SMPH) are measures that combine information on mortality and non-fatal health outcomes to represent population health in a single number. While such summary measures have many potential uses (see part 2), there are two that are particularly important for public health policy: (1) comparisons of the average health levels in different populations or subgroups, or in the same population over time; and (2) assessments of the relative contributions of different diseases, injuries and risk factors to overall population health. These two key uses may best be served by different forms of SMPH.

For reporting on the health of WHO Member States, SMPH provide a convenient and useful summary of the vast array of components of population health. SMPH do not replace the more detailed reporting of data on specific aspects of health and mortality or on the specific causes of health problems; rather they supplement these data with more comprehensive indicators that can be used to monitor trends and compare levels of health across populations. During the 1980s and 1990s, and particularly since the publication of the first results of the Global Burden of Disease Study in the 1993 *World Development Report*, there has been a growing debate on numerous aspects relating to the development and application of summary measures of population health. We hope that this book will provide a major contribution to that debate by assembling the views and arguments of health policy-makers and experts from a wide range of disciplines including epidemiology, demography, health statistics, health economics, philosophy and ethics. In this concluding chapter, we summarize the important conceptual, empirical and ethical issues identified and debated by contributors, and draw some conclusions and recommendations for the future evolution of summary measures of population health.

Concepts

Definition of health

The conceptual basis for summary measures of population health begins, logically, with the definition of health. The Constitution of the World Health Organization famously defines health as "a state of complete physical, mental and social well-being and not merely the absence of disease or infirmity", and notes that the "health of all peoples is fundamental to the attainment of peace and security" (WHO 1948). In the broadest terms, this definition sets forth a lofty ideal for health as an integral component of well-being and, further, expresses the notion that good health is a necessary condition for attaining the highest possible levels on all other aspects of well-being. In defining health in terms of an ideal, the WHO Constitution provides the first building block for an operational definition of health. Over the half-century since this definition was set forth, there have been continuing efforts to develop more precise conceptualizations of health that may be linked to operational measures.

From these efforts, one common theme that has emerged is that health may be viewed naturally as an intrinsic, multi-dimensional attribute of individuals; there is an intuitive understanding of health that crosses cultural boundaries, such that when we talk about a person's health, we are understood to be referring to his or her levels on the various components or domains of health. It is important to note that this view distinguishes health states from pathologies, risk factors or etiologies, and from encounters with health services or the application of health interventions. This conceptualization preserves the spirit of the WHO Constitution definition: rather than equating health with diseases or diagnostic categories, it recognizes a causal chain through which risk factors are determinants of diseases, and diseases in turn are determinants of health states.

A formal framework for cataloguing the multiple domains of health has been developed by WHO in the International Classification of Functioning, Disability and Health (ICF; WHO 2001a; also chapter 7.3). The ICF replaces the concepts of *disability* and *handicap* in the International Classification of Impairment, Disability and Handicap (ICIDH) with the concepts of *capacity* and *performance*. *Capacity* refers to an individual's ability on a domain as it would be manifested in a uniform environment (assuming motivation to perform the task), for example, the ability to walk 100 metres on a level, well-lit, non-slippery surface. *Performance* describes an individual's ability on a domain as it is manifested in his or her current environment. The gap between capacity and performance therefore reflects the impact of an individual's actual environment (and perhaps motivation) relative to the uniform environment. Both performance and capacity may be measured either with or without an individual's personal aids.

Given this distinction between capacity and performance, which construct do we aim to capture in summary measures of population health? To the extent that performance reflects an individual's unique environmental setting, which may also vary with time and as individual circumstances change, it is probably not congruent with most notions of health. We would not want to characterize the same cognitive impairment differently in two individuals simply because they have different vocations that call upon different types of cognitive tasks. Similarly, we would not say that an individual with a hearing impairment is healthier simply because she avoids noisy gatherings. These examples point to a common-sense understanding of health that does not correspond to performance because it excludes the idiosyncracies of an individual's environment.

The notion of capacity corresponds more closely to this common-sense interpretation of health by defining external environmental factors in a uniform way. More specifically, we believe that capacity *with* an individual's currently available personal aids is the most appropriate construct, as many societies commonly understand personal aids such as crutches, glasses or hearing aids to improve health levels on relevant domains. There remains a degree of arbitrariness in defining the boundary between personal aids and individual-specific environmental factors, but we believe that the inclusion of simple personal aids that should in principle be available to all people is most consistent with the intuitive societal notions of what constitutes health.

KEY DOMAINS OF HEALTH

In conceptualizing health as a multi-dimensional construct, we recognize that health domains constitute a subset of all of the domains of well-being. Having postulated this conceptual boundary, there are likely some core domains of health that almost all people would agree upon, while other domains might be less universally accepted as health domains. We may also identify domains of well-being that are not strictly health domains but can serve as good proximate measures of the experience of health (*health-related* domains). For operational purposes, there are some instances in which the best or only measurable indicators of the levels on certain health domains may in fact be consequences that are outside the realm of health.

In order to operationalize the measurement of health, we need to define a parsimonious set of domains that capture the components of health that are generally considered most important to people in determining their overall assessments of health levels. Although domains of health may overlap, the aim is to identify a set of domains that is exhaustive as well as generally acceptable as the content of the ordinary meaning of health. Chapter 7.1 proposes that key domains of health should be:

1. valid in terms of intuitive, clinical and epidemiological concepts of health;

2. linked to the conceptual framework of the ICF;

3. amenable to self report, observation or measurements;

4. comprehensive enough to capture all important aspects of health states that people value; and

5. cross-population comparable.

Although existing health state measurement instruments have differed considerably in their content in an attempt to arrive at a set of domains that covers the universe of health adequately, there are several domains that have been included in nearly all generic measures of health states, including pain, affect, cognition, mobility, self-care, usual activities (including household and work-related activities) and interpersonal relationships. Among these, it may be argued that some are core domains of health (e.g. mobility, pain, cognition) while others may be considered as proxy measures of multiple domains (e.g. self-care, usual activities).

THE BOUNDARIES OF GOOD HEALTH

Another issue that needs to be addressed in operationalizing a definition of health is whether all increments and decrements on a domain are understood as improvements and losses of health, respectively, or whether there is some threshold above which increments and decrements are not perceived as changes in a person's health state. For example, should one consider a person with an IQ of 180 as being healthier than another individual with an IQ of 150? Or should one say that the former is not necessarily healthier by virtue of a capacity that exceeds some norm for cognitive excellence? We believe that the concept of a threshold for full health accords better with commonly held societal views of health than an allowance for unbounded improvements in domain ability to be considered as improvements in health. The "supra-health" levels are perhaps better referred to as talent.

Some have argued that the threshold for full health can be identified purely in biological terms by examining the statistical distribution of functioning in the domain (Boorse 1977), but it seems clear to us that the domain threshold for full health is a normative choice: there is no criterion that would allow us, *a priori*, to choose a particular point on the population distribution of domain ability as representing the threshold for full health. We therefore suggest that the identification of thresholds for domain ability should be empirically-based and linked to health state valuations (described below). In intuitive terms, the threshold for a particular domain is the level of ability below which a majority of people generally recognize decrements as departures from excellent health. In practice, average health state valuations for levels of ability close to or above the threshold level will be extremely close to the value for full health, so that it is not necessary to explicitly delineate each domain threshold.

HEALTH STATE VALUATIONS

Thus far, we have elaborated a conceptual framework for health, in which health states are described in terms of levels on multiple dimensions such as mobility, pain, hearing and seeing. Health state valuations, in relation to these multidimensional profiles, constitute scalar index values for the overall levels of health associated with different states, measured on a cardinal scale that ranges from zero (for a state equivalent to death) to unity (for a state of ideal health). These valuations formalize the intuitive notions that health levels lie on a continuum and that we may characterize an individual as being more or less healthy than another at a particular moment in time. Health state valuations quantify departures from perfect health, i.e. the reductions in health associated with particular health states. It is important to emphasize that these weights *do not* measure the quality of life of people with disabilities and *do not* measure the value of different people to society.

In fact, there have been a variety of different conceptual interpretations of health state valuations that have led to considerable confusion in defining the basis for measuring and understanding these valuations. It is useful for us to contrast our conceptual definition of health state valuations with these other concepts.

Many health economists have defined health state valuations as measures of the utility associated with health states (see chapter 10.2). Our notion of health differs from utility in two important respects. Firstly, utility represents a broader construct, corresponding more closely to well-being than to health, strictly defined. Further, utility in the health context is typically defined in terms of the von Neumann-Morgenstern axioms of expected utility—i.e. conceptualized on the basis of choice under uncertainty. The use of the standard gamble technique for elicitation of valuations is linked to the expected utility framework, and therefore invokes both assessments of health levels associated with different states as well as attitudes towards risk and uncertainty. Thus, the notion of utility in the context of health state valuations combines our concept of health with the separate concept of risk aversion, which we do not believe is relevant for characterizations of health levels in summary measures (see chapter 9.4).

Another common interpretation of health state valuations has been as measures of quality of life (QoL), a term that has been used widely in various social science contexts to refer to the overall, subjective appraisals of happiness or satisfaction experienced by individuals. In health, the term QoL has been used often in a more particular way to refer to a multi-dimensional construct relating to symptoms, impairments, functional status, emotional states and what we have labeled as health domains. This use of QoL is clearly inconsistent with the general use of the term, so health researchers have taken to referring to this construct as "health-related QoL." To the extent that an individual's health-related QoL is conceived of as a vector of levels on "health-related" dimensions of life, it is similar to our conceptual framework for measuring health, albeit with less precisely articulated boundaries. Where health-related QoL is viewed as a summary measure of the contribution of an individual's health to her overall well-being, on the other hand, conceptual problems emerge from the fact that well-being is not clearly separable into independent health and non-health components, as Broome has argued convincingly (see chapter 3.1). In other words, when we compare the well-being or "quality of life" of individuals with different health levels, these relative comparisons may change depending on their levels on non-health dimensions of well-being. It is in this sense that a person with a long-term disability may say that their health-related quality of life is better than that of another person with no long-term disabilities.

We may avoid these difficulties if we define health state valuations to be simply indices of overall levels of health. Unlike the notion of utility, we do not believe that it is necessary to define this construct explicitly in terms of choices or preferences. Almost everyone can agree that a person with one amputated leg is healthier than a person with two amputated legs, all else being equal, without resorting at all to either the language of choice or to statements about the overall well-being of either person. While this is a simple case of a dominance ordering (because the difference is in the level of only one domain), the same intuitive notions apply to more complicated examples: if we say that somebody with a mild sore throat is, *ceteris paribus*, healthier than somebody with two broken arms, perhaps not everyone would agree, but most people could at least understand our statement through some common-sense notion of health. Indeed, this common-sense notion extends beyond ordinal comparisons, for example, allowing us to say that going from good health to having a sore throat is a smaller change in health than going from a sore throat to quadriplegia. In all of these cases, we submit that there is an intuitive understanding of the meaning of health that is not based on the concept of choice. Sen (1992) has similarly argued that welfare values do not need to be choice-based.

It is important to emphasize that, in defining health without reference to choice or preferences, we also distinguish our notion of health from Broome's broader notion of the "goodness" of health (chapter 3.1). In so doing, we avoid the problem of the separability of health and non-health components of well-being. Broome is undoubtedly correct to question whether the "goodness" of health—whether it is for comparative judgement or for some ultimate policy use—is truly separable from the "goodness" of non-health well-being. As Hausman argues in chapter 3.2, however, almost every culture has some notion of health that is distinguished from overall well-being, and it is this intuitive notion of health that we aim to capture in summary measures of population health. The World Health Organization is fundamentally concerned with the improvement of health as distinct from aspects of well-being that are not intrinsic determinants of health, and therefore requires an appropriately defined measure of population health.

AGGREGATION ACROSS TIME AND INDIVIDUALS IN POPULATION HEALTH MEASURES

In chapter 3.1, Broome raises some fundamental issues about the aggregation of health (more specifically the goodness associated with health) across time and across individuals. As we have emphasized here, our notion of health focuses more directly on the levels on a set of domains, rather than on the goodness associated with health, or overall well-being or utility. This focus, together with our careful consideration in chapter 1.3 of the different meanings of the term "healthier than" at the individual level, allows us to address the issue of aggregation in a fairly straightforward way.

Moving from the measurement and valuation of health at a moment in time, chapter 1.3 describes two other key perspectives that may be used in answering the question "Is person A healthier than person B?" The first is to compare the totality of health states experienced by person A and person B over their entire lifetimes. The second is to consider only the current health and future prospects of the two individuals. The latter perspective is probably closest to a common-sense notion of whether one individual is healthier than another. In this view, the past is excluded, but the influence of the past on current or future health is captured. The comparison of individual health in this perspective is based on each individual's health expectancy—the expectation of years of healthy life.

Aggregation across individuals presents another set of challenges, and different approaches may be required depending on the intended use. For example, health expectancies rely on a life table approach in which a hypothetical birth cohort is exposed to population rates of mortality and non-fatal health outcomes. In this case, there is no real aggregation across any real set of individuals. We may, however, construct a measure of the average health expectancy in the population which does result from an aggregation of the currently living members of the population (see below). For health gaps, a range of approaches are possible (see chapter 5.1), in which different sets of individuals and different time horizons are used as the basis for aggregation.

One important question is whether to include distributional concerns directly in summary measures of population health as part of the aggregation rule, or whether, on the other hand, to produce separate measures of average levels of health and distribution of health. Chapters 3.1, 3.8 and 3.9 address various viewpoints on this issue, and we discuss it further below.

HEALTH EXPECTANCIES

As summary measures of the overall level of health of a population, health expectancies have two advantages over other summary measures. The first is that it is relatively easy to explain the concept of an equivalent "healthy" life expectancy to a non-technical audience. The second is that health expectancies are measured in units (expected years of life) that are meaningful to and within the common experience of non-technical audiences (unlike other indicators such as mortality rates or incidence rates).

We can categorize health expectancies into two main classes: those that use dichotomous health state weights and those that use health state valuations for an exhaustive set of health states. Disability-free life expectancy (DFLE) is an example of the first class (Robine et al. 2001). Healthy life expectancy (or HALE) is an example of the second class (Mathers et al. 2001b; WHO 2001b). Health state expectancies such as DFLE give an implicit value of zero (equivalent to the valuation of death) for disability above a certain threshold; below this threshold the valuation is 1. This means that the summary indicator is not sensitive to changes in the severity distribution of disability within a population (criterion 5 of Murray et al.—see chapter 1.2). Additionally, the overall DFLE value for a population is largely determined by the prevalence of the milder levels of disability, and comparability between populations or over time is highly sensitive to the performance of the disability instrument in classifying people around the threshold. For these reasons, health state expectancies are not appropriate for use as SMPH.

In contrast, HALE is sensitive to changes in the distribution of health states, and thus meets one of the key criteria for an acceptable SMPH. Although healthy life expectancy cannot be additively decomposed with respect to causes or population subgroups, it is additively decomposable into health expectancies for specified levels of disability severity. Health state expectancies should thus be better understood as decompositions of summary measures than as SMPH in themselves. This interpretation is consistent with the usual ways in which families of health state expectancies are presented for a population (see chapter 4.1).

The calculation of health expectancies requires explicit choices about the time perspective adopted for defining event rates for the various input parameters, namely incidence, remission, prevalence and mortality. Thus, for example, one could calculate health expectancies as a pure *cohort* measure, where all events are based on observed events in a cohort. This would require tracing a birth cohort until every member had died. Alternatively, cohort event rates by age could be estimated based on projections.

Health expectancies could also be pure *period* measures, analogous to the standard demographic approach to calculation of life expectancies, where all event rates are calculated for a hypothetical cohort which is assumed to experience current age-specific event rates throughout life. These event rates would be the complete set of age-sex specific transition rates between all health states (including death).

The three perspectives identified in chapter 1.3 (health at a moment in time, health over the entire lifespan, or current and future health) provide a basis for constructing aggregate health expectancies across time and cohorts for populations. In principle, the population health expectancy defined as the average of all the *future* individual health expectancies for the people comprising the population at a given point of time satisfies all five criteria for SMPH (see chapters 1.2 and 4.1). This is because the future individual health expectancies are dependent not only on current and future transition rates (incidence) but also on the current health status (prevalence) of each individual.

Future individual health expectancies require assumptions about future incidence, remission and mortality rates that the individuals will face, whereas currently computed period health expectancies provide a measure based only on currently measurable aspects of health. For this reason, we may choose to define and estimate individual health expectancies by assuming that future incidence, remission and mortality rates that the individuals will face reflect current health conditions only. This would be an analogue of the well-known period life expectancies and health expectancies. We can then calculate a population-based aggregate health expectancy that satisfies the five criteria. For some comparisons, the average health expectancy could be based on a standard population to remove the effect of differences in age structure between populations.

The simplest method is to base the calculation of healthy life expectancies on the currently observed period information—particularly mortality rates and health state prevalences. This allows us to compute health expectancies for populations using Sullivan's method (see chapter 4.1). This approach requires only the data required for the period life table together with population prevalences for health states which can be measured using cross sectional population surveys and/or burden of disease analyses for prevalent disability in populations.

If sufficient data were available, it would be possible to use a multi-state life table based on the current observed period transition rates between all health states (and death), but to adjust these transition rates to reflect current risk exposures. Thus for example, the risks of lung cancer at each age could be based on current patterns of exposure to tobacco smoking, rather than on currently observed incidence or mortality of lung cancer (which reflects exposure 20 years or more in the past). This would be an extension of the concept of a period measure to include current risk exposures. Note that whereas a true period measure must be based on incidence rates (transition rates) for health states, it should reflect prevalence (rather than incidence) of relevant risk exposures, since it is the prevalence and duration of exposure that determines risk of transition between health states.

Health gaps

The second main use of summary measures of population health is to assess the relative magnitude of the contribution of different diseases, injuries and risk factors to levels of population health. Such information is a useful input to debates on priorities for research and development, priorities for focused attention of government for policy formulation and for identifying which interventions should be further evaluated. When using summary measures to look at different causes of population health levels, the critical question is different: Is cause A or B a more important contributor to levels of population health? To be comprehensible for the broader public, a summary measure used for such causal attribution should fulfill two important requirements: it should be easily understood and it should have the property of additive decomposition. In other words, the summary measure should be partitionable into causes or subgroups such that the sum of the SMPH across a set of mutually exclusive and exhaustive categories equals the total.

In general, health gaps can be decomposed into the contribution of various causes in a more intuitive and easily communicated fashion than health expectancies. DALYs are additive across causes to give the total health gap for a population. A health gap measure such as the DALY thus fulfills different needs for SMPH to be used for causal attribution. Part 6 of this book presents a series of viewpoints on the two possible approaches to causal attribution: categorical attribution and counterfactual analysis.

Since the primary purpose of measuring health gaps is to disaggregate them into the contributions of component causes, they should be formulated to capture the relative magnitude of causes of population health currently and in the near future. The simplest method is to base the calculation of health gaps on the currently observed period information— particularly mortality rates and health state prevalences and transition rates. This allows us to compute health gaps for populations using only period data for mortality and health states in populations. The most widely used implementation of this approach is DALYs.

The key conceptual issue relating to health gaps is the choice of the normative goal for health against which current conditions are compared. Chapter 5.1 discusses three different types of normative functions that may be defined: a population norm, an unconditional individual norm and a conditional individual norm. A population norm simply specifies a reference healthy life expectancy, allowing the calculation of a population health gap as the difference between the realized healthy life expectancy and this reference. Like healthy life expectancy, this type of health gap is not easily decomposed into the contributions of different causes. Furthermore, because it represents a life-table type measure aggregated across ages, it does not distinguish between different age patterns of health levels that produce the same overall health expectancy, even though norms for health may vary considerably by age.

An unconditional individual norm defines a set of age-specific target levels for health that do not change depending on the age an individual has attained, while a conditional individual norm may vary as individuals advance in age. For example, an unconditional norm may be defined as survivorship in full health up to age 100. An individual who lives to 101 in full health thus exceeds this norm and contributes nothing to the health gap measure. In contrast, a conditional norm, such as the two-part norm implemented in the DALY, may set a survivorship goal that is specific to the age that has already been attained. In this case, an individual who lives to age 101 in full health may still contribute to the health gap, given a norm for healthy life expectancy at age 101 that is greater than 0. The conditional norm allows for all individuals in the population to contribute to the total health gap, no matter what age they attain.

Criteria for selection of a specific normative loss function might include biological plausibility (in principle, the normative goal should be biologically achievable), desirability and, perhaps, some notion of fairness (for example, the fair innings concept described in Williams 1999). Based on the observed experience across countries, a reasonable normative survivorship function to select as the basis for defining a standard loss function would be one that equals the highest national life expectancy observed across populations, at present a life expectancy at birth of around 85 years. Loss functions based on local survival curves should not be used for international comparative health gap analyses, although such loss functions may be used for various other types of national studies.

ETHICS

THE ROLE OF EMPIRICAL ETHICS

In the conference behind this book and in subsequent discussions, one of the most lively debates has revolved around the question of empirical ethics (see part 12). Some authors have argued that any values that are incorporated, either implicitly or explicitly, in summary measures should be based solely on the empirical measurement of these values in the public, and that the entire enterprise of constructing summary measures is threatened by heterogeneity in values. For example, Mooney states in chapter 12.3:

> If the two (or more) populations are genuinely comparable in terms of their value bases, then comparing their health status might well be justified. The occasions on which such genuineness will be present, however, seem rather few and the larger the population groupings involved, the less likely that genuine homogeneity will apply.

The extreme version of this argument would suggest that all comparisons are impossible because of differences in individual values. Despite assertion by proponents of empirical ethics that there is extreme heterogeneity of values, empirical evidence suggests otherwise, at least in relation to health. Valuation studies carried out with deliberative small groups in 12 different countries have found surprising consistency in valuations across cultures (Murray and Lopez 2000). More recently, valuation studies carried out as part of the WHO Multi-Country Survey Study (Üstün et al. 2001) also have found remarkable consistency in health state valuations. This result is not, perhaps, a major surprise, given the fundamental importance of the core health domains to all human beings, irrespective of their social or socioeconomic circumstances. It is possible, though again the empirical evidence is not apparent, that there may be more heterogeneity in values around well-being outcomes than health outcomes, conceptualized as described above, as a set of domain abilities. Given the fundamental importance of the core health domains for the achievement of the things that people commonly value, we believe that comparison of health levels through SMPH is not only meaningful, but operationally achievable.

In fact, even if there is heterogeneity of values, other disciplines have found very straightforward ways to address this issue. For example, consumer price indices are computed in reference to a standard basket of goods, even though individual consumption patterns may vary widely. In descriptive epidemiology, where the age structures of populations differ, we use one common standard in order to make comparisons. This does not conflict with use of local standards for other purposes. Similarly, even though there may be variation both within and across countries on values that are incorporated in SMPH, for purposes of international comparison, it is quite appropriate to use a common standard.

Hausman in chapter 12.2 presents a compelling critique of empirical ethics, concluding as follows:

> Although there is a great deal to be said for finding out what people value, there is little to be said for empirical ethics... The main problem is that the defender of empirical ethics poses a false dichotomy:

either statisticians and health professionals decide, or the values of the target population rule... [T]here should instead be a dialogue between the values of the target population and the moral arguments of those who have laboured long over these issues. If the moral arguments of the statistician or health analyst are conclusive, then they should transform the social consensus. If there is wisdom in the social consensus (and the experts are sensitive and open-minded enough to recognize it), then the values of the population will reveal narrowness or flaws in the arguments of the experts. If the values within a society are genuinely moral values, then they must be both sensitive to rational argument and rationally defensible. Nothing should prevent the analyst from influencing the population's values and being influenced by them. Those who study health should have no authority beyond that conveyed by their arguments. But on moral issues those concerned with health should defer only to arguments, not to mere consensus. Empirical ethics is not a kind of ethics, and it is not an acceptable replacement for ethics. Population values have an important place *within* ethical reflection; they should not compete with it.

Of course health policy-makers are interested in people's values, and for WHO, in average global health state valuations and variations across populations. Where relevant, these empirical values may be modified in light of UN values relating to basic human rights. For values relating to age weighting and discounting, there are ethical and theoretical concerns that must be taken into account as well as empirical data. In particular, it is not possible to ask people in the future about their health values, though future health states contribute to health gaps in particular.

One notable exception to the argument against a strictly empirical approach to defining key value choices in summary measures relates to the understanding of health state valuations as reflecting different weights on the core domains of health. Unlike values such as time preference, there are no compelling philosophical arguments as to the relative importance of mobility versus cognition in overall assessments of health levels. Thus, we believe it is reasonable to use global average health state valuations in the construction of summary measures and to perform sensitivity analyses using the empirical range of valuations across Member States.

GOODNESS AND FAIRNESS

Part 14 of this volume presents an overview of some of the key debates around fairness concerns in applications of summary measures in health policy. While our view of summary measures as pertaining strictly to levels of health tends to exclude problems of equity and fairness from the actual measures themselves, there are a host of vital philosophical questions relating to the interface between goodness and fairness in societal decision-making. Chapter 14.1 and the commentaries that follow provide a brief introduction to these issues, and we refer readers to a forthcoming volume entitled *Fairness and Goodness* for a much more extensive treatment of the subject (Wikler and Murray, forthcoming).

TIME AND AGE

The incorporation of time preference and age weights in summary measures of population health has been controversial (see part 13). The following section summarizes some of the key arguments and recommendations that emerge from the various debates on these values.

Discounting health

When health gaps are calculated in order to assess the contribution of different diseases, injuries and risk factors to patterns of population health, a major purpose is to inform priorities for policy debate. Decisions on resource allocation require information on many other things as well such as the costs and benefits of specific intervention options, considerations of reducing health inequality or enhancing responsiveness and procedural fairness (see below). Nevertheless, the magnitude of different causes can guide the direction of policy debates about research and development and policy attention itself. As such, the time horizon of the assessment of health gaps should map to the time horizon of the impact of current decision-making. Given this linkage, it is reasonable to focus on the contribution of diseases, injuries and risk factors to health gaps in the near future as opposed to the distant future. The focus on the near future needs to be operationalized by defining a clear time cutoff beyond which health events are not included in the calculation and/or the inclusion of a discount rate in the calculation of health gaps.

In the Global Burden of Disease Study 1990, a 3% discount rate was used in standard DALY calculations (Murray and Lopez 1996). Given the simplicity of a constant time discount rate, and its standard use in discounting of health outcomes in cost effectiveness analyses, it seems prudent to continue to use for incidence-based health gaps measures, the constant 3% time discount rate embodied in the DALY. We recommend, however, given continuing debate about this value, that sensitivity analyses be included in the routine calculation and reporting of health gap measures in order to examine the impact of alternative choices regarding discounting.

For health expectancies, particularly period measures which encapsulate the experience of a representative individual who experiences current period transition rates and/or health state prevalences at each age of their life, time discounting is not appropriate. Likewise, when SMPH are reformulated as averages of individual healthy life expectancies or of individual expected gaps, then there appear to be few reasons to apply time discounting. The most cogent argument for time discounting, the research paradox, can be accommodated by applying generational discounting to future generations, and adding up health or health losses for individuals currently alive without discounting.

Age weights

Standard DALYs in the GBD 1990 included non-uniform age weights in order to reflect the dependency of children and older people on young adults. This argument, however, revolves around the contributions of young adults to societal well-being, perhaps outside of the realm of population health, strictly defined. Nevertheless, there are other arguments for non-uniform age weighting based on the intuitive notion that lifetimes have a shape, reflecting the way that individuals attach different values to different periods of their own lives. The available evidence does support the proposition that individuals attach different value to different periods of their own lives. In particular, in terms of the comparative judgement of whether population A is healthier than population B, individuals appear to place more weight on the health of individuals at middle ages than at older ages, and possibly at very young ages. While the exact shape of the age weighting function may be disputed, it seems to us useful to continue to compute health gap measures with non-uniform age weights for continuity in comparisons, but to adopt uniform age weights as the standard formulation for health expectancies. As with discounting, we recommend that sensitivity analyses be included in the routine calculation and reporting of health gap measures in order to examine the impact of alternative choices regarding age weights.

MEASUREMENT

The ultimate inputs into summary measures of population health are estimates, by age and sex, of the distribution of the population across different states of health, including full health, on the causes of states of ill-health by age and sex, as well as age-sex-cause-specific mortality rates for each population of interest. This section describes the basic requirements for the calculation of health expectancies and health gaps, and discusses some of the over-riding measurement challenges, in particular relating to the need for cross-population comparability.

MEASUREMENT OF MORTALITY

Reliable estimates of population numbers and mortality rates by age and sex are required for calculating both health expectancies and health gaps for a population. The "gold standard" for population-level data on the numbers of deaths in a population is complete registration of all deaths, by sex and age, and by year of occurrence for the normal resident (de facto) population. Each death recorded in a vital registration system should be medically certified by a qualified medical practitioner using the latest version of the International Form of Medical Certificate of Cause of Death. Selection of the cause to be coded as the underlying cause of death should be based on the rules and procedures specified in the 10th Revision of the International Classification of Diseases, Injuries and Causes of Death (WHO 1992), or on subsequent revisions. Where vital registration is incomplete, standard demographic techniques may be used to adjust for under-reporting of deaths (e.g. intercensal analyses or the Brass Growth-Balance method).

Other data collection systems have also been used successfully to compile data on the level of mortality in the absence of good national vital registration systems. Modules on child and adult mortality can be added to household surveys to estimate mortality levels either directly or indirectly. For example, the Demographic and Health Survey programmememe (DHS) has yielded comparable estimates of infant mortality and child (under 5) mortality for more than 60 countries since 1985. At other ages, mortality, particularly among working age adults, is a much rarer event than child deaths and hence larger samples are generally required. As for child mortality, levels of adult mortality can be estimated either directly from questions about deaths in the household over the past 12–24 months or indirectly from questions about orphanhood and the survival of siblings. Indirect methods for adult mortality are strongly prone to under-estimate mortality levels, frequently by up to 50–60%. Great care is therefore required when interpreting the results of these methods to estimate adult mortality and direct methods, with appropriate interview probes for misreporting, are likely to yield more useful estimates.

Finally, in situations where vital registration covering the entire population is not feasible, sample registration systems, or networks of disease surveillance points have been used to collect data on defined populations. Provided these "catchment" populations are chosen so as to be nationally representative, and provided the routine demographic and epidemiological surveillance is suitably rigorous, sample surveillance schemes can yield very useful data on age-specific death rates and on causes of death. Sample-based schemes have been successfully used for demographic surveillance in India (0.6% sample) and for epidemiological surveillance in China (1% sample). In the case of the Disease Surveillance Points system in China, cause of death is assigned on the basis of medical records for the deceased, where they exist and/or a structured questionnaire about symptoms experienced prior to death ("verbal autopsy").

MEASUREMENT OF NON-FATAL HEALTH OUTCOMES
Cross-population comparability

The health state measurement field has dealt rather well with issues of validity and reliability of instruments (see chapter 8.1), and this book does not attempt to add to this body of work. Ensuring the cross-population comparability of results adds a third dimension to survey instrument development. The difference between comparability on the one hand and validity and reliability on the other hand can be illustrated using the example of two thermometers, one of which measures temperature in Celsius and the other in Fahrenheit. Both thermometer measures give valid and reliable measurements of temperature. However, 26 degrees on the Celsius thermometer is not comparable to 26 degrees on the Fahrenheit thermometer. Comparability is fundamental to the use of survey results for development of evidence for health policy but has been under-emphasized in instrument development.

Some people may argue that there is no need for comparability in population health measurement. But the basis of science is comparable measurement: comparison creates possibilities of investigating broad determinants at national and cross-national levels. There is a strong demand at national and international levels for comparisons for these reasons, whether consciously articulated or not. Even where there is no interest in cross-national comparison, there is a need for comparison within countries over time, or across different sub-populations delineated by age, sex, education, income or other characteristics. Health measurements, particularly for policy-makers, generally only have meaning in context, and context means comparison. For example, a decrease in mortality of 10% over 10 years for a particular cause in a country, may be "good" or " bad" (e.g. if other comparable countries have achieved a 50% reduction with fewer resources). While it is possible to assess health progress purely with time comparisons within a country, relating this progress to health and other social interventions and trends is extremely difficult in the absence of comparison with other populations, simply because there is only one data point (the set of interventions that actually occurred).

We thus conclude that comparison is extremely important, and fundamental to all uses of SMPH. Population health information is largely irrelevant (i.e. uninterpretable) if we do not have it. This is a new and fertile area that SMPH bring into sharp focus, because mortality is comparable, but most measures of health states are currently not.

The fundamental challenge in seeking cross-population comparable measures is that the most accessible sources of data relating to health are self-reported categorical data. When categorical data are used as the basis for understanding quantities that are determined on a continuous, cardinal scale, the problem of cross-population comparability emerges from differences in the way different individuals use categorical response scales (see chapter 8.3). Response category cut-point shift can make crude comparisons of results across populations nearly meaningless, even when exactly the same questions are used, as illustrated by some of the examples provided in chapter 8.1. Recent analyses of surveys containing both self-reported and measured health status levels have documented systematic differences in the interpretation of self-report survey questions according to age, sex, socioeconomic disadvantage and other individual factors (chapters 8.2 and 8.4).

WHO has developed new approaches to solve the problem of comparability of self-report data, and results from the WHO Multi-Country Survey Study carried out during 2000–2001 provide strong evidence that the methods improve cross-population comparability (Üstün et al. 2001).

Health state valuations

Health state valuations provide the critical link between information on mortality and information on non-fatal health outcomes in summary measures. As reviewed in parts 9 to 11 of this book, the empirical basis for health state valuations has been relatively limited to date, and research has been conducted primarily in the United States and European countries. A key objective for WHO has been to enhance the empirical basis for health state valuations by collecting population-based measurements throughout the world using a set of standardized instruments and protocols based on the best current methods.

During 2000–2001, WHO conducted household and postal surveys on health in more than 60 Member States (Üstün et al. 2001) including a health state valuation component in the 10 large-scale household surveys. Because the available instruments are imperfect, a two-tiered data collection strategy has been used. Many of the techniques developed for the measurement of health state valuations have been designed to be implemented among highly educated respondents, as they rely on abstract and cognitively demanding thought experiments. The only appropriate valuation tool for respondents across a wide range of levels of educational attainment is the visual analogue scale, which has been implemented in diverse cultural settings, including Cambodia, Colombia, India, the Philippines and the United Republic of Tanzania, and has been demonstrated consistently to have higher reliability than other methods (see, for example, chapters 9.3 and 11.3). Based on long-standing results from both psychophysics and psychometrics, however, it is necessary to rescale valuation results obtained though visual analogue scales in order to obtain interval-scaled valuations for construction of summary measures. This rescaling should be empirically-based and therefore requires a second avenue of data collection using deliberative protocols based on multiple states and multiple valuation methods.

While we noted above that it is not necessary to conceptualize health state valuations using the language of choice, preferences do provide a convenient way to elicit information on these valuations. Choice-based elicitation techniques, such as the standard gamble and time trade-off methods, allow inference about levels of health by having respondents weigh changes in these health levels against other quantities, such as mortality risks or length of life. The analytical challenge lies in recovering the underlying assessments about health levels from these responses, which requires a parsing out of the different values behind individuals' answers to these various questions. We have implemented this approach as part of the WHO surveys in 10 countries, using groups with higher levels of educational attainment. The results of the deliberative, multi-method exercises are currently being used to estimate the relationship between responses on a visual analogue scale and the cardinal scale of health state valuations that is required in summary measures (see chapter 9.4).

A number of measurement challenges relating to health state valuations provide a fertile area for continuing research. Examination of variation in valuations across and within countries remains a key priority. To that end, WHO will continue to pursue an ambitious range of data collection activities in representative population samples in diverse settings. Thus far, these efforts have indicated minimal cross-country differences, but we await further results from additional countries. Comparisons between large population-based surveys and small, deliberative convenience samples should be undertaken in order to evaluate the relative measurement characteristics of these alternative modes.

The work summarized in this volume highlights several other important areas for methodological development, including the use of multi-method protocols to estimate the underlying valuations informing responses on standard elicitation techniques, alternative modes of presenting health states as stimuli for valuations, and estimation of the mapping functions that link multi-dimensional health state descriptions and health state valuations. A range of statistical problems must be addressed, including the proper specification of measurement error on health state valuations, the correct model specification for the valuation function and more sophisticated Bayesian modelling strategies for understanding heterogeneity in individual responses to different measurement methods.

Combining health surveys with epidemiological estimates

Health expectancies require information on the prevalence and severity distribution of various health states in the population, by age and sex, which may be obtained, in principle, from suitably large, nationally representative surveys covering the key domains of health. For the causal decomposition of health gaps, it is necessary to map prevalence (and incidence) of health states to disease and injury causes. It is not possible to do this using self-report health survey data, since respondents are often not aware of the causes of their health states, particularly when there are multiple health conditions.

For this reason, it is necessary to collect epidemiological data on specific diseases and injuries in order to ensure internal consistency with mortality data and population level health state prevalence data. Ideally, estimates of the prevalence of disease and injury outcomes (sequelae), by age and sex, would be built up from age-specific incidence, remission and case-fatality rates for each sequela in a given population.

The selection of specific diseases and injuries, the data sources for which might be given greater priority in a broader epidemiological data system, needs to be based on a set of clear criteria. Foremost among these would be diseases or injuries which *a priori* are considered to be major causes of disease burden and/or which are likely to collectively account for, say, two-thirds or more of the disease burden in a population. For each such disease or injury, a consultative process among epidemiologists, health statisticians and other public health personnel concerned with data collection should be organized to agree upon the ideal and minimal data sources required for calculating summary measures of population health. Sources of such information and their advantages and limitations are discussed in chapters 7 and 10 of Mathers et al. (2001a). Typically, these will include:

1. household surveys of prevalence (e.g. smear positive sputum for tuberculosis, infertility, affective and anxiety disorders, lung function tests, etc.) or of episodes of illness (e.g. diarrhoeal diseases) or seroepidemiological surveys (e.g. for hepatitis B/C);

2. sentinel sites (e.g. antenatal clinics for HIV), incidence of complications of disease (e.g. liver complications, cerebral malaria, amputations and neuropathies);

3. population-based incidence registries (e.g. for cancer, cerebrovascular disease, congenital anomalies, homicide); and

4. hospital discharge data (e.g. for cirrhosis of the liver, fires, road traffic accidents).

Recommendations about the key diseases and injuries for which data are required in order to calculate SMPH are under development by WHO in consultation with Member States. Both the ideal data sources and the minimal data sources are being identified to guide countries to determine priorities for health information systems to facilitate the calculation of these measures.

APPLICATIONS

MEASURING LEVELS OF HEALTH: THE NEED FOR BOTH TYPES OF SMPH

Improving overall levels of population health is a clear priority for WHO Member States. Healthy life expectancy is a readily understandable positive measure that is appropriately sensitive to survival rates and to the prevalence and severity distribution of health states among the population. As healthy life expectancy is based on a severity distribution of prevalence of health states, it is more comparable across populations than other measures based on dichotomous prevalence measures, since distributional data imply that the measure is much less sensitive to the threshold chosen for defining ill-health.

Neither life expectancy nor healthy life expectancy provide information on the leading causes of death or non-fatal health status in populations. It is not possible to disaggregate these measures in an additive fashion by cause (see chapter 4.1). Health gaps are additive across causes and across population groups and hence provide a more appropriate and useable SMPH for reporting on causes of loss of health for Member States (see chapters 5.1 and 6.1).

Summary measures are only one component of a coherent and integrated statistical framework. SMPH should be viewed as the apex of a hierarchy of related measures, rather than a piecemeal set of unconnected measures. The macro measures at the apex of the system, such as health expectancies and health gaps, provide a broad population-based overview of levels and causes.

SMPH AND SUMMARY MEASURES OF HEALTH INEQUALITY

Information about average levels of health in a population is important for health policy formulation, as is knowledge about inequalities in health within a population. Should there be one summary measure of population health that reflects both average levels of population health and the distribution of health within the population, or should there be separate summary measures of average population health and health inequality?

Some values such as concern for the distribution of health outcomes may figure prominently in public decision-making, but it is still debatable whether such fairness concerns should be integrated directly into the summary measure of population health or rather measured independently. The advantages of including fairness concerns in a summary measure is that it places these issues firmly in the health agenda. The disadvantage is that including fairness considerations directly in a summary measure of population health can complicate the summary measure profoundly and does not allow for different trade-offs between goodness and fairness.

Perhaps more importantly, it is clear that there may be fairness concerns that are central to the choice of interventions but are not as relevant to the comparative use of summary health measures. Nord (chapter 14.4) has drawn attention to a preference for giving health resources to the sick to some extent irrespective of their capacity to benefit, a form of distributional concern. One cannot argue that such a priority to the sick would be relevant to measuring population health even if it is critical to the debate on resource allocation across interventions and beneficiaries. Keeping fairness and goodness considerations distinct in the construction of summary measures of population health allows us to keep track of these different uses and needs. In general, a much sharper distinction needs to be made in the debate on the construction of summary measures of population health and the ethical dimensions of intervention choice. Some values such as discounting or age-weighting may be considered types of fairness considerations (discounting is related to intergenerational fairness and age-weighting to fairness across age groups). Or they may be seen as components of goodness (in this case amount of health). If the latter, there is a much stronger case that they be incorporated into a summary measure of population health.

Precedents for separate summary measures exist from other sectors. For example, in the case of income measurement, the common practice is to report average income per capita for a population and separately to report a measure of income inequality such as the Gini coefficient. There is, nevertheless, a rich literature on composite measures of average income and its distribution (e.g. Kolm-Atkinson measures, etc.). For health, it is simpler, closer to the tradition of health statistics and more easily communicated to the general public to have separate summary measures of average population health and health inequality. Consequently, we believe that WHO should develop and report on separate summary measures for level and distribution of health in WHO Member States.

The desirability of two distinct measures for summarizing the average levels of population health and health inequalities has implications for methods used to measure the valuations for time spent in health states less than full health. These methods should not incorporate distributional concerns. Rather, these distributional concerns should be directly captured in the summary measure of health inequality.

SMPH AND RESOURCE ALLOCATION

What is the use of summary measures of population health decomposed into the contributions of diseases, injuries or risk factors to prioritising investments in different interventions? Williams (1999) and Mooney (chapter 12.3 in this book) have claimed that a purpose of SMPH is to set health funding priorities and argued that this is inappropriate. Neither we, nor our colleagues, have ever claimed that resources should be directed toward health problems solely on the basis of their relative contributions to premature mortality and non-fatal health outcomes. Williams and Mooney are constructing a straw man by implying that we advocate using SMPH alone to select funding priorities.

While nearly everyone agrees that one very important input to prioritising resources for interventions is the cost-effectiveness of interventions, nevertheless, debates on priorities for health action can be informed by summary measures of population health. To estimate the benefits of an intervention at the population level and to monitor the impact of specific interventions when implemented, a valid assessment of the epidemiology of the disease, injury or risk factor addressed by the intervention is required. There are very few instances where marginal change in health at the population level can feasibly be measured in any way other than in terms of the difference between two assessments of level of health using SMPH. Additionally, where there are non-monetary fixed assets limiting the feasible combinations of interventions that can be delivered, such as the attention of senior Ministry of Health decision-makers, then these assets should be devoted not just to the most cost-effective interventions but to those cost-effective interventions with the potential to effect substantial improvements in population health status.

Information on the contributions of diseases, injuries and risk factors to summary measures of population health is also necessary for the health intelligence function of governments. If a disease, injury or risk factor is not yet recognized as a major problem, there will be no attempt to formulate intervention strategies or even to assess the benefits and costs of alternative intervention strategies. For example, one consequence of the GBD 1990 study has been to focus policy attention on intervention strategies for depression in low and middle-income countries, resulting in efforts to analyse the cost-effectiveness of interventions for depression. If decomposition of summary measures into the contributions of diseases, injuries and risk factors is necessary, this has significant implications for the design of summary measures, favouring health gaps over health expectancies (see Murray et al. chapter 5.1 in this volume).

The argument made by Williams and Mooney—that only incremental changes through intervention, and not the level of population health, matter—appears strange when extended by analogy to national income and product accounts. As Jamison (1996) writes on this analogy, "The most natural comparison [to the GBD] is to the development of National Income and Product Accounts (NIPAs)." (p. xix) Original pioneering efforts on NIPAs were followed by the codification of international standards in the System of National Accounts (SNA 1993). Despite codification, debate has continued unabated on the conceptual and empirical basis for national accounts—should environmental degradation be included in capital depreciation, should household production be included, etc. National accounts measure the level of economic activity in a country. Williams and Mooney must surely argue that this is unnecessary; they must argue that resources wasted on measuring national accounts could be better spent on calculating the incremental gains in national income that could be achieved through various policy options or interventions. Today, the myriad uses of national accounts have so enriched the field of macroeconomics that little energy is spent on questioning their utility. Summary measures of population health are, for the health sector, a natural analogue to national income and product accounts.

It is essential to distinguish clearly efforts to quantify the health gains from interventions for cost-effectiveness analyses from efforts to apply summary measures of population health in cross-national comparisons or other uses. Imagining that the most desirable summary measure of population health has been identified, one could argue logically that the benefits of a health intervention should be measured as the expected difference in this summary measure for a population with and without the intervention (Murray and Lopez 2000). At minimum, there should in general be consistency between the approach used to develop summary measures and that used to estimate the benefits of interventions, without necessarily formally defining the benefits as the change in the summary measure. Thus, for example, health state valuations might be the same for both uses, but the benefits of interventions could be measured directly as the increase in healthy years of life lived.

Concluding remarks

In this concluding chapter, we have attempted to bring together the various issues and viewpoints raised by the contributors to this volume in a way that will be helpful for policy and further scientific debate. These issues range from the conceptual underpinnings of summary measures of population health, to the technical and practical details of their construction and use, and to the various ethical considerations that such measures unavoidable entail. We have not tried to be prescriptive on all issues: indeed from the diversity of views and opinions expressed in this book, it would be premature to do so. Rather, in this chapter we have tried to draw together these opinions into coherent scientific argument around each of the key themes we have identified in the construction and use of summary measures. This should greatly facilitate the application of this body of work in public policy and better focus the agenda for future research. Where there is consensus, or virtual consensus, we have tried to be very explicit about the implications for summary measures of population health, and where there is not, we have tried to lay out the issues in a constructive and objective fashion. Transparency will increase confidence that a broad spectrum of legitimate scientific opinion has been canvassed and thus enhance the policy relevance of its content.

The Global Burden of Disease project, and subsequent work on burden of disease analysis and the use of healthy life expectancy to measure population health attainment in the analysis of health system performance of WHO Member States (WHO 2000; WHO 2001b) has stimulated broader interest in the design, calculation and use of summary measures of population health. The body of work on the burden of disease and comparative risk assessment has also demonstrated the feasibility of estimating health gaps and their key role in quantifying the contribution of diseases, injuries and risk factors for population health. Notwithstanding these contributions, there is clearly further scope for improvement in all aspects of the development and use of SMPH. The World Health Organization through its commitment to routinely assessing the global burden of disease, to regularly assessing the performance of health systems of Member States, and to leading an international dialogue on the development of summary measures of population health, has laid the scientific and institutional foundations to foster and advance this agenda. Meanwhile, we trust that the substantive debate and presentation of ideas collected in this volume will serve to promote greater understanding of the scope and potential of summary measures of population health to inform public health development and health policy.

REFERENCES

Boorse C (1977) Health as a theoretical concept. *Philosophy of Science,* **44**:542–573.

Jamison DT (1996) Foreword to the global burden of disease and injury series. In: *The global burden of disease: a comprehensive assessment of mortality and disability from diseases, injuries and risk factors in 1990 and projected to 2020. Vol 1*, Murray CJL, Lopez AD, eds., Harvard School of Public Health on behalf of WHO, Cambridge, MA.

Mathers CD, Vos T, Lopez AD, Salomon JA, Ezzati M, eds. (2001a) *National burden of disease studies: a practical guide.* 2.0., World Health Organization/ Global Programmememe on Evidence for Health Policy, Geneva. *www.who.int/ evidence/nbd*

Mathers CD, Sadana R, Salomon J, Murray CJL, Lopez A (2001b) Healthy life expectancy in 191 countries, 1999. *Lancet,* **357**(9269):1685–1691.

Murray CJL, Lopez AD, eds. (1996) *The global burden of disease: a comprehensive assessment of mortality and disability from diseases, injuries and risk factors in 1990 and projected to 2020. Vol 1.*, Harvard School of Public Health on behalf of WHO, Cambridge, MA.

Murray CJL, Lopez A (2000) Progress and directions in refining the global burden of disease approach: a response to Williams. *Health Economics,* **9**(1):69–82.

Murray CJL, Lopez AD (1999) On the comparable quantification of health risks: lessons from the global burden of disease study. *Epidemiology,* **10**(5):594–605.

Robine JM, Jagger C, Romieu I (2001) Disability-free life expectancies in the European Union countries. *Genus,* **57**(2):89–101.

Sen A (1992) *Inequality re-examined.* Russel Sage; Harvard University Press, New York; Cambridge, MA.

SNA (1993) *System of national accounts 1993.* European Communities, International Monetary Fund, Organisation of Economic Cooperation and Development, United Nations, World Bank. *http://esa.un.org/unsd/sna1993/*

Üstün TB, Chatterji S, Villanueva M, Bendib L, Sadana R, Valentine N, Ortiz J, et al. (2001) *WHO multi-country household survey study on health and responsiveness, 2000–2001.* GPE discussion paper no 37. World Health Organization/ Global Programmememe on Evidence for Health Policy, Geneva.

WHO (1948) *Constitution.* World Health Organization, Geneva.

WHO (1992) *International statistical classification of diseases and related health problems (ICD 10).* 10th edn, World Health Organization, Geneva.

WHO (2000) *The World Health Report 2000. Health systems: improving performance.* World Health Organization, Geneva.

WHO (2001a) *International classification of functioning, disability and health (ICF).* World Health Organization, Geneva.

WHO (2001b) *The World Health Report 2001. Mental health: new understanding, new hope.* World Health Organization, Geneva.

Wikler D, Murray CJL, eds. (Forthcoming) *Fairness and goodness: ethical issues in health resource allocation.* World Health Organization, Geneva.

Williams A (1999) Calculating the global burden of disease: time for a strategic reappraisal? *Health Economics,* 8(1):1–8.

Glossary of terms

ADAPTATION

Any change in true levels of functioning with reference to one or more domains of health. For example: improvement in ambulation following physical therapy. It is one of three phenomena (adaptation, adjustment and coping) describing changes in individual assessments of health levels.

ADJUSTMENT

Any change in the relative importance of different components of health in an individual's overall assessment of a multi-dimensional health state. It is one of three phenomena (adaptation, adjustment and coping) describing changes in individual assessments of health levels.

ADL: ACTIVITIES OF DAILY LIVING

Any of the tasks such as eating, getting in/out of bed, getting around inside, dressing, bathing or using the toilet, used in disability assessment instruments to measure performance.

AIDS: AQUIRED IMMUNODEFICIENCY SYNDROME

ALE: ACTIVE LIFE EXPECTANCY

A form of DFLE (q.v.) based on survey questions on limitations in activities of daily living (ADL).

BMI: BODY MASS INDEX

A measure of underweight and overweight calculated as weight (kg) divided by height (m) squared.

CEYLL: COHORT EXPECTED YEARS OF LIFE LOST

A form of health gap (q.v.) that measures mortality gap using the projected cohort life expectancy for the population to specify years lost due to death at each age.

CHD: CORONARY HEART DISEASE

Note: this is synonymous with ischaemic heart disease (q.v.).

CVD: CEREBROVASCULAR DISEASE

CHI: CHINA

Regional grouping used in the Global Burden of Disease study 1990.

COPING

Any change in reported health relating to shifts in norms and expectations that influence the mappings between true health levels and reported levels. It is one of three phenomena (adaptation, adjustment and coping) describing changes in individual assessments of health levels.

CRA: COMPARATIVE RISK ASSESSMENT

A systematic counterfactual approach to estimating health gaps (q.v.) (or changes in health expectancy) causally attributable to a risk factor or a group of risk factors.

DALE: DISABILITY-ADJUSTED LIFE EXPECTANCY

Synonym for HALE (q.v.) or healthy life expectancy.

DALY: DISABILITY-ADJUSTED LIFE YEAR

A health gap (q.v.) measure developed for the GBD (q.v.).

DFLE: DISABILITY-FREE LIFE EXPECTANCY

A form of HSE (q.v.) which gives a weight of 1 to states of health with no disability above an explicit or implicit threshold and a weight of 0 to states of health with any level of disability above that threshold.

DBP: DIASTOLIC BLOOD PRESSURE

EME: ESTABLISHED MARKET ECONOMIES

Regional grouping used in the Global Burden of Disease study 1990. Includes Western Europe, North America, Australia, Japan and New Zealand.

EQ5D: *See:* EUROQOL EQ-5D

EU: EUROPEAN UNION

EuroQol Group

A network of international multidisciplinary researchers originally from Europe, which now includes members from Canada, Japan, New Zealand, South Africa and the United States. Its objective is the development and application of a single, generic index value describing health-related quality of life.

EuroQol EQ-5D

A standardized instrument for use as a measure of health outcome based on 5 domains: mobility, self-care, usual activity, pain/discomfort, anxiety/depression. It can be used in the clinical and economic evaluation of health care as well as population health surveys.

FSE: former socialist economies

Regional grouping used in the Global Burden of Disease study 1990. Includes former socialist countries of Eastern Europe and Central Asia.

GPE: Global Programme for Evidence on Health Policy

The department within the WHO cluster Evidence and Information for Policy (EIP) responsible for work on summary measures of population health.

GBD: global burden of disease

A project to estimate health gaps (q.v.) for a comprehensive set of disease and injury causes, and for major risk factors, in the populations of the world using all available mortality and health data and methods to ensure internal consistency and comparability of estimates. The original Global Burden of Disease project estimated health gaps using DALYs (q.v.) for eight regions of the world in 1990 (see chapter 5.1). The WHO Global Burden of Disease 2000 project is updating these estimates for 14 subregions of the world for the year 2000 and subsequent years.

HALE: health-adjusted life expectancy

Any of a number of summary measures which use explicit weights to combine health expectancies for a set of discrete health states into a single indicator estimating the expectation of equivalent years of good health. Also referred to as "healthy life expectancy".

HE: health expectancy

Generic term for summary measures of population health, which estimate the expectation of years of life lived in various health states.

Healthy life expectancy

Synonym for HALE (q.v.) or health-adjusted life expectancy.

HeaLYs: HEALTHY LIFE YEARS

A health gap (q.v.) measure (see chapter 5.2) calculated on the basis of the incidence of pathological processes and the future non-fatal health outcomes and mortality from those processes.

HG: HEALTH GAP

A generic term for summary measures of population health; estimates the gap between the current population health and a normative goal for population health.

HOPIT: HIERARCHICAL ORDERED PROBIT MODEL

A statistical model developed by WHO to estimate response category cutpoints for self-reported items on health domains using information from measured tests or anchoring vignettes (see chapter 8.3).

HRQL OR HRQoL: HEALTH-RELATED QUALITY OF LIFE

HSE: HEALTH STATE EXPECTANCY

A form of HE (q.v.) which gives the expectation of years lived in a specified health state (which is given a weight of 1, while all other health states are given a weight of 0).

HUI: HEALTH UTILITIES INDEX

A standardized system for classification of health states (see chapter 7.2).

IADL: INSTRUMENTAL ACTIVITIES OF DAILY LIVING

Normative roles and activities such as heavy housework, light housework, laundry, shopping for groceries, getting around outside, travelling, managing money, taking medicine, telephoning, etc.

ICD: INTERNATIONAL STATISTICAL CLASSIFICATION OF DISEASES AND RELATED HEALTH PROBLEMS

A classification of diseases and other causes of mortality that was entrusted to the World Health Organization in 1948, along with the constitutional mandate to have it periodically revised as necessary. The current tenth revision was issued in 1992 to come into effect on 1 January 1993. The ICD is a member of the WHO family of international classifications.

ICF: INTERNATIONAL CLASSIFICATION OF FUNCTIONING, DISABILITY AND HEALTH

An international classification published by WHO in 2001 as endorsed by the 54th World Health Assembly in resolution 54.21. As a revision of the ICIDH (q.v.), the ICF is a member of the WHO family of international classifications (see chapter 8.3).

ICIDH: INTERNATIONAL CLASSIFICATION OF IMPAIRMENT, DISABILITIES AND HANDICAPS

A classification published by WHO for trial purposes in 1980 in accordance with the 1975 International Revision Conference and World Health Assembly resolution WHA29.35 of 1976. It has now been superseded by the ICF (q.v.).

IHD: ISCHAEMIC HEART DISEASE

Any of a number of heart conditions associated with deficiencies of the coronary arteries. Note: this is synonymous with coronary heart disease.

IND: INDIA

Regional grouping used in the Global Burden of Disease study 1990.

IRT: ITEM RESPONSE THEORY

Psychometric approach that uses statistical models to establish response category cut-points for different items in a survey instrument by comparing each response category to the underlying factor in the data.

LAC: LATIN AMERICA AND THE CARIBBEAN

Regional grouping used in the Global Burden of Disease study 1990.

LE: LIFE EXPECTANCY

Generic term for summary measures of population mortality that estimate the expectation of years of life lived. See also: period life expectancy.

LED: LIFE EXPECTANCY WITH DISABILITY

A form of HSE (q.v.) which gives a weight of 0 to states of health with no disability above an explicit or implicit threshold and a weight of 1 to states of health with any level of disability above that threshold.

LHE: LOST HEALTH EXPECTANCY

Expected lost years of equivalent full health, defined as the gap between total life expectancy and healthy life expectancy (LHE = LE – HALE).

LIFE EXPECTANCY: *see*: LE

MEC: MIDDLE EASTERN CRESCENT

Regional grouping used in the Global Burden of Disease study 1990. Includes countries of North Africa, Middle East and West Asia.

NHIS: NATIONAL HEALTH INTERVIEW SURVEY (US)

OAI: OTHER ASIA AND ISLANDS

Regional grouping used in the Global Burden of Disease study 1990. Includes countries in South Asia, South East Asia, North Asia and the Pacific region apart from Australia, China, India, Japan and New Zealand.

OECD: ORGANISATION FOR ECONOMIC CO-OPERATION AND
DEVELOPMENT

PERIOD LIFE EXPECTANCY

A summary measure of population mortality that calculates the expectation of years of life lived in a fictitious birth cohort assuming that at each
age the cohort experiences the age-specific mortality rates observed in the
real population during a specified time period (such as a given calendar
year). See also: life expectancy.

PEYLL: PERIOD EXPECTED YEARS OF LIFE LOST

A form of health gap (q.v.) that measures mortality gap using current
period life expectancy for the population to specify years lost due to death
at each age.

PTO: PERSON TRADE-OFF

A method for valuation of health states that asks respondents to choose
between hypothetical interventions that offer health benefits to groups of
individuals in different health states.

PYLL: POTENTIAL YEARS OF LIFE LOST

A form of health gap (q.v.) that measures mortality gap using an arbitrary
normative age (e.g. 70 years).

QALE: QUALITY-ADJUSTED LIFE EXPECTANCY

A form of HALE (q.v.) based on a question on activity restriction in the
Canada Health Survey.

REVES: RÉSEAU DE L'ESPÉRANCE DE VIE EN SANTÉ

International network on healthy life expectancy.

SD: STANDARD DEVIATION

SEYLL: STANDARD EXPECTED YEARS OF LIFE LOST

A form of health gap (q.v.) that measures mortality gap using a standard
life table to specify years lost due to death at each age.

SF-36: SHORT-FORM 36 HEALTH SURVEY

STANDARD GAMBLE (SG)

A method for valuation of health states based on the axioms of expected
utility theory. The standard gamble asks respondents to make choices that
weigh improvements in health against mortality risks.

SMPH: SUMMARY MEASURES OF POPULATION HEALTH

Indicators that summarize the health of a population into a single number. SMPH combine information about mortality and population health states. They may summarize either average health level or inequality for a population.

SSA: SUB-SAHARAN AFRICA

Regional grouping used in the Global Burden of Disease study 1990.

STD: SEXUALLY TRANSMITTED DISEASE

SULLIVAN'S METHOD

A method of calculating health expectancies using data on current prevalence of health states in a population (see chapter 4.1).

TTO: TIME TRADE-OFF

A method for valuation of health states that asks respondents to make hypothetical choices that weigh improvements in health against reduced longevity.

VAS: VISUAL ANALOGUE SCALE

A method for valuation of health states that asks respondents to assess the health levels associated with different states by locating them on a scale representing a continuum of health levels between endpoints referring to good and bad states of health.

WHO: WORLD HEALTH ORGANIZATION

WHODAS-II: WHO DISABILITY ASSESSMENT SCHEDULE-II

WHOQOL: WHO QUALITY OF LIFE ASSESSMENT INSTRUMENT

USBODI: UNITED STATES BURDEN OF DISEASE AND INJURY STUDY

YHL: YEARS OF HEALTHY LIFE

A form of DFLE (q.v.) based on two questions collected in the United States National Health Interview Survey, which are concerned with activity limitations and perceived general health.

YLD: YEARS LIVED WITH DISABILITY

The component of the DALY (q.v.) that measures the lost years of healthy life through living in states of less than full health.

YLL: YEARS OF LIFE LOST

The component of the DALY (q.v.) that measures the years lost through premature mortality.

Index